DATE DUE

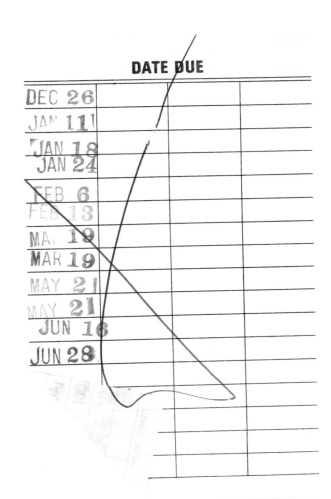

DEC 26		
JAN 11		
JAN 18		
JAN 24		
FEB 6		
FEB 13		
MAR 19		
MAR 19		
MAY 21		
MAY 21		
JUN 16		
JUN 28		

D1318859

CULTURE & COMFORT

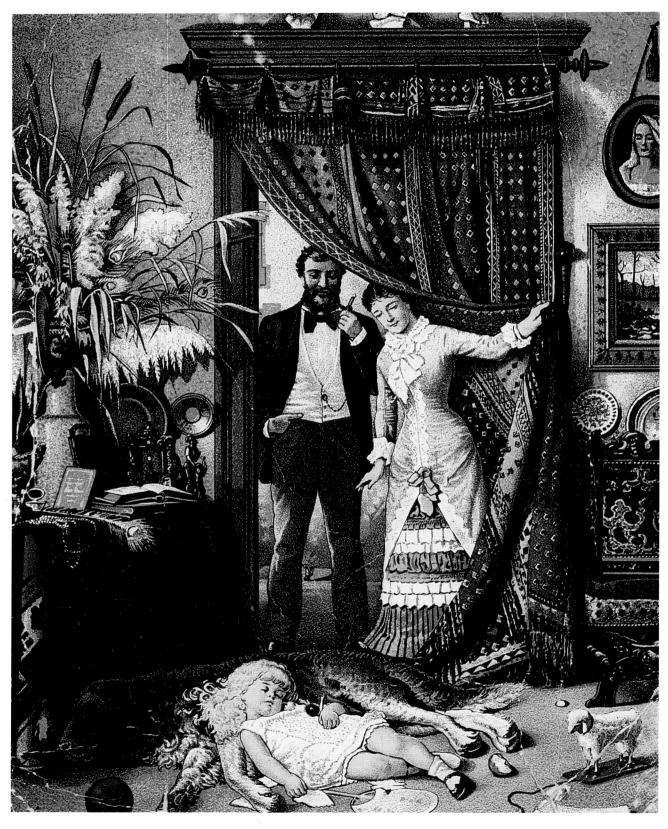

Plate 1. *Chromolithographed trade card for Waite Photographic Art Studio, United States, about 1885.*

CULTURE & COMFORT

People, Parlors, and Upholstery
1850–1930

Katherine C. Grier

The Strong Museum
Rochester, New York

Distributed by the University of Massachusetts Press

Copyright © 1988 by the Strong Museum

Culture and Comfort: People, Parlors, and Upholstery, 1850-1930 was published by the Strong Museum in conjunction with an exhibition of the same name, on view from 8 September 1988 to 16 January 1989.

The Strong Museum
Kathryn Grover, director of publications and editor
Kenneth H. Townsend, cover design
James Via and Michael Radtke, photography

Book Marshall Productions, Rochester, New York, page design
Rochester Mono/Headliners, Rochester, New York, typography
Flower City Printing, Inc., Rochester, New York, printing

Library of Congress Cataloging-in-Publication Data
Grier, Katherine C., 1953-
   Culture and comfort: people, parlors, and upholstery / Katherine
C. Grier
      p.   cm.
Published in conjunction with an exhibition at the Strong Museum,
Sept. 8, 1988 to Jan. 16, 1989.
Bibliography: p.
Includes index.
ISBN 0-940365-01-4: $27.95
1. Material culture—United States—Exhibitions. 2. Living rooms—
United States—History—Exhibitions. 3. Upholstery—United
States—History—Exhibitions. 4. United States—Social life and
customs—19th century—Exhibitions. 5. United States—Social life
and customs—1865-1918—Exhibitions. 6. United States—Social life
and customs—1918-1945—Exhibitions. I. Margaret Woodbury
Strong. II. Title.
E166.G83 1988   88-20112
392'.36—dc19   CIP

ISBN 0-940365-01-4

University of Massachusetts Press
P. O. Box 429
Amherst, Massachusetts 01004

cover: detail of lounge, oak and tapestry carpet, Martyn Brothers, Jamestown, New York, about 1885.

CONTENTS

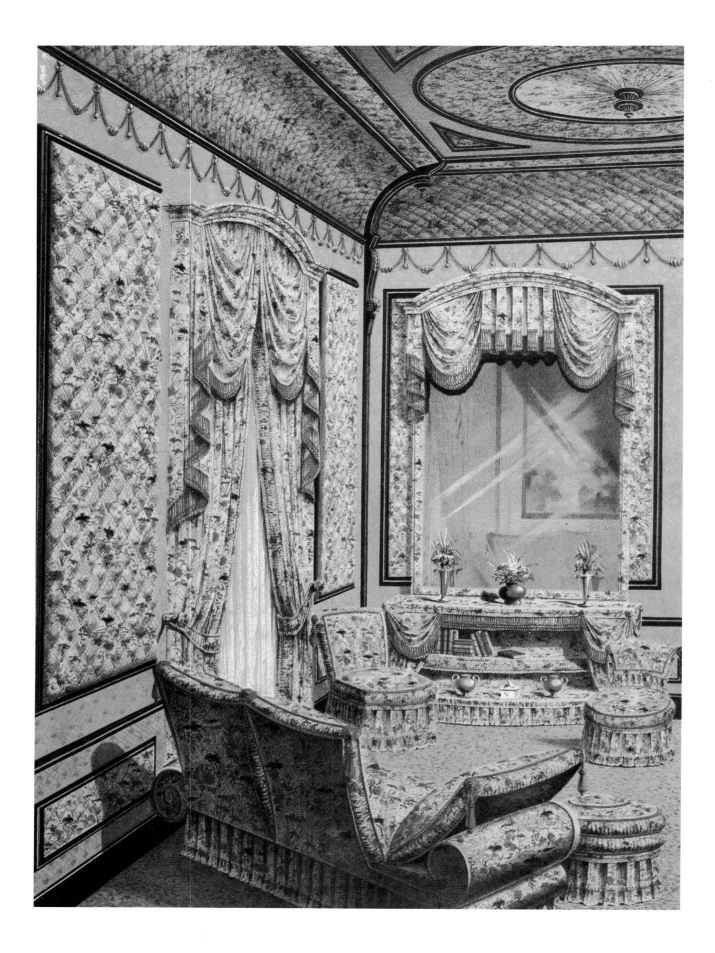

Plate 2. "Interior Decorations. United States," chromolithograph by Cosack and Co., Buffalo, New York, published by the American News Company, New York, New York; plate tipped into Frank H. Norton, Illustrated Historical Register of the Centennial Exhibition, Philadelphia, 1876, and the Exposition Universelle, 1878 *(1879).*

ACKNOWLEDGMENTS

This publication is one element of a larger project for the Strong Museum, comprising an exhibition, a videotape, and a conference that will result in a volume of papers. I want to thank the board of trustees, William T. Alderson, former director, and G. Rollie Adams, president and CEO of the Strong Museum. Thanks also to my coworkers at the Strong for supporting and participating in this work, including Richard Sherin, chief conservator; Patricia Tice, curator of household furnishings; and Melissa Morgan Radtke, collections coordinator. I especially want to acknowledge the help given to me by the staff of the museum's library during the months of research, as well as the hours spent by history division volunteers Rita Kuder and Wanda Lodico answering the research queries left on their library desk. Heartfelt thanks go to fellow Strong Museum historian William Siles for his interest in my work and support at critical moments and to Judy White, secretary for the history and exhibits divisions, for her hours of good-natured work on manuscript and grant drafts (and for scores of peanut butter cups shared during moments of tribulation). Harvey Green, chief historian and vice president for interpretation at the museum, brought me to the Strong and enabled me to develop this project, which grew out of my Ph.D. dissertation for the Program in the History of American Civilization at the University of Delaware. In his triple role as boss, colleague, and friend, he assisted my preparation of successful planning grant and implementation grant applications to the National Endowment for the Humanities. He also read and offered useful suggestions on all the chapters of the manuscript.

Preparing an author's rough manuscript for publication— especially one as heavily illustrated as this one—is a collaborative venture. I thank the individuals who played so important a role in this process, the staff of the Office of Publications and Technical Services at the Strong Museum. The photographs made by James Via and Michael Radtke, with the occasional assistance of Jonathan Bregman, not only revealed the visual qualities of the objects in new ways to me (and, I hope, to the reader); sometimes they made artifacts with very real conservation problems look much as they must have when originally purchased and used. Kenneth Townsend designed the cover and developed the graphic standards for the book, and Book Marshall executed the design. Kathryn Grover, the Museum's editor and head of the Office, took me patiently through many drafts of some chapters; I appreciate her continued, even passionate, support of the project and editorial expertise. Her assistant, Catherine Romano, kept careful track of photographs, figure lists, and footnote citations.

I am grateful to the National Endowment for the Humanities for its generous support of my research and this publication, along with the other components of the Culture and Comfort project. I received research assistance from staff members at a number of institutions, including the Winterthur Museum and Library; the Hagley Museum and Library; the Division of Domestic Life at the National Museum of American History, Smithsonian Institution; the Library of Congress; the Grand Rapids (Michigan) Public Museum and Grand Rapids Public Library; Old Sturbridge Village; the Gibson House Society, Boston; the Society for the Preservation of New England Antiquities; the Victoria Society of Maine; Castle Tucker, Wiscasset, Maine; The Free Library of Philadelphia; the Goldie Paley Design Center, Philadelphia College of Textiles and Science; and the Department of American Decorative Arts, Metropolitan Museum of Art, New York.

I have been the recipient of generous encouragement and thoughtful criticism from scholars working both in museums and in colleges and universities. Rodris Roth, curator of the Division of Domestic Life at the National Museum of American History, Smithsonian Institution, contributed substantially to my early interest in historical textiles and helped me learn how to look at the artifacts I have chosen to study. Kenneth L. Ames of the Office of Advanced Studies at the Winterthur Museum guided my study of domestic material culture at the University of Delaware. George Basalla of the history department at the University encouraged me to think very widely about material culture; he will demur, but his stamp is on much of my research, including this project. Lawrence Taylor of Lafayette College, whom I had the great good fortune to meet during his year in residence at the Winterthur Museum as a National Endowment for the Humanities Fellow, helped me employ the perspectives of cultural anthropology in my work. I have received substantive comments and encouragement from many others, including Carol Hoffecker, Elizabeth Lahikainen, Glenn Porter, Grace Seiberling, Dell Upton, Dorothy Washburn, and Susan Williams. I am honored to be able to call these individuals my friends, as well as my colleagues and teachers.

Finally, I want to thank my adviser and mentor Richard H. Bushman. Over the course of six years, in long hours of general discussion and through his comments on my written work, his open, speculative turn of mind has encouraged my own. During my years at Delaware, I discovered that becoming a historian of society and culture is a lifelong process of discovery and that the intellectual balancing act of interdisciplinary study can be particularly rewarding, if occasionally hazardous. One rarely hears the labors of writing history described as either an adventure or a long-term affair of the heart, but I think of my chosen work in those ways, and I owe much of my enthusiasm to Richard Bushman.

Melding the close study of artifacts with social and cultural history sometimes makes for difficult research and writing. Still, it is exciting, as well as a privilege, to have the opportunity to contribute to an approach to the study of history that is so new, where there is so much exciting research in progress. There are very few history museums with the means of fostering scholarly research and publication. The Strong is one of these. I hope that it will continue in developing its institutional commitment to supporting financially and nurturing research, giving scholars the time that allows them to take chances. Where this book has lapses in its argument or gaps in its information, the responsibility for these is my own. I hope that my readers will still find *Culture and Comfort* both informative and thought-provoking.

I dedicate this book to my family.
Katherine C. Grier

A NOTE ON THE TEXT

Although *Culture and Comfort: People, Parlors, and Upholstery, 1850-1930* is being published in conjunction with an exhibition of the same name, it is not an exhibit catalog per se but a work of social and cultural history that illustrates and analyzes artifacts and images to make its argument. The photograph captions do not constitute complete catalog entries; captions identifying objects name the visible materials only, rather than listing all secondary or invisible, structural elements (except where such normally invisible materials are the subject of the image). Readers interested in obtaining complete catalog information on any object depicted in the book should contact either the Strong Museum or the institution that owns the illustrated object.

While I have developed some expertise in the subject of historical upholstery fabrics, I am not an expert on the weave structure or dying and printing of such textiles and have not included this level of information in either captions or text. Rather, I have tried to use identifying names that would have been used in the decades between 1850 and 1930. Further, I have included as an appendix a brief glossary consisting of the names and descriptions of upholstery fabrics as dry goods merchants themselves used them. Here, bracketed information, usually other names by which fabrics have been known, has sometimes been added; any information that appears within parentheses appeared either in brackets or parentheses in the original texts used to compile the glossary. I hope that my research will stimulate more technical research and writing on upholstery fabrics of the late nineteenth and twentieth centuries, work that would help with both preservation and accurate reproduction of these textiles.

Figures are numbered consecutively in each chapter; color plates are numbered consecutively throughout the entire text. In keeping with Strong Museum practice, a country of origin for the complete object often is included in the photo captions. This is not necessarily the country of origin for the materials composing that object. For example, most horsehair used in the second half of the nineteenth century for manufacturing haircloth or as stuffing material in the United States was imported from South America. Most of the upholstery textiles dating before 1900 that are illustrated in the figures and plates are of European origins, particularly from France and England.

Special effort has been made to illustrate domestic upholstery in its original condition. Where replacement textiles have been used to repair pieces, this fact has been noted in the captions. I consider nineteenth- and early twentieth-century upholstery to be valuable historical evidence, meriting as careful consideration as any old, well-used, and damaged historical document. Just as damaged documents are not simply copied and the originals destroyed, historical upholstery should be preserved, even in a damaged state, and students and collectors must learn to see through its present condition and appreciate the information that does survive about its original qualities.

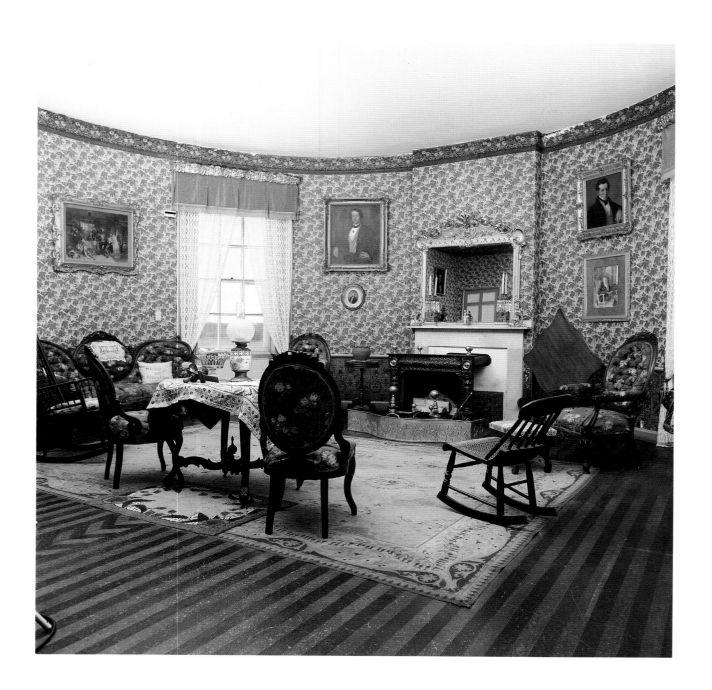

INTRODUCTION
SYMBOLS AND SENSIBILITY

In her 1881 advice book *Home Decoration*, Janet Ruutz-Rees informed her readers that bare doorways, walls, and window frames distressed the refined sensibility. "Some rooms seem to be all doors," she wrote; "in whatever direction one turns, the eye is confronted by an opening; and it is becoming very usual to drape the entire room in a way that shall make such necessities, as far as possible, parts of an harmonious whole." Draperies, Ruutz-Rees pointed out, allowed "the skillful hiding of defects..., the softening of angles, and happy obliteration of corners," just as the etiquette so important to respectable Americans in the nineteenth century softened the "angles" and "defects" of human character.[1] *American Etiquette and Rules of Politeness*, an inexpensive manners book published around the same time as *Home Decoration*, explained the "Value of Etiquette" by reminding its readers, "That culture only is valuable which smooths the rough places, harmonizes the imperfections, and develops the pure, the good, and the gentle in human character... Politeness in the hourly intercourse of life...smooths away most of the rudeness that otherwise might jar upon our nerves."[2]

It is no accident that the author of a book on interior decoration and another on manners chose to use similar language and concepts—"harmonizing," "smoothing," "softening" the defects or "rough places"—to describe the effects of both upholstery and etiquette. Both were believed to express the progress of civilization; both were described with a vocabulary that revealed a popular taxonomy, a way of choosing language that reflects the presence of some mental framework for organizing many kinds of human experience.

This book investigates the culture commonly known as "Victorian" by exploring how its parlors were furnished (figs. 1 and 2). The parlor was one of several spaces in houses (the other most commonly being the dining room) intended to serve as the setting for important social events and to present the civilized facades of its occupants. Its conventions of furnishing represented two poles of thought about the little world of the parlor—its domesticity ("comfort") and its cosmopolitan character ("culture"). The terms "culture" and "comfort" concisely designate two complex collations of ideas, attitudes, and assumptions that represent a critical tension in Victorian culture. "Culture" is used here as shorthand for the cultivated world view of educated, genteel, and cosmopolitan people whose habits of consumption (including furnishing a gala parlor) were intended to create an expressive social demeanor. On the other hand, "comfort" signals a group of ideas and beliefs not simply associated with a pleasurable physical state. It also designates the presence of the more family-centered, even religious values associated with "home," values emphasizing perfect sincerity and moderation in all things. Social commentators claimed comfort to be a distinctively middle-class state of mind.

Together, aspirations toward culture and comfort composed a cultural framework that set the terms for questions about personal cultivation and social progress. They also framed questions about consumption, including both dress and domestic furnishing. Such questions focused particularly closely on the act of setting aside space for and devoting family resources to the making of a parlor. The ideal parlor of culture presented a family's cultivated facade, but the ideal parlor of comfort at once discounted the value of that appearance. In fact, middle-class commentators insisted that the room be homey, not theatrical. Similar tensions existed in the realm of manners. Was a parlor person pious and domestic, or a cosmopolite, an American aristocrat?

Between 1850 and 1910, even though their contents were commercially available to everyone having money for furnishings, parlors in ordinary households retained their association with gentility, a set of personal attributes that supposedly was beyond the reach of commerce. People preferred to set aside spaces for formality when it was possible, although they adapted their own "gala apartments" to such special uses as funerals and the display of Christmas trees. In Anglo-America, the term "parlor" had described the best room, but this room was supposed to retain the identity of a family sitting room even as it also served more public and formal uses. For ordinary consumers, the problem lay in how to combine the domestic and the gala, how to create a "comfortable theater" for middle-class self-presentation.

Victorianism, as Daniel Walker Howe has defined it, was an Anglo-American, transatlantic, bourgeois culture of industrializing western civilization.[3] Not all nineteenth-century Americans were Victorians. Many immigrants, such as the millions of Irish Catholic peasants who arrived beginning in the 1840s, certainly were not Victorian, nor were several generations of their descendants. Yet even though Victorian Americans did not call themselves by this name, they knew who they were, and Victorianism embraced a set of symbols to which all other cultural groups in the nation responded. Non-Victorian Americans had on some level to be conversant with this dominant culture even if they retained their own cultural forms. They could scarcely avoid participating in some of its aspects, especially those associated with the burgeoning consumer society. The domestic goods that proliferated so dramatically after 1850 could potentially serve as a means of participating in Victorian culture. To own a home

Figs. 1 and 2. Parlor of Harriet B. and Samuel A. Stevens, 492 Cumberland Street, Portland, Maine, by unidentified photographer, about 1890. Like most parlors in ordinary households, the Stevens parlor blended old and new possessions gathered over time. The elaborate swag draperies were "French," a nod to the parlor as gala apartment. The overstuffed chair was "Turkish"; the tea table set for service was "colonial" and also signaled the rituals of parlor sociability. The mantel, its mirror another echo of past furnishing practice, surrounded a hearth that was not functional; it was instead a necessary decorative focal point as well as symbolic of the heart (continued on next page)

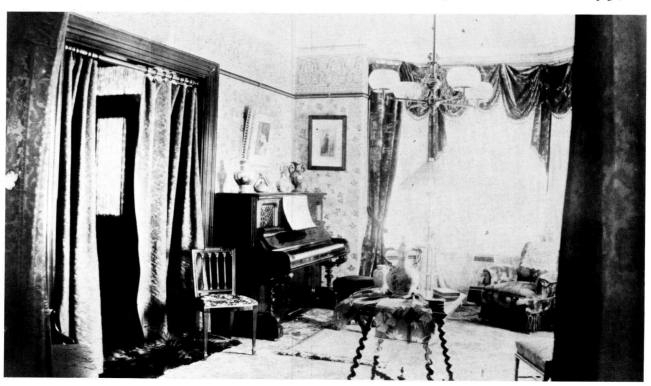

and purchase the proper furnishings for it meant that one shared, in some measure, the culture's vision of the formal characteristics of respectable family living.

"Home" was one of Victorian culture's most important and complicated symbols, a web of ideas, objects, and images that was powerful partly because it seemed so basic, even mundane. Even the apparently familiar word "home" is itself complex, bearing meanings that are both psychological and locational. To be "at home" not only means being present in one's place of residence; it also implies being at ease in some place or in the company of a like-minded person or group of people. To cultivate and demonstrate good manners, in the words of one nineteenth-century advice writer, was to be "at home" in all society.[4] "Home" also can connote a particular place, as large as a nation state. However, as their descendents do today, Victorian Americans usually thought of home as an actual physical site, composed of a building and its furnishings, peopled by the members of a family. Popular prints, sheet music, advice literature, and fiction all attest the concreteness of the ideal—a single-family residence, separated from its neighbors by a green strip of lawn or the fields of a farm (fig. 3).[5]

The corporeal quality of the symbol "home" even extended into the realm of popular religiosity. In the 1879 best seller *The Complete Home: An Encyclopædia of Domestic Life and Affairs*, Julia McNair Wright wrote, "Between the Home set up in Eden, and the Home before us in Eternity, stand the Homes of Earth in a long succession. It is therefore important that our Homes should be brought up to a standard in harmony with their origin and destiny. Here are 'Empire's primal springs;' here are the Church and State in embryo; here all improvements and reform must rise. For national and social disasters, for moral and financial evils, the cure begins in the Household."[6] The concept of "Heavenly Home" domesticated the "Pearly Gates" into a white picket fence around a real location where a person could be reunited with deceased relatives and create anew

of family life. The portières, or door curtains, made the room simultaneously cozy and theatrical, framing each doorway with drapery like the stage curtains at a play. One of the photographs, made through the door curtains, takes advantage of this framing effect. The room could be illuminated brightly with its large gas chandelier and a floor-standing kerosene piano lamp. The center table, deprived of its function as the gathering place for night reading, sewing, and play, was still an important convention of parlor furnishing. It presented to visitors a summary still life of what the owners valued—here, books and choice examples of their pottery collection, elaborated with scarf drapery.

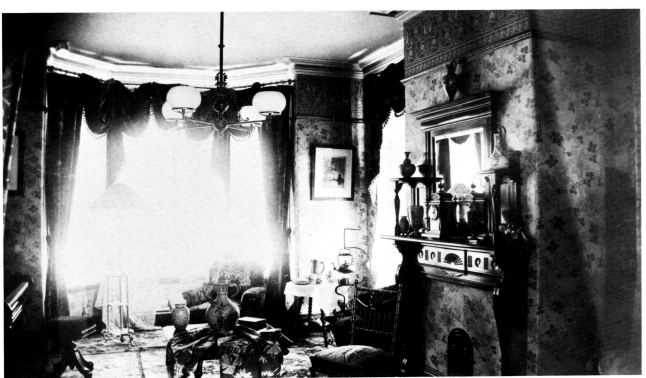

the earthly family circle. The Reverend W. K. Tweedie elaborated on these connections in a collection of pious essays titled *Home; or, The Parents' Assistant and Children's Friend* (1873). Chapter 3 was an exegesis on "Names for Home," including "the Eden of Home," "God's First Church," "A Miniature of Heaven," "a Copy of Heaven," and "a Nursery for Heaven."[7] Even so original an intellect and talent as Emily Dickinson employed a version of this formulation in writing of her father's death, comparing the grave to a house and, by implication, death to going home: "Father does not live with us now—he lives in a new house. Though it was built in an hour it is better than this. He hasn't any garden because he moved in after gardens were made, so we take him the best flowers."[8]

In books of household advice throughout the nineteenth century, the concept of the Christian household was a powerful one in discussions of home life. This concept enhanced the symbolic meaning of "home" by blending religiosity and domesticity. Catharine Beecher, devoting a chapter apiece in her *American Woman's Home* to "The Christian Family" and "A Christian House," argued that the "family state" was designed "to provide for the training of our race...with chief reference to a future immortal existence"; it was, she felt, "the aptest earthly illustration of the heavenly kingdom." As its "chief minister," each woman required "a home in which to exercise this ministry." Beecher believed that the physical qualities of each house should support "a style of living...conformed to the great design."[9] Hence, the private dwelling, rather than the public church building, became the most important sanctuary, and its contents also could serve as religious symbols.[10]

"Home" as a specific physical place also implicitly contained an ideal of ownership, possession, and permanence. In a world of little employment stability for ordinary people, without guaranteed pensions or financial security, such practical considerations necessary to family survival underlay the physicality of the symbol "home." Historian Richard L. Bushman has observed that while the complicated exchange network of rural American society between 1750 and 1850 provided some level of subsistence for almost everyone, the rural economy "worked much better...for people with land...Property and children were the only means of support when strength and health eventually failed."[11] Yet urban living became increasingly the dominant mode, whether by choice for the comparatively high wages and freedom it offered, or by necessity because some laborers could not sustain themselves in the rural economy. Families, Bushman has argued, began to "erect defenses in their urban homes against layoffs, wage cuts, illness and old age" through the uses that they applied to their dwellings. Workers who did not bounce from city to city accepted heavy mortgages and sacrificed their children's educations to be able to own a small house in the city. Through a variety of strategies—accepting boarders, providing shelter for relatives, and taking into the home piece work such as shoe finishing—the house became the "urban surrogate for the self-sufficient family farm." Such strategies were not confined to working-class families; middle-class families also resorted to taking in boarders and working out of their houses as financial circumstances required.[12]

Home in this particular context provided a real alternative, in economic terms, to the dangerous, unreliable, "outside" world of commerce and work. The Victorian understanding of the economic and social roles occupied by men and women incorporated and further developed the distinction between home and the world beyond its doors. In the nineteenth century, the old conception of

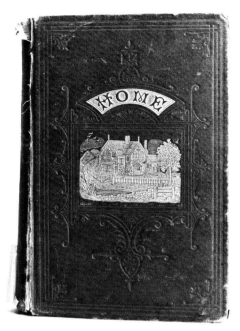

Fig. 3. Detail of cover, *Rev. W. K. Tweedie*, Home; or, The Parents' Assistant and Children's Friend *(1873). The cover of Tweedie's collection of pious essays was embellished with a picture of the ideal home, his "Miniature of Heaven."*

separate but complementary "spheres" of work occupied by men and women in pre-industrial economies became the "cult of domesticity," in which women became the guardians of the finer human feelings as well as the administrators of the household. In this vision of appropriate domestic life, "home" became not the resource for minimum subsistence but the space for psychological refuge from the rigors of economic life as well as the proper site for the expression of familial love and guidance.

Domestic Environmentalism

During the first half of the nineteenth century, popular thinking, widespread enough that it was regarded virtually as common sense, attributed great power to the family environment in the shaping of personal—and, by implication, national—character. This determinism was often expressed in the works of widely published authors who addressed themselves to women—Lydia Sigourney, the author of *Letters to Mothers* (1838); Harriet Beecher Stowe, the prolific author of domestic fiction and advice; Emma Willard, advocate of women's education; and Sarah Josepha Hale, editor of *Godey's Lady's Book*. The family, they argued, was the strongest and best antidote to the temptations and poisons of the commercial world. Although men provided the means of each family's material existence, women set the tone of that existence. As mothers, each nurtured the development of proper character in her children. A mother did this not only to enable them to succeed as adults but to perpetuate the very future of the American republic. Sigourney urged her readers to consider their vital role in quelling a tide of increasing public disorder:

> A barrier to the torrent of corruption, and a guard over the strong holds of knowledge and virtue, may be placed by the mother, as she watches over her cradled son. Let her come forth with vigour and vigilance, at the call of her country…like the mother of Washington, feeling that the first lesson to every incipient ruler should be "how to obey." The degree of her diligence in preparing her children to be good subjects of a just government, will be the true measure of her patriotism.[13]

Other authors of domestic advice and fiction expanded upon this vision of the feminine sphere in American society by suggesting that the masculine world of politics and business had become heartless and needed the gentle guidance of feminine morality. They justified this position through an argument that the State itself was, as Harriet Beecher Stowe put it, "but a larger family."[14] Almira Seymour, a less well-known author who published a small collection of essays titled *Home: The Basis of the State*, argued that domestic reform—that is, the proper ordering of "the hidden source of all growth and expansion…the organization of the Family, the institution of Home"—provided the bulwark against the chaos that rapid industrial and social change threatened.[15]

Popular thinking about child rearing and domestic life in pre-Civil War America continued to stress the example set for young children by the behavior and good character of family members. By the 1830s, discussions of domesticity and society also were infused with a second strain of deterministic thought that assigned to the house's physical setting and details the power to shape human character. Fully articulated by the 1830s, this "domestic environmentalism" conflated moral guidance with the actual appearance and physical layout of the house and its contents.[16]

Authors who stressed the concepts of the Christian family and republican motherhood also described the operation of the domestic environment upon an individual's sensibility. Catharine Beecher cautioned that although the "aesthetic element must be subordinate to the requirements of physical existence…it contributes much to the education of the entire household in refinement, intellectual development, and moral sensibility."[17] The article "The Domestic Use of Design" in the first issue of *The Furniture Gazette*, a London-based trade journal with transatlantic readership, described the effect of "domestic scenery" on sensibility in some detail:

> There can be no doubt that altogether, independently of direct intellectual culture, either from books or society, the mind is moulded and coloured to a great extent by the persistent impressions produced upon it by the most familiar objects that daily meet the eye…That a carefully regulated and intelligent change of the domestic scenery about a sick person is beneficial is obvious, and yet there are few who correctly apprehend to how great an extent the character, and especially the temper, may be affected by the nature of ordinary physical surroundings.

> Philosophy, however, is rapidly becoming practical, and the mechanical action which the objective world of nature exercises on the subjective universe of man's mind is at least clearly perceived, even if all the useful lessons deducible thence have not as yet been mastered. What architecture is to the mass, furniture in its domestic application is to the individual; and though the cathedral may produce an immense impression on a crowd, and even for the time on the human minds composing it, it will often happen that a comparatively utterly insignificant article in the house really does more in the way of impressing, or even moulding, the human intelligence with which it is in almost persistent contact…The practical deduction naturally to be taken from all this is, that the study of domestic furniture should become more aesthetic.[18]

The indirect, gentle influence that objects were thought to exert on the individual sensibility was very much like the kind of influence that authors of tracts and fiction about domesticity expected women to have on their families inside each private household and, eventually, on the political and social world beyond the home. In the household, worldly goods served as the communicative medium for higher ends. How this communicative chain—from women to things, thence from things to family members and selected outsiders—was believed to function can be found in one of Harriet Beecher Stowe's lesser novels, *We and Our Neighbors*. Describing the preparations of the newlyweds Eva and Harry Henderson for a series of "social reunions" in their small house on an unfashionable New York City street, Stowe digressed to explain how the character of a woman was made manifest in her home: "Self begins to melt away into something higher…The *home* becomes her center, and to her home passes the charm that once was thrown around her person…Her home is the new impersonation of herself."[19]

In the context of the Christian household, the fullest expression of the ideal of comfort, the selection and arrangement of possessions personified the nature of the woman who served as "priestess and minister of a family state."[20] Other Beecher family publications, including *The American Woman's Home*, restated this notion of a woman's proper occupation in the "Christian household." Properly selected and arranged interiors were analogs or material equivalents of the moral state of the household, just as genuine manners were considered the manifestation of morality in the realm of behavior. A woman as "minister of a family state" could serve moral purposes by manipulating the chain of associations that domestic objects inspired.

The influence that objects could have on the development of character was sometimes direct and easily perceived, as when a child was exposed to art objects or books in the household. Clarence Cook argued that the family "living room" (he objected to "parlors") was "an important agent in the education of life...It is no trifling matter, whether we hang poor pictures on our walls or good ones, whether we select a fine cast or a second-rate one. We might almost as well say it makes no difference whether the people we live with are first-rate or second-rate."[21] While Cook held a more secular view of the impact of possessions than other domestic critics, he still believed in the importance of shaping character by exerting a form of quality control on domestic possessions.

Increasing emphasis on the positive influence on character of rooms and personal possessions themselves had the effect of tying the formation of character to correct habits of consumption. This linking of consumption to the expression and formation of character helps explain the vehemence of much nineteenth-century domestic advice literature on interior decoration. Decor did not simply express culture but made it; objects were culture in tangible form, and possessions that were inappropriate to the social class of the family who owned them were a potential source of danger because they sent conflicting messages. The debate on this point was most strongly expressed in the opposition of "aristocratic" and "middle-class" models of parlor decoration and domestic comfort in both advice literature and a genre of popular fiction that may be called "moral tales of furnishing." The same authors who offered advice on the domestic economy of true comfort also often wrote these parables, which appeared in women's magazines and even in the form of lengthy novels.

The relationship of home to the commercial world was paradoxical, however. While the "cult of domesticity" made the absolute separation of the domestic and business worlds one of its major tenets, real considerations of labor and calculations of economic advantage and future security were tied to house ownership. On a level that touched even those families who could not own their own house, furnishings were also marked by an ambiguous tension between their symbolic value and their commercial origins. The continued vitality of domestic environmentalism as one component of Victorian popular thought was supported by this connection to the emergence of mass consumer culture. As Gwendolyn Wright has suggested, the ideal house was steadily viewed as a place for promoting family privacy, protection, and security despite its increasingly complex ties to consumer culture. The products of industrialization and commercialization, from factory-made furniture to commercially canned soup, permeated the site that was supposedly the haven from these forces during the last quarter of the nineteenth century.[22]

Yet the proliferation of consumer goods that were industrially produced and commercially marketed does not imply that their symbolic richness was necessarily cheapened or, as Siegfried Giedion has suggested, "devalued."[23] While "society" is the set of institutions that groups of human beings develop in order to keep daily life operating with some degree of smoothness, "culture," in the sense that anthropologists use the word, lies in the realm of the mind. It is an historically transmitted "pattern of meanings," as anthropologist Clifford Geertz has put it, "a system of inherited conceptions" about the nature of the world "by means of which men communicate, perpetuate, and develop their knowledge about and attitudes toward life." A culture expresses meaning by manipulating symbols; in so doing, it expresses to itself as much as to outsiders what it thinks is important to know about life.[24] The commercialization of objects that served as the vehicles for symbolic meanings was in fact one of the fundamental ways in which Victorian culture worked, the means through which its forms became the dominant mode of cultural expression in the United States in the nineteenth century. The objects that bore meaning within the overarching symbol "home"—its various furnishings—generally predated Victorian culture, although their availability was limited to families of means in the United States. The processes of commercialization—the creation of a national framework of distribution, marketing, consumer credit, and sales—made versions of these furnishings readily available to the ordinary members of American society. Victorian culture's longevity and vitality was due in part to this process. Such commercialization moved symbolic values throughout the culture, inviting broader participation in already established conceptions.

Symbols and Sensibility

The building, the miniature Eden of its grounds, many of the objects that filled its rooms, and even the family members residing there all potentially served as aspects of the symbol "home" because the meaning of each could be enriched by complicated chains of association. Ordinary people used objects to create rich personal connections to larger spheres of cultural meaning, a process that continues to shape the interior life of people today. Some of the associative chains engendered by particular objects people own and carefully save are strictly personal or even idiosyncratic, the product of individual experience: the handful of beach pebbles and shells collected on a vacation always suggest that time to the person who has saved them, but they are meaningless to outsiders. By contrast, symbols that predominate in a culture capitalize on agreed-upon sets of associations. These conventional meanings are culturally produced and reinforced through a wide variety of channels, including the popular media, informal learning from family members or associates, or formal instruction in schools and other institutions. Many chains of association blend the personal and the conventional: a miniature Statue of Liberty purchased on Liberty Island blends the qualities of patriotic icon and personal memento. A woman who is the mother of children in a household can be understood both in the uniqueness of her relationship to her family ("my mother") and as a representation of the idea of loving familial care.

In Victorian culture, "home," with its complex chains of association, made symbols out of domestic objects; today, the concept of home seems less capable of conferring the same symbolic weight to household furnishings. Many of the objects that acquired symbolic weight were utilitarian and common. As conventions of culture, these domestic symbols seem generally to have been understood by Victorian Americans, although some individuals might understand more nuances of meaning than others. In an analysis of Victorian mementoes of mourning, Lawrence Taylor has used the subjects and imagery of sentimental mourning poetry in *Godey's Lady's Book* to demonstrate how series of symbolic associations were believed to work: "This increasing importance of ritual objects—from locks of hair and empty cradles to gravestones—was a natural outcome of the prevalent 'theory of associations.' Put simply, objects, by virtue of their cultural form and/or specific history, were thought to be packed with meanings" for those individuals with "sensitive souls, or souls made sensitive by the impress of a properly ritual setting, whether church, cemetery, or museum."[25] Sentimental poetry and fiction not only helped to demonstrate the way in which such chains of association worked in connection to objects such as furniture, but they probably also served to perpetuate conventional associations.

"The Old Arm-Chair," a four-stanza poem by Eliza Cook that appeared in the popular magazine *Godey's Lady's Book* in March 1855, illustrates the actual structuring of associative thinking, as well as how popular literature supported the process. In it, an armchair served as a symbol within the larger symbol of home and neatly encapsulated its own range of meanings. The poem ascribed to this single piece of furniture a chain of associations that many, if not all, of her readers could have appreciated.

> The Old Arm-Chair
> I love it, I love it; and who shall dare
> To chide me for loving that old arm-chair?
> I've treasured it long as a sacred prize;
> I've bedewed it with tears, and embalmed it with sighs;
> 'Tis bound by a thousand bands to my heart;
> Not a tie will break, not a link will start.
> Would ye learn the spell? a mother sat there,
> And a sacred thing is that old arm-chair.[26]

Miss Cook's poem in *Godey's* employed the melding of personal and conventional, explaining that her deep feelings for the chair stemmed from its previous ownership by "a mother," a particularly honored social role. The next verse revealed that "a mother" was, in fact, Miss Cook's own mother, who gave her religious instruction from the chair and who passed through the stages of her life in it.

> In childhood's hour, I lingered near
> The hallowed seat with listening ear;
> And gentle words that mother would give,
> To fit me to die and teach me to live.
> She told me shame would never betide,
> With truth for my creed and God for my guide;
> She taught me to lisp my earliest prayer,
> As I knelt beside that old arm-chair.
>
> 'Tis past! 'tis past! but I gaze on it now
> With quivering breath and throbbing brow;
> 'Twas there she nursed me; 'twas there she died;
> And memory flows with lava tide.
> Say it is folly, and deem me weak,
> While scalding drops start down my cheek;
> But I love it, I love it, and cannot tear
> My soul from a mother's old arm-chair.[27]

Indeed, Miss Cook's memories of her mother were irrevocably tied to the simple presence of the chair. The poem moves from an explanation of a conventional association, the honor of motherhood, through a chain of personal meanings. A *Godey's Lady's Book* reader of 1855 would also be able to bring additional associations to the poem, especially the link between religion and domesticity. The symbol "home" incorporated both connotations, suggested in "Family Devotion," a popular print that depicted a family's regular devotional reading around its parlor center table (fig. 4).

Objects can express symbolic meaning in several ways. They can share messages in a comparatively direct way. The moral and aesthetic content of a popular print such as "Family Devotion" was

was easily legible; it triggered a set of popularly shared associations about the relationship of family life and moral growth and the emotional as well as physical closeness of the family circle. A verse such as "The Old Arm-Chair" can suggest a set of less directly perceived associations—the connection, for example, of a type of chair with mothers. Objects also can express symbolic meaning by possessing qualities that people consider analogous to larger cultural values.[28] For example, the soaring architectural space of a church is associated with the feelings worship is meant to inspire—awe, smallness in the face of divine truth—and its grandeur and size also "describe" the qualities of the Almighty. A set of lace curtains in a parlor window carried no overt message, as did a transfer-printed platter with a scene of Lafayette's visit to America. However, the way those curtains diffused and softened sunlight, the delicacy of the textile, and the patterns they might cast on the parlor's walls or the carpet all suggested the refined character of the parlor and the propriety of "softened" behavior there.

In this way, some symbols may be interpreted best as an expression of "sensibility," the distinctive form in which a culture's mental perception or awareness of itself is manifested. This awareness can exist in a realm of direct sensory perception, a recognition that is often expressed not directly but rather through actions or aesthetic choices.[29] Much of the sensory information that people receive is not easily described in words, nor is it processed at the level of conscious awareness.[30] Experience with things crosses a boundary between different modes of experience, between visual and tactile understanding and language.[31] However, even if it is often an inarticulate process, the act of choosing always makes a statement about one's personal and cultural values.

Exploring the history of sensibility and its symbols requires what might be called a "leap of faith" between the forms of evidence that do survive—the conventions of description and the objects themselves, often now bereft of their original contexts. Still, it is possible to determine some of the meanings that some people ascribed to sensory experience by comparing the language used to describe valued cultural concepts and experiences with the language used to describe objects. When certain descriptive terms cut across categories of experience, they are arguably evidence of a particular

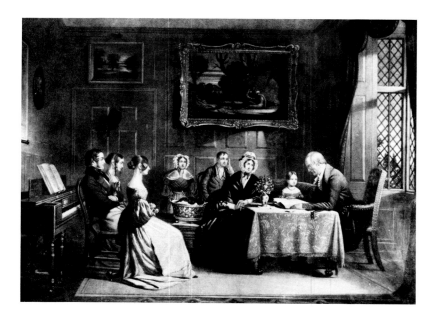

Fig. 4. "Family Devotion, Evening," engraving by James Scott for Tilt and Bogue, London, England, 1842, after a painting by Eduard Prentiss (1797-1854). Godey's Lady's Book for May 1842 published a small engraving after this print, a depiction of the ideal Christian home that the magazine promoted in its articles, fiction, and editorials.

way of organizing the world—what anthropologist Daniel Biebuyck has called "semantic taxonomy."[32]

Symbolic Languages: Furnishings as Rhetorical Statements

As they are found in sentimental fiction and books of furnishing advice, the nuances of use and meaning associated with domestic objects and household furnishing are sometimes astonishingly complex. Not every person can have appreciated equally all the possible chains of association connected to the domestic artifacts of their households. Probably, people were variably compelled by some meanings and unaffected by others. Furnishings in the Gothic style may have contained deep meaning for very pious people, suggesting the link between religion and domesticity; for others, they may simply have conveyed shallow associations with a specific church building.

However, popular literature (including fiction, poetry, and advice books) and popular imagery (published prints, pictures in periodicals, and photographs) provide considerable reason to believe that many ordinary Americans were seriously interested in learning the conventional meanings of things (fig. 5). Entire chapters of domestic manuals were devoted to explicating the meaning of finger-rings or the "language of flowers" (a term used in the period). Richard Wells' *Manners, Culture and Dress*, an advice manual that was reprinted often in the 1890s, listed in one chapter the meaning of 318 flowers and plants presented as gifts. A deep red rose signaled "bashful love"; an iris signaled "melancholy." The language of flowers, Wells pointed out, was "no new thing," having originated in the ancient East.[33] For those with a taste for them, the nuances of Victorian domestic life lay in this juxtaposition of cultural associations and personal experiences—for example, in the juxtaposition of the *idea* of "the mother's chair" with the chair favored by one's own mother.

As their interest in the "language of flowers" suggests, Victorian Americans were taken with the possibility of non-verbal kinds of expressive "languages" structured by "grammars." They found a highly nuanced language in the practice of etiquette. As Mrs. H. O. Ward, author of *Sensible Etiquette*, noted, "Society has its grammar as language has, and the rules of that grammar must be learned."[34] In 1902, the author of *Social Culture* declared that "manners constitute

Fig. 5. "Drawing Room," stereograph in the Popular "Five Cent" Series published by Stevens' Bookstore, Lewiston, Maine, about 1870. A few stereographs, such as this one illustrating an anonymous and typical pair of middle-class parlors, may have been published to initiate new consumers into the mysteries of furnishing modern parlors. Courtesy Smithsonian Institution; private collection.

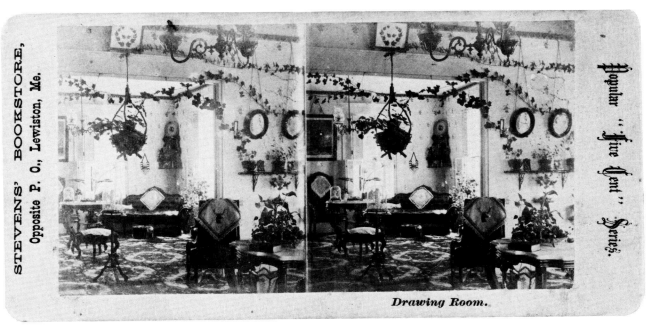

STEVENS' BOOKSTORE, Opposite P. O., Lewiston, Me.

Popular "Five Cent" Series.

Drawing Room.

the language in which the biography of every individual is written."[35]
Owners of furnishings also understood their symbolic, communicative
possibilities and consciously used them to make symbolic assertions
that could be understood, with varying degrees of clarity and
comprehension, by people who confronted them. In a fundamental
way, carefully planned rooms were designed to be rhetorical
statements in the sense that they consciously or unconsciously
expressed aspirations, what a person believed or wished to believe.[36]

Historians have long interpreted architecture as rhetoric. The
exclusively neoclassical public building campaign in the first decades
of American independence is a case in point. Aware that their
buildings would be judged by posterity, and believing that a nation's
public building and monuments were a statement of its character,
American intellectuals found classicism "a perfect style to express the
pastoral ideal" of republican virtue.[37] Thus, Greek Revival buildings
were a rhetorical statement of belief. The domestic critics of parlor
furnishing also understood and were troubled by the rhetorical ends
to which consumption of furnishings in the mid-nineteenth century
was put. Like critics of clothing fashions, they recognized that as the
commercialization of society proceeded and attractive clothing and
domestic furnishings became available to new groups of people, no
correspondence was guaranteed between what a person "said" he was
through the "language" of his possessions and what he really was;
one could no longer tell the players without a program. The use of
objects as a structured form of communication is more analogous to
language than to literacy, to rhetoric than to text.[38]

Further, it is possible to think of users of this language of objects
as being more or less successful in the act of communicating through
their manipulation, to be "artifactually competent" just as they were
linguistically competent. Because Victorian culture's symbols were so
often "real" in the sense that they were material and were often
available for ownership by individuals, we can describe the process of
gaining knowledge, fluency, and ease in their manipulation as a
process of gaining competence in communication. A wide range of
communicative skill was demonstrated through domestic furnishings,
from new consumers just learning the basic elements of furnishing to
"professional interpreters," the interior decorators.

The expanding universe of available consumer goods was like the
universe of words available in a language. The choices made by
individual consumers, which might have been highly idiosyncratic or
highly conventional, are comparable to the ordering of the
vocabulary they employed in speech.[39] In the furnishing of houses,
then as now, ordinary consumers were provided with a constantly
expanding range of choices, but specific room types were governed by
a "grammar" that indicated how comprehensible statements were to
be made. Some of the customs of furnishing had function as their
basis—dining rooms require tables, for example. But many of the
nuances of furnishing each type of room had other sources, historical
in origin and metaphorical in content. In the nineteenth century, for
example, dining room furnishings continued to employ a masculine
iconography of the hunt, even though few of the men who headed
dinner tables in these settings ever brought dinner home to their
families in such a direct manner.[40] Employing images of the violence
of the hunt, its conquests, and the abundance resulting from skill at
hunting reflected the sense of self as well as the economic competence
that good masculine providers were supposed to have. Placed inside a
family's house, such images were also a metaphorical statement of the
difference between the harsh world outside the home and the softer
one within its walls (fig. 6).

While each type of room could have been furnished in infinitely

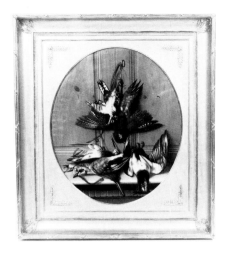

Fig. 6. Still Life with Game Birds, *oil on canvas by unidentified artist, United States, about 1840. Paintings and prints depicting trophies from the hunt were considered dining room subjects, along with depictions of fish, fruits, and vegetables. This painting hung side by side with one entitled* Still Life with Fish *in the dining room of Rochester, New York, journalist Joseph Curtis.*

various ways, certain elements were essential in order that any given room be understood as one of its type—a parlor, a dining room, or a library, for example. People furnishing a room not only made a set of selections based on the constraints of economics and the dimensions of interior space; they also made selections based on an understanding of what that room was supposed to include and signify. Ordinary consumers studied "ideal" statements that existed in the world—rooms in the houses of rich people opened for auctions, the "model" interiors at world's fairs—and followed cues in a variety of printed sources, including novels, magazines, and, by the 1890s, mail-order catalogs. They tried to recreate these ideals to the extent that their time, money, space, and understanding would allow. Depending on their resources and competence, the rooms they made "paraphrased" the ideal more or less exactly.[41]

Other terms have already been attached to the process by which individuals who are not perceived as social tastemakers make consumption decisions. Most typically applied is the term "emulation," "the endeavor to equal or surpass others in any achievement or quality...the ambition to equal or excel."[42] Thorstein Veblen associated "emulation" with the process of "social comparison of persons with a view to rating and grading them in respect to relative worth or value," what he termed "invidious comparison."[43] Viewing consumption decisions solely as a competitive process is, however, too narrow. For ordinary people, consumption for the purposes of parlor making may have been less competitive than demonstrative. By working toward some attainable version of a parlor, they proclaimed membership in the respectable middle classes. However, the idea of paraphrase seems particularly appropriate, because it implies that when a message is restated it experiences some change, often in the direction of compression or economy; it is reduced to its most concise elements.[44] Indeed, paraphrase of the parlor sometimes involved ingenious sets of compromises in the way it used the parlor vocabulary. At the lower end of the furniture-buying market, purchase of a single inexpensive lounge, with its intricate interplay of wood frame and rich-looking, brightly colored carpet upholstery, could serve as a paraphrase of an entire parlor suite. The idea of paraphrase is also useful in analyzing the economics of the design and production of less expensive lines of consumer goods. The production of inexpensive upholstery demanded, by the last quarter of the nineteenth century, that those elements of an object that indicate its style and its adherence to aesthetic standards be pared down to some minimally acceptable level.

Decorative Arts as Symbols: Upholstery

Within this study of parlor making and use, one type of parlor furnishing serves as a focal point because it seems particularly expressive of the tension between culture and comfort. Upholstery defined in its traditional sense—all the loose textile furnishings of rooms, draperies as well as seating furniture—was employed often and ingeniously in Victorian parlors. The levels of detail employed on both seating furniture and myriad forms of drapery suggest that both professional upholsterers and ambitious do-it-yourselfers found furnishing textiles rich in expressive possibilities (figs. 7 and 8). Further, upholstery in all its forms was increasingly available over the course of the nineteenth century to wholly new groups of consumers.

What Victorians labeled the "decorative arts"—furniture, textiles, ceramics and glass, silver, and all the other ornamental yet ostensibly functional objects that filled their rooms—were an integral part of the group of symbols contained within the larger symbol "home." Their complex character as objects was the source of pleasure—or, among design reformers, discomfort. As utilitarian objects, their perfected materials and workmanship and increased serviceability were products and emblems of advancing technology. The variety of their forms reflected civilization's improved understanding and "scientific" categorization of domestic activities. Their forms and their aesthetic qualities also were expressive of the highest human intellectual faculties, just as the "fine arts" of painting and sculpture were. As the anonymous author of "A Visit to Henkels' Warerooms in Chestnut Street above Fifth" in the August 1850 issue of *Godey's Lady's Book*, exclaimed, "Few things are better calculated to give pleasure to the patriot than those evidences of advancement, which are witnessed here and there in our country, in those arts that unite physical comfort with intellectual pleasure…Upholstery and cabinet-making…merit, we think, a high regard, as they call into action many of the most ingenious faculties of him who engaged in them practically."[45] In the view of this "patriot," the decorative arts were admirable for the inventive solution they offered to the relationship between the practical mechanical arts, domestic comforts, and the "intellectual pleasure" that the fine arts were capable of providing.

Because they bridged the realms of practical work and art, decorative arts also offered the possibility of creating long, complex chains of cultural associations and meanings in addition to the

Fig. 7. "Reading the Scriptures," colored lithograph by Alfred E. Baker, New York, New York, after a painting by English artist Benjamin Robert Haydon (1786-1846). The interior and woman's clothing date the image from the 1830s. Apart from the table cover, the room is devoid of upholstery, and it does not express the ideal of planned, matching interior decor.

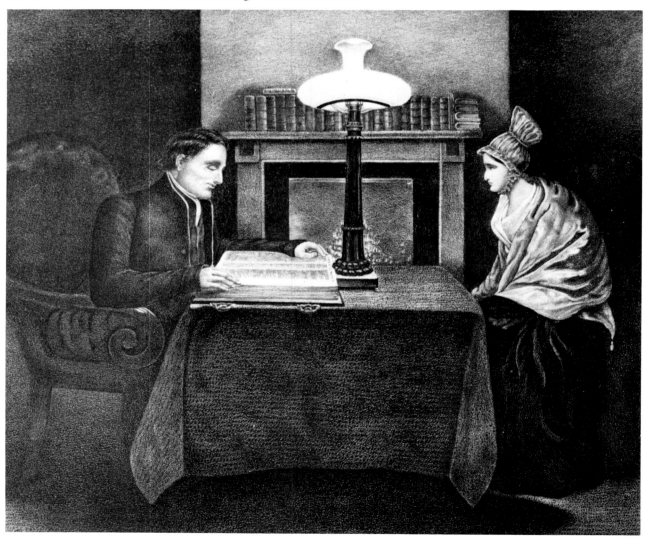

personal associations such objects could develop in the context of the private house. In this, rather than in the historical associations that "Gothic revival" or "Renaissance revival" furnishings bore in their ornamental detail, lies much of the Victorian *popular* fascination with furnishings. Ownership of decorative objects presented the possibility of the private house as a "memory palace" of culture, where the potentially dangerous outside worlds, not just of commerce but also of secular knowledge, could be tamed and made domestic by bringing them under the softening hand of familial influence.

The chain of historical and cultural associations attached to one type of furnishing—textiles—illustrates this point. All forms of household textiles, from simple domestic dress cottons to elaborate furnishing damasks, were the objects of considerable fascination throughout the nineteenth century because the industrialization of textile production changed their availability and cost so profoundly. The process of producing even simple sheeting for household use had always been time consuming, making all textiles comparatively expensive. Historically, beautiful printed, pile, and pattern-woven textiles used both for dress and furnishing enjoyed an association with wealth and power because their production was so labor and skill intensive, and some of the raw materials, such as silk and threads made from precious metals, were always scarce and expensive. In the mobile courts of feudal Europe, textiles—like precious metals and ivory—were an easily portable and tangible sign of the wealth and power of a prince.[46] This state of chronic scarcity and expense began to change in the second half of the eighteenth century with the invention of the spinning jenny in 1770. Mechanization of spinning and weaving affected the daily lives of ordinary people in profound ways, altering the nature of the family as an economic unit as well as changing the experience of work through the setting of the textile

Fig. 8. *"Reading the Scriptures," colored lithograph published by Nathaniel Currier, New York, New York, about 1855. Whoever reworked "Reading the Scriptures" transformed the couple into fashionably dressed parlor denizens and their room into a coordinated draped and upholstered setting that employs substantial yardages of decorative fabrics. The print suggests the power that a new conception of fashionable parlor decor and living held for middle-class people, as well as their changing access to furnishing fabrics. This room has been "softened" through textiles; the evident civilized and moral demeanor of its residents suggests their own "softening."*

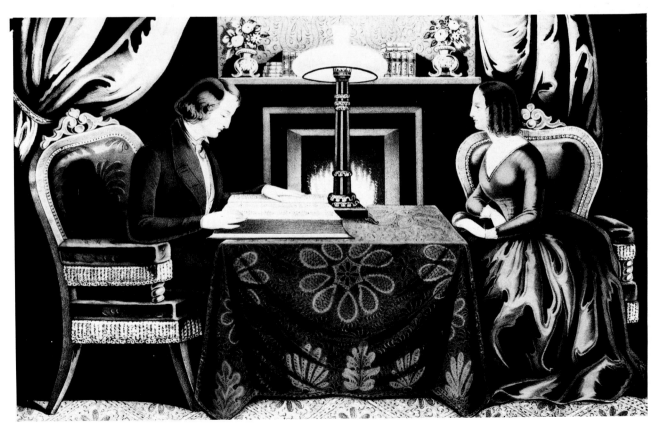

mill in the 1820s and 1830s.[47]

Throughout the first half of the nineteenth century, textile technology was as vibrant an arena for innovation as small computers are today; many talented individuals in both Britain and America devoted their lives to textile innovations. Like the computer industry, textile technology was also the object of considerable appreciation and comment because of its effect on ordinary lives. In 1836, Daniel Webster considered "the use of the elastic power of steam, applied to the operations of spinning and weaving and dressing fabrics for human wear" as "the most prominent instance of the application of science to art" for the benefit of mankind. In 1860, another author interested in technological progress could still call the manufacture of domestic cottons "a most beautiful and complicated art."[48]

There were other, peculiarly American, aspects to the public interest in textiles that made them a particularly meaningful part of domestic consumption. The eighteenth-century debate about the effects of fashion and luxury upon the citizens of the colonies and the young republic, which decried domestic consumption of foreign "finery," had often focused upon imported textiles for furnishing and clothing rather than upon other imported consumer goods. Textile production and consumption had first been politicized through the Stamp Act controversy, when non-importation and non-consumption resolutions directed to English goods led to a craze for "spinning bees" among fashionable young women and to the fad for wearing garments of homespun fabric at the public events of local high society. Boosters of domestic textile production developed a "rhetoric of homespun" that linked household spinning and weaving to republican virtue well into the nineteenth century. The editor of *Niles Weekly Register* noted in 1821:

> We never reflect upon the progress and prospects of that portion of the national labor which is applied to household manufactures, without feeling our hearts warmed with a national pride; for all the virtues, moral, religious and political, are interested in it. Tens of thousands of amiable, respectable and lovely young women...of those ranks and conditions in life which, a few years since, almost as much despised a distaff as they did a field-hoe, are now engaged to drive away the diseases and distresses of inanity, and keep themselves in health and cheerfulness, render themselves good wives, and estimable mothers, while they add to the comforts and conveniences of their parents, and make a "plentiful house" by a diligent attention to spinning, weaving, bleaching, dyeing, etc.[49]

The dramatic proliferation of factory-woven plain household textiles after the introduction of the power loom in America in 1815 was accompanied by an equally dramatic decline in their prices. Between 1815 and 1830, the price of a yard of unbleached shirting material dropped from forty-two to seven and a half cents.[50] The author of *Eighty Years' Progress of the United States* (1867) described the drop in textile prices in common parlance: "The price of a good calico is now twelve yards to a bushel of wheat. Forty years ago it was one yard for a bushel of wheat. The quality of goods at the same time has improved in a greater ratio. The handsome prints that now replace the 'factory checks' of that day, show as great a change as does the price."[51]

The first successes of fully mechanized textile production affected the cost of plain and printed fabrics for clothing and such basic domestic uses as bed linen. However, the development of the lace net loom and the jacquard loom attachment in the first decade of the nineteenth century began the process of adapting mechanized production to fabrics for drapery and upholstery. Bobbin net grounds for laces that could be embellished by hand embroidery were produced by machine beginning in 1809. Entire lace curtains were made by machine by the 1840s. Machine-made tapestries for upholstery uses were in production in Great Britain by the 1850s; carpet upholstery—tough, brightly colored, and inexpensive—was a commonplace on inexpensive furniture by 1870.[52] The development of new classes of factory-woven furnishing textiles such as velvets and plushes with sturdy and inexpensive cotton grounds brought further change to furnishing textile consumption. While most upholstery production remained European until the 1890s, and many beautiful furnishing fabrics continued to be handmade and expensive, ordinary consumers gained access to a range of furnishing fabrics that had, in the scope of living memory, been reserved for individuals of wealth.

Careful study of upholstery can illuminate the continuing power of conceptions of parlor life established decades earlier, conceptions that seem to have survived even when the context that inspired their initial articulation no longer existed. If many surviving upholstered chairs still seem "uncomfortable" to modern eyes, were they ever meant to be so? Or did they serve other functions more important to parlor makers, symbolic functions or uses that expressed some connection to eighteenth-century ideals of self-presentation? Were draperies more important as aesthetic statements than as fabric barriers to keep out the heat or cold? If upholstery is one medium that embodies the tension between culture and comfort, do changes in its forms and uses also help chart evolution in these two poles of thought?

This book will follow Americans' interest and understanding of parlor upholstery and drapery from their early exposure to it in a variety of commercial settings to their growing ability to imagine and then realize themselves creating and living in such spaces in their own homes. It traces the effect of two competing models of domestic life on the development of the middle-class parlor and the ways in which consumers learned the fundamental vocabulary for furnishing these spaces. The complexities of the concept of comfort are explored, including the cultural limits on getting comfortable and the rationale behind the popularity of spring-seat upholstery. The book explores the sensibility that found meaning in the formal visual and tactile qualities of upholstery, and how such preferences were one facet of larger patterns of thought embracing the concept of "refinement." It analyzes how the upholstery trade interpreted these aesthetic preferences and notions about seated comfort. Within the economic compromises that manufacturers were able to achieve in design and production, they made parlor furnishings that satisfied the sensibilities of Victorian Americans and were accessible to a broad range of incomes. The associations Americans made between objects and the world around them—in fact, their very connections with that world—are exemplified by the vast popularity of furnishings promoted as "French" and "Turkish," as well as in objects that had no apparent connection to historical revivals, such as parlor suites, lounges, and door and window drapery. Such goods and the values they symbolized were pervasive and popular enough that they became ultimately accessible through do-it-yourself projects in countless advice books and magazines. Americans could even turn barrels into upholstered chairs, creating for themselves virtually from nothing a symbol of middle-class gentility. Finally, *Culture and Comfort* examines the replacement of the parlor by the modern living room. Surprising continuities and significant changes became apparent by the 1920s, suggesting that Victorianism waned slowly and unevenly in early twentieth-century America.

CHAPTER ONE
IMAGINING THE PARLOR

In 1853, the New York daguerreotypist M. M. Lawrence opened his new heliographic establishment on the upper floor of 381 Broadway. Prospective clients first entered a 25-by-40-foot "reception room" which was described in *Humphrey's Journal of Photography* as "furnished with rich, heavy Brussels carpet...the walls handsomely papered, window shades, and appropriate lace curtains, gilt cornices and ornaments, rosewood furniture, upholstered and covered with green velvet." Gentlemen waiting for admission to the "operating room," the site of the actual picture-making, remained in this elegant interior. Women, however, were invited to prepare themselves for their portraits in a 25-foot-square "ladies' parlor" which was "carpeted with rich tapestry...walls covered with richest blue velvet and gold paper—rose wood furniture, covered with blue and gold brocatelle—reception, easy and rocking chairs, tête-à-têtes, &c...Marble-top centre table, rose wood book-stand..."[1]

M. M. Lawrence furnished his photography studio's reception room and ladies' parlor as if they were drawing rooms in a well-to-do private household. Beginning in the third decade of the nineteenth century, publicly accessible "commercial parlors" like Lawrence's were a new kind of interior space that proliferated in several kinds of businesses with which ordinary Americans had periodic contact. Between 1830 and 1880, Americans who were invited to patronize these establishments sought, consciously or unconsciously, specific things from these fashionable public facades. Beyond their ostensible purposes, these interiors were an intermediary between the sources of tasteful furnishings and new consumers who were themselves deeply interested in having parlors and in furnishing them appropriately. Many of the mechanisms that now inform people about new fashions in furniture and interior decoration—mass magazines, which devote much of their space to photographs of exemplary rooms; books devoted to furnishing advice; and showroom model interiors—did not exist in the middle decades of the nineteenth century or were new commercial developments, located in only the largest urban centers. Thus commercial parlors not only supplied furnishing information in three dimensions and glowing color; they also provided the experience of simply being in a parlor. In so doing, they implied that parlor gentility was accessible through the great engine of American commerce—and that the temporary inhabitants of the rooms were themselves (or could become) "parlor people," comfortable with the room's social ceremony and at home in its special middle-class milieu.

All these forms of commercial parlor predated the agencies typically given greatest credit for changing and educating public taste—the department store and the international exhibition.[2] At least a century before the 1851 Crystal Palace Exposition, a "consumer revolution" had been underway; citizens with new means to purchase what historian Neil McKendrick has termed "decencies"—and, in time, luxury goods—were also eager seekers of information to guide their consumption.[3] Between 1830 and 1880, they found model parlors in hotels, on steamboats and railroad cars, in photographers' studios, and in the meeting rooms of various voluntary associations. These "public parlors" in commercial spaces had symbolic functions as well. Such elegant settings captured the imagination of at least those segments of the public that were middle class and urbane in their aspirations, if not yet in their actual means.

The commercial parlors in hotels, steamboats, photography studios, and railroad cars usually were not copied exactly by aspiring parlor makers, although many of them could have been reproduced. They were model interiors that allowed people to try on the idea of having a parlor; they were settings in which people could picture themselves. The model interior between 1830 and 1880 was not necessarily created with the goal of creating or changing taste, although some creators of these interiors, such as George Pullman, actually believed that the spaces they furnished would make their clientele more refined. Most of the model rooms played a role in the creation of consumer demand merely by providing an experience—that of being in a carefully decorated room that looked like a parlor and suggested its suitability for similar purposes. Commercial parlors stimulated demand by provoking a process of imagining, providing access to a setting that made it possible to imagine oneself owning and using such a room.

How might this process of individual imagination have taken shape in the minds of thousands of American consumers? Before demand for ownership of objects can be aroused in the minds of potential buyers, they must not only learn that the objects exist; the possibility of owning them must also be perceived as *real*. Not only must per capita income or productive capacity be sufficient, but there must also be a change in attitudes about spending. People must believe that spending income on consumer goods can make an actual difference in their lives, either in terms of greater physical comfort or in terms of expressing one's self or social relationships. In other words, they must perceive the possibility of economic and social mobility to be real—that society is fluid, to some degree, without the restraints of ironclad castes.[4]

Using furnishings to make social claims was not confined to relatively flexible social structures; as historian Penelope Eames has argued, furnishings expressed political power in England, France, and the Netherlands between the twelfth and fifteenth centuries.

> When social and political power was exercised through continuous contact between the seigneurial lord and his men of every rank, as it was in the feudal societies of the Middle Ages, that power was sustained, re-enforced and advertised by ceremony. Court ceremonial was structured by elaborate rules of precedence and behaviour in which the position of each individual, in any given situation, was apparent, not only in what he *did*, but by what he *used* in terms of his clothing, his food and his furnishings. Certain forms of furniture, and indeed furnishings in general, reflected those degrees of honour, or precedence, which were termed *estate*...[and] which might govern use, form, ornament and fabric.[5]

In the court life of Burgundy during this period, the degree of excellence permitted in specific furnishings—the number of shelves permitted in the stepped buffets used to display the concrete wealth of plate owned by the lord or the number of coverings on state beds—was regulated by written rules. These rules for furnishings were the equivalent of sumptuary laws for clothing by rank.[6] Possession of clothing or furnishings of particular quality was not simply a function of wealth but also a reflection of caste-like social status. Imagining ownership—the creation of desire and hence of demand—was beyond the realm of possibility for most individuals.

By the eighteenth century, however, to aspire to own furnishings became plausible for new groups of people, a circumstance that coincided with changing concepts of decor. The idea of furnishings as a created setting for display of social power was indeed medieval; however, as royalty consolidated its claims to power and lords were no longer required to maintain portable households in order to retain control of their holdings, concepts of architecture and decor also changed.[7] Although it clearly had roots in the seventeenth century, the idea of creating self-consciously decorated rooms as personal settings for the display of cultivation (a highly refined form of social competition) in addition to political power gained force in the eighteenth century. It attained its highest refinement in the French concept of *civilisation* but also held sway in England and its colonial territories.[8] It is possible to think of the tastefully decorated salons of men and women of cultivation as extensions of their dress, which also, within the dictates of fashion, became more personally expressive. Thus, the habit of mind that perceived furnishing as a means of expressing social status (whether real or desired) was long-standing, but, by the second half of the eighteenth century, it was linked firmly to the developing notion of changing fashion and "taste," an association that remained strong through the nineteenth century.

The motivation to furnish was in place as Victorian culture developed, but processes of consumer access to information about durable goods such as furniture were underdeveloped until the last decades of the nineteenth century. By the 1870s, furniture producers and various kinds of professional mediators (decorators, home economists, and retailers) stepped up their efforts both to make information about furnishings available and to influence consumer taste. Furniture trade periodicals such as *The American Cabinetmaker, Upholsterer and Carpet Reporter*, new in the 1870s and 1880s, were part of this effort. These professional periodicals demonstrate that furnishing trades continually introduced "decorative novelties" to keep consumers active in the marketplace, which suggests that the wheels of consumer interest had been set in motion and had been well greased some decades earlier.[9] Another information source new to the late nineteenth century was the "model room" created by furniture manufacturers or interior decorators for commercial demonstration purposes. It seems to have been a product of the 1876 Centennial Exhibition in Philadelphia. Before this time, furniture warerooms were conglomerations of merchandise organized by price line or type. Although many exhibitors retained the old techniques of typological display of goods, a number of model rooms at the Centennial seem to have suggested to furnishing manufacturers the efficacy of presenting what would now be termed "a total look" to potential buyers. Grand Rapids, Michigan, furniture companies, particularly Berkey and Gay, were the first to set up "rooms" offered for sale on the show floor (although the company's marketing strategy was aimed at sales not to individual consumers but to store owners during the semi-annual furniture markets).[10] Popular decorating advice books and articles were also largely a product of the 1870s and later, although earlier domestic economy manuals often included a chapter on furnishing.[11] Specific decorating advice in mass magazines appeared sporadically until the 1870s and was usually not illustrated or included pictures of single objects out of context. Mass publications sometimes included images of exemplary parlors, as when *Gleason's Pictorial Drawing-Room Companion* published an engraving of the parlor of a New York merchant in 1854 (fig. 1). Occasionally, the costume prints in magazines also included enough detail of room furnishing to provide useful information to fashion-conscious readers (fig. 2). But extensive photomechanical illustrations of domestic interiors did not appear in periodicals until the 1890s.

For consumers, information on personal fashion—clothing styles, modes of hair-dressing, and the like—seems to have been the easiest of all types of advice to obtain and the most widely disseminated, even among those who could not read or afford to subscribe to magazines with fashion plates. Information about new styles in clothing and hair dressing was readily transmitted through face-to-face contact between social classes, which in nineteenth-century America occurred in the mingling of street life. On her first visit to New York in 1832, British actress Fanny Kemble commented on the quality of clothing worn by lower-class people, including Afro-Americans on Broadway: "After dinner, sat looking at the blacks parading up and down; most of them in the height of fashion, with every colour of the rainbow about them."[12]

However, such casual mingling did not extend to socializing within the houses of the fashionable, at least in cities. New members of the middle classes there probably knew less about the style of living of the wealthy (who received their fashion news directly from European émigré decorators and through networks of contacts with Europe) than rural Americans who entered the houses of small-town leading citizens for special occasions such as funerals. Over the course of the nineteenth century, city neighborhoods that once contained an economic cross section became increasingly stratified and too large to encourage socializing among the elite and the professionals,

Fig. 1. *"A Parlor View in a New York Dwelling House," engraving after a drawing by A. Kimbel in* Gleason's Pictorial Drawing-Room Companion *(11 November 1854). The brief article accompanying this image described the parlor as "the interior of an apartment in a magnificent mansion uptown, where one of the most eminent of our merchants has surrounded himself and family with all the elegancies and luxuries to which years of successful enterprise entitle him....The room looks like a fitting abode of a man of refinement—a drawing room where a lady of elegant manners and educated tastes might appropriately receive her guests."*

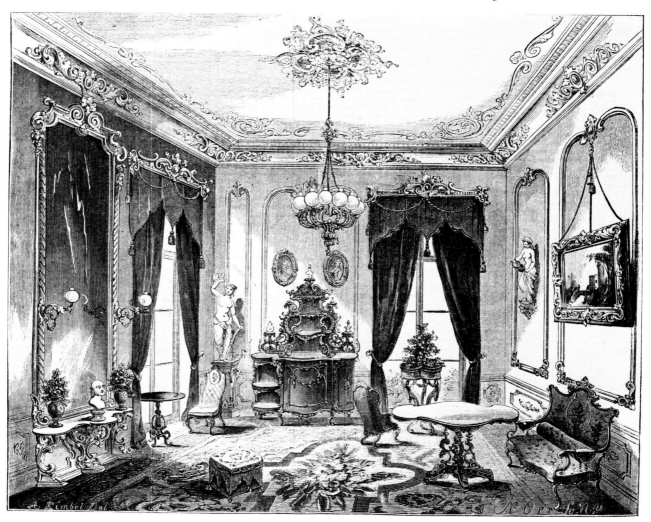

substantial merchants, small business people, and "respectable" skilled artisans that constituted the middle class. It is likely that the upper classes and lower classes intermingled in the homes of the wealthy more often than did the rich and the middle classes, since working-class people were employed as domestic help. Moreover, the execution of various charitable activities sometimes brought the well-heeled to the residences of the poor.[13]

Ordinary Americans with modest incomes and aspirations to fashion could occasionally gain admittance to the homes of the fashionable. One of the most important ways may have been the household auction, which provided not only furnishing information but also the possibility of ownership of furnishings that would otherwise have been beyond their means (fig. 3). The story "A Bargain: Is a Penny Saved, Twopence Got?" in an 1854 issue of *Gleason's Pictorial Drawing-Room Companion* described a New York City auction preview in "an elegantly furnished private mansion" owned by a man named Lyons.

> [The house] looked as if the owners had only gone out for morning calls, and might be expected back at any moment. The curtains, mirrors, suites of elegant furniture, set forth in the catalogue...were arranged as if for an ordinary reception day, instead of the press of an ignoble crowd,—second-hand furniture

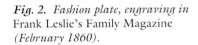

Fig. 2. Fashion plate, engraving in Frank Leslie's Family Magazine *(February 1860).*

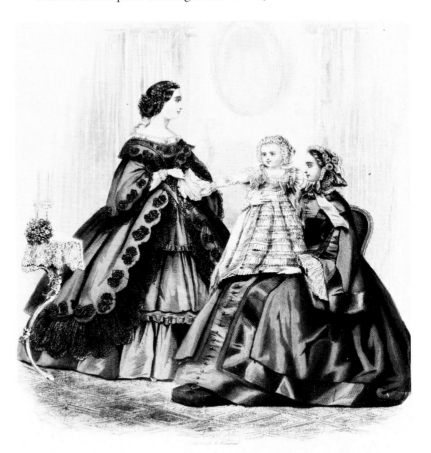

FEBRUARY 1860.

men, small boarding-house people, ladies, porters, idle spectators, and busy-bodies thronging around.[14]

The heroine of the story, a country girl visiting city friends, was appalled at the crowds who "swarmed from the kitchen to the servants' rooms," "scanned the furniture," "tried the springs of the sofas and chairs," and "plunged themselves up and down in the library chairs." She was chided, however, by an acquaintance who described the benefits of auction sales:

> "That's it, you see," Mr. Allen said…"That's the way so many people of moderate means have their houses so handsomely furnished. A man of taste like Lyons or yourself, collects books, and pictures, and furniture, to be dispersed eventually after this fashion. The next owner 'declines housekeeping' in turn, and the things being a little more tarnished by removal or use, are purchased a shade cheaper by a class a grade lower in the scale, and so *decencus averni*."[15]

Household auction catalogs confirm that these sales offered the public contact with beautifully planned and furnished parlors, as well as elegantly appointed dining rooms and chambers. A catalog for a sale of "Handsome Household Furniture" in New York City on April 22, 1841, described the "Front Parlour" furnishings as including a "large pier glass," "royal Wilton carpet," "2 rosewood couches, covered with fawn coloured striped satin, with figured blue silk border," two divans to match, and "4 chairs, with stuffed backs, to match, with figured blue chintz covers for all." The room's windows were curtained with "very elegant window curtains, fawn colored,

Fig. 3. *"An Auction of Splendid Household Furniture, To Be Sold without Reserve," engraving in* Harper's Weekly *(3 April 1858).*

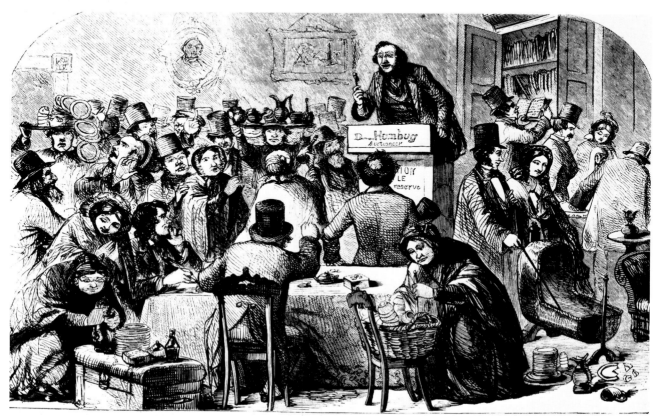

AN AUCTION OF SPLENDID HOUSEHOLD FURNITURE, TO BE SOLD WITHOUT RESERVE.

with blue trimmings"; all the furnishings were listed as being "good as new, made by Ellcau." An 1853 sale of "Genteel Household Furniture," also in New York City, included in its inventory of the front parlor an eight-piece suite upholstered in "crimson plush," "rich tapestry Carpet," and two windows with gilt cornices from which hung "very rich crimson and maroon drapery and lace window Curtains, &c." The room was also furnished with a variety of mirrors, candlesticks, sofa tables, and two "Ptgs Landscape and cattle."[16]

For most Americans, commercial parlors provided incipient parlor makers their first contact with consciously "designed" interiors—or even with as simple a novelty as spring-seat upholstery and lace curtains. In her popular novel of 1854, *High Life in New York*, Ann S. Stephens described one such encounter in the parlor of the Howard Hotel through the eyes of the book's "author," the Connecticut farmer Jonathan Slick. Upon being invited to take a seat on a "cushioned bench," Slick did not demur.

> "Wal," sez I, a bowin, "I don't care if I du, just to oblige you;" so down I sot, but the cushion give so, that I sprung right up on eend agin, and when I see it rise up as shiney and smooth as ever, I looked at her, and sez I—"Did you ever!" "It's elastic," sez she, a puckerin up her mouth. "I don't know the name on it," sez I, "but it gives like an old friend, so I'll try it agin."[17]

We cannot know how many people developed a taste for parlor life through their contact with parlors in commercial buildings, but articles and advertisements in newspaper and magazines suggest that the public was very interested in these rooms. The presence of a properly genteel parlor or a parlor-like setting became a selling point for photographers' studios, hotels, and steamboat and railroad lines. Parlors in commercial spaces were an integral part of the web of ideas and images about the rapid advance of civilized living in America that resulted from commercial activity, a set of ideas that crystallized in the concept of "palaces of the people." The New York City "dry goods palace" of the period 1845 to 1875 was a specific architectural type whose exterior featured specific palatial iconography . The prototype was A. T. Stewart's "Marble Palace" (1846) on Broadway and Chambers Street, the largest and most famous dry goods palace of the period.[18] Hotels and other commercial buildings, the kinds of steamboats commonly called "palace steamers," and railroad cars such as "Wagner's Palace Parlor Car" were all "palaces of the people" whose parlors were publicly accessible rooms of state. In a series of articles on new "first-class hotels" in America in the early 1850s, publisher Frederick J. Gleason associated the proliferation of hotels with "the advancements of civilization and refinement in our growing country" and claimed that, by 1852, "nearly every city in this Union boasts of a first-class hotel, which though devoted to the accommodation of the public, is yet equal to a European palace" (fig. 4).[19] In 1854, journalist Reuben Vose articulated the popular equation between commerce and civilization's progress that supported the creation of New York City as a "city of palaces" when he claimed, "Commerce is the great civilizer of nations, and where merchants flourish, there all that adds charm to social existence will be found in the greatest abundance."[20]

The concept of the commercial palace and its related interior space, the commercial parlor, were visible symbols that carried real power among commercially minded Americans. By frequenting these places, middle-class Americans could become "parlor people," even if only for a short time; they could imagine themselves possessing that space. Reuben Vose described the pleasures of taking a seat in the "marble hall" of New York's Fifth Avenue Hotel in terms of imaginary ownership:

> If slightly fatigued a seat may be occupied in the hotel, and before him will pass more of the real beauty and wealth of the nation than in any other spot in the city. Here we recover from the toils that recur with every rising sun. Here as we gaze on the wealth of the world we feel at "home." *Yielding to the illusion of the place, and to a suggestive imagination, we often fancy that we are the happy owner of all that glides in beauty before us—except the ladies.*[21]

Contemporary commentators even blamed the American taste for hotel living at least partly upon the public's enthusiasm for the spurious gentility access to hotel parlors offered, the very access Vose found so seductive in his imaginings of financial success.[22]

Commercial parlors were created and recognized as such because they featured furnishings that, placed in any kind of setting, seemed unequivocally to denote the presence of a "parlor." During the first half of the nineteenth century, a specific set of elements came to be

Fig. 4. "La Pierre House, Broad Street, Philadelphia," engraving in Gleason's *(8 October 1853).*

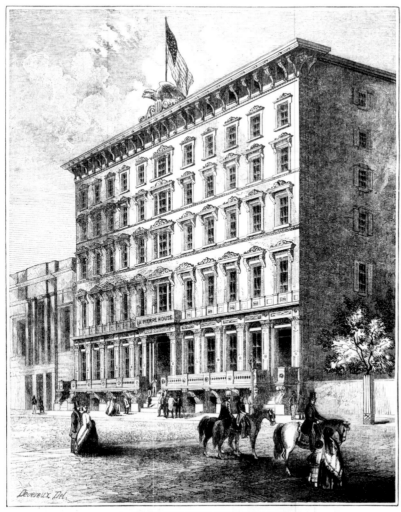

LA PIERRE HOUSE, BROAD STREET, PHILADELPHIA.

viewed as essential to such a room—carpets, window draperies with lace curtains, a parlor suite, "reception" or "fancy" chairs, a center table, a piano, a decorated mantel, and myriad smaller objects. Moreover, certain terms for fabrics, carpets, and even wood types were so emblematic of ideal parlor decor that they provided a descriptive shorthand for authors or journalists describing rooms, as in the words "damask" or "satin" and descriptions such as "richly carved" for furniture and "velvet" for carpets. Finally, in order to attain the parlor ideal fully, the room had to give the appearance of having been furnished all at once; even if furnishings did not match exactly, the room should seem to have been furnished in a coordinated—hence more expensive—manner. In M. M. Lawrence's elegant heliographic establishment, *Humphrey's Journal* noted, "every article here is selected with the greatest care to uniformity."[23]

Although the largest and most elaborate parlors in commercial spaces expressed a scale of expenditure that was beyond the means of most consumers, the elegant interiors of first-class hotels, steamboats, and the largest photographers' studios still used a vocabulary of furnishings that was comprehensible to middle-class consumers, at least through midcentury. A description of the ladies' drawing rooms of Philadelphia's Girard House in 1852 set out the terms of this vocabulary:

> The floors are covered with painted velvet carpets, that echo no footfall; the curtains, yellow damask, relieved by rich lace hangings, and the most costly trimmings; sofas, lounges, étagères, tables, rosewood, *inlaid*; the sofas, &c., seated and backed with yellow satin, the chairs entire gilt, and yellow satin. The walls, from which gigantic mirrors blaze and multiply on every side, are decorated, and each parlor furnished with a massive chandelier of new style.[24]

The Girard House's decor, while grand, seems very close in appearance to the parlors in the Philadelphia home of Mrs. Israel Pemberton Hutchinson, on Spruce above 10th Street, as they appeared in this description of ten years earlier:

> Their rooms are the most beautiful I ever saw. *All* the furniture [is] from Paris of the most costly description and admirable taste and keeping. The front room is in rosewood and some rich fawn colored stuff for drapery and sofas, with immense mirrors and splendid chandelier, candalabra, lamps, bronze ornaments, etc.; the back room, which is the dress room, is in blue and white damask and gold. The woodwork of chairs is massy gilt, the chandelier, candalabra etc. ormolu of exquisite taste and execution.[25]

The first commercial parlors seem to have taken their appearance from their domestic counterparts in the homes of wealthy Americans. Because they were new kinds of places—ones in which socializing was an element of the "product" being sold, whether accommodations, transportation, or likenesses—there existed no real precedent in America for the appearance of spaces that commingled social and commercial functions in quite this fashion. However, parlors in well-to-do private houses in the late eighteenth and first decades of the nineteenth centuries served as a social space which brought together sizable groups of the "best people," the select company rather than the more constricted domestic group of the middle-class parlor later in the nineteenth century (fig. 5). Some of the first commercial parlors may have served this function.[26] Because the "best men" of communities such as New York and Boston were also the first to finance first-class hotels and steamboat companies, they appear to have chosen to furnish their commercial parlors along familiar lines, hiring firms who also provided furniture for their residences. Other later commercial parlors probably took their decorating cues from public interest in these first rooms.

Fig. 5. The Tea Party, *oil on canvas by Henry Sargent, Boston, Massachusetts, about 1824. Courtesy Museum of Fine Arts, Boston; gift of Mrs. Horatio A. Lamb in memory of Mr. and Mrs. Winthrop Sargent.*

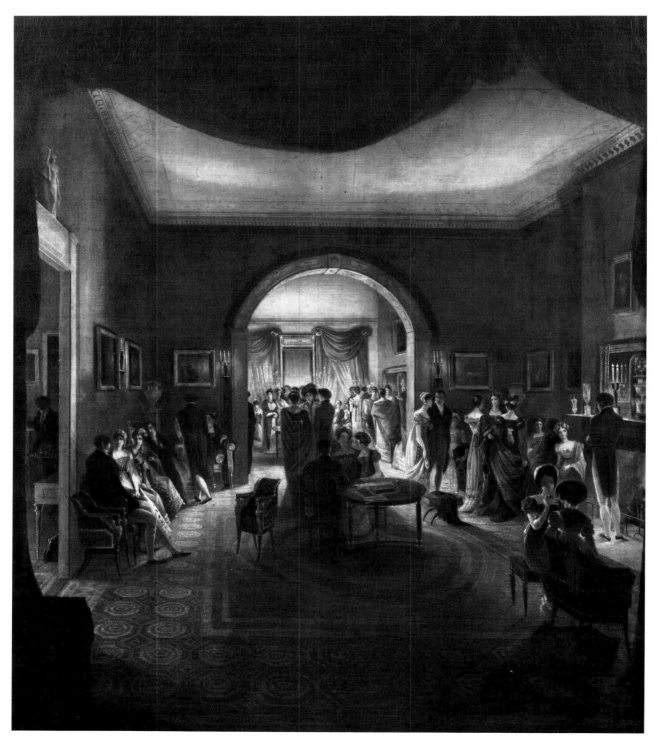

Hotels as Model Interiors

The public rooms of city hotels were perhaps the most influential form of commercial parlor between 1830 and 1860. In urban settings, the power of fashion was greatest, and consumers could directly translate the information on room-making that such interiors provided. The range and number of public rooms in good hotels varied. Francis J. Grund, a German scientist and mathematician who wrote a travelogue in 1837 about his trip to the United States, considered a typical hotel in a larger American city to contain "besides the bar a ladies' and a gentlemen's drawing-room, a number of sitting and smoking rooms for the gratuitous use of boarders, a newsroom, and one or two large dining-rooms."[27] With the exception of the bars and service areas such as barber shops, hotel public rooms were analogous to specific-use rooms in the homes of upper middle-class and wealthy Americans—for example, the reading room or newsroom was similar to the private house's library. Grund noted that the "elegantly fitted up" public rooms were intended to "supply, in a measure, the want of private parlours," which were few in number and expensive in hotels.[28]

As Reuben Vose's fantasy of "owning" the public room suggests, nineteenth-century hotels appear to have been even more open for the public's perusal, use, and informal instruction in civility than are such spaces today. Anthony Trollope was astonished at the number of local people who passed time in hotel public rooms: "[There] is always gathered together a crowd, apparently belonging in no way to the hotel…In the West, during the months of this war, the traveller would always see many soldiers among the crowd,—not only officers, but privates. They sit in public seats, silent but apparently contented, sometimes for an hour together."[29] He considered such spontaneous but companionable crowding into public places a peculiarly American characteristic.

In this social meeting-place role, the hotels Trollope described were carrying on a function that taverns had served in the eighteenth century, but with changes in their scale, appearance, and pretensions. Eighteenth-century inns were generally private houses that had been converted, but between 1790 and 1830, entrepreneurs in East Coast cities opened larger structures built specifically as inns, in order to meet the needs of increasing numbers of transients. These larger inns continued the eighteenth-century inn's role as a social gathering place with "gaudy Long Rooms and Bar Parlors," rooms that could be leased for social events such as balls.[30]

Not only did the appearance and size of hotels change, but the way people thought about them also seems to have evolved. The notion of the "palace hotel" developed, denoting a first-class hotel offering individual accommodations for guests, a variety of special services, and leasable space for public social gatherings.[31] The first published appearance of the term "palaces of the people" in reference to hotels probably occurred in a Washington, D.C., newspaper article about the opening of that city's National Hotel in June 1827. The first-class hotel was a publicly accessible site that could still be associated with social ceremony and power and a kind of public civility—and, best of all, this social power and refinement was located in the world of commerce, a sphere of activity that seemed open to every man.

Between 1830 and 1860, large hotels were constructed in all major American cities and in communities with aspirations toward size and commercial greatness. In 1836, for example, the same year that John Jacob Astor opened New York City's first palace hotel, the Astor House, Buffalo, New York (population 16,000), welcomed the opening of the American Hotel, which was built in the "Grecian" style, a term which in this case included a center stained-glass dome. Civic boosters freely acknowledged that the presence of a first-class hotel was associated with the progress of civilized living in America and believed citizens should be educated by them. Frederick Gleason, publisher of *Gleason's Pictorial Drawing-Room Companion*, was a particularly avid hotel enthusiast. In 1852, the periodical presented a series of descriptions of palace hotels and views of their facades, "not only for the amusement of our readers, but also for their real benefit."[32] Foreign visitors observed the power of the hotel as a concrete symbol of aspirations for a society that was both open and refined. In the 1860s, Anthony Trollope wrote that Americans still were obsessed with hotels: "They are quite as much thought of in the nation as the legislature, or judicative, or literature of the country; and any falling off in them, or any improvement in the accommodation given, would strike the community as forcibly as a change in the constitution, or an alteration in the franchise."[33]

The Tremont Hotel of Boston, which opened in 1829, is generally considered to have been the first palace hotel. Its architectural plan and details, its provisions for privacy and security, its pioneering inclusion of systems for heating and rudimentary plumbing, as well as the size and grandeur of its public rooms, attracted so much interest that a book was published containing its plan and selected details, along with a brief history and description of the interior finishes.[34] The Tremont's public rooms included two parlors for receiving new arrivals, two more "appropriated to the use of families," two sets of rooms for parties and clubs, six parlors attached to suites of rooms (promptly taken by permanent residents), and a large reading room with an attached "public Drawing-room for gentlemen."[35] The reading and drawing room was free to hotel guests; "a small annual subscription" allowed any male citizen to use it as a library and club.

No images of the Tremont's first public parlors appear to have survived—if any were ever drawn or photographed. The appearance of its interior and those of other pre-Civil War palace hotels can be pieced together, however, through what is known about the tradespeople who provided fittings for both hotels and domestic interiors in major American cities. Hotel furnishing was not yet a separate specialty in the furniture business, and the hotel parlors were furnished by warerooms and upholsterers who supplied domestic furnishings for middle-class and wealthier clients.

Twenty-one cabinetmakers, upholsterers, and importers of carpets, mirrors, and lighting devices supplied furnishings for the Tremont as well as for the houses of the well-to-do Bostonians. Because the hotel was paid for by a stock company of the city's "better men," its furnishings probably reflected their upper-class preferences, informed through contact with imported furnishings and publications. Sherlock Spooner, one supplier, advertised his firm in the 1829 Boston city directory as "constantly manufacturing every article in the CABINET, CHAIR, AND UPHOLSTERY hue." He offered "Spring-seat Rocking Chairs, Couches, Sofas, Mahogany Chairs, Music Stools" as well as a range of specialized tables "in superior style."[36] Another supplier, upholsterer and furniture merchant William Hancock, included a woodcut of a fancy Grecian couch in his advertisement that same year. Several examples of furniture made around 1830 with Hancock's paper label survive, including an elegant sofa with upholstered cylindrical arms in the collections of the Metropolitan Museum of Art (fig. 6).[37] The Tremont House parlors in 1830 may, in fact, have looked much like the large parlors of around 1824 depicted in Henry Sargent's painting *The Tea Party.*

The furniture of the LaPierre House, which opened in Philadelphia in 1853, was supplied by George A. Henkels' sizable furniture warerooms, which provided furniture for middle- and upper-class households in the Philadelphia area between 1850 and 1876.[38] Henkels' stock of furniture fell well within the canons of middle-class taste as interpreted by *Godey's Lady's Book,* which promoted the firm's current offerings in several articles in 1850.[39]

A sixteen-page catalog for Henkels' warerooms, dating from around 1855, suggests the types of furnishings the LaPierre's public rooms—a ladies' parlor, a "reception parlor," another for gentlemen, the main dining room, and several tea rooms—might have contained (fig. 7).[40] With the exception of a group of comparatively inexpensive "Plain style" furnishings (probably late neoclassical "pillar and scroll" style) and a passing mention of "Elizabethan" style on the title page, the listed furniture was all based on fashionable French revival styles. The catalog offered "Drawing-Room" furniture as a type distinct from "Parlor Furniture." While the range of forms offered in each of these lines was the same, the distinction between them was cost and degree of ornamentation. Drawing room furniture (which may have been imported) was offered in the "antique" style, an interpretation of sixteenth-century furniture highly carved in the "grotesque" style with animal and plant imagery. The French called the style of such furnishings "Renaissance."[41] The drawing room "Trio Tête-à-Tête" in the group ("elaborately carved, Satin covering") was offered at the breathtaking price of $350. Less expensive ($60 to $75) but still fashionable "Têtes" listed under "Parlor Furniture" were offered in a plainer (probably less highly carved but retaining the basic shapes and ornament of the style) version of the antique style or the popular Louis XIV taste. All three options offered customers "Tête-à-tête" sofas, matching arm chairs, ladies' chairs and side chairs—the grouping of forms that, sold together, comprised the typical seven-piece parlor suite of the 1860s through 1880s. "Consol" and "Center" tables, étagères, and reception chairs rounded out the basic parlor line.

More is known about the appearance of the draperies in the La Pierre's public rooms, thanks to an illustrated article that appeared in the February 1854 issue of *Godey's.* The magazine touted the "celebrated depot" of W. H. Carryl, which supplied curtains, furniture coverings, window shades, and "all kinds of parlor trimmings" for the La Pierre (fig. 8). The plates were one of a series of images of "parlor window drapery" furnished by Carryl that appeared over the course of several years in the magazine. The article

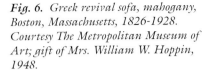

Fig. 6. Greek revival sofa, mahogany, Boston, Massachusetts, 1826-1928. Courtesy The Metropolitan Museum of Art; gift of Mrs. William W. Hoppin, 1948.

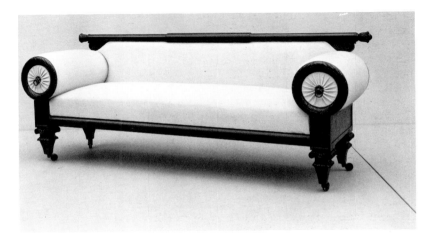

marked no difference between the kinds of draperies used in houses and in commercial parlors, and the materials and forms listed correspond to middle-class interior decoration. Among these were "heavy green lambrequins" in the parlor and tea room, whose "rich bullion fringe" was praised for being so close in appearance to real gold bullion that "it would take a practiced eye to detect it." Reading and drawing room curtains were made in brocatelle, an upholstering fabric which, at midcentury, was either all wool or had a linen warp and wool weft and was woven in damask patterns with the figures formed by the warp in a satin weave. It was a middle-class substitute for expensive brocaded fabrics and damask made of silk.

The parlor window drapery in *Godey's* ("Fig. 1" in that magazine) was claimed to be "nearly identical" in style to the window treatments found in the hotel's principal drawing room. They were "draped with crimson, garnet, and gold brocatelle, finished by heavy cornices and the richest corresponding decorations," along with "exquisite lace curtains, as in the plate, falling below." "Fig. 2" represented the draperies of the "elegant suite of parlors on the second floor," which were "curtains of brocatelle, crimson, yellow, and green and gold, equally rich and suited to the style of the apartments, as in the drawing-room below." *Godey's* congratulated Carryl for the part his curtains played in giving the hotel "a cheerful welcome and homelike feeling."[42]

Interiors that probably bear a close resemblance to public parlors in first-class hotels of the mid-nineteenth century are to be found today in what was, until the 1940s, a summer residence in Portland, Maine. Known today as the Morse-Libby Mansion, or Victoria Mansion, the brownstone Italianate villa was constructed between 1858 and 1861 by Ruggles Sylvester Morse, a self-made man whose entire career was devoted to hotels.[43] Morse was born in Leeds, Maine, in 1813, but family history (otherwise undocumented) holds that he left the state in the early 1830s to work first at the Tremont House in Boston and then at New York's Astor House. A father-and-son team named Boyden, who managed the Tremont and later the Astor, may have brought the evidently able Morse along as an assistant manager. After a brief sojourn to California to look for gold in 1849, Morse wound up later that year and in 1850 as an employee of the St. Charles Hotel in New Orleans, perhaps serving as manager. Between 1853 and 1870, Morse became proprietor of three New Orleans "caravan-seris"—the Arcade, City, and St. James Hotels.

Morse, who lived until 1893, became a wealthy man through the

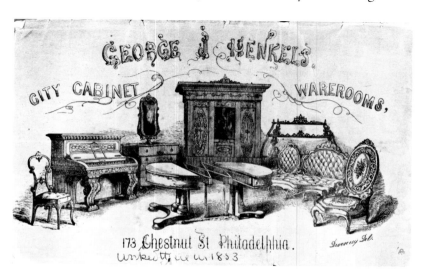

Fig. 7. Cover of Catalog of Furniture, George J. Henkels, City Cabinet Warerooms, 173 Chestnut St., *Philadelphia, Pennsylvania (about 1855). Courtesy Henry Francis du Pont Winterthur Museum Library; Collection of Printed Books.*

hotel business, so much so that he was able to own a house in New Orleans, a "plantation" some miles outside of town, and the Portland villa. It seems safe to assume that Morse's tastes (and those of his wife, who was also a Maine native) were formed by his knowledge of hotel decor, especially in his adopted city. The floor plan of the house, with its grand central staircase and large drawing and reception rooms, the elaborate and brightly colored rococo revival interior painting and architectural details, and the furnishings in the French taste all recall the descriptions of first-class hotel parlors, especially the description of Philadelphia's Girard House (plates 4 and 5). Two photographs of the drawing room from the end of the Morse era (taken about 1890) show wall-to-wall carpet of a large rococo pattern with center medallion of roses, chair upholstery of satin with bullion fringe and, on the seats of gilt reception chairs, what was probably a brocaded silk (figs. 9 and 10). The windows were hung with satin valances and draperies, embellished with fringe and tie-backs in contrasting colors, with lace undercurtains. A slightly later photograph, of the reception room during the ownership of the house by the Libby family (who left the interiors substantially unchanged), shows a button-tufted easy armchair in the French taste as well as a *bourne* or ottoman, the large round fabric-covered couch designed to occupy the center of rooms. The *bourne* was a French innovation, its design a reflection of the "Turkish taste" that was an element of French decor throughout the nineteenth century.

What is also striking about the Morse-Libby Mansion's public rooms, as they are depicted in turn-of-the-century photographs, is the absence of personal memorabilia and the restrained use of ceramics and other decorative accessories. When they appear, as in the mantel garniture of the reception room, it is because they are considered

Fig. 8. "Fashion Plates for Decorating Parlor Windows," engraving in Godey's Lady's Book *(February 1854).*

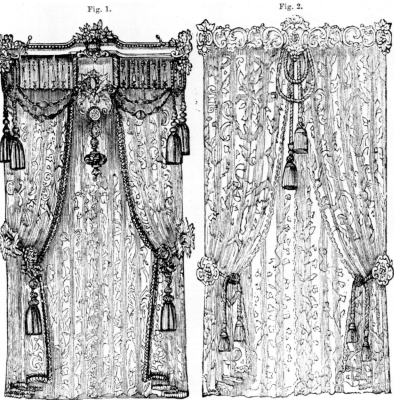

elements of the decorative scheme. This absence of knick-knacks and *bibelots*, the scale of the rooms, their exuberant decoration, and their French furnishings, suggest their fundamentally public character. At the same time, they are furnished with what, to the mid-nineteenth-century sensibility, were recognizably parlor furnishings.

Public parlors in hotels also seem to have served as sites for parlor-like entertainments. Some evidence suggests that the kinds of socializing that took place in the public parlors of the Tremont House may have been much like the convivial receptions and tea parties given in large private houses. *Sayings and Doings at the Tremont House in the Year 1832*, a two-volume miscellany of dialogs, sentimental and comic stories, and "letters" written pseudonymously by "Costard Sly," described several social gatherings in the hotel's public parlors, including formal calls and large parties. The participants were residents of the hotel and other Bostonians. A story called "No Mistake About That" described a large after-theater party:

> The play was over. As the ladies were putting on their bonnets, or calashes, and shawls, &c—a whisper went round, "Do—do, pray, come over to the TREMONT, and take some refreshment—a little chocolate, for instance,—DO!"

That *do* was irresistable. The ladies laughed, and accepted the invitation. In a few seconds, to their great surprise, they found themselves in a magnificent saloon, (the ladies' dining and drawing rooms in the TREMONT had been thrown into *one*,)

Fig. 9. Drawing room, view toward rear of house, Morse-Libby House, Portland, Maine, by unidentified photographer, about 1890. Courtesy Victoria Society of Maine.

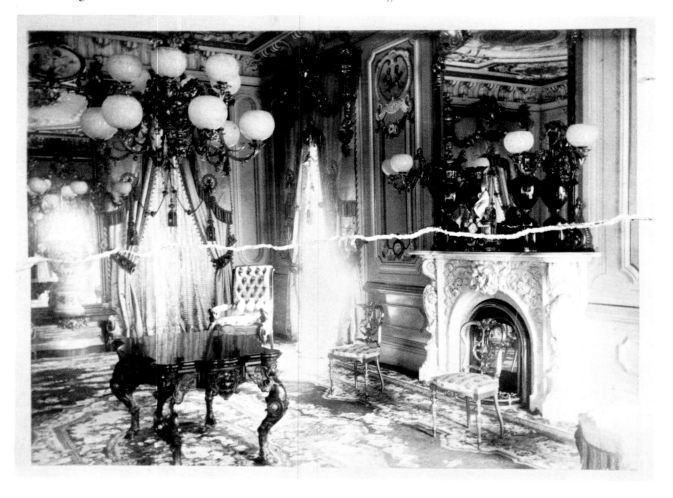

brilliantly lighted, and so forth,—and already occupied by a large party of ladies and gentlemen,—their friends and acquaintences;—of course, the most approved fashionables of Boston. A band of music was in attendance.[44]

Another story, "A Second Scene in the Ladies' Drawing Room," drew all the characters in the book together for a party whose tone was decidedly domestic. The participants provided their own amusements: "The doings were simple—common-place enough. There was some dancing—some singing—and a good deal of eating and drinking between heats."[45]

An article on life along the Mississippi, published by the *Illustrated London News* in 1858, devoted considerable space to a description of social life at the St. Charles Hotel. Its author's comments suggested that such socializing was simultaneously public and commercial in character, yet "domestic" enough to be suitable for the wives and daughters of planters.

The most prominent public building in New Orleans is the St. Charles Hotel, an edifice somewhat after the style and appearance of the Palace of the King of the Belgians at Brussels. During the twelve days I remained under its hospitable roof it contained from seven hundred to seven hundred and fifty guests...The southern planters, and their wives and daughters, escaping from the monotony of their cotton or sugar plantations, come down to New Orleans in the early spring season, and, as private lodgings

Fig. 10. Drawing room, view toward front of house, Morse-Libby House, Portland, Maine, by unidentified photographer, about 1890. Both photographs were damaged, which accounts for the horizontal breaks across the images. Courtesy Victoria Society of Maine.

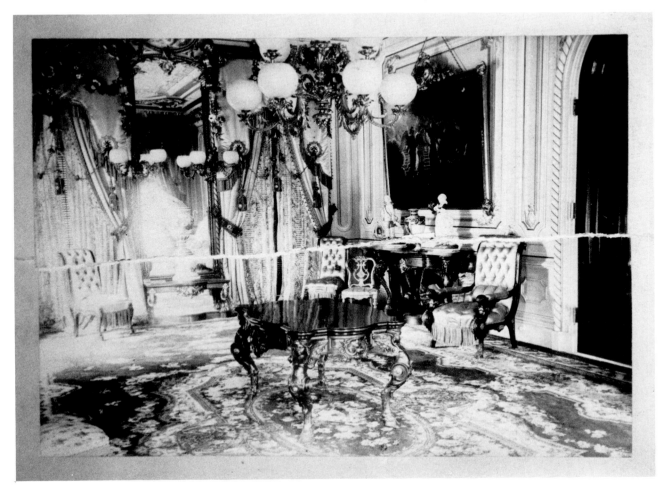

are not to be had, they throng to the St. Louis and St. Charles Hotels, but principally to the St. Charles, where they lead a life of constant publicity and gaiety...After dinner the drawing-rooms offer a scene to which no city in the world offers a parallel. It is the very court of Queen Mab, whose courtiers are some of the finest, wealthiest, and most beautiful of the daughters of the south, mingling in true Republican equality with the chance wayfarers, gentle or simple, well-dressed or ill-dressed, clean or dirty, who can pay for a nightly lodging or a day's board at this mighty caravanseri.[46]

To this commentator, as to "Costard Sly," hotel parlors presented interesting possibilities for social life in a new setting, a commercially fostered version of the "select company."

More modest hotels, in both the largest urban centers and provincial cities, also tried to provide their clientele with elegant parlors for socializing. Anthony Trollope noted that all the hotels he frequented during his 1861 visit, even in the West, contained the complete range of public rooms—"two and sometimes three" ladies' parlors (which in the West were rarely used, he noted), as well as "reading rooms, smoking rooms, shaving rooms, drinking rooms, parlors for gentlemen in which smoking is prohibited."[47] In 1848, the Waverly Hotel in Rochester, New York, contained "Reading, Receiving and Bar Rooms" on its first floor, "public Drawing Rooms," private parlors and bed rooms, and the dining room on its second, and a leasable ball room or lecture hall on its fifth floor. The local newspaper commented, "All are remarkable for their neatness, order and convenience, and are furnished in elegant style...The whole arrangement of the house is such that all will feel at home."[48]

But was it possible for a middle-class American to be properly at home in the commercial parlors and sitting-rooms of hotels? Although only a small percentage of American families probably lived in hotels, their number was significant enough to inspire comment among European travelers and American commentators. These observers disagreed about the effects that hotel living—and its gentility—had on the domestic sentiments of their residents, especially women. Francis Grund thought boarding "commendable on the score of economy" both for single men and newly married couples, not only because it permitted marriages to take place "a little sooner than their means would otherwise allow them" but because it saved expenses on servants as well as rent.[49] Thirty years later, the author of *Eighty Years' Progress of the United States of America* claimed that hotels provided "an unrivaled combination of the applications of human ingenuity to the improvement of domestic life" with their "splendid furniture, elaborate food, economical yet liberal housekeeping, labor-saving machinery."[50]

Even when observers deemed hotel life close enough to more traditional domestic arrangements to be safe and suitable for women, the open character of hotel parlors created special etiquette problems. How could residents negotiate the important middle-class ceremonies of daytime social calling, dining, and evening entertainments in parlors and dining rooms that were public? These concerns were common enough that the sensible Miss Eliza Leslie, author of domestic economy manuals and cookbooks, offered several chapters of very specific advice on "Deportment at a Hotel, or at a Large Boarding House" in *The Ladies' Guide to True Politeness and Perfect Manners* (1864). The nature of her commentary illustrates the real difficulties that socializing in public parlors sometimes entailed, while demonstrating that hotel parlors were indeed used for the same purposes as their domestic counterparts. Leslie devoted particular attention to the problems of social calling and parlor pastimes:

> In a public parlour, it is selfish and unmannerly to sit down to the instrument uninvited, and fall to playing or practising…If you want amusement, you had better read, or occupy yourself with some light sewing or knitting-work…Should a visitor come in to see one of the boarders who may be sitting near you, change your place, and take a seat in a distant part of the room…It is best for the visited lady to meet her friend as soon as she sees her enter the room, and conduct her to a sofa or ottoman where they can enjoy their talk without danger of being overheard.[51]

Some middle-class commentators worried that hotel life was dangerous because resident families were also members of the middle classes upon whose domestic sentiments the continuing development of republican virtue depended. As did even more modest boarding houses, family hotels provoked this kind of criticism in both editorials and moralizing short stories. For example, in the supposedly factual account "American Homes in New York Hotels" by "William Brown" in an 1857 issue of *Harper's Weekly*, newlyweds encountered firsthand the negative effect that living at the "St. Thunder Hotel" had upon domesticity (fig. 11). Even the new styles of fashionable furniture had a bad effect upon their lives: the spring bed was so noisy that it prevented sleep, and an untied spring poked through the yellow and purple brocatelle cover of the showy but shoddy spring seat sofa, ruining the bridegroom's trousers. In "Boarding Out," published in *Harper's Weekly* that same year, the author pinpointed access to parlor life as a common yet spurious motive for choosing the hotel "mode of living."[52]

Apart from the convenience of travel, the most common motive which persuades to the mode of living alluded to is economy. But it is quite clear that this idea of economy is founded upon a false

Fig. 11. "How We Sit in Our Hotel Homes," engraving in Harper's Weekly (26 December 1857). This illustration accompanied the story by "William Brown," "American Homes in New York Hotels."

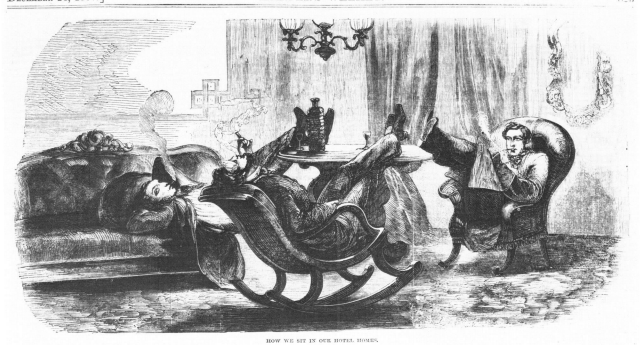

HOW WE SIT IN OUR HOTEL HOMES.

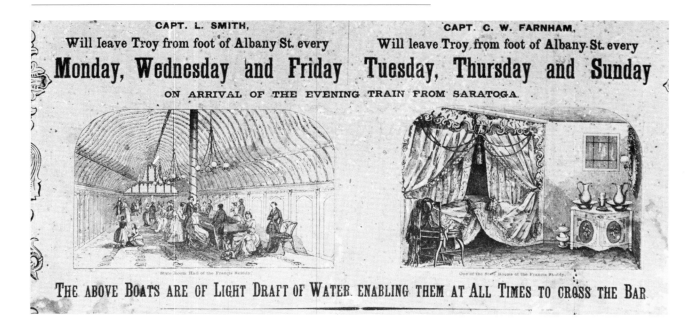

standard of the necessities of life. If the tastes of our people were better regulated, and mere show was not preferred to substance, there would be less resort to the hotel or boarding-house on the plea of money-saving. If gingerbread furniture, damask curtains, tapestry carpets and a French cook are essential to happiness, there is no doubt they can be secured in greater perfection and at a less price by the gregarious hotel system than by individual effort. Such luxuries, however, as we all know, are not essential to happiness, and however permissible as superfluous enjoyments, they certainly are too dearly paid for when at the expense of domestic virtue and happiness.[53]

To these critics, hotel parlors and their "superfluous" luxuries dangerously blurred the necessary separation between the domestic haven and the world outside. They appeared domestic on the surface, yet they exposed young women in particular to lives of "publicity and indolence" rather than to the privacy, permanence, and well-regulated round of household management that a home offered, attributes that encouraged their moral development. Hotel parlors were nothing more than a facade, "a theatrical mockery of society, where the characters and scenes, always varying and shifting, can only present a passing show and produce a temporary excitement."[54] The "passing show" of the hotel parlor and the opportunity to participate in the facade of commercial gentility was, of course, precisely what Reuben Vose and the mixture of planters and traders at the St. Charles enjoyed.

Fig. 12. Detail of broadside, printed by Francis Hart, New York, New York, 1857. This popular poster advertised the superior accommodations offered by the Francis Skiddy, a night boat that ran between New York City and Saratoga. The image of the "State Room Hall" showed a group of genteel passengers enjoying informal music entertainment. Courtesy Mariners' Museum, Newport News, Virginia.

Steamboats and Railroad Cars as Model Interiors

Contemporary reporting and commentary about the glamorous interiors of eastern and western river steamboats and coastal packets appeared in the mid-1820s, soon after fare competition for profitable passenger traffic began on the Hudson River and the Long Island Sound/Providence-to-Boston Lines. Initially, this kind of genteel travel was expensive—the elegant Hudson River paddle steamers "having a bar and a ladies' cabin and perhaps a band of music" charged up to three dollars for the New York-to-Albany run. By the 1840s, however, even fancy boats charged as little as a dollar for the same route.[55]

The history of Hudson River steamboat travel, which at its peak involved regular runs by approximately one hundred vessels, demonstrates the ways in which line operators made use of the growing preoccupation with fashion and creature comforts in their competition for passengers. Between 1825 and 1864, competition often centered on the issues of safety and speed, and improvements in boat and steam engine design decreased upstream running time from seventeen hours to about seven.[56] Yet as early as 1825, Hudson River steamboat companies already had begun to advertise the accommodations they offered as an added inducement to passengers (fig. 12). Some lines experimented with the concept of the "safety barge," a towboat arrangement which featured the same range of public rooms and amenities that would soon be offered by first-class hotels. In 1825, an advertisement for the Steam Navigation Company's barges the *Commerce* and *Lady-Clinton* noted that each was "fitted exclusively for passengers, with a dining Cabin of nearly 90 feet in length, a deck Cabin for the accommodation of ladies, a range of state rooms for private families, a reading room, and all the usual accommodations found in the best steam boats."[57]

By the late 1830s, paddle steamers plying the western lakes and rivers also featured parlor-like public rooms and even separate sleeping cabins for passengers who could afford a higher fare.[58] Steamboats tended to have at least one large, general-use room known almost uniformly as the "saloon," a popularization of the term "salon," which was used to describe very large reception rooms in grand houses. Saloons were also features of early ocean-going steam vessels; some of these interiors were so notable that their image was central to the transfer-printed china series "The Boston Mails" of about 1842 (fig. 13). Although constrained by limited space and the

Fig. 13. Detail of platter, "The Boston Mails" series of transfer-printed earthenware by James and Thomas Edwards, Burslem, England, about 1842. The series included five views of interiors from the four transatlantic steamships operated by the Cunard Line. In the June 1936 issue of The Magazine Antiques, *Ellouise Baker Larsen discussed the series and illustrated all five interior views.*

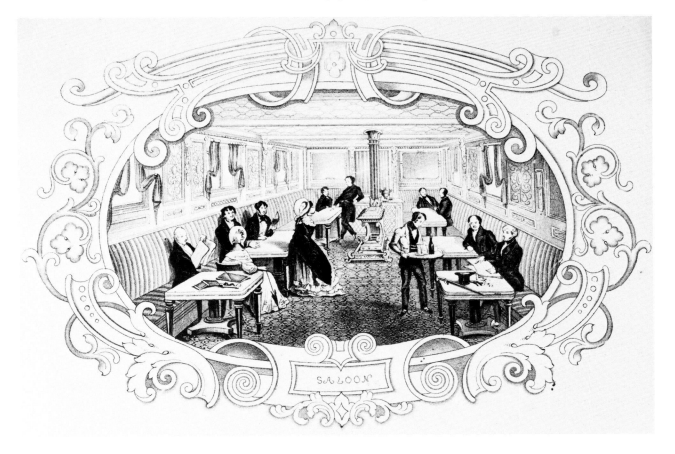

need to provide sleeping berths and furniture that would be stable during rough weather, the rooms illustrated in this series paraphrased parlors as much as possible by using upholstered couches built into the wall (called *banquettes*), mirrors, carpets, and decorative mantels and woodwork. Sometimes the main saloon served as men's sleeping quarters and featured convertible furniture. The gentlemen's cabin on the *Empire State*, which entered service on the Fall River line in 1848, doubled as the dining room, and its berths were concealed from passengers by the use of "drapery of different colors mixed with lace shades," a reflection of window fashions for houses.[59]

Ladies' parlors also doubled as their sleeping quarters, except on boats large enough to have separate staterooms (fig. 14). In her short story "Mrs. Pell's Pilgrimage," Mrs. C. M. Kirkland described the ladies' cabin on a Hudson River steamer as containing rocking chairs and settees, which doubled as sleeping couches. An illustration accompanying the story revealed an elaborately draped doorway and wall-to-wall carpet (fig. 15).[60]

In keeping with parlor furnishing conventions, the main saloon of the *City of Boston*, one of the Norwich and New York Transportation Company's small fleet of steamers used on Long Island Sound in the early 1860s, was furnished with wall-to-wall carpet, center tables under gas chandeliers, and a large set of furniture designed in some variation of a "Louis" style (fig. 16). The furniture, shown in "summer dress" with striped slipcovers, included a type of circular sofa that was designed as an expanded version of a parlor sofa. It had extra sets of arms, and the back probably was upholstered on two sides.[61]

Just as first-class hotels in the antebellum period were christened palace hotels, the biggest and best of the domestic steamboats were dubbed "palace steamers." Describing a trip on the *Bay State*, which ran between New York and Newport between 1847 and 1863, Philadelphian Sidney George Fisher wrote that its interiors were "another wonder of modern art": "The saloons, cabins & staterooms are all painted and gilded in the most splendid style & sumptuously

Fig. 14. *"Interior View of the Ladies Saloon of the Steamer* Atlantic,*" colored lithograph by C. Parsons, United States, published by G. and W. Endicott, 1846. Courtesy Mariners' Museum, Newport News, Virginia.*

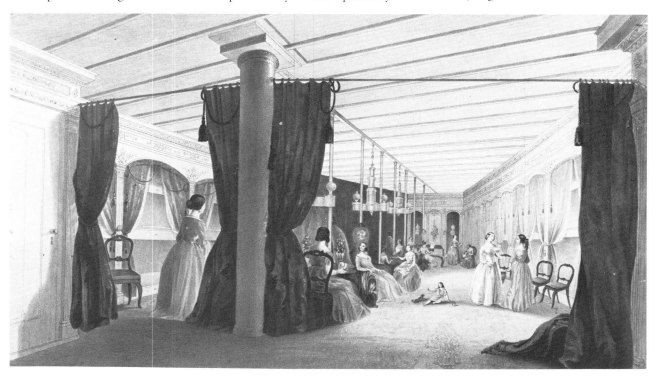

furnished. Brilliant Saxony carpets, chandeliers, marble tables, sofas, armchairs of every pattern, well-cushioned and covered with the richest stuffs, silk curtains, French china, cut glass, mirrors fill every apartment."[62] Added to the fleet of the Boston Newport and New York Steamboat Company in 1865, the *Old Colony's* saloon featured a mixture of French-inspired parlor chairs, their show covers (the term for the decorative fabric) made of what appears to be a printed velvet and silk stripe rep or terry, ribbed fabrics that were typically found on parlor suites of the period (fig. 17).

The Great Lakes also was home to a fleet of increasingly luxurious passenger steamboats from 1838 to 1857, when financial panic forced many lake shipping lines into bankruptcy. By the time prosperity returned, railroads had obviated the need for these large and expensive vessels. The *City of Buffalo*, admittedly the most luxurious as well as the last of the breed, was the object of much public curiosity during its construction. Before the inaugural voyage, the boat was opened to public inspection, and the local press published a lengthy description of its appointments.

> The ladies' private cabin, on the after main deck, is excellently arranged; it is handsomely furnished with rich brussels carpets, rosewood furniture, upholstered with fine plush...Passengers, upon going on board, enter a fine reception room furnished with sofas, marble-topped tables, etc., and in the centre is a pretty fountain...
>
> Proceeding up the grand stairway, at the first landing, on the floor, we notice a large brass buffalo, and overhead a handsome mirror and splendid landscape painting. This introduces us to the grand cabin, lighted by sky-lights, and a splendid stained glass dome at the further end. On either hand the doors open up into the state-rooms. The cabin has an arched ceiling, which, together with the panels, are ornamented by gilt mouldings, the white and gold making a very rich appearance. This cabin is like a gallery as

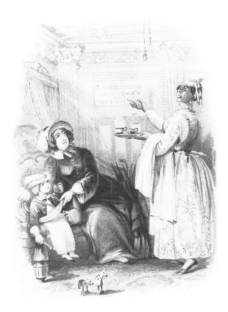

Fig. 15. "*Mrs. Peli's Pilgrimage,*" *engraving by C. Bart in Mrs. C. M. Kirkland,* A Book for the Home Circle *(1853).*

Fig. 16. Main saloon, City of Boston, *by unidentified photographer, about 1865, reproduced in J. Howland Gardner, "The Development of Steam Navigation on Long Island Sound,"* Historical Transactions 1893-1943, The Society of Naval Architects and Marine Engineers *(1945). Courtesy Steamship Historical Society Collection, University of Baltimore Library.*

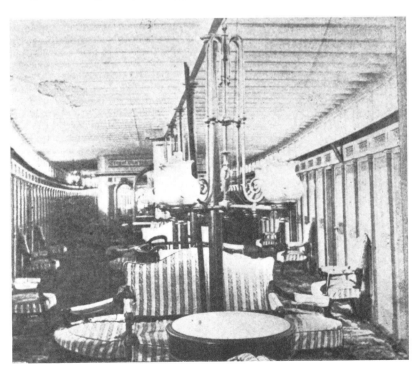

we look into the cabin below. Several splendid chandeliers light it by night, the centre one of which is double, the lower portion lighting the ladies' cabin. The furniture is of richest rose-wood, with damask and plush upholsterings; the carpets are costly brussels, and the 'tout ensemble' magnificent.[63]

The description of the *City of Buffalo's* decor closed with the note that all carpets and upholstery had been purchased from A. T. Stewart and Co. of New York. Appropriately, the first and most famous "dry goods palace" in the United States provided the interior fittings for the palace steamboat.

Thinking back on his riverboat piloting days, Mark Twain was aware of the symbolic power of "floating palaces," especially in communities far from cities. He reminisced that Mississippi steamboats were "indubitably magnificent" when compared to midcentury "superior dwelling-houses and first-class hotels in the [Mississippi] Valley."

To a few people living in New Orleans and St. Louis they were not magnificent, perhaps; not palaces; but to the great majority of those populations, and to the entire populations spread over both banks between Baton Rouge and St. Louis, they were palaces; they tallied with the citizen's dream of what magnificence was, and satisfied it.

Fig. 17. Saloon of Old Colony, *by unidentified photographer, 1865. Courtesy Mariners' Museum, Newport News, Virginia.*

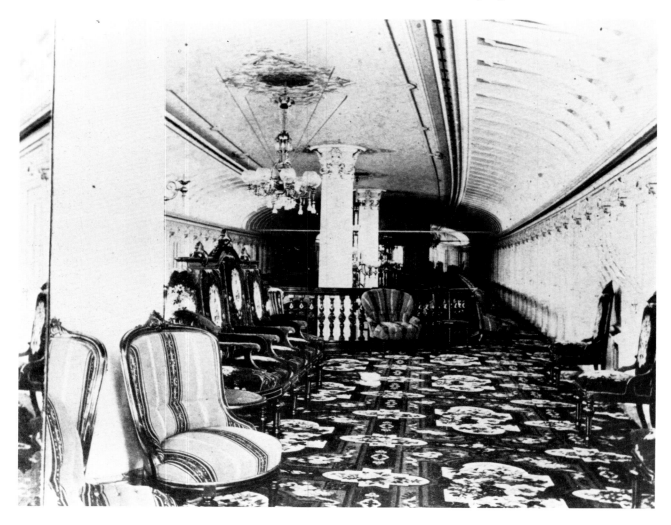

Their interior fittings, from the "far receding snow-white 'cabin;' porcelain knob and oil-picture on every state-room door" to the ladies' cabin with its "pink and white Wilton carpet, as soft as mush, and glorified with a ravishing pattern of gigantic flowers," provided visitors "a bewildering and soul satisfying spectacle!"[64]

According to one 1889 history of railroading in America, the comforts available on steamboats inspired George Pullman to attempt to upgrade sleeping and travel accommodations on railroad trains.[65] By the 1840s, as railroad lines grew longer and the possible length of trips was extended, passenger cars began to be equipped with more elaborate creature comforts.[66]

As early as 1842, a fancy railroad car containing upholstered seats, curtains, and carpeting was placed on public display in Rochester, New York, and received notice in local papers. The *Rochester Evening Post* described four of the six cars, destined for service on the Auburn and Rochester Railroad, as containing separate rooms for ladies, with "luxurious sofas for seats and…a washstand and other conveniences."[67] Following the practice of hotels and steamboats, most railroads provided separate accommodations for women by the mid-1840s, either in the form of a small ladies' parlor in a section of a passenger car or an entirely separate ladies' car. They usually contained a sofa in addition to the typical bench seating.[68]

First-class passenger cars appeared on trains by the late 1830s, and luxury sleeping cars and parlor cars had proliferated by the 1850s. The latter usually appeared on short lines between large cities and cost one to two dollars per day more than normal coach fares, although access to parlor-cars was sometimes offered free of charge on competitive routes. In a large advertisement for its western routes, the Chicago, Burlington and Quincy Railroad offered passengers from Buffalo use of "B. & Q. Palace Drawing-Room Cars, with Horton's Reclining Chairs" at no additional charge.[69] Such parlor cars featured reclining chairs for passengers as early as the mid-1850s, when the Illinois Central Railroad introduced its new "Gothic" stateroom cars (fig. 18).[70] The design of reclining chairs on railroads was related to the design of barber chairs, as well as to patent reclining chairs for domestic interiors.

Even ordinary railroad cars were embellished with window curtains and decorative painting and featured comforts that were associated with parlors, especially spring seating (fig. 19). Most probably, they provided many Americans with their first contact with luxurious-looking, deep-colored pile upholstery fabrics in the form of sturdy mohair plush, one of the most popular furniture covers of the late nineteenth century. Beginning in the 1850s, mohair actually was chosen by railroad companies for seating because of its resistance to dirt and its long-wearing qualities.[71] In an 1881 technical manual for the textile trade, the entry under mohair noted, "The best mohair plushes are almost indestructible. They have been in constant use on certain railroads in this country for twenty years without wearing out." Wool and mohair plushes (the latter also were called "Utrecht velvet") had been used on some good-quality furniture throughout the century; mohair gradually supplanted wool because of its superior luster and colors as well as its sturdiness. Until the 1880s, plush made from mohair was still comparatively expensive because it was imported. By the 1890s, domestically woven mohair plush had become a luxury fabric for ordinary people and was featured in the parlor-suite offerings of Sears, Roebuck and Co.'s catalogs.[72]

Fancy railroad cars captured the public's imagination, just as steamboats had several decades earlier, because they combined symbols of refined living and domestic comfort with mobility. The humorist Benjamin Franklin Taylor described parlor cars, which he called "flying drawing-rooms," as "home adrift" and pronounced "flying bedrooms" [sleeping cars] to be "among the crowning achievements of railroad travel" in their ingenious planning.[73] Even Americans who could not afford to pay for travel in "flying bedrooms" or "flying drawing-rooms" were able to get a firsthand look at their interiors through public exhibition of the newest and fanciest cars. In 1876, the Jackson and Sharp Company of Wilmington, Delaware, sent two such cars, built for private clients, to the Centennial for display. One, the "Brazilian car of State," contained a drawing room with "a sofa and two tête-à-tête chairs, covered with silver bronze leather with claret rep puffing [a loosely pleated decorative technique used on both seat fronts and backs] and silk fringe and tassels" and window curtains of "green figured rep."[74]

The decorated interiors of railroad cars continued to represent popular furnishing taste through the last decades of the nineteenth century (fig. 20). Their elaborate dark woodwork, button-tufted seats, portières, and figured carpets reflected the parlor furnishing preferences of ordinary Americans and expressed the popular understanding of upholstered refinement and comfort. In fact, railroad upholstery epitomized so powerfully the middle-class parlor of the late nineteenth and early twentieth centuries that later furnishing advice books sometimes employed it as a case in point of "old-fashioned" bad taste. *The Modern Priscilla Home Furnishing Book* of 1925 dubbed the common parlor-furnishing practices of its readers' youths "the Early Pullman period of home decoration."[75]

Photographers' Studios

The description in *Humphrey's Journal of Photography* of the two elaborate parlors in photographer M. M. Lawrence's New York City portrait studio demonstrates that their appointments were remarkable, but not unique. By the late 1840s, many daguerreotype operators went to great expense to create separate reception areas that included lavish draperies, suites of upholstered furniture, wall-to-wall carpeting, large mirrors, and center tables. Some, such as Ball's Great Daguerrian Gallery of the West in Cincinnati, furnished reception rooms with pianos to encourage informal parlor musicales among

Fig. 18. Advertisement for Chicago and Alton Railroad, 1882, reproduced in John White, The American Railroad Passenger Car *(1978). Courtesy The Johns Hopkins University Press.*

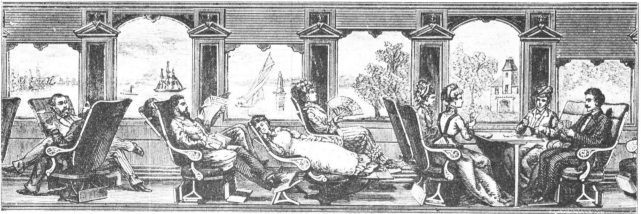

INTERIOR VIEW OF RECLINING CHAIR CAR, (DR. HORTON'S PATENT)

These Luxurious Cars are run in All Through Trains, Day and Night, between St. Louis and Kansas City, St. Louis and Chicago, and Kansas City and Chicago, Without Change,

—VIA—

Chicago & Alton R. R.

NO EXTRA CHARGE FOR SEATS IN THESE CARS.

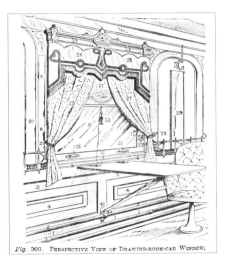

Fig. 300. Perspective View of Drawing-room-car Window.

Fig. 19. *"Perspective View of Drawing-Room Car Window," engraving in Mathias N. Forney, ed.,* The Car Builder's Dictionary *(1879; reprint, 1974). Courtesy Dover Publications.*

waiting patrons. Mr. Ball's gallery was the subject of a half-page illustration and descriptive article in *Gleason's Pictorial Drawing-Room Companion* for April 1, 1854 (fig. 21). The gallery consisted of five rooms, the largest of which was the "Great Gallery," which displayed paintings, prints, allegorical figures representing the arts, and a handsome selection of Mr. Ball's half- and full-plate daguerreotypes. The author of the article described the decor as "replete with elegance and beauty."[76]

Articles describing and praising such photographers' studios appeared in both middle-class periodicals and photographic journals such as *Humphrey's Journal of Photography* and the *Photographic Art-Journal* throughout the 1850s. They tended to focus on the most elaborate and elegant studios as examples of what could be achieved by photographic practitioners of vision and ambition. However, parlor making among photographers spread through all but the cheapest studios from the 1840s to the 1860s in cities and larger towns across the United States. In the Rochester *Daily Advertiser* for March 3, 1848, the daguerreotypist T. Mercer advertised the opening of a new set of "Branch Daguerrian Rooms" to accommodate the rapidly expanding city:

> These Rooms are fitted up in a style of unusual splendor—are supplied with every thing the extravagant could desire, the luxurious sigh for. After naming *Sofas, Divans, Ottomans,* and *French Chairs,* comes one of *ELDER'S* splendid *Golden Pier Tables,* with a Glass, (the first completed in Rochester) in which, 'tis said, the *Fair,* look more lovely still, and assume that pleasing expression so much coveted by Artists, and their friends. Carpets of downy softness are spread beneath the feet, and hush the noisy tread. Statuary from Italy, of *pure marble,* adorn the Rooms at various points; the walls are hung with some of the finest works of Art, both of pencil and engraver.[77]

Only after extolling the beauty of his receiving room did the advertisement's text mention "*premium* DAGUERREOTYPES," taken by Mercer himself, for a fee ranging from one to twelve dollars each depending upon the size of the image and the case chosen for it. A competitor advertised in the same issue the addition to the firm's receiving gallery of "a new and magnificent SERAPHINE [a type of reed organ], of fine tone, for the amusement of visitors."[78]

By the 1860s, Rochester's photographers emphasized the range and prices of photographic practices available in their studios—ambrotypes, photographs on paper, "Imperial" enlargements which could be painted over into "oil portraits." Attractive rooms, while still important, were no longer a novelty worth much advertising copy. Powelson's "new and elaborate Photographic Rooms" in 1864 simply encouraged prospective patrons to "take a look at the new Gallery, which is acknowledged by everyone to be the best fitted up, finest carpets and most elegant furniture, the most commodious toilet room for the ladies to be found in the country."[79] In the western United States, examples of reception parlors fitted up with lambrequins (window valances of fabric), parlor suites, decorative chairs produced by the firm of George Hunzinger of New York City, and potted palms survived at least until 1900, with style changes reflecting new fashions in parlor decor such as wicker "fancy chairs" (fig. 22).[80]

By the 1870s, the efforts of ordinary studio photographers working in provincial cities to provide elegant parlors for waiting patrons had become so common that the activity was burlesqued in the photographic advice literature. H. J. Rodgers' *Twenty-Three Years*

under a Sky-Light, published in 1872, was directed both to
photographers and prospective customers. Rather than presenting
technical advice, Rodgers used anecdotes on good and bad clients
encountered in his business to address etiquette questions related to
behavior in the studio and to advise both photographers and patrons
on how to obtain the best possible portraits. He depicted the
commercial portrait photographer as a long-suffering "working stiff"
whose efforts at presenting a genteel public face were frequently tried
by onslaughts of boors, rubes, and ignoramuses. In one such
anecdote, Rodgers illustrated the trials of keeping up a refined
reception room by describing the entry of a group of young men:
"They step carefully over the door rug, and having approached the
middle of the room, wipe their feet on the Brussels carpet...When
told that they must wait five or ten minutes, and after roughly
handling specimens of art, especially selections framed in gold-leaf,
they 'set down,' elevating their muddy *under-standings* (which are
suitable for a Connecticut River fishing smack) into the best and most
expensive upholstered chair."[81]

Historians estimate that three million daguerreotypes were made
annually in the 1840s. This suggests that the experience of passing
time in a photographers' studio was common by then; it grew even
more ordinary in the next decade. Photographers encouraged their

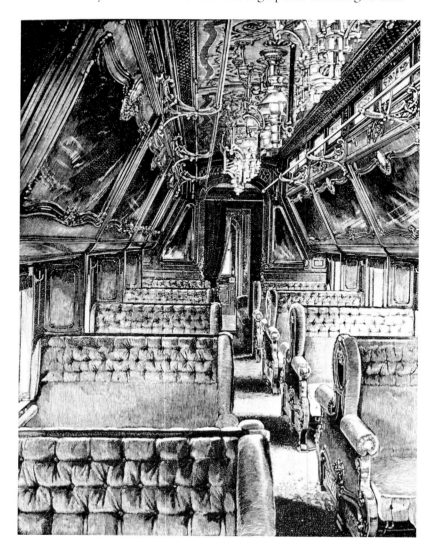

Fig. 20. *"Pullman Sleeper on a
Vestibuled Train," engraving in Thomas
C. Clarke et al.,* The American Railway
(1889).

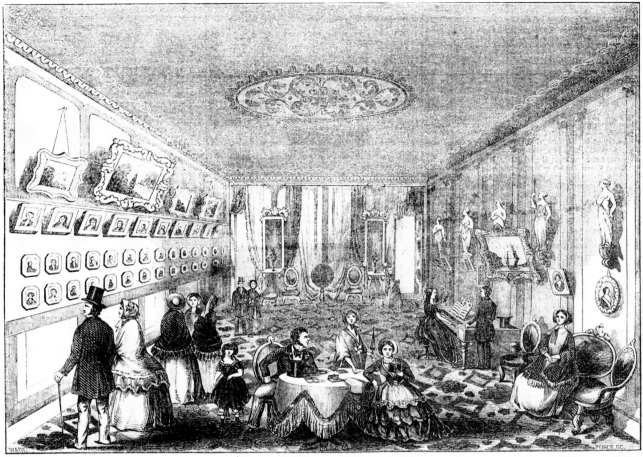

BALL'S GREAT DAGUERRIAN GALLERY OF THE WEST.

Fig. 21. *"Ball's Great Daguerrian Gallery of the West," engraving in* Gleason's *(1 April 1854).*

prospective patrons to visit newly redecorated studios for inspection and to pass a pleasant hour or two in the reception rooms.[82] A properly decorated studio located in St. Louis in 1851 was praised as "a most agreeable place to spend a leisure hour," and an 1848 advertisement for Rochester's Emporium Daguerreotype Gallery invited "ladies and gentlemen" to visit the gallery "whether they desire to sit for portraits or not."[83]

Both commercial pressures and commercial or social aspirations led to the creation of quasi-public spaces that used the material vocabulary of gentility—the artifacts of the parlor—to attract and keep audiences. Historian of photography Richard Rudisill has offered the hypothesis that such settings "allowed the photographer to control his clients more effectively" because the setting differed from their homes "only in degree."[84] Indeed, some advice literature directed to photographers did proffer similar arguments. M. A. Root's influential photography advice book *The Camera and the Pencil* (1864) devoted a whole chapter to the "Fitting Up of Heliographic Rooms." He noted that the experience of waiting needed to be pleasant in order to awaken "proper moods" in sitters and suggested that furniture that reproduced Hogarth's curving "line of beauty" was most effective to this end.[85] Six years earlier, in a series of articles for the *American Journal of Photography* entitled "Expressing Character in Photographic Pictures," E. K. Hough had noted, "Almost every operator is ambitious of having what is called a 'nice place,' and he fits up his room as richly as he can afford, but he usually makes one fatal mistake: he puts his wealth and beauty in his

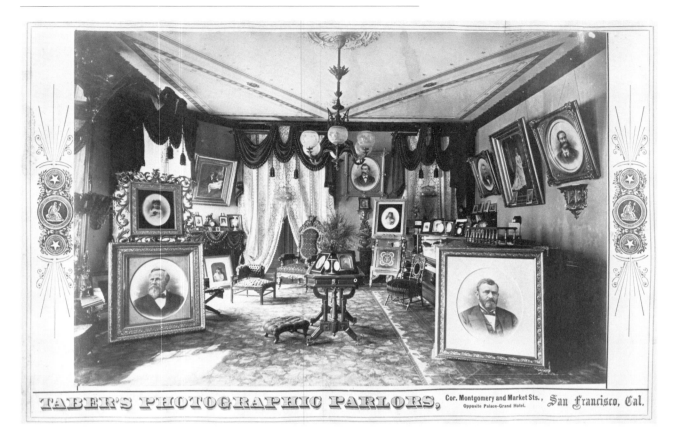

reception room, while his operating room is left comparatively unfurnished, and comfortless, with the dirty paraphernalia of the art scattered about, and a strong disagreeable smell of chemicals."[86]

Getting the best out of sitters was only one motive for parlor-making activity, however. Photographers sought to attract and hold patrons for repeat visits, even offering their reception rooms as an agreeable and socially acceptable site for spending leisure hours. The illustration of Ball's Great Daguerrian Gallery showed patrons socializing and enjoying an informal musicale. Additionally, displaying their own photographs alongside art in parlor-like settings suggested that photographs were both artistic and appropriate elements of parlor decor. Photographers thereby guided new habits of consumption by suggesting that photographs themselves were genteel, as was the photographer who owned the parlor setting.

The Model Room at Expositions and Fairs

Attendance at fairs—international expositions, mechanics' fairs, and state and county fairs—was a regular event among Americans in the second half of the nineteenth and the early years of the twentieth centuries.[87] The Centennial clocked ten million visits in 1876, while the White City of the World's Columbian Exposition of 1893 in Chicago recorded about twenty-five million. Fair goers learned what has been termed "the lesson of things" as they passed through the enormous buildings that categorized the works of man by country of origin, by degree of transformation by man's hand—from raw materials and agricultural products to consumable goods—and by their place in the scale of human intellectual achievement, from applied and mechanical arts that grouped machines and the "minor arts" by categories to the perceived apex of civilization, the "fine arts."[88]

Fig. 22. Advertisement for Taber's Photographic Parlors, San Francisco, California, about 1880. Courtesy The Bancroft Library, University of California.

Household furnishings exhibited in international expositions had been displayed as merchandise with visible prices as early as 1855.[89] The organization of these manufacturers' exhibits was much like those in stores of the period, simple groupings by category or displays of material abundance, such as "waterfalls" of textiles.[90] Even displays of furniture sometimes followed this simple, abundant style of display. Gardener and Co.'s exhibit of perforated veneer seating furniture at the Centennial was organized as a pyramiding cascade of chairs.[91] Published images of exemplary furniture, household accessories, and textiles from the numerous illustrated accounts of fairs also tended to concentrate upon isolated objects or groupings with no backdrop to suggest appropriate sites for their display. The accompanying texts usually concentrated upon simple description of materials and techniques of manufacture, their costliness, and their design.

The notion of the overtly didactic or exemplary model room setting was not completely alien to fairs before the Centennial. Beginning with the Sanitary Fairs of the 1860s, "New England Kitchens" were a popular attraction, exposing visitors to settings that were furnished with a miscellany of "colonial" furnishings and memorabilia and were populated by women in "quaint" costumes. The New England Kitchen at the Centennial consisted of two buildings which contrasted a colonial kitchen of 1776 with a "modern" example of 1876. The colonial kitchen was dominated by a large fireplace whose mantel shelf was covered with candlesticks and other paraphernalia. It was furnished with spinning wheels, cradles, a settle, and various pieces of furniture with "Pilgrim century" provenance, such as a small desk "which John Alden brought over with him on the Mayflower." Ironically, the idea of constructing a separate colonial kitchen building seems to have been realized first not in the United States but in the "primitive woodland village" built for the International Exhibition in Vienna in 1873. This village included furnished examples of Hungarian and Austrian regional architecture, populated with residents in appropriate native costume, as well as several ethnic restaurants.[92]

Model room settings created specifically for the purpose of selling their contents were an innovation of the Centennial (fig. 23). These vignettes, created by elite British, French, and American furniture and interior decoration firms, occasioned enthusiastic remarks in a number of books about the fair, although only a few examples were illustrated. For example, the Philadelphia decorating firm of Smith and Campion exhibited four settings—a parlor, a library, a dining room, and a bedroom. Several books of commentary on the Centennial Exhibition discussed what was, by all accounts, a new approach to selling and displaying furnishings:

> An interesting feature of the Exhibition is the method which the upholsterers, decorators, and furniture-dealers have chosen by which to display their goods to the best advantage. This method consists in dividing the sections allotted to them into rooms, which are afterwards fitted up as parlor, library, boudoir, dining-room, or any special apartment.[93]

James D. McCabe, author of a lengthy illustrated history of the Centennial, noted that "makers of the finest grades of furniture in New York and Philadelphia went to great expense" in recreating "rooms of the usual size, which were handsomely carpeted, provided with curtains, doors, frescoed ceilings and walls, and superb gas fixtures and mantel-pieces. The rooms were open on one side. With the homelike surroundings thus provided the furniture showed to the

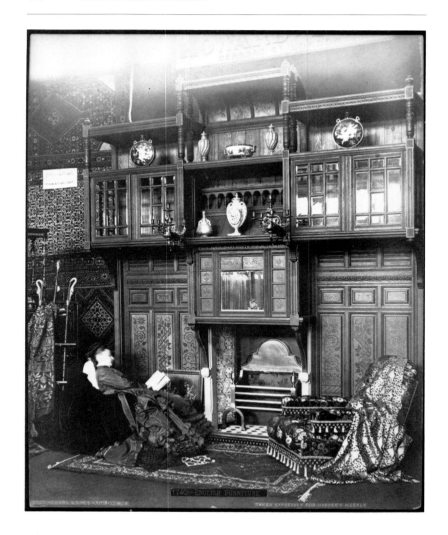

Fig. 23. "English Furniture," Howard and Sons Exhibit, Centennial Exhibition, Philadelphia, Pennsylvania, photograph by Centennial Photographic Co., 1876. This print was reproduced as an engraving in Harper's Weekly *during that year as well. Courtesy The Free Library of Philadelphia, Print and Picture Department; photograph by Joan Broderick.*

best possible advantage. It was of the most elaborate description, and was richly upholstered."[94]

The room that may have represented the height of taste and luxury to the popular imagination (although the firm received no prizes) was a "boudoir" in the Turkish/French taste exhibited by Philadelphia upholstering supply firm Carrington, deZouche and Company. The room was a tour de force of button tufting in cretonne (unglazed printed cotton fabric which often was printed with the same floral designs as glazed chintz), reflecting the kind of fabric-swaddled interior that made its appearance in France as early as the first decade of the nineteenth century.[95] A black-and-white plate of the room appeared in Walter Smith's *Industrial Art*, volume 2 of *Masterpieces of the Centennial International Exhibition*, and was reproduced three years later in Frank H. Norton's *Illustrated Historical Register* of the 1876 Philadelphia and 1878 Paris Exhibitions, this time in glowing color (plate 2).[96]

Some observers found these model rooms fascinating because they seemed to offer a peek into the mysterious households of the rich (settings that lost their mystique, if not their attraction, through the publication in the 1880s of vanity books such as *Artistic Houses*).[97] One commentator enthusiastically noted that the rooms offered "glimpses of the surroundings of the classes who set the fashions, such as could be had in no other way. We look into the most private apartments, the boudoirs and bed-chambers, which are so artfully arranged as to suggest occupancy. Bric-a-brac and knick-knacks are disposed about in studied carelessness so as to make the effect as natural as possible."[98] The rooms were theatrical sets awaiting the entrance of fashionable people. The Shoolbred displays heightened this effect by raising the rooms on platforms and framing the views with drapery, including lace curtains (fig. 24).

Parlor Making by Voluntary Associations

Between 1830 and 1880, other kinds of commercial parlors occasionally appeared in cities, in assembly rooms and "drawing rooms" attached to theaters.[99] However, a particularly telling form of parlor making that was public but not commercial was undertaken by voluntary associations for their own use. Some men's clubs, such as the Atheneum of Philadelphia, were organized by members of social elites, but others were largely made and occupied by groups of respectable young working men and took the form of reading rooms, athenaeums, or parlors. The "New York Atheneum" rooms described in detail in *The Daguerreian Journal* of November 15, 1850, were a typical example. For the modest fee of $12 per year, the member gained access to "three very spacious apartments" located under the galleries of the Academy of Design in New York City. Although the "great size and height" of the rooms made them unusual, the anonymous author felt that these qualities heightened "the imposing effect of interiors devoted to social intercourse." He went on to marvel at the effect of the coordinated decor (executed by "Mr. Patterson of London"):

> We are familiar with immense concert halls and public ballrooms, but our residences are generally too small to admit of very spacious saloons or drawing rooms. In addition to this peculiarity, the colors used in the furniture and decoration are harmonious; the prevailing tint of one of the apartments being green, of another crimson, and the third neutral.[100]

The author described the reading room as having green flocked wallpaper, "heavy green curtains," and floral patterned carpets which "had a costly look." The descriptions suggest that contact with this kind of planned interior, the kind that might be found in well-to-do households, was a new and pleasant experience for the author—perhaps one he might try to repeat at some future date.

The urge to create and congregate in such respectable-looking interiors was so strong that associations of fire fighters, groups long known for their roughness and competitive brawling at the scenes of fires, also created for themselves what seem to modern eyes astonishingly elaborate and expensive session rooms by the 1850s. An illustration from the *Illustrated London News* series "Transatlantic Sketches"—this one devoted to the firemen of New York City—depicted a "Parlour Belonging to New York Firemen" (fig. 25). Not only were the firefighters depicted as top-hatted, waist-coated gentlemen, but their depicted setting featured many of the elements that by this time were recognized as essential for a parlor. "C. M."—the author Charles Mackey —noted that firemen's parlors were furnished "with a degree of luxury equal to that of the public rooms of the most celebrated hotels."

> At one of the central stations, of which I send you a sketch, the walls are hung with excellent portraits of Washington, Franklin, Jefferson, Adams, and other founders of the Republic; the floor is covered with velvet-pile carpeting, a noble chandelier hangs from the centre, the curtains are rich and heavy, and the sideboard is

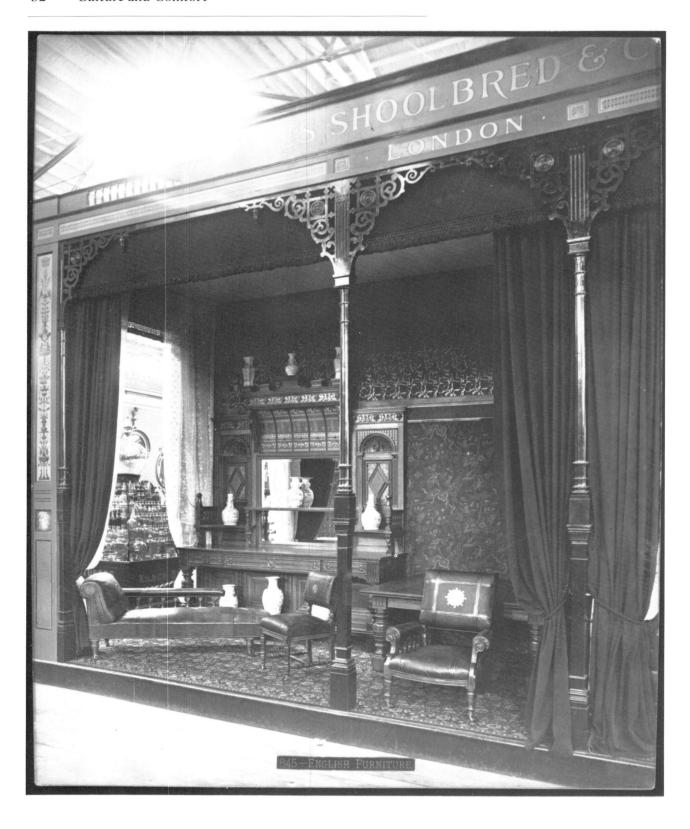

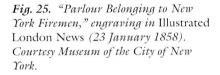

Fig. 24. Model interior, exhibit of James Shoolbred and Co., London, England, main building, Centennial Exhibition, Philadelphia, Pennsylvania, photograph by Centennial Photographic Co., 1876. Courtesy The Free Library of Philadelphia, Print and Picture Department; photograph by Joan Broderick.

spread with silver claret-jugs and pieces of plate, presented by citizens whose houses and property have been preserved from fire by the exertions of the brigade; or by the fire companies of other cities, in testimony of their admiration for some particular act of gallentry or heroism which the newspapers have recorded.[101]

The reporter was impressed by the willingness of volunteer firefighters, "mostly youths engaged during the day in various handicrafts and mechanical trades, with a sprinkling of clerks and shopmen," to engage, on behalf of the company, in "an amount of expenditure which is not the least surprising part of the 'institution'," money that went to uniforms, decorated fire equipment, and to "furnishing of their bunk-rooms and parlours at the fire stations."[102] While the brawling and spontaneous street processions depicted in the article have been considered expressions of working-class, urban folk culture, the same firemen expressed their allegiance to middle-class respectability by adopting clothing associated with status, such as top hats, and creating a genteel setting for themselves which incorporated the standard trappings of a parlor as well as a sideboard, another symbol of respectability borrowed from the dining room and used to display the company's award silver. In comparing its furnishings to those of a hotel, Mackey may have offered a clue to the model followed by the fire company in its parlor furnishing. Fire companies in other cities also created elaborate parlors for themselves (fig. 26).

A World Full of Parlors

The appearance of the parlor in steamboats and trains is partly due to the increase in the number of Americans traveling during the first half of the nineteenth century for business and pleasure. Improvements in transportation technology and the development of canals, better roads, and railroad track beds encouraged long-distance travel by making it less grueling. Some way of accommodating travelers on long journeys without stopping for overnight accommodations made sense to companies, since they could make money on the service and offer the fastest trip.

The increased presence of women and children travelers was also a factor in the process of making such mobile and commercial "domestic interiors," and at least part of the traveling public's interest in the interior arrangements of such vessels was stimulated by the presence of women and children on board. An account by Thomas L. McKenney of a barge trip up the Hudson River in 1826 praised

Fig. 25. "Parlour Belonging to New York Firemen," engraving in Illustrated London News *(23 January 1858). Courtesy Museum of the City of New York.*

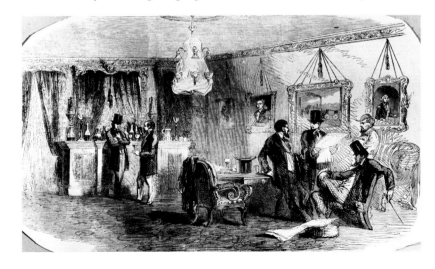

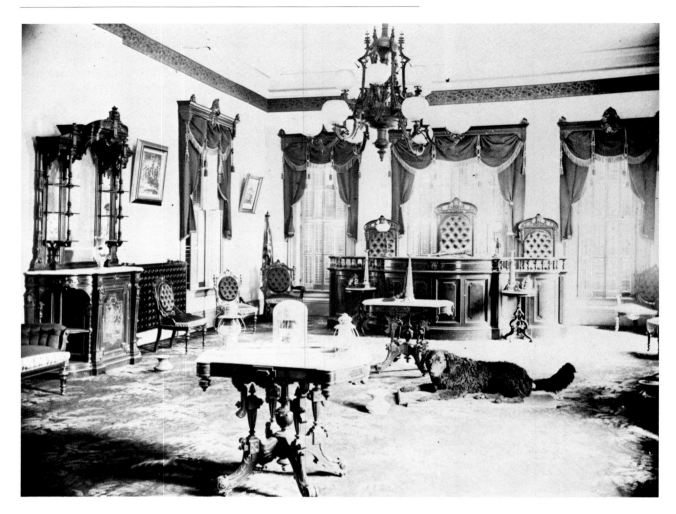

the "ladies cabin and apartments" not only for their "splendid" furnishings but because "a lady has all the retirement and comfort which the delicacy and tenderness of her sex requires."[103] Apart from the practical considerations associated with tending small children or women's special sanitary needs, the concern of operators and commentators may have been stimulated by the increasing power of the cult of domesticity. Internal public transportation of such an unprecedented physical scale needed to be made suitably domestic, in both its actual physical arrangements and the associations carried by the decoration of at least some of its interior spaces. But the realities of domestic life sometimes overwhelmed steamboat gentility. English actress Fanny Kemble considered the atmosphere of the ladies' cabins far from genteel, despite their parlor pretensions, because so many women with small children were confined there in bad weather:

> The ladies' cabin, in winter, on board one of these large steamers, is a right curious sight. It is generally crammed to suffocation with women, *strewn* in every direction…what with the vibratory motion of the rocking chairs and their contents, the women's shrill jabber, the children's shriller wailing and shouting, the heat and closeness of the air, a ladies' cabin on board an American steamboat is one of the most overpowering things to sense and soul that can well be imagined.

Fig. 26. *Session rooms, probably Active Hose Company, Rochester, New York, by unidentified photographer, about 1873. The session rooms of this hose company doubled as a men's club. The dog is stuffed and is presumably a mascot. Courtesy Rochester Public Library, Local History Division.*

Separate women's parlors on steamboats (by the late 1820s) and railroad cars (from the 1840s) and separate family parlors and women's dining rooms in hotels allowed women to relax their public decorum temporarily. They also separated women from the coarse behavior of many traveling men, particularly their drinking of spiritous liquors and the smoke and tobacco spittle (fig. 27). European travelers such as Fanny Kemble in the 1830s and Charles Dickens in the 1840s were appalled at the public behavior of "these very obnoxious chewers of tobacco." Kemble complained: "It has happened to me after a few hours' travelling in a steam-boat to find the white dress, put on fresh in the morning, covered with yellow tobacco stains; nor is this offensive habit confined to the lower orders alone. I have seen *gentlemen* spit upon the carpet of the room where they were sitting, in the company of women, without the slightest remorse."[104] This separation was not absolute—women could and did participate in mixed-sex social life in the saloons of steamboats, on railroad coaches, and in the large parlors of hotels. But they could escape to the ladies' parlors on steamboats and railroad cars, mobile islands of domesticity.

On the railroad cars of the 1850s and 1860s, before the appearance of the parlor car, women's parlors may also have been the most domestic in appearance, using fabric draperies and plush upholstery, while areas of cars open to men used leather seat cushions and other materials sturdy enough to stand the onslaught of mud from boots on the seats and tobacco juice on every conceivable surface. In his 1873 *World on Wheels*, Benjamin Franklin Taylor even suggested that "women sprinkled through the cars keep a train upon its honor, if not upon the track, and elevate the lumbering things from a common carrier to an educator."[105]

Some of the businesses that engaged in the practice of making parlors—steamboat companies, hotels, and photographers—do not seem to have much in common on the face of things. However, all three were engaged in trying to sell their service or product in an intensely competitive market. After 1825, for example, five different steamboat lines were already in competition for the passenger traffic between New York City and Albany. Selling comfort and genteel

Fig. 27. *"Reading Room, Astor House," watercolor by Nicolino V. Calyo, about 1840. Because the men who used hotel reading rooms ruined the furnishings with their tobacco spitting, even elegant hotels used leather upholstery and no carpets in these masculine retreats. Courtesy Museum of the City of New York.*

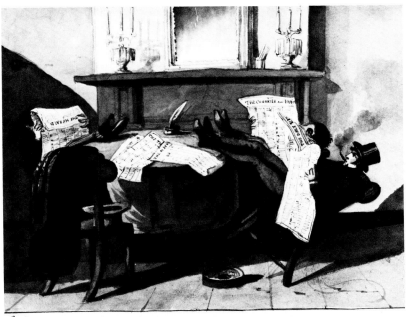

surroundings in a travel setting (when most travel was a dirty, uncomfortable, tiresome process at best) offered a service in addition to basic transportation that could create the competitive edge for a steamboat line. Hotels such as the Tremont House of Boston offered a rare service to travelers—comfortable, clean, and genteel accommodations—and, to attract a clientele with money to spend, they provided an experience which was, to America of the 1830s, uniquely urban and refined. Finally, the photographer's studio was a commercial setting that grew out of a combination of factors. The pressures of economic and professional competition and the artistic aspirations on the part of certain members of the community of photographers stimulated parlor-making effort, as did the willingness of Americans (including middle-class women with leisure hours to spend) to patronize such refined commercial settings.

Commercial parlors also grew out of the assumption that the appearance of the refined commercial parlor would discipline and civilize its clientele, which also justified the expenditures to create parlors. The most articulate statement of this position appeared in an "interview" with George Pullman from the early 1890s.

> Putting carpets on the floors of cars, for instance, was considered a very useless piece of extravagance, and putting clean sheets on the beds was even more an absurdity in the minds of many. They said that men would get in between the sheets with their boots on. But they did not. So it was with the more elaborate and costly ornamentation and upholstery which has been steadily developed. It was criticised…as useless extravagance—a waste of money on things which passengers would only destroy. It has not proved to be the case. I have always held that people are very greatly influenced by their physical surroundings. Take the roughest man, a man whose lines have always brought him into coarsest and poorest surroundings, and the effect upon his bearing is immediate. The more artistic and refined the mere external surroundings, in other words, the better and more refined the man. This goes further than the mere fact that people will be more careful in a beautifully decorated, upholstered and carpeted sleeping car than they would were not such surroundings above them. It goes, when carried out under other conditions, to the more important matter of a man's productive powers and general usefulness to himself and society.[106]

The Select Company in the World of Commerce

An explanation of the development and proliferation of public parlors in commercial spaces between 1830 and 1880 is incomplete without reference to the symbolic and rhetorical power commercial parlors had because they were both commercial and genteel. Victorianism, the bourgeois culture of industrialization and commercialization in Anglo-America, did not suddenly appear full blown, wielding a new and untried vocabulary of symbols. Instead, the culture emerged first in the commercialization of existing symbols, as well as in the articulation of new symbolic forms peculiar to a modernizing, commercial world. Two powerful metaphors permeated descriptions of the commercial spaces under investigation here—the palace and the parlor. Palaces, symbols of the concentration of royal power, existed outside the world of commerce, in the realm of power divinely ordained and inaccessible to ordinary people. When Americans appropriated the symbol of the palace to describe the "palace hotel," the "palace steamboat," or the "dry goods palace," they were grafting an old symbol to a new situation, suggesting the simultaneously leveling and uplifting effects of

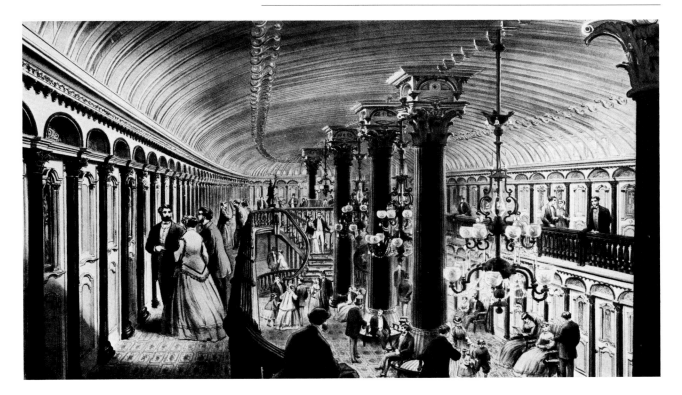

Fig. 28. *"Grand State Room Saloone/Steamer DREW/Of The Peoples Line," chromolithograph by Parsons and Atwater, published by Endicott and Co., New York, New York, about 1867 (the date of the boat's first run). Courtesy Mariners' Museum, Newport News, Virginia.*

democratic society ("every man a king") and commercially derived money. The second symbol transplanted into the commercial sphere, the parlor, was the site of formal social ceremony in the household and the room that most clearly bespoke the notion of gentility—of personal cultivation in appearance, etiquette, and education. The commercial parlor represented the commercialization of the concept of gentility, and its presence in commercial "palaces" may explain why elegant, gala furnishings rather than homey, modest versions of parlor decor appear to have been preferred for them.

Middle-class gentility also required appropriate settings in which it could be expressed. The parlors in the best hotels were locations for entertainment and social ceremony for guests, residents, and outsiders; they were a commercial version of the beau monde of cultivated people in the decades after 1830. At the same time, ladies' parlors in particular provided a domestic haven that buffered their interactions with the broader public in commercial spaces and provided an interim solution for a society still looking for a place (in both the psychological and spatial sense) for women in the public sphere. Finally, because anyone with the money and desire could create a commercial parlor, as photographers did, anyone could attempt to imply membership in the world of refinement and cultivation.

For several decades after 1830, most first-class hotel parlors (and probably the more modest examples of respectable hotels) were essentially large-scale versions of the fashionable drawing rooms in private houses.[107] But beginning in the 1850s, some commercial parlors grew more grand and less home-like. The public rooms of some first-class hotels and the most lavish steamboat interiors became so elaborate that their original relationship to domestic parlor furnishing became blurred (fig. 28). For example, with the remodeling of the *Isaac Newton* and the *New-World* in 1855, the grand saloons of Hudson River palace steamers began to take on a theatrical appearance, extending through several decks with gallery-level promenades.[108] The interiors of the most elaborate hotels, such as the Palace in San Francisco and the St. Nicholas in New York, were, as Russell Lynes has called them, fantasy settings.

Americans experienced difficulties in controlling the uses of the public parlor, because it was open to such uncultivated individuals as tobacco chewers and ill-behaved photographers' clients. They also expressed ambivalence about the effects some commercial parlors had on domestic life, because new members of the middle classes seemed to relish parlor life, even in hotels, over a more sparse yet more private domestic environment. Still, commercial parlors served to stimulate interest in creating gala parlors in the private households of new members of the middle classes. In a world that provided few models for interior decor, commercial parlors introduced people to the vocabulary—the forms of parlor furniture, carpets, draperies, and wall decoration. They also showed the observant the nuances of that vocabulary—matching color schemes and the use of certain woods, fabrics, and, as Jonathan Slick discovered, the newest techniques of upholstery construction. Public parlors both expressed the aspirations of commercializing American society and provided models for the aspirations of new participants in Victorian culture, creating demand by priming consumer imagination during the first decades of public parlor making.

CHAPTER TWO
THE COMFORTABLE THEATER:
PARLOR MAKING IN THE MIDDLE-CLASS
VICTORIAN HOUSEHOLD, 1850-1910

The word "parlor" is rarely used to describe a type of room anymore, and when it is, it is usually in the context of hair-cutting salons that have no particular pretense toward high fashion or deliberately quaint restaurants that specialize in serving ice cream. As a descriptive term, "parlor" has little in the way of cultural power.

This was not always the case. For Victorian Americans, the word "parlor" carried a wealth of associations. "Parlor" usually denoted a space within a private household in which families could present their public faces (fig. 1). It was used for the purposes of social ceremony—the place in which calls and social visits by friends were received and the setting for entertainments such as tea parties and musicales. For many families, parlors also were the location of such rites of passage as small weddings and laying out the dead, for meetings of women's clubs, for the Christmas tree, for courting, and for visits from local dignitaries. Over the course of the nineteenth

Fig. 1. "Parlor of Mr. F. P. Appleton Residence," stereograph by S. Stowe, Lowell, Massachusetts, about 1879. Courtesy Society for the Preservation of New England Antiquities.

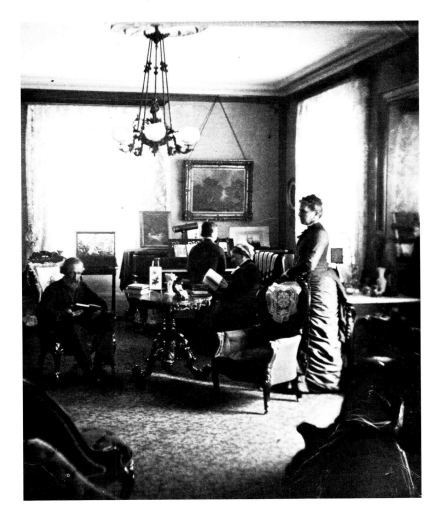

century, even as critics decried parlors as "these ceremonial deserts...useless and out of place in the houses of nine-tenths of our Americans," average people who aspired to be identified as members of the middle classes focused some of their energy and financial resources on making a parlor for themselves.[1] Setting aside a specific room for the purposes of social rituals and furnishing it for that use—once a prerogative only of families of means—became an activity that denoted membership in, or aspirations to belong to, the respectable middle classes.

If the term "parlor" has little meaning today, one has only to add the descriptor "Victorian" to achieve quite a different effect. Victorian parlors were "stuffy," "crowded" with useless and bizarre objects, and "dirty" because of the dust their myriad contents collected. They were also "uncomfortable," which is the most damning kind of modern criticism. In her memoir of middle-class life in Pittsburgh at the turn of the century, Ethel Spencer criticized the uncomfortable quality of her family's parlor from the perspective of the 1950s:

> The house was square. To the right of the central hall as one entered was the library and to the left the parlor. The parlor went through many transformations and toward the end of our occupancy of the house it became a living room, but in our childhood no one could have lived in it happily. It was meant for occasions—for formal calls, for receptions, for Sundays, but not for everyday living. No one could have relaxed in its overstuffed rocking chair of vast proportions or felt at home with its tall china lamp, a Victorian monstrosity of the first order (fig. 2).[2]

Indeed, as the second half of the nineteenth century passed, parlors were stuffed full of increasing numbers of things. As Clarence Cook complained in 1878, "What with easels, chairs not meant for use, little teetery stands, pedestals, and the rest of the supernumerary family filling up the room left by the solid and supposed useful pieces, it is sometimes a considerable test of one's dexterity and presence of mind to make one's way from end to end of a long New York drawing room."[3] This multitude of things was often hard to clean, and to maintain a parlor required a certain degree of dedication. While many women relied on the services of at least a visiting laundress, most cleaned their own houses. But for most incipient

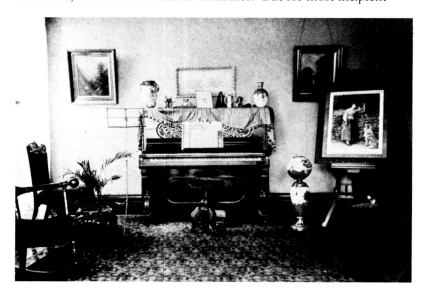

Fig. 2. The Spencer parlor, 719 Amberson Avenue, Pittsburgh, Pennsylvania, about 1910, photograph by Charles Hart Spencer in Ethel Spencer, The Spencers of Amberson Avenue *(1983). Courtesy Elizabeth Ranney.*

parlor makers in the second half of the nineteenth century, anticipated maintenance problems seem not to have stifled the impulse to furnish and embellish. For example, when Mr. and Mrs. George Ware Fulton built and furnished their Second Empire-style "dream house" near Rockport, Texas, in the mid-1870s, they purchased furniture, drapery, and carpets for most of the rooms from companies in Cincinnati and New York. The parlor was furnished in a manner reflecting typical conservative upper middle-class good taste for the time: a seven-piece suite and several window chairs covered in silk were included in the room, as well as a number of other fancy chairs, wall-to-wall Brussels carpeting, and window lambrequins made of cretonne (a heavy, unglazed cotton, printed with large figures as was chintz). The Fultons furnished their parlor this way despite the fact that all the furnishings were in constant peril from the ravages of moths, beetles, roaches, and Gulf Coast humidity and mold. In a letter written when she and her husband were out of town, Mrs. Fulton reminded her daughter to shake out the lambrequins and handle the parlor furniture weekly to discourage vermin. Residents of the Gulf Coast still tell outsiders that constant use and handling of textiles is necessary to prevent infestations.[4]

Housekeepers in the urban Northeast did not have to worry about weevils in their lambrequins, but they faced their own special trials, particularly soot from burning coal and gas. Ethel Spencer recalled that her mother "spent hours pinning ten-foot long [lace] curtains to stretchers when they had to be washed—which was about twice a month in those days of uncontrolled smoke."[5]

Despite the unrelenting labors involved in maintaining parlors and the criticisms of parlors as coldly formal, uncomfortable spaces that wasted family resources and saw little daily use, it is clear that thousands of Americans devoured parlor furnishing advice from books and periodicals. For these consumers, the equation between comfort and ceremony in the parlor was balanced in favor of as much formality as their limited resources could muster. Middle-class American families who made such rooms often chose to use rooms other than the parlor—the kitchen, the dining room, a second parlor, or a sitting room—as the place where they gathered daily. Sometimes the motivation for limiting parlor use to special occasions was associated with practical concerns: it was expensive, for example, to heat an extra room. However, most families who saved their parlor for social purposes seem to have been motivated by the desire to give due respect to the scale and gravity of the events they knew were expected to take place there.

The middle-class parlor between 1850 and 1910 was the descendant of two different kinds of best rooms of the eighteenth and early nineteenth centuries. Edith Wharton and Ogden Codman, Jr., described this "mixed ancestry"—from the gala apartment and the "family sitting room"—in *The Decoration of Houses* (1897):

> In modern American houses both traditional influences are seen. Sometimes, as in England, the drawing-room is treated as a family apartment, and provided with books, lamps, easy-chairs and writing tables. In other houses, it is still considered sacred to gilding and discomfort, the best room in the house, and the convenience of all its inmates, being sacrificed to a vague feeling that no drawing-room is worthy of the name unless it is uninhabitable. This is an instance of the *salon de compagnie* having usurped the rightful place of the *salon de famille*; or rather, if the bourgeois descent of the American house be considered, it may be more truly defined as a remnant of the "best parlor" superstition.[6]

In many pre-Georgian American house plans of the seventeenth and eighteenth centuries, the name "parlor" designated one of two rooms on the house's ground floor, the other being the hall. Like all rooms in such houses, the parlor was a multi-purpose space. It was where the family's best possessions, including the best bed in the household, were stored and displayed. Although company was received there, the parlor was not what might be termed a "gala apartment," a room designed for socializing. Beds disappeared from parlors in more expensive homes during the second half of the eighteenth century, but in modest houses they continued to be found there well into the nineteenth century.

The second source for the parlor of the mid-nineteenth century was a result of two cultural imperatives. As etiquette became more formalistic and codified, well-to-do Americans increasingly favored house plans that more rigorously separated public and private regions of houses (fig. 3). In addition, a new conception of entertainment in households linked to the social and commercial demands of an urban bourgeois culture required the presence of a special apartment devoted to that purpose. Planning for special-use rooms in houses, called the art of distribution, was perfected by French architects in the late seventeenth century. In house plans, the major categories of human activity were segregated, and each specific function was allotted its own domestic space.[7] In grand houses, architects planned several kinds of public rooms to serve the needs of gatherings of varying size and intimacy. Salons were places where, according to the architect Alexandre Jean-Baptiste Le Blond in 1710, "people of quality are received and one may dine on grand occasions." "Grand cabinets" (later called *apartements de société*) were "very glamorous reception rooms of moderate size, where one could expect to find select company" in less formal circumstances than in salons.[8]

Fascinated with the ingenious French plans, English architects adapted these room divisions in the eighteenth century, but the requirements of English society were somewhat different. Robert Adam's plan for Syon House, remodeled in the early 1760s, included both private and public dining rooms. Next door to the public dining room was "a splendid with-drawing room for the ladies, or *salle de compagnie*, as it is called in Paris." Next to this was the gallery, "an admirable room for the reception of company after dinner, or for the ladies to retire to after it" and, finally, a circular "saloon" for public entertainments along the lines of balls or very large receptions.[9] The concept of the "drawing room" or "parlor" in fashionable houses of the late eighteenth and early nineteenth centuries combined the functions of the "with-drawing room" and the "gallery" (a term that was not used in America). It was closest in concept to the French *apartement de société* and was intended as a location for the display of social graces and personal cultivation. The function of the French *salon* had been split between Adam's saloon and the public dining room.

Members of the economic and social elites in America probably gathered their ideas about the function and contents of parlors both from their connections to English gentry and from time spent in France or in the company of French visitors to America. The French conception of what might be called the "social geography" of gentility seemed particularly seductive, however, and Francophiles in the last decades of the eighteenth century, such as Philadelphian Samuel Powel III, attempted to reproduce it. A native of Philadelphia, Powel was reared as a gentleman and traveled in Europe for seven years before his marriage in 1769. He served as mayor of Philadelphia during the Revolution, and his house was the site of lavish entertainments both for members of the Continental Congress as well as officers of the British Army.

When Powel returned from his European sojourn, carrying with him a collection of furnishings (now lost), he promptly remodeled his house on Third Street. The new front rooms on both floors reflected his understanding of the public facade of a gentleman; the presence of his children and evidence of domestic work were noticeably lacking. The first two floors of the house's primary block, facing the street, were devoted completely to "parlors" that were drawing rooms and an impressive second-floor ballroom for evening entertainments—rich

Fig. 3. "Design No. 19," engraving in Calvert Vaux, Villas and Cottages *(1857). Victorian houseplans typically included several rooms for visitors and outsiders on the first floor at the front of the house; and bedrooms and rooms for housekeeping—kitchens and pantries—were placed at the back of houses and upstairs.*

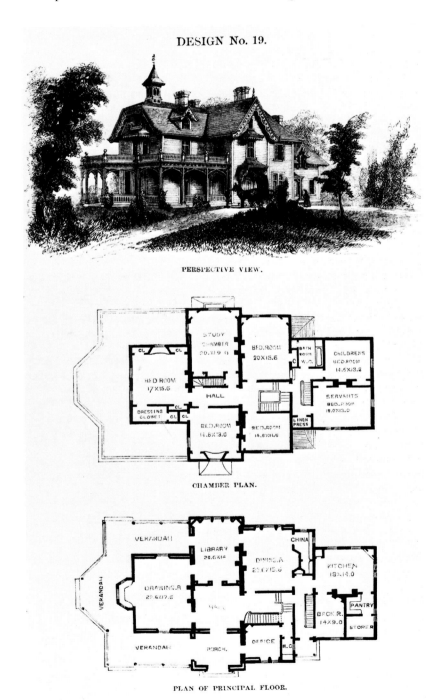

DESIGN No. 19.

PERSPECTIVE VIEW.

CHAMBER PLAN.

PLAN OF PRINCIPAL FLOOR.

suppers, music and dancing, card playing, and lively conversation. Sleeping and daily living were confined to the third floor of this block and to a simply furnished rear wing. The denizens of parlors such as Powel's were members of a "select company," not a cross-section of the entire society nor a close-knit family group but instead men and women of similar social class and breeding.[10]

By the mid-nineteenth century, the old term "parlor" was still in use in the United States. Yet, even in middle-class households, ideas about the function of parlors—and about the nature of the possessions appropriate to such rooms—had evolved toward the concept of the "drawing room," devoted to the presentation of the public self. Neither personal accounts nor published furnishing advice are consistent in using the term "parlor" as distinct from "drawing room." Books that use the term "drawing room" sometimes seem to be addressed to audiences who must have had enough rooms and resources to feature a gala space devoted only to entertainment. Other terms, including "salon" and "sitting room," also occasionally appear. The term "sitting room" presents another exercise in analyzing the ambiguities of domestic architectural terminology and actual patterns of use. In houses with adequate space, "sitting room" referred to a separate room that saw daily, casual use as a center for reading, sewing, and other family activities, as opposed to the parlor's more formal function as a site for social ritual. As case studies of room use indicate, the "sitting room" could be a back parlor, equipped with older, simpler furniture. Often the dining room or kitchen doubled as the sitting room if a house did not possess enough rooms. In these instances, families still chose to reserve their parlors for formality.

In the second half of the nineteenth century, the word "parlor" seems to have been commonly understood as the *Century Dictionary* defined it in 1890: "a room in a private house set apart for the conversational entertainment of guests; a reception-room; a drawing-room;...In the United States, where the word "drawing-room" is little used, *parlor* is the general term for the room used for the reception of guests."[11] Even in households that could not set aside a room for only occasional use, the parlor was the center of formal sociability. Catharine Beecher described it as the space "reserved for the reception-room of friends, and for our own dressed leisure hours."[12] The authors of *Beautiful Homes; or, Hints in House Furnishing*, an 1878 advice book directed toward new consumers of household furnishings, explained the purpose and appearance of the parlor by referring to the older understanding of the term. For members of the "middle classes," the parlor served "both as reception-room and that chosen apartment, which in olden times was the 'best room' of our grandmothers."[13]

For middle-class families, the modern parlor now had to be presentable enough—its furnishings sufficient evidence of modern tastes—to serve as the family's *apartement de société* even if it doubled as the sitting room. However, advice literature made plain that separate rooms were preferable: "With these requirements, it is in the parlor therefore that we find the choicest treasures that the house can afford, that will tend to the hospitable entertainment of guests," Mrs. C. S. Jones and Henry T. Williams wrote in *Beautiful Homes*, "just as in the sitting-room or living-room are gathered the dearest tokens of love of the family circle."[14] The 1882 edition of *Webster's Dictionary* noted this double usage when it described the parlor as the room "which the family usually occupy for society and conversation, the reception-room of visitors, &c...; sometimes, the best room of a house, kept for receiving company, as distinguished from the sitting room of the family."[15]

The impulse to make modern parlors in middle-class households gathered momentum steadily after 1830 and continued into the twentieth century, moving down through the economic strata as far as incomes allowed the purchase of appropriate furnishing. Architectural advice books published in the middle decades of the nineteenth century reveal that parlors became an important aspect of space and room use planning even in very modest structures, which is one manifestation of Victorian efforts to elaborate upon the eighteenth-century art of distribution.

In Victorian house plans for large and small suburban "villas," apartment houses, rowhouses, and many farmhouses, cooking was separated from eating by the inclusion of a dining room. A range of other private activities took place in the back regions of houses—sleeping, care of clothing, and children's play. A front hall provided a psychological buffer zone between the outside world and the domestic realm. And, ideally, the plan also designated a space that the family could reserve specifically for the presentation of its dressed-up social identity—the parlor.

Calvert Vaux's *Villas and Cottages* (1864) provided designs for suburban and rural houses in varying degrees of grandeur and expense, but almost all included a parlor. The related rooms, and the language Vaux used in naming each, reveal something about how the houses' owners might be expected to spend their time in the spaces. Small houses had a parlor and a living room (which was sometimes also the dining room); large houses had a parlor, a living room, a study or a drawing room, a morning room, and a library.[16]

Even house plan books addressed specifically to audiences with limited incomes revealed the importance placed on setting aside valuable domestic space for the purposes of the parlor. One such plan book was S. B. Reed's *House-Plans for Everybody*, first published in 1878 by Orange Judd and Co., the New York publisher of the weekly newspaper *American Agriculturalist* (which, at its peak of popularity in the late 1860s, had a circulation of 160,000).[17] *House-Plans for Everybody* was one of a variety of inexpensive advice books aimed at respectable members of the lower middle and middle classes, especially those living in rural areas. The book was a particular success for the firm, remaining in print at least until 1900. It was distributed by both Sears, Roebuck and Co. and Montgomery Ward and Co., whose catalog for spring and summer 1895 described *House-Plans for Everybody* as a "useful volume" for "persons of moderate means." It sold for $1.10 plus postage.[18]

The book consists of forty house plans arranged in order of increasing expense. Considerable space was devoted to modest single-family dwellings; ten of these were estimated to cost $1,100 or less to construct. Although the houses were often very small, the interiors were marked by the division of interior space into tiny rooms with their specific functions labeled. Parlors appeared as early as Design V ($650), which included an eleven-by-eleven-foot "Kitchen or Living-Room" and a thirteen-by-fourteen-foot "Parlor." Reed understood that having differentiated room spaces was more important to his rural and small-town audience than were generous, open spaces: "Conventional modes of living have established a system of household arrangement and economy requiring for every home of even moderate refinement, a house with a front hall, a parlor, a dining room, and a kitchen on the first floor, and a liberal suite of chambers on the second story."[19]

Within Reed's small houses, several architectural features helped define any particular room as a "parlor." Mantels were important, even though most of the houses would actually have been heated by stoves, because the hearth was an emblem of family. In the comments for Design IX, a "Country or Village Cottage," the parlor had a "marble shelf" but was warmed by a "radiator" beneath it, which communicated heat from the stove in the adjoining room.[20] Bay windows (available in prefabricated form for fifty to sixty dollars complete) were a second important parlor feature. Reed noted in passing that not only would such windows add space to parlors, but also that a bay window "indicates refinement."[21] Indeed, architectural details such as elaborate mantels could provide important cues about the type of decor appropriate in a room and were the focus of much furnishing effort and attention. However, parlors could in theory be made anywhere that a space could be found for them.

A variety of other sources attest the development of what might be termed "parlor consciousness" in both new members of the middle classes and individuals aspiring to that respectable, if not always well-defined, identity. Interest in having a modern parlor was not only an urban phenomenon, although the sources of news about changes in furnishing tastes were located in cities. The desire to make modern parlors reached into the economic and social elites of small-town and rural America by the 1820s and slowly moved into less urbane groups in such communities. In the 1850s and 1860s, women's magazines such as *Godey's Lady's Book* and *Peterson's* published articles that made explicit the assumption that their readers included women living "at a distance from cities, who wish to send orders" for up-to-date furnishings.[22]

The 1850 *Godey's* article "New Furniture" carefully listed the contents of the modern house room by room. The most up-to-date parlors or drawing rooms contained sets of "sofas and ordinary chairs, covered with satin damask, crimson and black, deeply tufted or knotted" or with velvet, plush or haircloth covers over rosewood frames. Modern parlors also incorporated "lounging or arm-chairs," pianos, sofa tables with oval marble tops, and étagères, which required explanation because of their newness. These freestanding sets of shelves were meant to be filled with "elegantly bound books and *bijouterie* [decorative accessories such as vases and ceramic figures] of all descriptions" in the parlors of elegant houses.[23]

"New Furniture" diagrammed the conventions or "vocabulary" of furnishing middle- and upper-class urban households, some of which would remain essentially unchanged for the rest of the century—at least at the level of popular, rather than fashionable, taste. Its description of old-fashioned parlors noted with evident scorn that some of the solid citizens of rural communities still did not understand modern tastes in furniture: "Now, this may cause divers groans from 'honest country folk,' where chairs, a bureau, a looking-glass, and a table, are still considered the essentials of parlor furniture; and a sofa or centre-table luxuries, that call forth the remark from visitors, that 'Squire Smith, or Major Jones' people are living quite too stylish!'"[24] In a fictional description of the rural owners of a new frame house, Mrs. C. M. Kirkland described the family's "parlour," which she clearly considered typical, as containing white "curtains" (from the description, actually decorated window shades) "with netting and fringe half a yard deep," a shelf of books, a rag carpet, and "the best bed, with volumes of white drapery about it." The special character of the parlor was confirmed by the fact that the kitchen was the room "in which the family usually lived."[25]

Even though information about the modern way to furnish parlors usually emanated from cities, differences in the tastes of ordinary urban and rural parlor makers were not extreme by the second half of the nineteenth century, at least in areas no longer subject to the roughness of frontier living or to extraordinary geographical or social isolation. In their abilities to create modern parlors, ordinary consumers in rural communities differed from their comparable urban peers chiefly in their initial difficulties in obtaining access to goods (problems that improved transportation, cheaper periodicals and books, and the arrival of the mail-order business eventually solved) and, among smaller farmers, in a shortage of cash (a chronic problem in the rural economy generally) with which to purchase consumer goods from faraway places. The penetration of the rural market by a national or regional consumer culture drew more people into a network of similar middle-class tastes and is one of the most important results of the commercialization of society. Once only elites were cosmopolitan, with access to national and international information about changing tastes in fashions. Over the course of the nineteenth century, ordinary people also became cosmopolitan in a modest way through the popular ideas, tastes, and goods of middle-class consumer culture.

As the western territories were settled in the second half of the nineteenth century, respectable families created up-to-date parlors for themselves in rough places where steamboats and railroads permitted shipping but where social calling was an impossibility. The Fulton family made determined efforts to transplant a middle-class parlor typically found in the East to Texas. The Kohrs family, a prosperous ranching family of Deer Lodge Valley, Montana Territory, purchased the furniture for a "magnificently furnished parlor" in their log ranch house in St. Louis in 1868; it was shipped as far as Fort Benton by steamer.[26]

The Household, a monthly magazine published between 1868 and 1903 in Brattleboro, Vermont, provides additional evidence that less prosperous rural women were interested in and knew about the furnishing practices of the urban middle classes by the 1870s. Published correspondence from *The Household's* readers and frequent firsthand accounts (some probably fictionalized) of parlor making indicate that farm wives knew what proper parlors ought to contain. Each issue included descriptions of homemade upholstered furniture, curtains and mantel lambrequins, "tidies and antimacassars" (ornamental needlework pieces used to protect furniture surfaces), and parlor ornaments such as homemade bracket shelves. Many of these articles suggested that attractive parlor furnishing could be attained without having to purchase all the elements ready-made. In one article, "How We Furnished the Parlor," the narrator helped a neighbor create a parlor with fifty dollars and elbow grease. The money was spent largely on upholstery fabrics (for curtains, shelf and mantel drapery, and chair cushions) and a twelve-dollar lounge. It represented the accumulation of years of savings that the farm wife had originally designated for a "raw silk [parlor] set"; she knew that a parlor suite was an essential component of conventional parlor furnishing.[27]

The Household also encouraged "parlor consciousness" by heading its articles with room names, including the "Drawing Room," "Parlor," "Library," and "Dressing Room." These "departments" also suggested the appropriate activities for each particular space. Although the majority of *The Household's* audience probably did not have more than a single parlor or sitting room, to organize content in this way addressed the ideal dimensions of social activity or women's work that took place in each. The "Drawing Room" section represented personal refinement and social interaction, containing brief essays of a sentimental or moralizing nature such as "Memory's Treasures," fiction of the same tone, and some discussion of the arts. It also included advice on etiquette; these bore titles such as "Courteous Manners" and "Visitors and Visiting." The "Parlor" concentrated upon the life of the family, including articles for or about children and suggestions for pastimes with titles along the lines of "Games for Winter Evenings." It offered instructions for guessing games with a literary bent—"The Shakespeare Game," the "Game of Mythology," and another called "Poetical Pot Pie." The "Library" division promoted self-improvement with articles on literature and music. Finally, the "Dressing Room" was the location of general advice on housework other than cooking (sewing in particular) and instruction in "fancy work" and homemade interior decoration. Through its organization, *The Household* provided readers both practical household advice and a vision of the possibilities that having rooms strictly for social purposes might provide.[28]

The various genres of advice book—etiquette and "parlor pastime" books—and a second category of information—personal reminiscences of parlor life as it was actually lived in a variety of urban and rural places—reveal how Victorians thought parlors should be used, and how these ideas differed from the ways in which parlors were actually used in the decades after 1850. In the first decades of the nineteenth century, prosperous families of the American elites continued to furnish beautiful parlors as the settings for entertainments for the select company, as Samuel Powel's had been. In a diary entry for March 4, 1839, Sidney George Fisher described one such theatrical setting and its participants:

> At 9 went to a small, but very beautiful recherche [refined] party at Mrs. Geo: Cadwalader's. It was made for Mrs. Harrison. The rooms are very rich and splendid, & also in excellent taste, tho I think too costly for our style of living and habits. Walls & ceiling painted in fresco by Monachesi [a Philadelphia portrait painter], curtains, chairs white & gold, beautiful carpets, etc. etc., in two large rooms, brilliantly lighted, and filled with about 50 well-dressed and well-bred men & women, sitting in quiet talk, made a pretty scene. The supper was in the same style of sumptuous elegance, without profusion. They have been accustomed to this thing all their lives, and do it with ease, propriety & grace. Very different from the gaudy show, crowded glitter and loaded tables of certain vulgar people here, who by mere force of money have got into a society to which they are not entitled by birth, education or manners.[29]

In their discussions of parlor social life, most nineteenth-century etiquette books echoed Fisher's description of the beau monde or aristocratic ideal of parlor decor, entertainments, deportment, and social grace of parlor people. Underlying their advice is the same concept of the parlor as a theatrical location for personal display that guided the remodeling and use of Samuel Powel's front rooms. Books that offered advice on etiquette described a world of parlor entertainment—receptions, musicales, and tea parties—that Sidney George Fisher would have recognized, even though many middle-class people might have been uncomfortable with the formality of behavior at such events.

For this reason, to use etiquette books as a guide to actual habits of middle-class living, especially in the second half of the nineteenth century, requires some caution. Manners books are a highly stylized genre of domestic advice literature, marked by repeated plagiarism over very long periods of time. For example, *Social Culture*, an 1903 etiquette manual common enough in libraries to suggest its wide circulation, borrowed heavily from Emily Thornwell's *The Lady's Guide to Perfect Gentility* of 1856, which in turn cribbed much of its material from *Etiquette for Ladies; with Hints on the Preservation,*

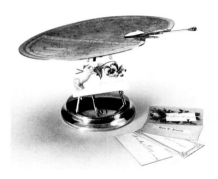

Fig. 4. *Calling cards and card receiver, Wilcox Silver Plate Co., Providence, Rhode Island, about 1880.*

Improvement, and Display of Female Beauty, first published in Philadelphia in 1838 and reprinted as late as 1856. *Etiquette for Ladies*, which employed several untranslated French terms and mentioned social life in Paris several times in its pages, may be a translation and American reprint of an earlier French work, as yet untraced.[30]

Etiquette books did describe at least some parlor social behavior as it really happened—the survival of large numbers of calling cards and card receivers certainly supports their concentration on this aspect of parlor ritual (fig. 4).[31] Perhaps much of their advice on the forms of social life is best considered as an expression of the range of social and personal possibilities that ordinary Victorian Americans envisioned in the mastery of etiquette and domestic ritual. Etiquette books represented a vision of the expressive possibilities of formal social life.

Manners books devoted particular attention to the rituals of formal calling, which had become more important in the first half of the nineteenth century. Their instructions indicate that calling was considered an urban activity, since it consisted largely of brief social visits, impractical and unnecessary in small communities or between rural households. The author of *Etiquette for Ladies* explained (using the term "visit" where other books use "calling") that "visits are a very important part of Etiquette: they are not merely the simple means of communication established by necessity, since they have at once for their object, duty and pleasure, but they enter into almost all acts of life." The author described several categories of visits, "on new-years-day," "of friendship," and the "half-ceremonious" and "ceremonious" visits of formal calling.[32] Formal calls ("ceremonious visits") were very brief. They sometimes entailed simply leaving a card and were largely a means of maintaining social acquaintance; "half-ceremonious" calls were more friendly visits. In all kinds of calls, authors informed their readers, visitors were received in the "reception room" of the house, the parlor or drawing-room where the occupants of the house, usually the women, waited and occupied their time with reading or fancy work. Many advice authors recommended that regular afternoons be set aside for being "at home" to callers so as to avoid missing callers while one was out calling oneself.

The authors of *American Etiquette*, an 1884 volume that may have a more authentic "voice" than *Etiquette for Ladies* because it seems to contain fewer plagiarized passages, tried to clarify the rituals of calling by explaining them in terms of social efficiency. The "system of calls," they wrote, was "one of the necessary inventions of polite society in thickly populated localities…where the circle of acquaintances is large [and] less time can be devoted to each…the social machinery is necessarily more complicated." The authors described a number of calling occasions, all of which were acted out in the parlor—general formal calls ("a mere device for keeping up acquaintance"); formal calls for special occasions, as after a party; "morning," that is, daytime calls; "evening calls," which were limited to friends of the family; "calls of congratulation"; and, finally, "friendly calls," brief visits among friends.[33]

Today it is difficult from reading about the practice and etiquette of calling to derive a real sense of its nuances and meaning for participants. However, as described in *American Etiquette*, the categories of "calling" were very much like a description of the occasions upon which individuals today would pick up the telephone; it seems no coincidence that use of the telephone has been designated "calling." Telephone calls, however, can be made when the caller is in a disheveled, less-than-presentable state; parlor calls required both controlled self-presentation on the part of the caller and an appropriate setting for the recipient of the call. Calling and other parlor activities—formal receptions, tea parties, balls, and other evening gatherings that etiquette books devoted considerable space to describing—may become more comprehensible if the parlor is thus viewed as a space that contained the necessary props, held in readiness, for formality. These props offered myriad possibilities for the temporary transformation of oneself into a parlor person.[34]

Around midcentury, another type of parlor social activity, the parlor pastime, developed its own genre of advice book. Parlor pastimes encompassed a range of games and activities including guessing and word games, amateur theatricals and similar entertainments, and activities that employed toys and objects to amuse, instruct, and encourage conversation among both children and adults—stereopticons, scrapbooks and photo albums, and board games.

Parlor pastime books can be grouped into two types. Dating largely from the 1850s and 1860s, the first emphasized adult activities. Some, as in Catharine Harbeson Esling's *The Book of Parlour Games*, featured old games (what may now be called folk games such as "Blind Man's Buff" and kissing or courting games) with rules set in print. They relied heavily on practical jokes and even upon physical humor (figs. 5 and 6). Such pastimes lay outside the rules for polite deportment outlined by manners books. Others, such as Frank Bellew's *The Art of Amusing*, published in 1866, emphasized genteel theatricals for adults.[35]

Some of the parlor pastime books went so far as to suggest that such activities were necessary because formal parlor entertainments were often so dull. Sidney George Fisher's diary entry comparing Philadelphia's genteel elite with the local parvenus also suggests that the lengthy and anxious preparation involved in presenting oneself in the parlor, along with the handicap of a less cosmopolitan education and world view, was actually too wearing for self-made members of the prosperous middle classes. The author of one pastime book noted, "We have seen a whole party of estimable people sit round the room for hours together in an agony of silence, only broken now and then by a small remark fired off by some desperate individual, in the forlorn hope that he would bring on a general conversation."[36] Another observed,

> There are not many refined miseries keener than the sufferings of a hostess who, in the fullness of her heart or from some conventional necessity, invites a few friends to spend a social evening at her house, and as a result sees them at last seated in a dismal semi-circle, all apparently animated, or rather deadened, by a full purpose not to enjoy themselves.[37]

While manners books usually described a world in which no children disrupted the smooth execution of parlor social ritual, the second type of parlor pastime book, which developed in the 1860s and 1870s, often described gatherings in middle-class households where young and old mingled. These books also suggested that such gatherings had long precedent: "It is a good old custom in New England, on Thanksgiving evening, for old and young to join in merry games," Mrs. Caroline L. Smith, or "Aunt Carrie," wrote in *The American Book of In-Door Games, Amusements, and Occupations* in 1873. "And now we are glad to see the same custom extends even to the Christmas holidays."[38] These games and activities could take place whether or not visitors were present. One game recommended

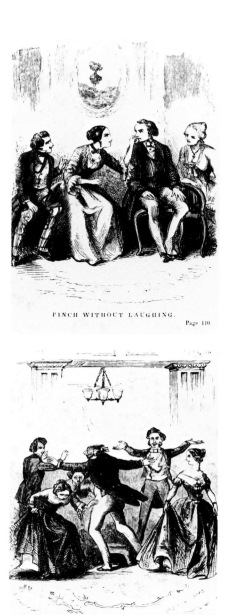

Figs. 5 and 6. "Pinch Without Laughing" and "Blind Man's Buff," engravings in Catharine Harbeson Esling, The Book of Parlour Games *(1854).*

to provide "life to a quiet company on a stormy winter evening," according to Aunt Carrie, was "menagerie," where each participant was given the name of an animal to imitate on signal.[39] Along with charades and tableaux, authors also recommended arithmetical puzzles, "The Game of Twenty Questions," games of memory, and "Musical Games or Home Dancing," including versions of musical chairs.[40] Diaries sometimes confirm that adults and children amused each other with such puzzles and riddles on long evenings and also drew pictures for each other. These activities seem to have taken place in rooms all over the house.[41]

Manners books and manuals of instruction for familial parlor pastimes from the second half of the nineteenth century described two poles of parlor social activity that correspond to the dual origins of the Victorian parlor—the drawing room and the multi-use parlor/sitting room of the hall/parlor type house. Yet in the daily rounds of real life, use seems to have been more complicated than both kinds of advice literature suggest. Because the piano was there, parlors were the locations of informal dances in the evening and of group singing (including hymns on Sunday). Because they were not in constant use, parlors were a good place for a private conversation, a solitary cry, or courting. All these activities took place in the formal parlor of Grove Hill in Virginia, according to the memoir of occupant Lucy Breckenridge, along with the more usual social gatherings.[42] Common and important rituals, which people understood through information passed along through a family or other informal networks, were staged here. One such practice was the custom of laying out the dead for viewing (fig. 7). Here the Victorian parlor became an appropriate setting for a traditional ritual whose importance eclipsed those of other social ceremonies in mid-nineteenth-century parlor life (fig. 8).[43]

The range of more lighthearted social activities taking place in any individual family's parlor varied depending upon the amount of space in houses (fig. 9). Victorian Americans nonetheless tried to keep one room from being used daily by the family. In larger households, a formal parlor or drawing room could be devoted only to the entertainment of callers and guests; in these houses, a family sitting room served as the everyday gathering place. For example, the formal parlor of the Tucker family of Wiscasset, Maine, was the site for temperance society meetings and similar ceremonious occasions, but children were not allowed to spend time in the room unsupervised or sit on its eight-piece parlor suite (fig. 10).

Some houses were planned with a pair of parlors, connected by wide doorways often fitted with sliding pocket doors. In this situation, a family might have a "front parlor" or "best parlor," the most formal and showy room, and a "back parlor." The back parlor could serve as a family sitting room, but the spaces could also be combined and used as one large space for the purposes of entertaining. Harriet Beecher Stowe's *We and Our Neighbors* (1875) chronicled life in a middle-class household on an "unfashionable" street in New York City and described the shifting use of double parlors, from informal family space to a setting for formal calling. The protagonists, Harry and Eva Henderson, kept house with the help of a cook-housekeeper and a part-time maid, the cook's daughter. Their house had a pair of small parlors, one of which doubled as a sitting room in the afternoons and evenings. At the couple's weekly "at homes" on Thursday evenings, the doors between the parlors were opened to accommodate the larger group, the room received special decorations, a tea table was set up, and the furnishings were rearranged to encourage conversation. Eva also

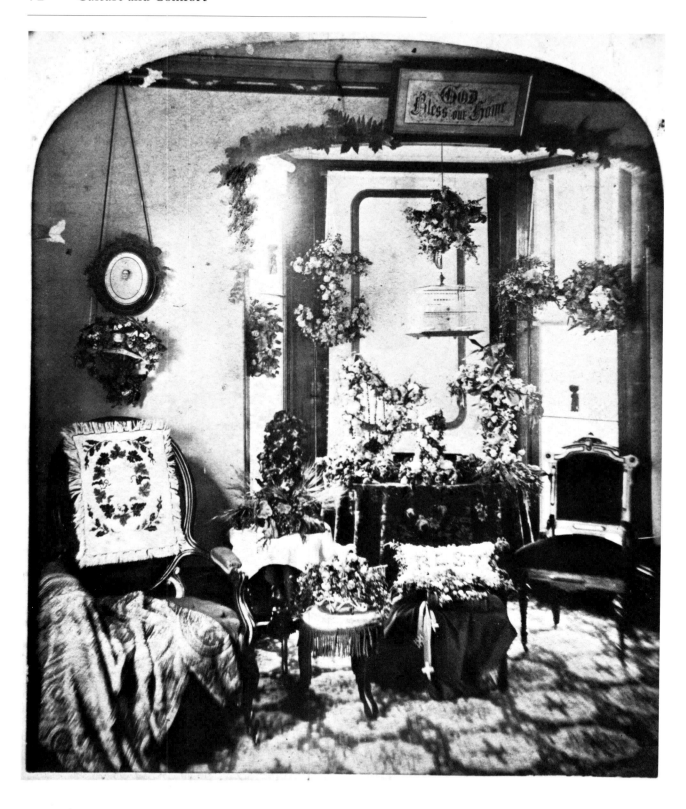

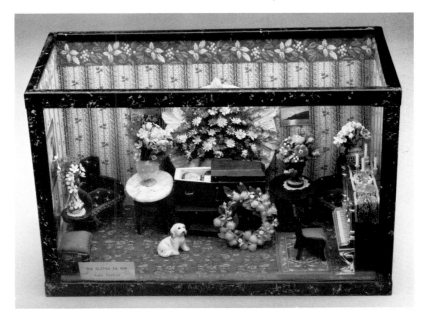

Fig. 7. *"Decoration of Flowers, at the Funeral of Clara Jane Treat, Residence of Dr. N. Q. Tirrell, East Weymouth. On Sunday April 16, 1876," stereograph by unidentified photographer. Courtesy Society for the Preservation of New England Antiquities.*

Fig. 8. *"The Coffin in the Home Parlor," miniature room by Alice C. Steele, Cummington, Massachusetts, about 1935.*

received occasional formal calls in the front parlor in its everyday arrangement.[44]

Even less prosperous households could be equipped with two parlors, with one reserved for special occasions such as courting or visits from teachers. In a memoir of growing up in a respectable, modestly prosperous Catholic family in Buffalo, New York, of the 1870s, Alice Hughes Neupert recalled the decoration and customary use of both the front and back parlors around 1880:

> The front parlor was for state occasions only, and for entertaining priests, nuns, and important visitors such as Charles Deuther, organist at St. Patrick's Church…The two front windows were hung with lace curtains and lambrequins or valances of dark red velvet heavily fringed and ornamented with long cords and tassels at the side. In each corner was a large easy chair, one with a paisley covering and the other a newer style of cinnamon brown. If you pushed a button on this latter chair, a foot stool slid out. The other corner of the room held a dark chair with a high back, upholstered with *high* green satin. It had slender arms, and we were never supposed to sit in it. There was a marble topped table in the center on which stood a carrara marble statue of "winter"…another little silver dish for cards and a bound book of *Great Musicians*, that smelled sort of leathery.[45]

The front parlor also contained the family's prized piano, over which hung a large print of Beethoven.

> Now the back parlor. In those days the carpeting of the double parlors was always the same, as well as the wallpapering. These carpets…were small patterned with dark red and yellow roses and much greenery. Because the back parlor was used more, this carpet was saved by putting a crimson colored rug with a gray border over it, which gave a cheerful aspect to the room. I remember a table cornerwise with a cover made of scarlet flannel, black fringe and black cut out dragons at each corner. This table also held a lamp and teakwood box which smelled like cinnamon and held a turtle that could move its legs. There was also a Chinese ornament made with brown and yellow shells. There

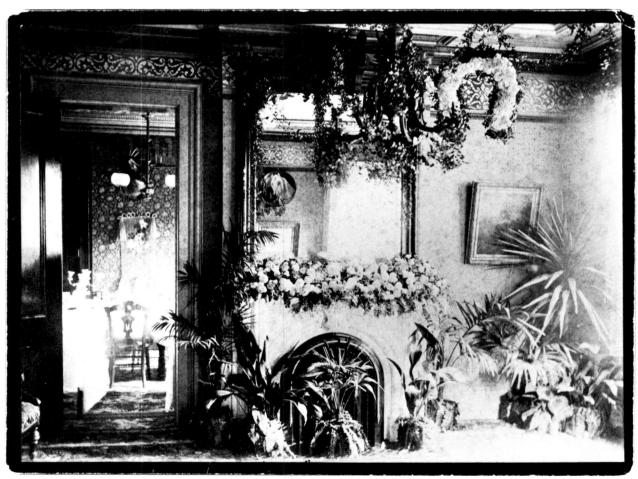

Fig. 9. *"Back parlor of the Otis House, for the wedding of Mary S. Otis and Fred W. Baker, June 19, 1889," by unidentified photographer, Rochester, New York. A handwritten note on the photograph mount states, "Back Parlor—married under the horseshoe—all white and green in back parlor." The open doorway offers a glimpse of the dining room, its table set for the reception afterward. Throughout the second half of the nineteenth century, weddings often took place at home. Photographs of such parlor ceremonies support the advice offered by Florence Hartley, the author of* The Ladies' Book of Etiquette *(1860): "When the wedding takes place at home, let the company assemble in the front drawing-room, and close the doors between that and the back room. In the back room, let the bride, bridegroom, bridesmaids, and groomsmen, the parents of the bride, and the clergyman, assemble....then open the doors and let the ceremony begin."*

were two side windows in this room hung with straight lace curtains. In one window hung the bird-cage with a Kentucky Cardinal in it...The other window held the goldfish bowl that never contained less than four little fish flashing around...In the center stood a great square black heating stove that furnished the heat for the two parlors, the front hall, and the bedroom off the back parlor...One corner of this back parlor held a whatnot which was used for a bookcase...On the top shelf there was a piece of amethyst colored quartz that we were never allowed to touch. In the corner near the dining room door was a sofa, horsehair, of course, that my mother had when she was first married. It was not large, and there was a throw over it of some kind of Roman striped material and a large yellow painted velvet pillow with yellow painted roses at each corner...After supper when there chanced to be company we all went into the back parlor where the stove was. Edgar and I would take down one of Dr. Kane's books [the family owned a six-volume set titled *Dr. Kane's Trip to the Arctic*], sit on this sofa, and pretend we were looking at the pictures, but in reality we were whispering awful things about the company.[46]

This passage not only suggests the special character of the front parlor; it is also rich in detail about the compromises that average families necessarily made in both furnishing and preserving parlors. Some furniture was so special that it had to be saved, especially if the family could not afford to replace it easily. Potential despoilers such as children were not allowed to use it.[47] Mrs. Neupert's mother, Mrs. Hughes, also had to employ furniture from the first, leaner years of her marriage—the haircloth-covered sofa—to be able to furnish both parlors completely. Not only was the sofa in the back parlor older, but its haircloth was exceedingly sturdy and could withstand use by Alice and her brother; it was there they sat during parlor evenings. Mrs. Hughes also preserved the matching carpet of both parlors by protecting the back parlor's with an additional rug. Because the back parlor had the heating stove, it seems to have doubled as the everyday sitting room for the family.

In some middle-class families, the parlor was reserved for special occasions such as Sundays or holidays, and the dining room doubled as the family sitting room. Alice Steele's memoir of her turn-of-the-century childhood in rural western Massachusetts noted that her family "lived mostly in the big dining room and between meals the

Fig. 10. *Richard Holbrook Tucker seated in the parlor of his house, Castle Tucker, in Wiscasset, Maine, 1894. Courtesy Castle Tucker.*

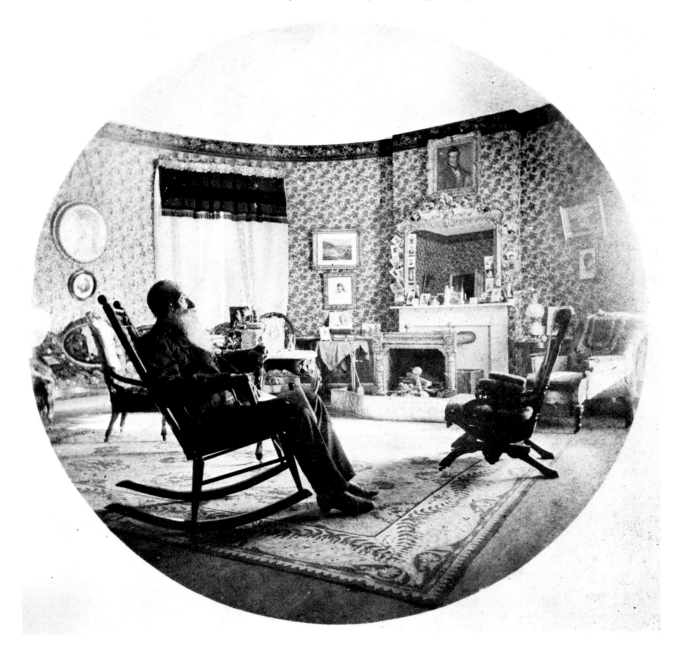

dining table was used for every purpose from my school work to dress making." Even though the family had another "sitting room," it was "used chiefly for writing letters and made a nice quiet place for the baby to sleep." The parlor was preserved unused, with shades "nearly always drawn except for Sunday afternoons when the minister or my sister's beau might call."[48] The Howard Yearick family of Konnarock, Washington County, Virginia, Pennsylvania-Germans removed to southwestern Virginia with a lumbering company at the turn of the century, also used the dining room as a family sitting room. Yearick was a boss carpenter, and the company housing for skilled workers and foremen provided both a dining room and a parlor. The Yearicks included a lounge and rocking chairs with their dining room furniture and used that room as the sitting room most evenings. The parlor, with its Brussels carpet, sofa, and lace curtains, was reserved for special occasions such as women's club meetings and the Christmas tree (fig. 11). Portières separated the parlor and the dining/sitting room; they were usually kept open.[49]

For some, the "library" was the family sitting room, as in the Hartford, Connecticut, house of Samuel Clemens, who lived there with his family between 1874 and 1891; the first floor also contained a formal parlor called the "drawing room." The Spencer family of Pittsburgh had a "library" across the hall from the parlor which was its family sitting room. It gained its name from the presence, in one corner, of "built-in bookcases with drawers below them in which games were kept."[50]

By the end of the nineteenth century, families who aspired to demonstrate some level of parlor gentility but who had very little room in their households—living in better tenement apartments or very small company houses—still might set aside some space for the purposes of what social worker Margaret Byington called the "front room"—despite the decrease it caused in precious living space or the necessity of family members sleeping in that room (fig. 12).[51] Byington's contemporary, Louise Bolard More, also described a number of parlors in respectable working-class households in her 1907 study *Wage-Earners' Budgets*: "The typical home of the wage-earners in this district is quite well furnished and fairly neat and clean. The 'parlor' is usually gaudy with plush furniture (sometimes covered with washable covers), carpet on the floor, cheap lace-curtains at the windows, crayon portraits of the family on the walls, and usually religious pictures of the saints, the Virgin Mary, or 'Sacred Heart,'

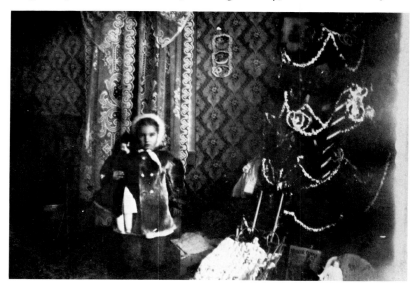

Fig. 11. Katherine Yearick at age five in her family's parlor, at Christmas, Konnarock, Virginia, post card by unidentified photographer, 1910. Author's collection.

Fig. 12. *"A 'Front Room',"* *photograph by Lewis Hine in Margaret Byington,* Homestead: The Households of a Mill Town *(1910; reprint, 1969). Courtesy Ayer Company Publishers.*

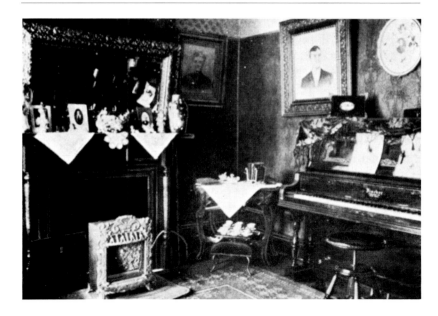

Fig. 13. *"Where Some of the Surplus Goes," photograph by Lewis Hine in Margaret Byington,* Homestead: The Households of a Mill Town *(1910; reprint, 1969). Courtesy Ayer Company Publishers.*

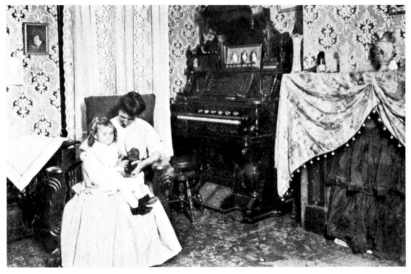

sometimes a couch, and the ubiquitous folding-bed" (fig. 13).[52]

In such crowded living conditions, elements of the recognized vocabulary of parlor furnishings often had to be adapted to signal that such a space existed. For example, convertible lounges, or flat beds disguised through the use of "Turkish couch covers" and piles of decorative pillows, signaled parlor during waking hours. A trade card for the Boston firm of Sidney Squires and Co., of the Squires Automatic Sofa Bed, advised, "See before buying a Parlor Bed," and the term survived well into the twentieth century in the advertising of the Kindel Bed Company of Grand Rapids, Michigan.

Other elements of parlor decor were also employed in these minimal parlors, particularly parlor-type portières, draped center tables, lounges upholstered with carpet or plush and decoratively upholstered "fancy chairs" or rockers (fig. 14). One 1894 photograph of a college boarding-house room in Norton, Massachusetts, suggests how such "parlors"—special spaces devoted particularly to social ceremony such as visiting—carved from single-room living spaces might have looked (fig. 15; see plate 6).

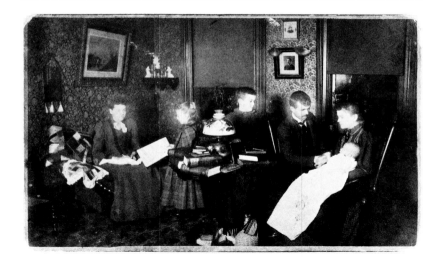

Fig. 14. Family in parlor, Rockland County, New York, by unidentified photographer, about 1895. This New York State family used a center table, a rocking chair, and an upholstered lounge to say "parlor." The halo effect was caused by the photographer's flash powder.

Variations from house to house, and the difficulties of labeling that sometimes accompany them, complicate efforts at making general statements about how middle-class parlors were used and furnished. They do not, however, call into question the parlor's function in middle-class households—presenting through its appearance the social identity of a family and serving as the site for domestic ceremony. The problem, for middle-class parlor makers, was how to accommodate comfortably the various functions of the parlor when there was only one room in which the family could congregate specifically for leisure. The domestic and formally social functions of such a room could seem quite incompatible in their requirements, a tension that could be resolved with a variety of compromises. The parlor, however it was used, was still the focal point of furnishing expenditures, and furnishing solutions depended upon the calculations of desire and necessity made by each family.

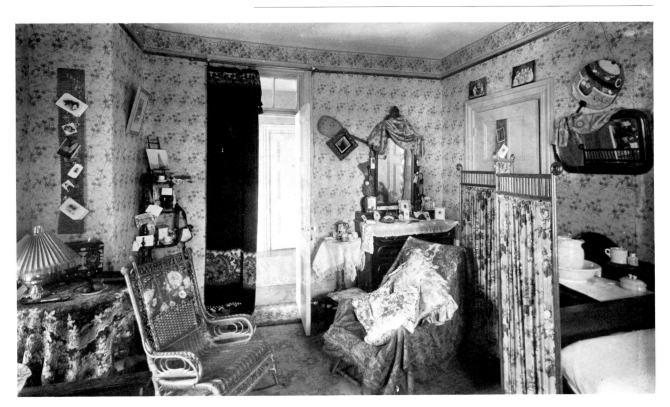

Fig. 15. Girls' room in boarding house,
Wheaton College, Norton, Massachusetts,
by unidentified photographer, 1894.
Courtesy Society for the Preservation of
New England Antiquities.

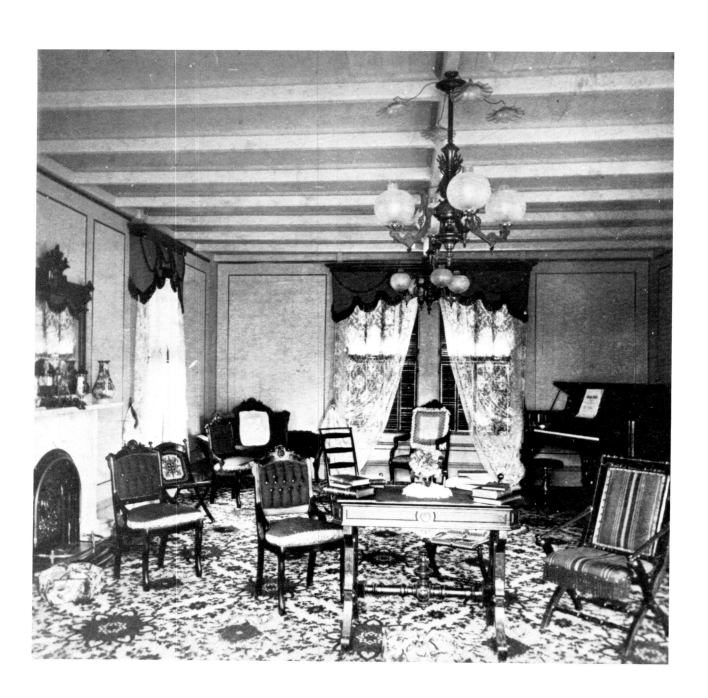

CHAPTER THREE
"ORTHODOX AS THE HYMN BOOK": THE RHETORIC OF PARLOR FURNISHING, 1850-1910

Fig. 1. Parlor of Dr. H. A. Tucker's summer cottage, Oak Bluffs, Martha's Vineyard, Massachusetts, stereograph photographed and published by C. H. Shute and Sons, Edgartown, Massachusetts, about 1875. Most of the "vocabulary" of middle-class parlor furnishing is visible in this image of Dr. Tucker's parlor—parlor suite, center table, folding chairs, wall-to-wall carpet, fancy window drapery, piano, carpet-covered footstools, and a fancy fireplace and mantel surmounted by an elaborately framed mirror. Courtesy Society for the Preservation of New England Antiquities.

No matter how a family resolved the tensions between social ideals and actual means and use of household space, middle-class parlors between 1850 and 1910 relied upon certain conventions of furnishing and arrangement in order to demonstrate and proclaim a family's understanding of what a parlor was and how it was ideally used (fig. 1). In creating such a room, a family not only created a rhetorical representation of itself but a statement about the nature of its relationship to cultural values as well.

Between 1850 and 1880, the recognized and ideal vocabulary of modern parlor furnishing encompassed an ornate matched set of parlor seating furniture, which might be augmented by such forms as upholstered "reception" chairs, parlor rockers, and decorative upholstered footstools. Wall-to-wall carpets and the fanciest window drapery in the house were also fundamental, as were decorative lighting devices, including fancy lamps and chandeliers; center tables that had marble tops or were elaborately covered; display shelves or cabinets; pianos; a mantelpiece (with a large mirror if possible), and wall decorations, including small wall-hung decorative shelves and objects in frames. Some women's handwork was displayed, while needlework in the form of decorative pillows, throws, and tidies contributed to the decorative effect of the upholstery. When the Fulton family of Rockport, Texas, purchased furniture for the parlor of its new house in 1876, the choices reflected typical tastes of the time—a "Fine Parlor Suite," according to the invoice, two parlor rocking chairs, two "Window Chairs" for the bay window, a marble-topped center table, several smaller tables, and a pedestal.[1]

After 1880, a number of additional elements—many embellishments upon earlier furnishings—became common parts of the parlor vocabulary. Often, these were textile furnishings, door curtains (called portières) and myriad additional forms of semi-permanent drapery—piano covers, mantel lambrequins, and tables having permanently affixed fabric coverings; forms of "scarf drapery"; and mountains of elaborately decorated sofa pillows. Parlor organs, which were less expensive than pianos, appeared as the newest bearer of parlor musical culture. Between 1880 and 1910, parlor suites were still common, but the number of pieces offered and their importance slowly declined. Some new forms of seating furniture, such as platform rocking chairs and a new range of unusual "fancy chairs" in wicker, faux (imitation) bamboo, and even metal tubing, could be purchased separately or as part of parlor suites. Lounges and backless couches, which occasionally appeared in parlors between 1830 and 1880 as parts of large expensive sets of furniture, became increasingly important ways for families of small means to participate in parlor making.

Communicating through parlor furnishing was a two-sided affair. In their selection and manipulation of furnishings, middle-class families demonstrated their fluency with the terms of this vocabulary. Their success could be measured by the degree to which the "messages" of parlor furnishings were legible to outsiders. Among the more conventional objects such as parlor suites, pianos, a center table, the best curtains in the house, and a decorative mantelpiece or mantel shelf, a family could include more personal objects—family photograph albums, or homemade objects such as needlework pictures. These familiar things communicated details of a family's particular character within that setting. (Such personal touches were missing from gala parlors in the first decades of the nineteenth century.) Finally, other accessories—natural specimens, paintings, ceramics or *bibelots* from foreign places—communicated further details of the cultured facade of the parlor's owners (fig. 2).

Within the range of furnishings available after 1850 that signaled the presence of a parlor, even consumers of ordinary means could create a room that emphasized the tradition of the gala apartment, the parlor as a theater of culture. French furnishings and upholstery, including the concept of planned unified decor, were popular expressions of the gala parlor. Or, through the styles of decoration and the upholstery they chose, they could opt to create a less ostentatious space, a comfortable parlor that expressed the middle-class ideal of virtuous civility. After 1880, some changes and additions to parlor furnishing also reflected the influence of what has been called the "aesthetic movement" in America; advocates of aesthetic furnishing urged abandonment of what they perceived as rigid formulas for matching furnishings, including the use of a single style and a single color in a room, and encouraged employment of

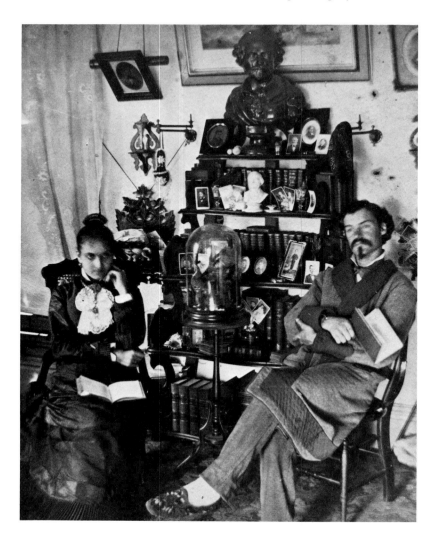

Fig. 2. "Our Home./ From Samp [?] and Abbie/ To Fannie Rich/ Minneapolis, Minn./Oct 8th 1878," stereograph photographed and published by M. Nowack, Minneapolis, Minnesota, 1878. The couple in this photograph took care to have themselves portrayed as cultured people with their art corner. The side stand or étagère displayed their modest library, natural specimens and other small treasures, and a large bust of Shakespeare perched precariously on the top shelf. The photographs displayed for visitors the couple's network of friends and kin. The needlework match holder shaped as a slipper, the front of the wall pocket, and Samp's fancy slippers probably were Abbie's own work. *Courtesy Smithsonian Institution; private collection.*

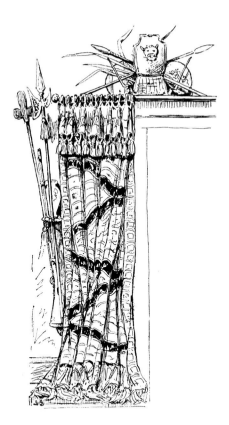

Fig. 3. "Portière for Hall," engraving in Constance Cary Harrison, Woman's Handiwork in Modern Homes *(1881).*

"art needlework" in portières and other drapery (fig. 3). However, while ordinary consumers were certainly interested in the aesthetic taste, the movement affected popular choices in parlor furnishing only in a few specific ways. Portières did become extremely popular, although in the form of factory-woven chenille or "tapestry" rather than the designs recommended by advocates of aesthetic furnishing (fig. 4). (The art needlework that middle-class women turned out in enormous quantity—wall pockets, mantel lambrequins, embroidered Japanese fans, and artistic piano drapes—was also not exactly what aesthetic reformers had in mind.) Aesthetic taste in furnishing seems not to have affected the belief among many consumers that parlor suites (the pieces of which matched by definition) were the core of parlor furnishing, nor does it seem to have altered the common use of such elements as the center table.

The fact that aesthetic taste encouraged eclecticism, however, well suited most aspiring parlor makers. Usually, most families had to make do with mixed lots of furniture anyway—out-of-date parlor suites too good to throw away, favorite rocking chairs, upholstered chairs, simple wooden chairs, and recycled or homemade window curtains, table covers, and cushions. What one modest advice book called the "esthetic craze" dovetailed nicely with the financial necessities of most middle-class people, encouraging them to consider miscellaneous combinations of furnishings not as the pathetic result of financial necessity but as the ingenious expression of up-to-date furnishing taste (figs. 5 and 6).[2] In 1888, one author of furnishing advice offered this counsel to amateur decorators:

> The most popular view of the parlor is as a shrine into which is placed all that is most precious…this is really the most sensible view to take. Unless one has a very large establishment it is unwise to endeavor to give a distinct style—to make out of it Queen Anne, Louis Quinze, Marie Antoinette, a reminiscence of Pompeii, or a reflection of Japan. To indulge in a date, epoch, or national idiosyncrasy in surroundings implies a purse deep enough to gratify any passing caprice. Moreover, anything of this sort must be perfectly done…The safe plan is to make of your parlor a cosmopolite, equally at home with all nations and all ages.[3]

Although domestic critics carped about the impracticality and nonsensical character of much parlor furniture, some understood that the parlor was the most artificial—that is, the most cultural—space in houses, and that its furnishings expressed in rhetorical fashion both aspects of sensibility and ideals of social relationships. Ada Cone, a contributor to *The Decorator and Furnisher* in 1891, understood the power of parlor furnishing conventions even as she disapproved of many of them. In "Aesthetic Mistakes in Furnishing—The Parlor Centre Table," she wrote, "It cannot be contended that because a few persons of taste have discarded it, it is therefore out of fashion, it is an institution, as orthodox as the hymn book. It is practically universal; in expensive as well as in humble houses [it is] still the objective point and the *pièce de résistance* of the room…The fact that this piece of furniture holds so tenaciously its place, though contrary to convenience and taste points to an ideal in furnishing the parlor other than that of convenience and taste."[4]

The fact that Cone regarded the parlor center table to be "orthodox as the hymn book" indicates the degree to which parlor making was a learned activity burdened with conventions. Between 1830 and 1880, commercial parlors taught aspiring consumers something about modern parlor furnishing and "parlor gentility." Beginning in the 1870s, furnishing advice books, many with a didactic "household art" focus, proliferated. They were directed at those consumers who already had furnished their homes but were ready for a change in style, especially if it carried connotations of particular sophistication on their part. However, just as these authors of sophisticated architectural and furnishing advice urged readers to abandon the parlor for the "living hall" or "living room," other titles such as those published by Henry T. Williams in the late 1870s and Orange Judd and Co. in the 1880s addressed a different audience still interested in learning the standard conventions. These advice books were written to teach brand-new consumers what they should wish for. Williams outlined the typical contents of a parlor for his readers:

> The regular suite of parlor furniture consisting of chairs, table and sofa is generally accompanied by piano with its stool and stand for music, *étagère*, ottomans, and various knick-knacks or *bric-a-brac* as these are now termed; also pictures, brackets, tasteful wall-pockets perhaps, and the mantel which is now almost a piece of furniture, while the windows are draped as has been suggested, those who can procure them will find a charming natural adornment for simple muslin or lace curtains, in Ferns, Ivy-sprays, and other woodland productions.[5]

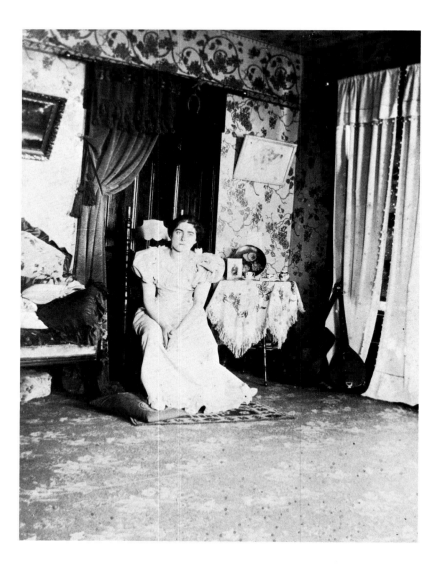

Fig. 4. Unidentified parlor, photographed by J. J. Henry, Chapinville, New York, about 1900. This modest room contains a factory-woven chenille portière, decorative sheer curtains, and the settee from a parlor suite. An older piece of furniture, the settee carried a message about proper parlor deportment in its formal lines, which were disguised with piles of soft cushions —a transitional moment in the gradual change to less controlling forms of seating.

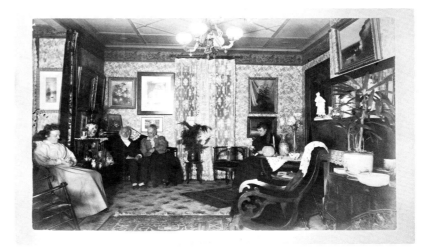

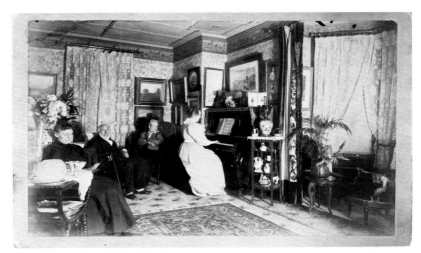

Figs. 5 and 6. Two views of McGonegal family parlor, 44 1/2 Vick Park A, Rochester, New York, by unidentified photographer, about 1895. The parlor of Mr. McGonegal, Rochester's superintendent of the poor, used a mixture of artistically arranged new and old upholstered furnishings, including a parlor suite of the 1870s. Courtesy Rochester Public Library, Local History Division.

At the turn of the century, mail-order catalogs also introduced new consumers to the vocabulary of parlor furnishing, both through the typologies of merchandise they presented in their pages and through concise statements of standard decorating advice in their descriptions of curtains, carpets, and furniture. *Sears, Roebuck and Co. Catalogue No. 104, 1897* was filled with furnishing advice for its rural and small-town audiences, not only in the choices offered but also in tidbits that could be gleaned in the hours spent pouring over the printed descriptions. Under "Rattan Chairs," the aspiring parlor maker learned that rattan was suitable "for parlor or library at all seasons of the year" and that "odd pieces" (chairs, shelves, and small tables that did not match the rest of the room's furnishing) were "sought after more largely than ever." A caption under "Princely Parlor Furniture" informed readers, "The prevailing style in furniture is to have the various odd pieces upholstered in harmonizing colors of different shades," although the caption offered to send matching sets.[6]

The conventional elements of parlor furnishing contributed in several ways to the rhetorical statements that the complete room setting was capable of making. For example, objects containing imagery or mottoes often provided easily legible clues to a family's values (fig. 7). Engravings of cultural heroes at critical moments in their lives or in typical instructive moments, such as the common prints of George Washington, Abraham Lincoln, and other statesmen as good family men, made such statements. The parlor of Alice Hughes Neupert's German Catholic family contained an engraving of Charles I going to his execution (an appropriately pious and popular Catholic historical subject) and, over the piano, a scowling portrait of Beethoven, whose presence indicated both the family's interest in music and their Germanic identity.[7]

Some objects that had no narrative content still were quite readily understood as symbols because of their use. Pianos suggested hard-won, usually feminine accomplishments and the family's appreciation of music. Elaborate family albums suggested the owners' ties to a network of other like-minded individuals and documented the bonds of sentiment.

Other parlor furnishings operated as symbols even less directly because they operated at the level of sensibility, shaping sensory experience in parlors. Deciphering the symbolic qualities in their forms and materials is necessarily a more speculative enterprise. Seating furniture provided cues about seated posture and deportment that suggested the appropriate character of parlor social life. Carpets hushed the sound of footfalls and helped to muffle other sounds (a quality that received special notice from authors describing commercial parlors).

The center table, which Ada Cone described as the *pièce de résistance* of typical parlors, is an example of the ways in which symbolic meanings are crafted from the conjunction of necessity and desire in furnishing practices.[8] In a world where artificial light was precious, provided for most families by kerosene lamps rather than municipal systems, parlor center tables were the location of the brightest pool of light in the room, and the brightest and most decorative lamps. They were a natural gathering place after dark for families whose means required thrift in the use of lamp fuel. However, the image of gathering around a table was also a common and powerful visual trope symbolizing the close ties and unity of purpose for voluntary associations, and tables in portraits also were associated with scholarly study. Tables draped with "Turkey work" carpets in portraits from the seventeenth and eighteenth centuries displayed wealth. In the Christian context, draped tables also were related to iconography of the Last Supper, representing here the ceremony as well as the unity of religious belief (fig. 8). Draped tables, located in the front of churches, were the location for the

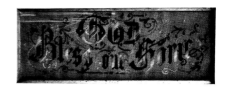

Fig. 7. Wall motto, wool thread and punched paper, United States, 1860-1880.

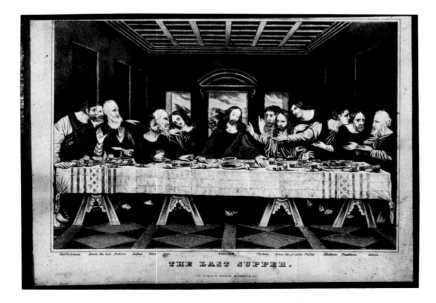

Fig. 8. "The Last Supper," colored lithograph published by Nathaniel Currier, New York, New York, 1845.

Fig. 9. *Cover of* The Ladies' Repository and Home Magazine *(January 1869).*

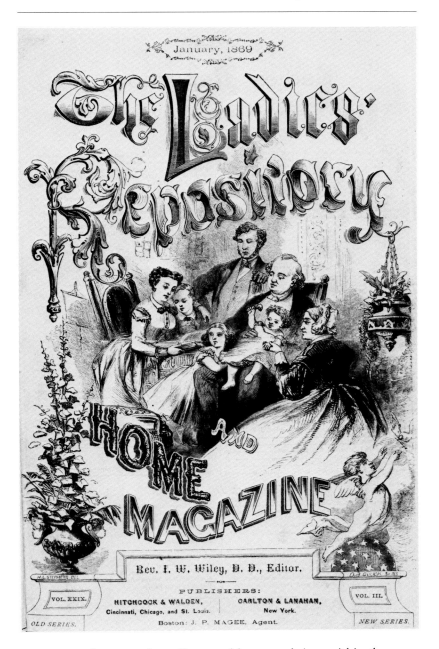

sacrament of communion. Center tables were shrines within the ritual space of the parlor, the sites of carefully edited selections of familial possessions—family Bibles, other important books (including family albums, which both organized family pictures and made them historical by encapsulating them in a book), calling card baskets, and a miscellany of other items such as stereoscopes. The "Christian family" gathered closely together around the closed circle of the center table symbolized the ideal of middle-class family life (fig. 9).

The center table's cover increased and elaborated the table's ceremonial character (fig. 10; plates 6 and 7). A table cover could qualify any table for center table use, even one that was roughly made or damaged. By being voluminous and elaborate in its design, it emphasized the importance of the table. If hand worked, the table cover both reflected a woman's accomplishments in the household and further emphasized the table as one focal point in the room (fig. 11). Textile furnishings created a sense of ceremony for the parlor's

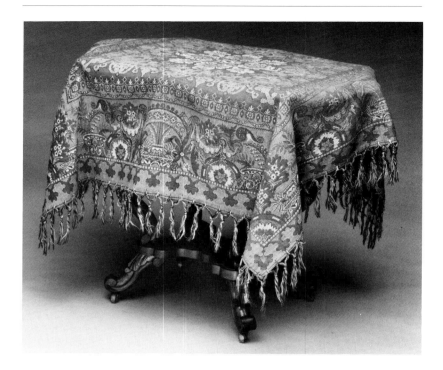

Fig. 10. *Center table cover, reversible figured cotton with metal threads, United States, about 1895. In the mid-1890s, manufacturers added metallic "tinsel" threads to cotton center table covers and marketed them as a fashionable novelty.*

important, if small-scale, domestic rituals. As the health and happiness of the domestic world required constant embellishment and attention to detail, so the presence of objects that represented hours of attention, especially ornamental needlework, signaled the watchful attention of family members, women in particular, to its maintenance. Draping could thus emphasize the separateness of the parlor from the world outside. Overtly religious artifacts in and around the center table cued the equation of religion and home, an aspect of the concept of comfort. These references included framed religious mottoes embroidered on perforated paper, or wax crosses under glass domes. In time, this relocation of religion in the home became a kind of secular equation in which the religion was of the family itself, a more subtle reference that, of all possible seats of meaning, the parlor center table with its decorative drapery and selection of valued objects expressed most profoundly.

In the last quarter of the nineteenth century, some advice writers on domestic interiors were so familiar with the common equation of the parlor and the shrine that they could treat the formulation ironically, as Ada Cone did in her discussion of the center table as a "mistake" of parlor furnishing. Shrine building continued in more than one location in the parlor, however. "Art corners," decorated mantels, draped shelves, and small tables were also shrines, dedicated to the secular values of civilization or culture, the other axis of parlor values made manifest in furnishings (see fig. 11). The displays of exotica, souvenirs, minerals, and books on the étagère of the Hughes family parlor in Buffalo created a shrine to civilization.

The pole of values expressing an interest in culture reflected the best qualities of civilized living in the domestic world, represented *in toto* and in microcosm by this most cultural of interior spaces—its refinement, its highly artificial quality, and, somewhat paradoxically, its connection with (and control through consumption of) the cultural goods of the world outside its walls. Here the parlor and its contents became a memory palace for the best aspects of the world outside. Etagères, hanging shelves, piano tops, and the art corners of the 1880s and 1890s were miniature museums. To this end, the textile furnishings of the parlor operated in two ways. They contributed to the room's cultured facade through historical revival styles and offered an analogy to popular understanding of civilization's action on human character. In the latter instance, upholstery operated by influencing the sensory character of the parlor, affecting vision and tactile sensation in particular. Textile furnishings softened the world of sensation. They obliterated the edges of hard furniture surfaces and mediated, through structural padding, the contact of the body with seats. Heavy door and window curtains muffled sound, literally softened light, and enhanced domestic quiet. Thus textiles could serve as a metaphor for the softening benefits of civility, which was evidence of the progress of civilization.

Once aspiring parlor makers owned the appropriate trappings for a modern parlor, they faced another challenge. In order to be considered genteel, a parlor person was required to be comfortable with the manipulation of the furnishings of the parlor, to demonstrate the ability to pick up the cues offered by their appearance and proper use. Pianos, paintings, furnishings—in theory, all these offered opportunities to communicate in ways that other parlor people could appreciate. This shared self-display among appreciative peers was the essence of gentility in the parlor, but mastering the requirements for self-presentation apparently seemed difficult enough that thousands of Americans turned to etiquette books for advice.

While eighteenth-century English guides to conduct suggested that gentility was not a closed stratum of society but a set of standards for living, the idea that gentility was a potentially inclusive standard found its fullest expression in American etiquette books.[9] Becoming genteel by dint of personal effort was a corollary to the American belief that individual economic progress was possible. The titles and opening pages of inexpensive etiquette books suggested to readers that do-it-yourself gentility was possible. Arthur Martine's *Hand-Book of Etiquette, and Guide to True Politeness* (which sold in 1866 for fifty cents) billed itself as "A Complete Manual for Those Who Desire to Understand the Rules of Good Breeding, The Customs of Good Society, and to Avoid Incorrect and Vulgar Habits," while the first

Fig. 11. This unidentified Upstate New York parlor displayed much art needlework, including the appliquéd felt table cover and the Battenburg lacework covering what may be a box of stereographs on the center table. The lace curtains at the window, too good to shorten, were folded down at the top and fashioned into a swag arrangement.

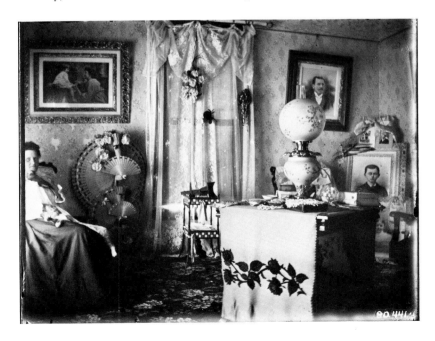

sentence of *Decorum* (1881) promised that "high birth and good breeding are the privileges of the few; but the habits and forms of the gentleman may be acquired by all."[10]

Several serious, unresolved tensions are evident in the explanations of etiquette and parlor behavior promulgated by manners books published well into the 1870s. What historian Karen Halttunen has labeled "sentimental culture"—middle-class culture in the first decades of what we call the Victorian era—valued sincere emotion and believed in the importance of mutual correspondence between feelings and behavior. But etiquette books argued that deep feelings were inappropriate to the parlor and required restraint in their expression. To succeed in the domestic theater of the parlor, parlor people had to be models of self-control, able to conduct their self-presentation with disciplined restraint of both feelings and body. A parlor person knew how to enter a room, how to sit gracefully, how to control the hands and feet, and how to modulate the voice. "Let your carriage be at once dignified and graceful," Florence Hartley wrote in *The Ladies' Book of Etiquette, and Manual of Politeness.* "To sit with the knees or feet crossed or doubled up, is awkward or unlady-like. Carry your arms, in walking, easily; never crossing them stiffly or swinging them beside you. When seated, if you are not sewing or knitting, keep your hands perfectly quiet...Never gesticulate when conversing; it looks theatrical, and is ill-bred; so are all contortions of the features."[11] Physical self-control was to be accompanied by control of the feelings. *Etiquette for Ladies*, a manners book that was plagiarized a number of times in the nineteenth century, warned that "excessive gaiety, extravagant joy, great depression, anger, love, jealousy, avarice, and generally all the passions, are too often dangerous shoals to propriety of deportment...It is to propriety, its justice and attractions, that we owe all the charm of sociality."[12] The restrained physical self was meant to be the harmonious expression of restrained parlor feelings.

The popular belief that anyone could learn perfect politeness created problems, however, because taken to its logical extreme it suggested that the socially polished legions could contain multitudes of bad but very mannerly people.[13] Authors of etiquette books tried to circumvent this inconsistency by developing a "sentimental typology of conduct," which insisted that true manners were sincere, true intentions were always legible, and insincere manners could be detected.[14] They also took care to identify a second, negative pole of parlor etiquette. Authors of manners books warned their readers to avoid manners that were slavish in their adherence to fashion, hence ridiculous and "affected." Affectation, "looking, speaking, moving, or acting in any way different when in the presence of others," Florence Hartley wrote in the *Ladies' Book of Etiquette*, "especially those whose opinion we regard and whose approbation we desire..., is both unsuccessful and sinful." Not only was it hypocritical, hence sinful, but affectation exposed its perpetrator to contempt because it was "the false assumption of what is not real."[15] Insincere manners were not heartfelt, nor were they consistent in their efforts at civility. "A well-bred gentleman or lady will sustain their characters as such at all times, and in all places—at home as well as abroad," one 1857 volume advised. "If you see a man behave in a rude and incivil manner to his father or mother, his brothers or sisters, his wife or children...you may at once set him down as a boor, whatever pretensions he may make to civility. Good manners should always begin at home."[16] In sum, middle-class manners were to be sincerely felt, moderate and controlled in their forms of expression, and the manifestation of a consistent method and point of view for interacting with the world.

The nineteenth-century thinking that identified two poles in etiquette—the "sincere" manner as opposed to the empty forms of affected and insincere etiquette—actually appeared in discussions of manners before in the eighteenth century, in both England and on the Continent. The dichotomy developed first as part of the European rhetoric of middle-class self-definition. Sociologist Norbert Elias has argued that *civilisation*—the process of improving standards of education, behavior, and economic growth by which human society progressed—emerged from the courtly ideal of the "civil man" or "man of honor," a term that members of the French courts used to describe and distinguish themselves from the rest of the rude, uncivil populace. The "courtly bourgeoisie," those members of the French middle classes involved with the administration of the regime during the second half of the eighteenth century, further developed the concept.[17] Members of these middle classes joined members of aristocratic classes in the social and intellectual life of the salons of Paris. To these bourgeois thinkers, the process of "true civilization" contained, in addition to increasing means and refinement in knowledge and behavior, one other component—"the ideal of virtue." Members of the courtly bourgeoisie claimed virtue was essential to a true understanding of the concept of civility. Virtue, they also argued, was a necessary attribute of character among members of their own class. Without virtue, all forms of civility were empty and false. To Elias, the concept of true civilization was the way in which the middle class could define itself in relation to an aristocratic society whose behavior and customs it did not necessarily respect but did not completely reject.

A similar process of middle-class self-definition was occurring in seventeenth- and eighteenth-century England—and also in its Anglo-American colonies. The middle-class model of civilized behavior separated the forms of manners—etiquette—from a general code of behavior that could be developed in children through example and the cultivation of childhood proclivities. In *Good Manners* (1711), Jonathan Swift characterized the distinction in this way: "I cannot so easily excuse the more refined critics of behaviour, who having professed no other study, are yet infinitely defective in the most natural parts of it...On the other hand, a man of right sense has all the essentials of good breeding, though he may be wanting in the forms of it."[18] England's bourgeoisie was larger and its society more fluid; however, it still created a set of distinctions between the "fine gentleman of intellectual and social accomplishment," whom contemporaries identified as having strongly continental, especially French, origins, and its own version of true, virtuous civility—the "Christian gentleman."[19]

In America, the distinction between fine and virtuous manners that appeared in etiquette books was employed to somewhat different ends than it was in England. In the political culture of the United States between 1790 and 1850, this set of distinctions was a counterpart to debates about republican virtue, and it was employed both to identify the desirable characteristics of republican citizens and to ferret out real or imagined threats. Controversy and debate centered upon the alleged connections between economic and political systems. Jeffersonians tried to establish a link between republican virtue and agrarian life and used the squalid conditions of the English industrial working class as evidence that industrialization was one more threat to the ability of Americans to govern themselves.[20] Followers of Alexander Hamilton, on the other hand, argued that *only* through manufacturing could the nation and its government become independent and wealthy enough to survive.

Sincere manners were appropriate to republican America and

compatible with a number of other American characteristics, including political virtue, self-sufficiency, and virtuous, self-disciplined consumption. Empty and affected social forms were associated with servility and moral ruin, just as an unhealthy dependence on and infatuation with fashion, particularly European luxury, inevitably led to financial ruin. Thus, a family's life always contained, in microcosm, the risk of the larger cycle of rise and decline of an entire civilization. But like the American republic, virtue could enable both the individual and the nation to be free from what seemed an inevitable cycle. The unresolved tensions in parlor etiquette, between the demands of etiquette's forms and the desire to appear natural and sincere, resonated with an entire structure of thought about the nature of, and threats to, American virtue. This thinking dominated discussions of art and architecture in the first decades of the republic but also focused periodically upon the concept of "fashion."[21] The relationship between virtue, fashion, and luxury in the realm of manners and household consumption provided the stuff of debate in women's periodicals and manners books for decades. Manners that were merely fashionable were not republican manners. Consumption that was predicated only upon fashion's dictates was equally suspect.

The discomfort that authors of middle-class etiquette books expressed about the relationship of manners and character was related to another rhetorical position in the popular literature of household consumption and furnishing, domestic economy, and sentimental fiction. As manners demanded sincerity in self-expression, "sentimental fashion"—the discussion of middle-class sincerity as expressed in women's clothing—argued that "dress was an index of character" and identified "sincere" and "insincere" modes of dress.[22] The search for sincerity extended beyond dress because the possibilities of middle-class purchasing power increasingly included fashionable household furnishings. According to Lydia Sigourney, the author of *Letters to Mothers* (1838), "Simplicity of taste, extending both to dress, and manner of living, is peculiarly fitting in the daughters of the republic."[23] It was not simply fitting but absolutely essential, because "home and its virtues" were considered "the great conservative influence to which especially our country is to look for its security against anarchical disorder." Home provided the "best support" for the values upon which a republic was particularly dependent.[24] Yet the parlor was a source of temptation located inside the household because, in its guise as a gala apartment, it was particularly vulnerable to fashion's unholy sway (fig. 12).

A debate about the appropriateness of middle-class and aristocratic forms of parlor making in America—their etiquette, their furnishing, and their corresponding degrees of comfort—grew out of both the "mixed ancestry" of the parlor that Edith Wharton and Ogden Codman acknowledged in their 1897 volume *The Decoration of Houses* and the rhetorical demands for "sincerity" in furnishing. The descendants of the eighteenth-century drawing rooms of the beau monde were the spaces whose decoration middle-class domestic critics would later label "aristocratic." Unlike sitting rooms, these parlors were not homey, nor were they meant to be used in the family's moments of private leisure. Rather, their formal, matched furnishings—special accessories in sets such as mantel garniture and candelabra, large sets of furniture, elaborate upholstery, and examples of the fine arts—were symbolic of a more formal, even ceremonious, function and character. They were the theatrical settings for the fine gentleman and his feminine counterpart, the lady of fashion.

The genteel parlor type was identified with aristocratic or courtly taste in parlor furnishing. The view of "New York Merchant's Parlor" in an 1854 issue of *Gleason's Pictorial Drawing-Room Companion*

Fig. 12. *"Fashionable and Unfashionable,"* *the engraved frontispiece in Mrs. C. M. Kirkland,* A Book for the Home Circle *(1856),* *contrasted domestic virtue with the frivolity of parlor fashion.*

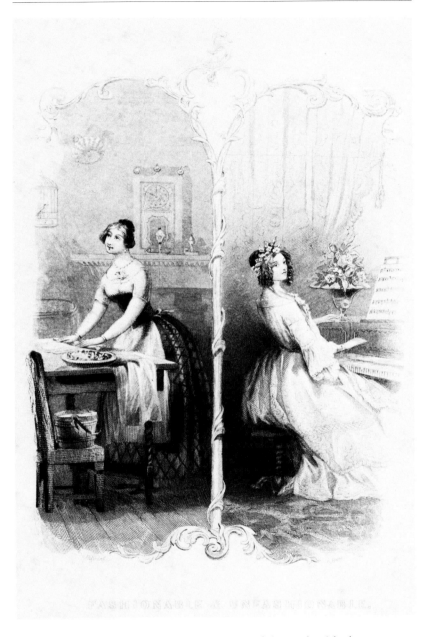

represents a typical "aristocratic" version of the parlor ideal at midcentury; its caption suggested that the room, owned by "one of the most eminent of our merchants,...looks like the fitting abode of a man of refinement —a drawing room where a lady of elegant manners and educated taste might appropriately receive her guests."[25] (It is no accident that, from its carpet to the chandelier, the room was furnished in the most flamboyant expression of the "French taste," including both rococo revival and "French Renaissance" furnishings.)[26]

In American cities, cosmopolites who modeled themselves on the eighteenth-century English and French beau monde participated in a genuine social "season," marked by a full round of balls or "routs," receptions, and card parties. In their parlors, as one late 1820s American reprint of an English etiquette book stated, "the graces of social intercourse are chiefly displayed;...learning relaxes from his gravity of feature; pedantry throws aside his gown and trencher; and wisdom, with the affability of benevolence, mingles in the amusements and shares the feelings of the young, the gay, and the lovely." The furnishing of such rooms was supposed to reflect the tone of the social life conducted there—"light and elegant."[27]

In the gala parlor, manners, humanistic education, and habits of consumption were united, because the concept of civilized living contained, by implication, the ideal of enlightened consumption. Material possessions were not only props for the social life of gentility but became outward expressions of inner gentility. This conception first appeared in eighteenth-century France, where, as Rosalind Williams has noted,

> To many enlightened thinkers of the eighteenth century, it seemed self-evident that enlightened consumption—patronage of the arts, the vivacious conversation of the salons, collection of paintings and books—was a necessary means to the advancement of civilization. With a little mental effort the habitues of the salons could equate their concrete social pleasures with the highest and most abstract social goals. The nature of "the civilizing process" remained mixed and ambiguous, a blend of idealism and materialism. In the eighteenth century the idea of civilization referred both to a general social and political ideal

Fig. 13. "*Front Parlor in Abraham Lincoln's House, Springfield, Ill.— Sketched by Our Special Artist,*" *engraving in* Frank Leslie's Illustrated Newspaper *(1860), reproduced in Peter Thornton,* Authentic Decor *(1984). In the article that accompanied this engraving, a reporter for* Leslie's *observed, "The house in which a man of mark dwells is, like his handwriting, interesting, as to a certain degree indicating his character. The sitting-room and parlor of Abraham Lincoln, in his house at Springfield, are...simply and plainly fitted up, but are not without indications of taste and refinement.*"

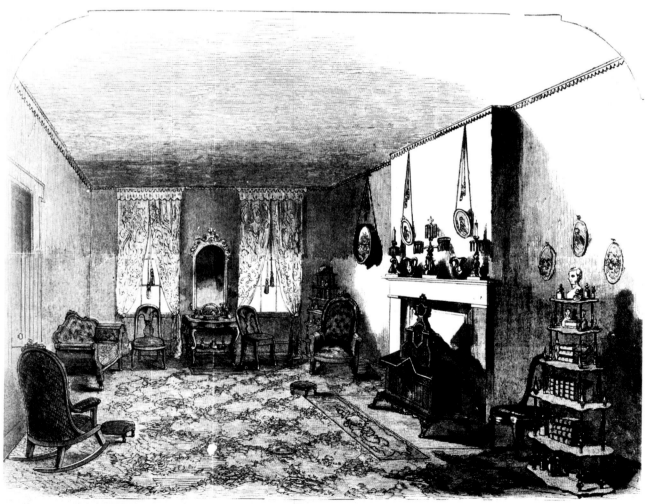

FRONT PARLOR IN ABRAHAM LINCOLN'S HOUSE, SPRINGFIELD, ILL.—SKETCHED BY OUR SPECIAL ARTIST.

and, more narrowly, to a comfortable way of life reserved for the upper classes.[28]

The same patterns of thought that associated consumption with quality in the eighteenth century could be applied to other groups entering the arena of consumer culture in the nineteenth century. If possessions could be outward expressions of the civility of the courtly world, they could also, by implication, become the outward mark of middle-class virtue—if middle-class people did not succumb to the temptations of fashion. Fearing the dangers that social ambition contained for middle-class people, advice writers promoted a vision of parlor life in opposition to the parlor of gentility, one that stressed moderation and family closeness. The engraving of Abraham Lincoln's parlor published by *Frank Leslie's Illustrated Newspaper* in 1860 is an emblem of the middle-class model of parlor furnishing, modest in ambition and appropriate for thrifty consumers with middling incomes (figs. 13 and 14).

Since the ideal of virtue was an aspect of middle-class identity, any vision of appropriate middle-class consumption had also to stress virtue. The origin of middle-class ideals of etiquette may lie in European society of the eighteenth century, but the vision of middle-class consumption seems, naturally enough, to have found its fullest expression in the middle-class century, the nineteenth century, and in the world's most middle-class nation, the United States. It appeared among members of the middle classes who did not have a permanent aristocracy of birth against which to react but who still fretted over the possible attractions of aristocratic fashion and its potentially debilitating effects on republican virtue. Middle-class ideals of appropriate etiquette and consumption forced a redefinition of the character of the parlor in the mid-nineteenth century, as concepts of political virtue had helped the European middle class define itself a century earlier. For much of the American middle class, parlor life

Fig. 14. Unidentified parlor in Boston, Massachusetts, stereograph by Holton and Robinson, Boston, Massachusetts, 1868-1870. This view suggests that the "plainly fitted up" Lincoln parlor may have been representative of middle class comfort in its time. Courtesy Society for the Preservation of New England Antiquities.

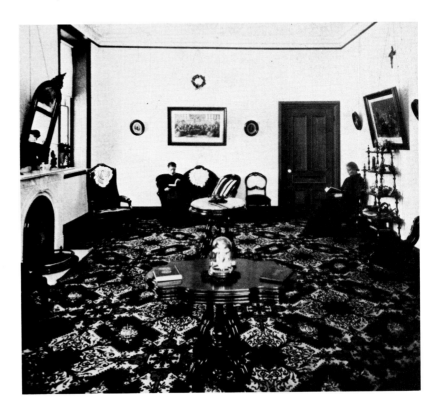

emphasized modest consumption and self-control. It took place, too, in a narrower social world—among members of a family and its intimate friends, not among the select company of social peers.

The middle-class vision of the parlor as the location for a family-centered social life probably arose from the conjunction of a number of circumstances of daily living in Anglo-America. Historian John Cornforth has suggested that, in the second half of the eighteenth century, England experienced the rise of a more home-centered culture among the well-to-do, middle-class and gentry alike. In these years, a new realm of domestic ritual developed among the gentry—calling, family dining, and intimate musical evenings rather than large-scale entertainments. An articulated preference for "homey" interiors existed in some English families of means at the end of the eighteenth century. In a letter written in 1799, Lady Louisa Stuart discussed Archerfield, a country house in which she then was a guest, by comparing it unfavorably with Dalkeith, another English country house. "It wants nothing but more furniture for the middle of rooms. I mean all is set out in order, no comfortable tables to write or read at; it looks a fine London house prepared for company; quite a contrast to the delightful gallery at Dalkeith, where you can settle yourself in any corner."[29]

Cornforth has connected the informal style of domestic comfort that came to characterize interiors in country houses during the first half of the nineteenth century to the taste for country life among the well-to-do, where family activities at home formed the center of social life, as opposed to the public socializing that took place in London during the social season. For those who could afford it, city houses provided the family's beau monde facade, while country living was where one really was at home. However, it would be erroneous to suggest that the homey parlor was a phenomenon simply of country living among the well-to-do. Such "homey" parlors were already in existence among middle-class families with adequate but more limited incomes on the Continent as well as in England.[30] Not having the resources for gala rooms, nor the cosmopolitan social life that required them, ordinary families had always experienced even their most public rooms as multi-functional, family spaces. Such rooms were formal on one occasion, less formal and more familial day by day. The homey interiors of English country houses may simply have provided additional confirmation of the desirability of "hominess"; bourgeois necessity may have intersected with new genteel preferences.

However, in the American context, middle-class hominess took on a unique and highly charged character because of the association of middle-class virtue with the future of the republic. The rhetorical banner under which the debate about domestic virtue took place was the concept of "comfort." At midcentury, the champions of comfort were domestic advisers and critics, mostly women whose outlets were nationally circulated periodicals and books of household advice and sentimental fiction (fig. 15). Their discussions of comfort not only claimed its appropriateness for middle-class people but also contended that only people unblinded by the demands of fashion could understand the concept. Mrs. C. M. Kirkland, author of *A Book for the Home Circle* (1853), staked out a typical position on the topic:

> Comfort is one of those significant and precious words that are apt to be much abused. It is so comprehensive that people try to make it everything, just as "religion" has been stretched to cover the burning of heretics, and "justice" the gratification of vindictive feelings or the vices of envy. It is so good a word, in its

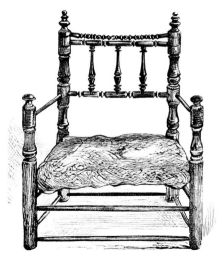

Solid Comfort.
No. 25.

Fig. 15. "Solid Comfort. No. 25," illustration in Clarence Cook, The House Beautiful *(1878).*

true character, that none but honest and true people can use it with propriety. It is, by tacit consent, banished from the vocabulary of Fashion; and if Ambition should make a dictionary, Comfort would find no place in it. The French, who are lovers of *pleasure*, have been obliged to transplant our word *comfort* bodily into their language, as they had before naturalized a correlative word—*home*, after they had adopted the idea. Strange that we, proud as we are of our right to it, should ever misuse it.[31]

By contrasting "comfort" and "fashion," Mrs. Kirkland suggested that comfort was both permanent and rational, while fashion was transient and capricious. By opposing comfort to "Ambition," she suggested that comfort was the stable, modest, and true result of self-knowledge. The very concept of comfort also was Anglo-American. Comfort was not the unrestrained "pleasure" of the French, who were the epitome of fashion, who were unhomelike, and who were, therefore, uncomfortable.

In ordinary middle-class households, American advisers charged, parlors conceived along the lines of the merchant's parlor illustrated by *Gleason's* were inappropriate for middle-class living. Such parlors were too formal for daily use, wasted family resources better spent on books and other tools for family education, exhausted middle-class housekeepers with their maintenance requirements, and restricted normal family living to one or two downstairs rooms in houses. In their most extreme criticism, they argued that the parlor of fashion damaged the formation of youthful character.[32]

The negative effects of parlor making on domestic comfort were often explored in moral tales of furnishing in popular books and magazines. In these stories, which were by turns wryly humorous or earnest and overwrought, domestic critics often attacked specifically the vocabulary of fashionable parlor furnishing as the public understood it and offered the middle-class "comfortable" parlor as an appropriate alternative. Harriet Beecher Stowe, the most famous of the sentimental domestic writers, drove home the message of middle-class comfort many times in the course of her long career. One of the most striking forums was a series of columns, *House and Home Papers*, published under the pseudonym and in the narrative voice of a man, "Christopher Crowfield." Stowe critiqued certain parlor furnishings as symbols of fashion and suggested that even innocent ambition led to wasted money, energy, and family happiness.

In the humorous opening story, "The Ravages of a Carpet," the Crowfield family was introduced to the reader in its homey but well-worn parlor. The family spent comfortable evenings there reading, sewing, or with friends who casually dropped in; the children played games with each other and with their pets. These evenings were disrupted, however, by the purchase of a brand-new Brussels carpet in a vivid floral print. The new prize made the rest of the furnishings appear even more shabby, and a general redecoration, done with the aid of a fashionable upholsterer, ensued. The effects of this change were disastrous at first:

> In a year we had a parlor with two lounges in decorous recesses, a fashionable sofa, and six chairs and a looking-glass, and a grate always shut up, and a hole in the floor which kept the parlor warm, and great heavy curtains that kept out all the light that was not already excluded by the green shades.
> It was as proper and orderly a parlor as those of our most fashionable neighbors; and when our friends called, we took them stumbling into its darkened solitude, and opened a faint crack in one of the window shades, and came down in our best clothes,

and talked with them there. Our old friends rebelled at this, and asked what they had done to be treated so, and complained so bitterly that gradually we let them into the secret that it was the great south-room which I had taken for my study, where we all sat, where the old carpet was down, where the sun shown in the great window, where my wife's plants flourished and the canary-bird sang, and my wife had her sofa in the corner, and the old brass andirons glistened and the wood-fire crackled,—in short, a room to which all the household had emigrated.[33]

The Crowfield family's new parlor was shut up, an unused, unwanted room that served as a daily reminder to the family of the follies of fashion and social convention. As Stowe described it, middle-class comfort had no facade; middle-class people, because they were naturally sincere, did not need to present a different public face to society. Her contention that the contents of the homey middle-class parlor reflected the family in its true character articulated an alternate conception of room decor that contrasted the parlor as a public reflection of, or aspiration toward, gentility with the room as a reflection of middle-class character. Store's distinction is analogous to the difference between empty rhetoric and sincere statement.

Other moral tales of furnishing were less good-natured, however, often conveying the message that consumption in the pursuit of fashion could and did lead to financial ruin, the tragic separation of families, and permanent damage to young, impressionable family members. In "Furnishing; or, Two Ways of Commencing Life," which appeared in *Godey's Lady's Book* in 1850, Alice B. Neal contrasted the parlor furnishing decisions of two young women to compare their moral characters. Neal's abbreviated descriptions of the two models of parlor furnishing suggested that her middle-class readers already knew something about the debate between the tendencies to create aristocratic and domestic parlors and that they knew both models well enough to be able to picture for themselves the settings, completing in imagination what was only sketched in the text.

"Furnishing" contrasted the consumption habits of two cousins as they prepared to begin married life. The profligate and fashion-conscious city cousin, Adelaide, had an unlimited budget with which to purchase furnishings for her parlor. Without looking elsewhere, she selected its contents from the warerooms of George B. Henkels of Philadelphia. The country cousin, Anne, who was soon to marry a poor young doctor, had only six hundred dollars (still a tidy sum) to purchase the entire contents of her house. She shopped carefully, comparing the prices at Henkels' (the site of her first expedition, undertaken with Adelaide) to the more reasonable prices for furnishings offered at smaller, less fashionable establishments.

Adelaide, whose taste followed the aristocratic ideal, chose a rosewood parlor suite with black and crimson silk damask covers, tables with Siena marble tops, an étagère, and a velvet carpet. Anne, whose tastes represented solid middle-class comforts, opted for a three-ply tapestry carpet, a single sofa instead of a suite, an "octagon center table" (emblem of her soon-to-expand family circle), and "mahogany chairs with cane seats" which were expected to wear well. Needless to say, Adelaide and her new husband George began their marriage on a standard of living which they could not maintain; George was eventually forced to sell the house and its contents and leave for California to begin life anew. Anne took in the bereft Adelaide, who learned to appreciate the true meaning of domestic life seated at her cousin's side, on one of the mahogany chairs at the octagonal parlor table, before George sent for her to join him.[34]

On occasion, Harriet Beecher Stowe could be equally hyperbolic in her condemnation of the parlor of fashion. In another of the *House and Home Papers*, titled "Home-Keeping vs. House-keeping," Christopher Crowfield described how the family of an old friend was destroyed by the burden of caring for possessions, especially a fashionable parlor containing furniture covered in "garnet-colored satin" and "heavy, thick, lined damask curtains, which look quite down to the floor." Because they had been a gift, these furnishings did not strain the couple's finances; still, their marriage was ruined and their children's dispositions embittered because "social freedom" had been "crushed under a weight of upholstery."[35]

The prescription for avoiding the moral and social disasters of fashionable furnishing was the necessary symmetry of economic resources and desire. In her *Domestic Receipt Book*, Catharine Beecher advised her audience of "young and inexperienced housekeepers" that good taste, "that nice perception of fitness and propriety which leads a person to say and do whatever is *suitable* and *appropriate* in all possible circumstances...leads a woman to wish to have her house, furniture, and style of living, in all its parts, exactly conformed to *her means*, and *her situation*."[36]

Symmetry also required consistent, orderly application of means to situation along rational principles. A woman with "good sense and good taste," Beecher noted, "will not, while all that is *in sight* to visitors, or to out-door observers, is in complete order, and in expensive style, have her underclothing, her bedroom, her kitchen, and her nursery ill-furnished, and all in disorder. She will not attempt to show that she is genteel, and belongs to the aristocracy, by a display of profusion, by talking as if she was indifferent to the cost of things, of by seeming ashamed to economise." Like the inconsistent man cited by etiquette writers, who treated his family badly while displaying fine manners to outsiders, attending only to a family's public face was the mark of a "vulgar, unrefined person."[37]

The authors of midcentury architectural advice books oriented to middle-class families made a point of concurring with the conceptual symmetry of means and situation. In *Village and Farm Cottages* (1856), Henry William Cleaveland and William and Samuel D. Backus urged the housewife to avoid the "folly of imitation." They wrote, "Good sense, good taste and good morals alike repudiate the paltry vanity which furnished a house not for its constant occupants to use and enjoy, but for occasional visitors to look at and admire."[38]

Keeping up with fashion reduced homeowners to being "only exhibitors" in their homes. Worse yet, the financial strain destroyed the carefully prescribed boundaries between the domestic realm and the heartless world of commerce. Almira Seymour noted, "Volumes might be written on the moral effects upon character of the home of assured comforts held in unquestionable possession, however simple in its details, compared with palatial show-rooms held by a more-or-less uncertain tenure, in the midst of which the husband knows no rest from pecuniary anxieties, and is constantly tempted into the business-gaming risks of the present; where the wife is overburdened with cares in which the heart has no place."[39] Emma Wellmont warned her audience that consumption that, by offering employment to artisans, "is commendable in a millionaire," was imprudent for "those who have only a comfortable competence; and we regret to add, the definition of this distinction often introduces imitators into a labyrinth of trouble, from which it is hard to become extricated."[40]

Finally, attaining true comfort required more than avoiding the allurements of "the absurd demands of ever-changing fashion."[41] Those who would seek true comfort also must avoid the misapprehension that comfort was simply a physical state, the "consolation" of the "mortal frame." Mrs. Kirkland and other conservative middle-class domestic critics questioned the evident popular preoccupation with bodily comfort, demonstrated at least in part by the efforts of thousands of aspiring inventors of furniture, heating and lighting devices, and other ingenious domestic improvements to enhance it. Critics alleged that increasing affluence, invention, and acquisition threatened the necessary and fundamental opposition of comfort and fashion and tried to guide women toward a "middle way," toward appropriate levels of domestic consumption and domestic comfort.[42] This middle way had to be carefully monitored. Kirkland suggested that "making present gratification [of sensory desires]" one's most important concern had a "hardening effect" on character.

To these advisers, comfort was a moral condition with requirements like those of sincere etiquette.[43] Almira Seymour made the connection explicit when she argued that making a home truly comfortable "demands that sublimest and most saving of all heroism,—*perfect sincerity*."[44] Unfortunately, knowing how much physical comfort was too much was very much like walking the fine line between natural and affected manners. As Kirkland warned her readers, "We are all more or less disposed to self-indulgence, and as some amount of it is proper enough, it is not always easy to determine where right ends and the wrong begins." Middle-class people in the world of increased creature comforts were not expected to abjure all its facets, but to select carefully and not neglect the inner person.[45]

If parlors were the rooms in a home most apt to mirror fashion, upholstery in that room was particularly prone to manifest this capriciousness. Among domestic critics, upholstery became a critical benchmark in the effort to define the material limits of middle-class comfort. The fashionable upholsterer interpreted new, usually foreign fashions in room decor and supplied these expensive conceits to frivolous consumers. He was to dressing rooms as the fancy dressmaker was to dressing women; he pandered to their most fickle impulses.[46] Moreover, although upholstery was the most important element in setting the tone of a room, its expense and comparative impermanence also disturbed advocates of thrift. In their attribution of moral content to furnishing, Cleaveland and the Backuses charged upholstery with "dishonesty," especially in the innovation of spring seating:

> Even the hardest and homeliest bench that was ever made of oak plank, is a more comfortable and more respectable article of furniture than many of the spring-seat and hair-cloth sofas and rocking-chairs, which we have met with,—soft plump and elastic to all appearance, but which when we, in good faith, accept their invitations, let us down with a sudden jerk, and make us painfully acquainted with their internal mechanism.[47]

Not only was parlor upholstery dishonest, but its transitory character broke the chain of domestic associations that made household furniture truly comfortable. In "The Quaker Settlement," chapter 13 of *Uncle Tom's Cabin*, Stowe compressed both of these criticisms into a brief passage describing a pair of rocking chairs: "a small flag-bottomed rocking chair, with a patchwork cushion in it, neatly contrived out of small patches of different colored woollen goods, and a larger sized one, motherly and old, whose wide arms breathed hospitable invitation, seconded by the solicitation of its feather cushions,—a real comfortable, persuasive old chair, and worth, in the way of honest, homely enjoyment, a dozen of your plush or brocatelle drawing-room gentry."[48] Some authors argued that the impact of a transient existence in constantly changing fashionable "theaters" such as hotels damaged "that strongest bond of society, the power of association." By extension, the fashionable furnishings of hotel interiors and elite parlors could have a negative impact on individual morals and, ultimately, upon the national character.[49]

Even though parlor making was both an urban and rural phenomenon (because it was a middle-class activity), the authors of moral tales of furnishing suggested repeatedly that rural people were the bastion of true comfort, just as they were the source of republican political virtue (fig. 16). Some authors simply compared city and rural people, as Alice Neal did in "Furnishing." Other "comfort theorists" employed the plot device of rural people lured by city fashion as a way to demonstrate the folly of fashion and the solidity of rural comfort.

An example of this formulation of "city fashion, rural comfort" may be found in *The Widow Bedott Papers*, a series of comic "letters," dialogues, and stories in the popular literary genre known as "Yankee papers," published serially in the mid-1840s. The Widow Bedott, a simple but ambitious woman who had always lived on farms, snared a second husband in the form of a Baptist preacher, the Reverend Sniffles.[50] The Reverend resided in a distinctly unfashionable parsonage. After their triumphant honeymoon tour through various rural outposts in Upstate New York, the new Mrs. Sniffles began a campaign to update the house, declaring that "'tain't fit for ginteel folks to live in." When the Reverend protested that he had always

Fig. 16. "*A New England Fireside,*" *engraving in* Ballou's Pictorial Drawing-Room Companion *(10 March 1855). The anonymous author of the article accompanying this illustration described this scene as the "interior of a good old-fashioned New England homestead, many of which yet exist, remote from cities and large towns, in all their primitive purity and attractiveness....We do not look with jaundiced eyes upon a brilliant ball-room, crowded with graceful forms...—but it is a relief sometimes to turn away from the contemplation of the highest social refinement and splendor, and see how comfortable and happy people may be with a few wants and no luxuries. From such firesides great and noble men and women have gone forth into the world.*"

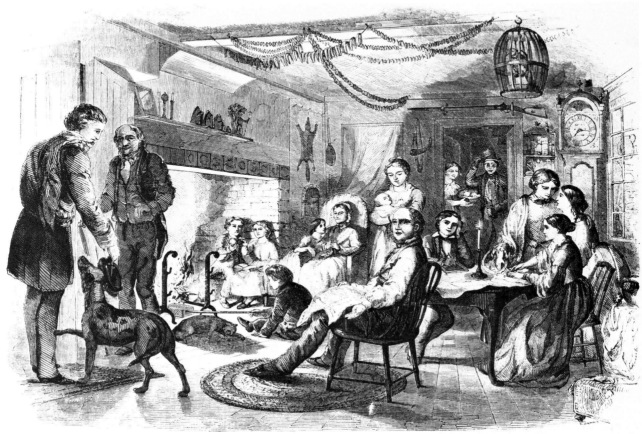

A NEW ENGLAND FIRESIDE.

found the house "very comfortable," Mrs. Sniffles displayed her understanding of the material signs of respectable parlor life, information gained through visiting parlors made by neighbors who had New York City contacts.

> Comfortable! who cares for comfort where gintility's consarned! *I* don't. I say if you're detarmined to stay in it, you'd ought to make some alterations in't. You'd ought to higher the ruff and put on some wings, and build a piazzer in front with four great pillars to't, and knock out that are petition betwixt the square room and kitchen, and put foldin' doors instid on't, and then build on a kitchen behind, and have it all painted white, with green winder blinds. *That* would look something *like*, and then I shouldent feel ashamed to have ginteel company come to see me, as I dew now…I say we'd ought to have new furnitur—sofys and fashionable cheers, and curtains, and mantletry ornaments, and so forth. That old settee looks like a sight. And them cheers, tew, they must a come over in the ark. And then ther ain't a picter in the house, only jest that everlastin' old likeness o' Bonyparte. I'll bet forty great apples it's five hundred years old. I was raly ashamed on't when I see Miss Curnel Billins look at it so scornful when they called here. I s'pose she was a counterastin' it with their beautiful new picters they're jest ben a gittin up from New York, all in gilt frames.[51]

The Widow's misguided preference for gentility over comfort provided a humorous lesson to middle-class readers. Moreover, to her mind, gentility was associated with novelty and fashion, not with the antique, the portrait "five hundred years old."

Through such fiction and essays, domestic critics argued that the courtly parlor, a public facade contained within a family's dwelling, was inappropriate for middle-class people, while the homey parlor of comfort, the parlor without a facade, reflected the best qualities of family life. They encouraged simplicity and sincerity in both parlor furnishing and parlor social life and judicious moderation in the pursuit of material goods rather than the heedless pursuit of fashion. They also argued that parlor display did not create true parlor people, an argument that the presence of parlors in commercial spaces everywhere contradicted by inviting participation. Critics' arguments disregarded a set of cultural priorities that gave birth to these models, among them the perceived need to set aside a space for social ritual. For consumers with the means and space, the way to give both social ritual and family life their due was to have both kinds of rooms, a "best parlor" or "drawing room" where they could express their hard-earned, hard-learned parlor selves, and a sitting room for their more private, familial selves.

CHAPTER FOUR
BODILY COMFORT AND SPRING-SEAT UPHOLSTERY

In the decades when domestic advisers were claiming comfort as a middle-class state of mind, a condition of internal and external harmony created through the symmetry of modest economic means and modest desires, the public at large was experimenting happily with a number of inventions designed to increase bodily comfort, inventions that these same critics considered of dubious value on moral and symbolic grounds. For example, architectural and domestic advice books voiced a common litany against parlor stoves, which made rooms considerably warmer and less drafty than did open fireplaces. Domestic critics disliked parlor stoves at least partly because of the symbolic meanings attached to the open hearth. Lewis F. Allen, author of *Rural Architecture* (1852), described an airtight stove in a farmhouse as "looking black and solemn as a Turkish eunuch upon us, and giving out about the same degree of genial warmth as the said eunuch would have expressed had he been there." Allen added, "A farmer's house should *look* hospitable as well as *be* hospitable, both outside and in, and the broadest, most cheerful look of hospitality within doors, in cold weather, is an *open* fire in the chimney fireplace."[1] The fireplace was "intimately connected with our ideas of domestic comfort," a symbol of family togetherness (literally so, when the hearth was packed with individuals struggling to keep warm).[2] Its replacement by the parlor stove seemed to signal a devaluation of family life.

These same critics found current fashions in furniture, particularly in the parlor, too "prinked up," to use Allen's words, too "gingerly" and "fatal to domestic enjoyment." Some singled out modern upholstery for special abuse. Concurring with the authors of *Village and Farm Cottages*, who considered "the hardest and homeliest bench" as "more comfortable and more respectable" than modern haircloth-upholstered furniture, Lewis Allen found "positive comfort" in a seat "by the wide old fireplace, in the common living room, comfortably ensconced in a good old easy, high-backed, splint-bottomed chair."[3]

At the same time that Allen offered his opinions on true comfort in seating furniture, American inventors patented a number of improvements in the physical support offered by both beds and seats through the use of resilient structures that incorporated coil springs or metal strips held in tension. Simultaneously, American upholsterers adopted new European techniques for building and fastening together increasingly deep layers of traditional stuffing materials. Even when resilient spring structures were applied to chairs that were in no way designed for seated comfort as we know it today, popular understanding seems to have been that these innovations were the newest and therefore best way of making comfortable seating furniture.

At first, spring-seat upholstery was expensive to produce because of the materials and skilled labor it required, but it became so desirable that a market for cheap versions seemed guaranteed. In the second half of the nineteenth century, particularly after 1870, large upholstery shops and manufactories explored a variety of production alternatives to reduce the cost of spring-seat upholstery. Makers of cheap upholstery tried to market furniture that had spring structures and that was properly "refined"—"softened" from a visual and tactile (but not necessarily physical) standpoint, "finished" in appearance, and visually complex.

However, much upholstered seating furniture made between 1850 and 1910 does not fit modern ideas about comfortable seating. Seating furniture that fulfills this definition of what constitutes a comfortable chair for home use (as opposed to a comfortable chair for working at an office desk, for example) typically has one or more of three characteristics. It is upholstered, especially where it is in contact with the hips, the thighs, and the back. It has a resilient structure, which now usually consists of foam (introduced as early as the 1930s but uncommon for several decades) but until the 1950s almost always consisted of an internal spring structure held in tension. In a few kinds of seats, analysis of the human body has affected the structure of the chair frame itself, and other specialized chairs are adjustable, allowing reclining as well as upright postures. However, the most popular "comfortable" furniture allows users to adjust their postures without changing its form. It permits sitting with feet curled underneath the body, sitting slumped, and lying down (fig. 1). In fact, some pieces of furniture are so large and soft that it is difficult to sit up straight in them, with one's feet on the floor.

Broadly, the trend in popular upholstered furniture between 1850 and 1930 was toward types of seating that we might consider comfortable today, although such furniture did not commonly enter the ordinary parlor until the 1920s. Overstuffed chairs with spring seats, and perhaps spring backs or wire frames, were expensive and unusual in the 1850s and 1860s (fig. 2; plate 8). Such chairs represented tours de force of American upholstery skills and were exhibition pieces, such as the "Turkish fauteuil" covered in "white brocade silk" displayed at the New York Crystal Palace in 1853.[4] Over the next three decades, similar chairs were introduced in factory upholstery catalogs, often as single reading chairs, and "Turkish" overstuffed suites were one middle-class alternative in parlor furniture in the 1880s (fig. 3). By the 1890s, much upholstered seating furniture was less posture controlling and larger in scale than were, for example, typical parlor chairs of the 1870s. However, this change was slow and uneven, and changes in consumption are difficult to chart. Individual households seem to have placed certain kinds of upholstered furniture in specific settings, with more "comfortable" chairs placed in libraries or sitting rooms and the furniture we now consider stiff placed in parlors (fig. 4). Just as families used parlors in different ways and combined the standard vocabulary of parlor furnishing to reflect personal preference, so too attitudes about what

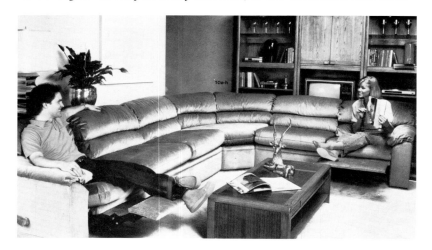

Fig. 1. "Modular System by Barclay," photograph in Sibley's Home Sale Catalog, *Rochester, New York (September 1985). Courtesy Sibley's Department Stores.*

Fig. 2. Armchair, walnut, printed cotton, Marcotte and Company, New York, New York, 1869. This chair, described in the 11 August 1869 bill as a "stuffed all over Bergere," was part of the Codman family's 1869 redecoration of the drawing room of the Grange. It was purchased "tufted without covering," perhaps directly from France, and cost seventy dollars. Marcotte covered it with ten yards of "garnet striped Cretonne Chintz," a brightly printed fabric without the sheen of true cotton chintz, and seven feet of red-and-white silk gimp; he then applied two "W. and S. [wool and silk?] rosettes," adding another $20.80 to the cost. The chair also was provided with "flounces," which may have been what is now called a "dust ruffle." With its loosely stuffed tufting and cotton upholstery, the chair represented a type of seating furniture that was not part of typical middle class parlor furnishing in America. Courtesy Society for the Preservation of New England Antiquities.

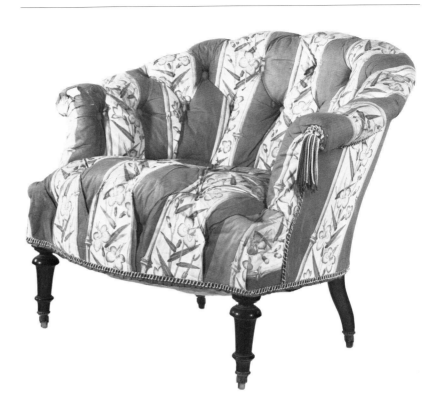

constituted comfortable seating and where it properly belonged demonstrated considerable variation. With the introduction of popularly priced "davenport" sofas in the 1910s, seats we now consider comfortable were included in the middle-class parlor.

This changing preference in upholstered seating also was influenced by a range of social and cultural customs and constraints that varied by room, by the demands of etiquette on social ritual, by the restraints upon posture and movement imposed by dress, and by the impact of gender roles upon furniture use. In these contexts, furniture that seemed to invite relaxation was not always relaxing. Logical deductions, based upon its structure and form, about how furniture was used may not be accurate indicators of how it was typically used, just as one's intuitive expectation that Victorians used heavy draperies in the parlor to block drafts is contravened by the knowledge that many people chose to use only lace curtains and valances year round. Like the parlor itself, upholstered parlor furniture had a mixed ancestry. Its functions were not dominated by simple utility alone but expressed long-standing notions about the symbolic functions of seats. Some chairs, such as parlor reception chairs, never were meant to be comfortable; instead they were props for social ceremony, or rhetorical devices, signals of a family's knowledge that such social ceremony was proper to parlors even if it never took place in its own house. Parlor seating furniture also communicated status, whether real or aspired.

The decorative covers of chairs were one way to make these rhetorical statements. Historically, richly decorated chairs, which had embroidered seats and fabric-covered legs and arms or were draped with "chair cloths" or padded with elaborate cushions, were concrete symbols of wealth and indicators of power in Europe between 1100 and 1500 (fig. 5). In the medieval world, where most furniture was rough and fine possessions were necessarily portable, such chairs were "seats of authority," emblems of power and precedence in

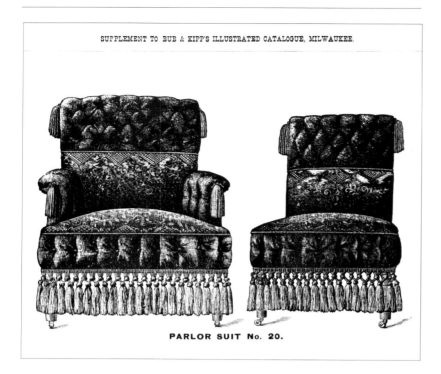

SUPPLEMENT TO BUB & KIPP'S ILLUSTRATED CATALOGUE, MILWAUKEE.

PARLOR SUIT No. 20.

Fig. 3. *Armchair and side chair from* *"Parlor Suit No. 20," engraving in* Supplement to Bub and Kipp's Illustrated Catalogue of 1885, *Milwaukee, Wisconsin (June 1885).* *While Bub and Kipp offered seven-piece* *parlor suites in American mohair plush* *for as little as $50 wholesale, No. 20, an* *overstuffed suite with spring edges, cost* *$110 with the same cover. The higher cost* *reflected both the additional upholstery* *materials and the labor involved.*

households. Seats of authority were signaled by their raised position on a dais, by the presence of backs and arms, and by the use of ornamentation, particularly textile coverings that could either be part of the seats' construction or a temporary drapery that might even include a canopy. Originally, chairs that were permanently upholstered with fabric were padded no more than were saddles (the upholstery trade originated with saddle-making). Cushions might be added to such chairs as a concession to bodily comfort, but they were not critical to the chair's symbolic status as an adjunct of state.

By the seventeenth century, upholstered chairs had evolved into a variety of forms, and well-to-do households might have many chairs with upholstered seats and backs, particularly the type known now as "farthingale chairs" (fig. 6). Still, the symbolic roots of these chairs lay in the idea that textile-covered chairs were emblems of status. Ownership of many such chairs tokened new expressions of wealth and power made possible both by economic and commercial development leading to the growth of cities, as well as the end of the political necessity for large households to move and transport valuable possessions frequently.[5]

The "reception chairs" commonly found in nineteenth-century parlors seem to recall the old symbolic function of chairs with decorative upholstery. Ostensibly reserved for formal social occasions, reception chairs did not match other parlor chairs. Their elaborate frames and covers often combined more than one fabric, multicolored trims, and decorative needlework including beading and tufted Berlin work that would have been destroyed if the chairs had seen much use (fig. 7). Reception chairs signaled the formal activities taking place in parlors; their intricate appearance and accepted function created one more metaphor for the refined, formal parlor (figs. 8 and 9; plate 9).

Upholstered chairs also were tied to the realm of symbolic behavior, whether it expressed political ideals or, by the eighteenth century, social ideals. In the eighteenth century, beautifully upholstered chairs served as symbols of another kind of power, the social power of the beau monde of gentility. Their forms and

Fig. 4. *Wire frame sofa in the library of the Voigt House, Grand Rapids, Michigan, about 1900. Two of the Voigt family's first-floor rooms, the drawing room and music room, contained sets of parlor furniture that were smaller in scale and more formal in character than the library's sofa, recently reupholstered with green wide-wale corduroy similar to the original cover. Large and extremely deep, this sofa is meant for long-term sitting, appropriate to the designated activity of the room; its corduroy upholstery was an "informal" covering. Courtesy Voigt Collection, Grand Rapids Public Museum.*

decoration made manifest ideas about the character of cultivated social life in the salon and signaled the presence not only of money but also of new forms of cultivated taste. All the furnishings of salons—writing tables, cabinets for display of small treasures, bookcases—manifested in their forms and ornament a vision of graceful social interaction based upon personal cultivation and upon manners and deportment that were polished yet effortless, not awkward and labored.

The "easy manner" was part of the behavioral typology of gentility. According to the *Oxford English Dictionary*, ease may mean the "absence of pain or trouble" and a condition of rest that is "comfortable, luxurious, quiet." However, ease is not a condition of relaxation per se; rather, the "easy manner" is characterized by freedom from "constraint or stiffness; chiefly of or in reference to bodily posture or movements. Also *transf.* of manners and behavior; Free from embarrassment or awkwardness."[6] The easy manner was

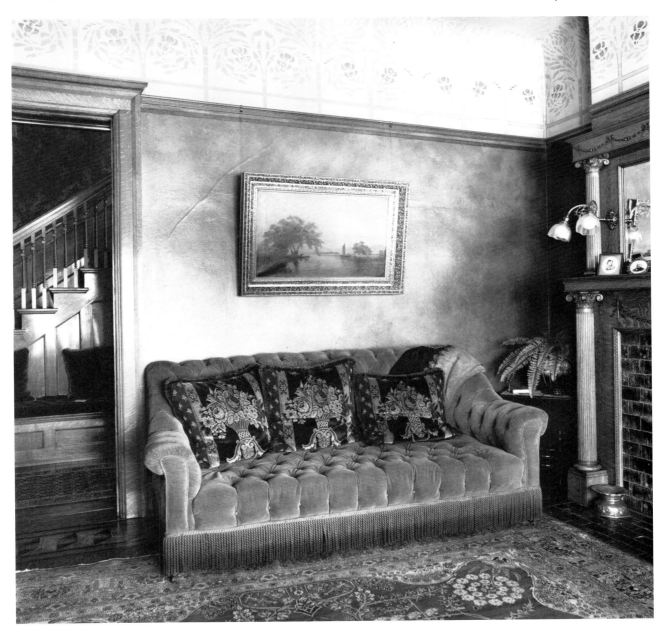

one in which genteel behavior was second nature, where deportment was characterized by effortless self-control. Its ideal was embodied in the social interactions of the salon, where cultivated minds, graceful deportment, refined manners, and beautiful settings and furnishings were in perfect correspondence. When we study eighteenth-century "conversation pieces" or portraits of gentlepeople, the postures depicted are upright and dignified, but not stiff (fig. 10).[7] The "easy" posture was not unconstrained; in fact, the heavy shaping of garments aided proper deportment. Women's corsets kept their postures straight, and the vests and coats of gentlemen were tailored so tightly that they helped shape their wearers' postures into a characteristic "S" curve. In their portraits, these epitomes of gentility often sit away from the backs of chairs, yet they seem comfortable and in harmony with their settings. The carved chair backs seem to be a decorative element in a composition of the seated person and the chair.[8]

Whatever they symbolize when unoccupied, chairs are most expressive in a context of use, where they are part of a communicative unit including the sitter, the dress of that occupant, and his or her deportment. Any examination of physical comfort in seating furniture must take into consideration this social and cultural dimension, not necessarily clear in even the most thoughtful, close scrutiny of the form of chair apart from its context of use. For example, posture had long been considered one indicator of rank and character. In medieval Europe, posture and bearing, as well as clothing, helped distinguish a person of rank. The world of gentility in the eighteenth century continued to employ a version of the historical connection between deportment and social rank, but deportment now signaled personal cultivation and was a critically important component of education.[9]

Judging from advice on deportment published after 1850, the Victorian ideal of bodily self-control in the parlor still relied upon the older conception of the "easy manner" of gentility, even though advice offered to middle-class people was given a different cast, and made more confusing for would-be parlor people, by the demand that their behavior be sincere. The sheer number of rules articulated by advice authors suggests that enterprising, self-improving individuals in quest of proper deportment faced a daunting task in their effort to appear both sincere and cultivated. Authors of etiquette books still argued that correct use of chairs, props in the theater of the parlor, should display both graceful, easy, and genteel deportment and, by extension, the character of the sitter.

Florence Hartley, author of *The Ladies' Book of Etiquette, and Manual of Politeness* (1856), urged her readers to "let the movements be easy and flexible, and accord with the style of a lady."[10] This ease, however, required extraordinary control of the voice, feet, hands, arms, and posture. Hartley did not automatically equate such labored composure with artificial manners. The goal was self-mastery so flawless that it became second nature. In the interim, as would-be gentlepeople learned etiquette, they had both to act naturally and guard constantly against displaying ill breeding, a painful exercise at best (figs. 11 and 12).[11]

The structure of parlor furniture could play an important role in advancing or sabotaging the efforts of parlor people to communicate their gentility through their deportment. Miss Leslie advised her readers to avoid purchasing sofas and chairs with "high and narrow" seats and backs that "incline forward," for "they allow little more than their edge to the sitter, who is also obliged to keep bolt upright, and remain stiffly in the same position."[12] Preference for chairs with slanted backs was not meant to imply that complete relaxation was

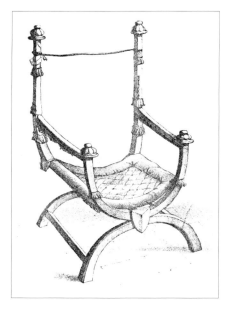

Fig. 5. *Armchair at York Minster, illustration in George Ayliffe Poole and J. W. Hugall,* York Cathedral *(1850), reproduced in* Furniture History *(1981). Courtesy The Furniture History Society.*

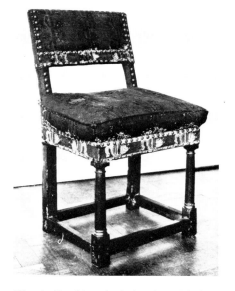

Fig. 6. *Farthingale chair, about 1615, in the collections of Victoria and Albert Museum, photograph in Oliver Bracket,* English Furniture Illustrated *(1950). Courtesy A. & C. Black Publishers, Ltd.*

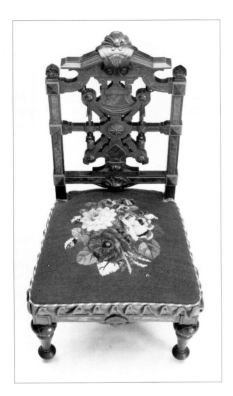

Fig. 7. Reception chair, walnut, wool rep and Berlin work, United States, 1865-1875.

permissible: Leslie also urged caution in sitting in rocking chairs. "Swaying backwards and forwards in a parlour rocking chair…," she wrote, "is a most ungraceful recreation, particularly for a lady…and very annoying to spectators, who may happen to be a little nervous."[13]

Other advice authors also warned readers against the temptation to relax completely in the parlor, even if the room was provided with furniture that seemed to invite repose. One cautioned, "Lounging on sofas or easy chairs, tipping your chair back on two legs, throwing your leg over your knee, or sitting in any unnatural position—these habits are always considered indecorous, and when ladies are present are deemed extremely vulgar."[14] Florence Hartley advised, "Avoid lounging attitudes, they are indelicate, except in your own private apartment. Nothing but ill-health will excuse them before company, and a lady had better keep [to] her room if she is too feeble to sit up in the drawing-room."[15] Popular fiction sometimes used the deportment of characters as a clue to their personal strengths or failings. In *High Life in New York by Jonathan Slick, Esq.*, Slick's parvenu cousin, Mrs. Beebe, exposed herself as an affected fraud not only by her "puckered up" appearance (she was adorned with ruffles, false hair, and a corset so tight that her waist "warn't any bigger round than a pint cup") but also by the way in which she sat in a parlor rocker: "She sot down in one of the rocking-chairs and stuck her elbow on her arm and let her head drop into her hand as if she warn't more than half live."[16]

Finally, along with its ability to imply genteel ease, erect posture was sometimes claimed to be essential to proper health. "Lounging, which a large number of persons indulge," and sitting "with the body leaning forward on the stomach, or to one side, with the heels elevated to a level with the head" was not only exemplary of bad manners but "exceedingly detrimental to health."[17]

Parlor etiquette tamed human behavior by binding it within certain boundaries. As parlor furnishing evolved, the forms of some upholstered furniture—lounges, couches, and parlor rockers in particular—created potential new sources of confusion about parlor deportment. In the 1880s and 1890s, new fashions for "Turkish" furniture, particularly low couches, apparently presented some parlor people with unanticipated deportment difficulties that some periodicals tried to assuage with advice such as "How to Sit on a Divan."[18]

Deportment's requirements aside, even with the gradual trend between 1850 and 1910 toward seating furniture that modern eyes can recognize as comfortable, another set of constraints on posture and seated comfort existed that affected women alone. Products of the centuries-old practice of corseting and employing padding and frames for skirts in undergarments, these strictures were designed to create fashionable body shapes and to aid deportment. Throughout the nineteenth century, the elaborate structure of undergarments compelled middle-class women in full dress (that is, in the clothing they would have worn for social occasions and in public) to limit their range of movement, constrained their ability to interact with furnishings, and harnessed their experience of their bodies in social settings.[19] The presence of corseted women in social situations served not only as a statement about fashion but also as a bodily metaphor for the larger setting of parlor social ritual. Women, the conservators of culture, experienced bodily constraints that were analogous to the restraining morals and manners of civilized living.[20] At least one nineteenth-century commentator noted a direct and necessary connection between corseting and morals: "It is an ever present monitor indirectly bidding its wearer to exercise self-restraint;

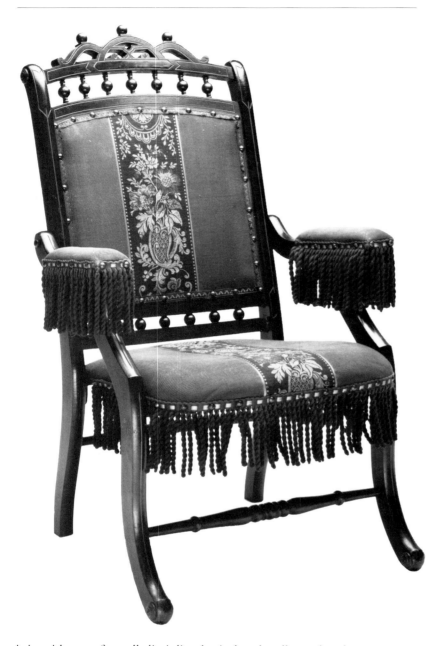

it is evidence of a well-disciplined mind and well-regulated feelings."[21]

The degree and kind of encumbrance offered by women's underclothes varied as fashions changed. In the 1850s and 1860s, wide skirts with stiff crinolines and hoops made contact with chair backs and sitting in chairs with full arms difficult. From this difficulty arose the parlor suite convention of the "ladies' chair." Although their legs were freed and corsets relatively short, women would have found it difficult—even if it had been desirable because of the problem of managing one's skirts gracefully and modestly in social situations—to assume relaxed posture in a full crinoline or "cage" (a petticoat stiffened by metal or whalebone hoops). Drawers, loose-fitting underpants with a split in the middle, still were not a universal element of women's dress in 1850. Crinolines speeded their acceptance.

Wide hoops disappeared by the mid-1860s, but cages for skirts

Fig. 9. Reception chair, walnut, figured wool rep and silk velvet, George Hunzinger, New York, New York, about 1875. George Hunzinger's advertisement in the 1874 edition of Cleary's Improved Commercial Directory of the Furniture, Carpet, and Upholstery Trades *described his chairs as "fancy"—that is, for use as decorative accents and reception chairs. Courtesy The Hudson River Museum.*

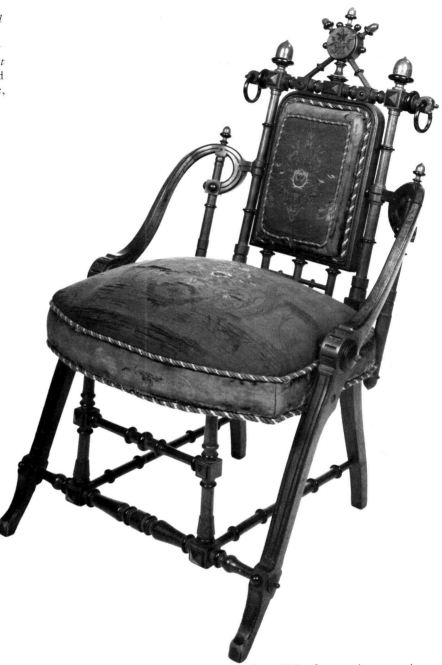

continued to be employed through the 1880s, for evening wear in particular (figs. 13 and 14). They were augmented by another form of encumbrance, the bustle, which survived in one form or another into the 1890s. Although ladies' chairs in parlor suites appeared through the 1870s, there seems to have been little real correspondence between the forms of upholstered parlor furniture and the advent of the bustle in women's clothing. Bustles first appeared as simple tie-on pads stuffed with horsehair or down or made from several ruffled layers of horsehair fabric. As the draping of women's derrières became more elaborate, large bustle structures, with a metal framework, were necessary. Like hoops, large bustles made sitting back in chairs difficult at best, inspiring a number of inventors to patent folding bustles (fig. 15).

Unlike the full skirts of midcentury, the longer, narrow lines of

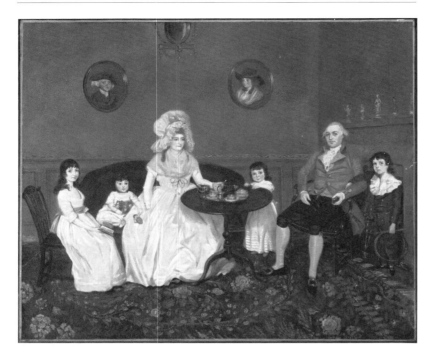

Fig. 10. The Samels Family, *oil on canvas by Johann Eckstein (1736-1817), United States, 1788. Erect posture, with the sitter's back held straight and away from the chair's back, was an important expression of genteel deportment reinforced by the structures of ladies' corsets and skirts and men's tightly fitting formal waistcoats. Courtesy Museum of Fine Arts, Boston; Ellen Kelleran Gardner Fund.*

dresses that appeared in the 1870s and again at the turn of the century required the use of very long corsets. Fashion advisers never discussed the simple logistical problems of negotiating one's way through the world laced tightly from sternum to pubic bone, but advertisements for corsets sometimes indicate that the simple act of sitting or bending could result in broken corset boning (and certainly abdominal bruises) (fig. 16). Lounging was almost impossible. Thus women were offered products such as the "Pearl Corset Shield," which the Montgomery Ward and Co. catalog for the fall and winter of 1894-1895 noted "prevents corsets breaking at the waist and hips…Will protect the body from the ends of broken stays."[22] Between 1870 and 1910, the "relaxed" pose of a fully dressed, corseted woman was one in which she rested her stiffened torso sideways against the corner of a sofa or propped her upper back (at the shoulder blades) against the back of a chair (figs. 17 and 18). "Turkish" overstuffed furniture, especially large, deep "pillow-back" chairs, must have presented particular challenges. And, as clothing historian Cecil Saint-Laurent has observed, just as overstuffed lounges and davenports became truly popular between 1900 and 1914, corsets reached their greatest length and "strangled" women "from the shoulder to the thighs."[23]

The limits a fully dressed woman experienced in sitting in a relaxed manner suggest that certain kinds of upholstered chairs, particularly the various forms of reclining, adjustable chairs, were sex specific in their use, whether they appeared in parlors or in other rooms (fig. 19). Advertisements for the Marks Patent Folding Chair, a popular and well-publicized recliner of the 1880s, always show men enjoying the chair's "Solid Comfort." Of course, women were not always fully dressed in their layers of chemise, drawers, corset, crinolines or bustle, and petticoats. Those who did their own housework or farm chores were less encumbered by necessity, and women who had servants also wore morning dresses that permitted "half-corsets" and no bustles. Parlor social life required full dress, however, a process of adornment onerous enough that etiquette books urged women to set aside one morning each week for receiving callers if "home duties make it inconvenient to dress every morning to receive visitors."[24]

Reconstructing patterns of use and meaning associated with upholstered parlor furniture is made more complex by technical and technological developments in the craft of seat upholstery during the second half of the nineteenth century. By 1850, much, perhaps almost all, parlor seating furniture was made with layered seat structures containing stuffings of horsehair and plant materials (tow from the waste of flax, dried Spanish moss and "sea moss," wood shavings, and cotton batting) underpinned by a layer of metal coil springs held in tension by tying them together and to the chair frame.

Figs. 11 and 12. *"Ungraceful Positions" and "Gentility in the Parlor," engravings in Thomas E. Hill,* Hill's Manual of Social and Business Forms *(1885; reprint, 1971). Courtesy The New York Times Company.*

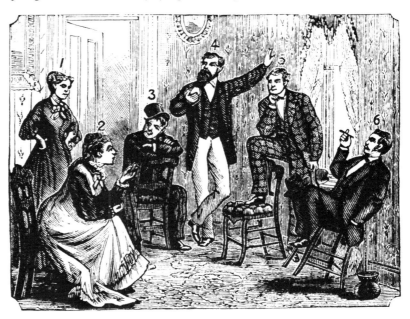

FIG. 6. UNGRACEFUL POSITIONS.

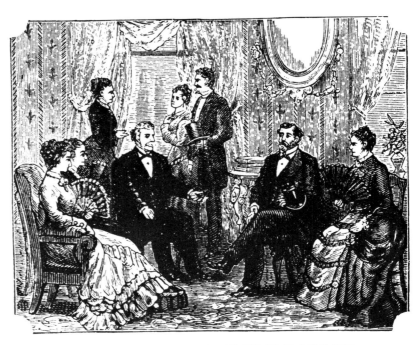

FIG. 7. GENTILITY IN THE PARLOR.

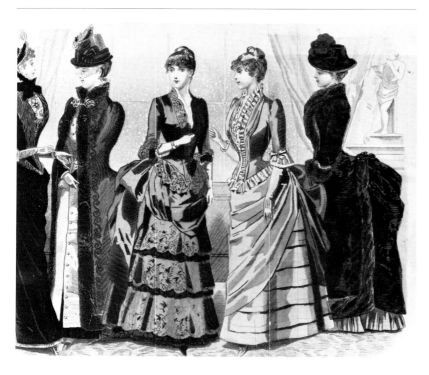

Fig. 13. *"A Snowy Reception Day,"* *hand-colored engraving in* Peterson's Magazine *(December 1885).*

Spring-seat upholstery changed the design of chairs because of the depth needed for the upholstered structure and the tension it put on frames. It required new skills on the part of upholsterers, set off a spate of new patents for furniture, and created a new sector of the furniture trade in spring manufacture. Spring seats also appear to have had an impact on popular thought about how bodily comfort in seating furniture might best be achieved. They were not an inevitable result of efforts to attain greater bodily comfort in furniture but represent a particular culture's singular technological solution to a perceived need. How that need was articulated and where spring-seat structures first appeared in ordinary furniture also provided some clues to changing popular thought about one's entitlement to certain kinds of comfort and about how such comfort might best be achieved.

Upholstered furniture provides bodily comfort through its resilient padding. Until the advent of foam upholstery, this padding was a "sandwich" of layers of stuffing and fabric held together and on the chair frame with stitching, ties, and tacks or staples. The history of chair upholstery techniques can be described briefly as the story of craftspeople's efforts to stuff more, thicker, and more resilient fillings into the upholstery sandwich contained within and wrapped around the frames of seating furniture. Until the advent of spring-seat structures, all upholstered furniture had "dead seats," seats that did not have the elasticity of interior springs.[25] Any resiliency dead seats provided was the result of natural elasticity in materials, as in the "give" of wadded or curled animal hair or the woven webbing attached to the underside of the seat frame. The stuffing material was stitched into place, and an undercover of cotton or linen was generally fastened to the seat frame. The "show cover," the decorative fabric selected for the chair, was then cut and sewed and tacked into place (fig. 20).

Although the layers of padding in upholstered chairs certainly mediated the contact of the sitter with the chair frame and provided more warmth than wood alone, most structural upholstery (as opposed to cushion seats) was stuffed to be quite firm rather than

Fig. 14. Skirt cage, engraving in
Daniell and Sons Catalogue, Spring and
Summer, *New York, New York (1885).*
In the 1870s and 1880s, bustles often
were incorporated into full-length cages
or wire frames (called "tournures") over
which petticoats and skirts were draped.
Such contraptions were meant primarily
for use with "walking suits" or evening
clothes. Although the steels were of small
diameter and very flexible, sitting
comfortably probably was quite difficult
given the combination of cage, petticoats,
and narrowly tailored skirt fronts.

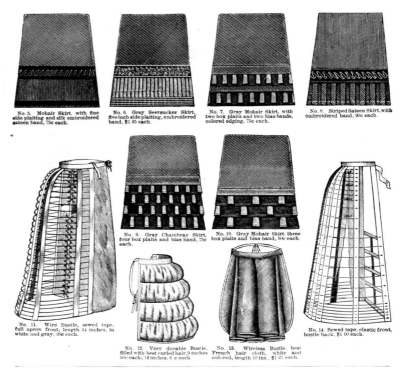

Fig. 15. Advertisement for Taylor's
Patent Folding Bustles, about 1880, in
Cecil Saint-Laurent, The Great Book of
Lingerie *(1983). Some bustles were*
constructed as small pieces of high-quality
upholstery themselves, with channel
tufting filled with resilient horsehair.
Others were large steel cages that
prevented women from leaning against
chair backs unless the bustles were
designed to fold up, as this patented
model was. Courtesy Vendome Press.

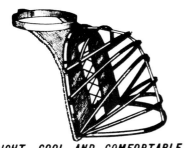

LIGHT, COOL AND COMFORTABLE.
The best Fifty Cent Folding Bustle in the
market. It is recommended by fashionable ladies
and leading dressmakers. PERFECT in shape and
ADJUSTABLE in size. The improved folding
principle used in this Bustle results in its always
regaining its shape after pressure. It is the easiest
and yet the most effective and durable spring ever
presented. Its superior finish and elegant style
make it a most desirable Bustle.

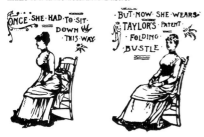

luxuriously soft. This was even the case with most pleated tufting in America until the end of the nineteenth century. Because stuffing in the arms and backs of chairs tended to get lumpy, upholsterers used tied stitches like those in simple unquilted comforters to hold the layers in place. Sometimes they were passed through the show cover as well and became a decorative element in the chair; thus they were forerunners of decorative button tufts. The other type of early padded upholstery, the loose or cushion seat (also called a "squab") sat on top of the chair seat and was a type often employed by amateur upholsterers in the nineteenth century.[26]

By 1830, upholsterers in Europe and America began to offer their customers the innovation that had the single greatest impact on the construction of upholstered furniture in the nineteenth century—the use of coil springs in seat structures. An 1822 patent taken out by Viennese upholsterer George Junigl stated that his "improvement on contemporary methods of furniture upholstery...by means of a special preparation of hemp, with the assistance of iron springs" resulted in a structure "so elastic that it is not inferior to horsehair upholstery," which set the standards for resiliency.[27] Coiled springs had appeared in a piece of furniture more than seventy years earlier: the "Chamber-Horse," an exercise apparatus, was advertised by Henry Marsh in the *London Daily Post and Advertiser* in 1739 and 1740.[28] These early uses were isolated, however, and seem to have had no real impact on the upholsterer's craft.

Construction of upholstered furniture became more complex and difficult to master as a craft with the adoption of springs, which changed the structure of the upholstery sandwich dramatically (figs. 21 and 22). Spring tying was a tricky proposition, as it is still, and early efforts probably failed frequently, exploding out of the seat frame or even cracking it. The first chair springs were made from copper, but that metal did not retain its resiliency long enough. Tempered steel eventually supplanted copper, but it also created

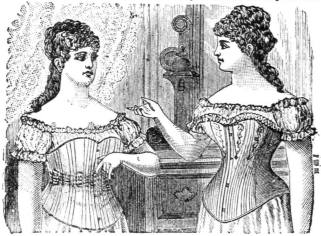

I have worn this Corset | I have worn the Flexible
three days and every bone | Hip Corset three months and
over the hips is broken. | every bone is still perfect.

The money will be refunded for every Flexible Hip Corset
which breaks over the hips. This corset is so comfortable
that a lady can lie down in it with ease, so flexible that it yields
readily to every movement of the body, and yet so firm that it
gives the requisite support to the sides. White or drab.

Price, $1.00.

Fig. 16. Advertisement for "Flexible Hip Corset," engraving in Edward Ridley and Sons' Catalog and Price List Fall and Winter 1882-1883, New York, New York. The caption guaranteed that a purchaser's money would be refunded if the corset "breaks over the hips"—that is, if the boning of the corset snapped when the wearer sat down or bent over.

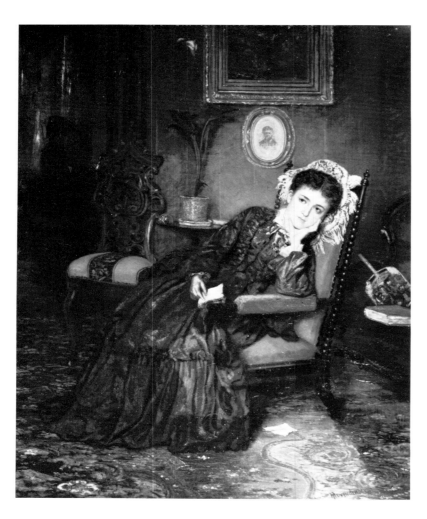

Fig. 17. A Reverie, oil on canvas by Thomas Hovenden (1840-1895), United States, 1873. The young woman in this painting has turned to the side and rests her upper shoulder against the chair back; her torso is stiffened from her corsets. Courtesy Bernard and S. Dean Levy, Inc.

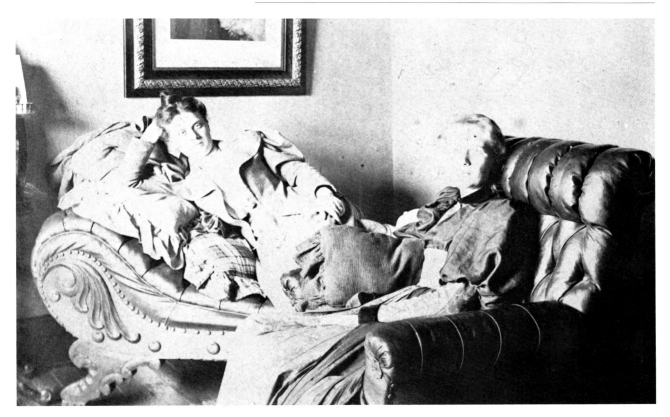

Fig. 18. *"Mrs. Mendenhall and Miss Zehuder," by unidentified photographer, United States, about 1895. Even though one woman is stretched out rather provocatively on a Turkish lounge, she is not slumped. Rather, her torso is held rigidly straight by her undergarments.*

problems. Apart from rust, which could eventually damage the twines, the first steel springs had an alarming tendency to break from brittleness caused by improper tempering. These difficulties contributed to the suspicion among critics that spring-seat upholstery was "insincere." In 1877, the authors of *Suggestions for House Decoration in Painting, Woodwork, and Furniture* still protested against the "'grins and grimaces' of modern upholstery," praising the softness of "honest horsehair and feathers" over "iron springs," which, they argued, were "always out of order and cannot have their anatomy readjusted without the intervention of the manufacturer, by whom alone the complexity of their internal structure is understood."[29]

Coil springs applied to furniture were introduced to Anglo-America in the late 1820s and early 1830s. John Claudius Loudon, author of the influential *Encyclopedia of Cottage, Farmhouse and Villa Architecture and Furniture* (first published in England in 1833), illustrated a spiral spring and explained its use in carriages and seats, but he devoted most of his discussion to its benefits in mattresses.[30] Indeed, before 1850, most American furniture patents that incorporated springs in furniture focused upon the eternal human quest for a good night's sleep. Bed springs were efforts to replace rope-bottom beds, which required frequent adjustment and allowed mattresses to sag in the middle; tying the ropes required so much strength that advice books such as *The Workwoman's Guide* recommended that women not tackle this chore without masculine help. Some early bed spring patents offered woven wire bed bottoms or variations much like the structure of trampolines, which employed small coil springs to hold fabric tautly in bed frames.[31] Bed springs were expected to provide even bodily support and to require little maintenance. At a time when bedbugs were difficult to control, such bed bottoms also were easier to keep clean.

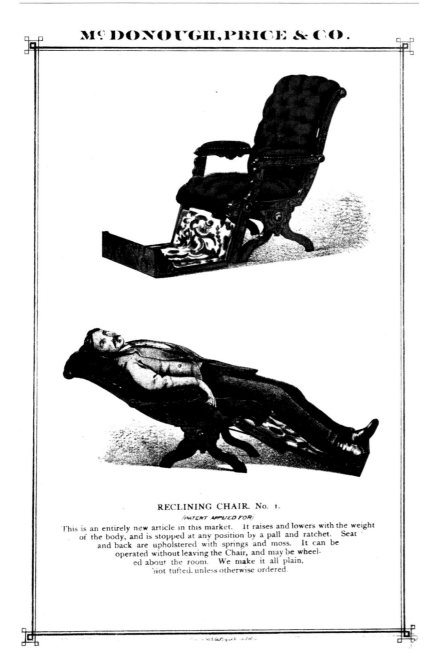

MᶜDONOUGH, PRICE & CO.

RECLINING CHAIR. No. 1.
(PATENT APPLIED FOR)

This is an entirely new article in this market.   It raises and lowers with the weight of the body, and is stopped at any position by a pall and ratchet.   Seat and back are upholstered with springs and moss.   It can be operated without leaving the Chair, and may be wheeled about the room.   We make it all plain, not tufted, unless otherwise ordered.

Fig. 19. "Reclining Chair No. 1," chromolithograph in McDonough, Price and Co. catalog, Chicago, Illinois (1876). Courtesy State Historical Society of Wisconsin.

Like their English counterparts, many of the first American patents exploring the use of springs in chairs described the inventions' benefits as aids to invalids. Springs not only were expected to support their bodies more evenly, but the inventors' specifications also recalled the provision for exercise that had been incorporated in the eighteenth-century chamber horse. Daniel Harrington's 1831 rocking chair patent incorporated springs to provide a "rocking and rolling motion," an "improvement for giving motion or exercise to invalids in their room of confinement."[32]

In their attention to the needs of the sick, these early chairs incorporating springs also reflected one of the historical circumstances that traditionally fostered upholstered seating furniture before the nineteenth century. In the houses of prosperous Americans in the seventeenth and eighteenth centuries, completely upholstered chairs such as wing chairs were typically employed for the comfort of ill or aged members of a household. Such chairs featured both padding and particularly supportive framing that not only blocked drafts but allowed weak sitters to lean to one side. On occasion, these invalid chairs were adjustable and often seem to have served as chamber potty chairs. Peter Thornton has noted that the earliest adjustable chairs "seem to have been those devised for some illustrious invalid." Upholstered chairs with reclining backs also were used in the chambers of pregnant women by the middle to late seventeenth century.[33]

Providing the most physically accommodating and warmest seat in the house for people with special physical needs remained one of the motivations for owning upholstered chairs throughout the nineteenth century. Loudon equated provision of certain "comfortable easy chairs" with family care of the aged and infirm. He even suggested that families of limited means might provide one by tying homemade back and seat cushions to ladderback arm

Fig. 20. Cross sections of a dead seat and a spring seat. A typical dead seat is composed of these layers: a platform of interwoven strips of linen or jute webbing, nailed to the underside of the chair frame; a piece of closely woven cotton or linen that keeps the stuffing from falling through the webbing; an edge roll, stitched in place to keep the seat edge from breaking down; a stuffing layer, called a "cake," of curled horsehair or less expensive plant material; and a cotton undercover. In spring seats of good quality, the spiral springs first were sewed to the webbing; they then were lashed in place in a state of tension with twines. Fabric was fastened over the tied springs. Drawings by Kenneth H. Townsend.

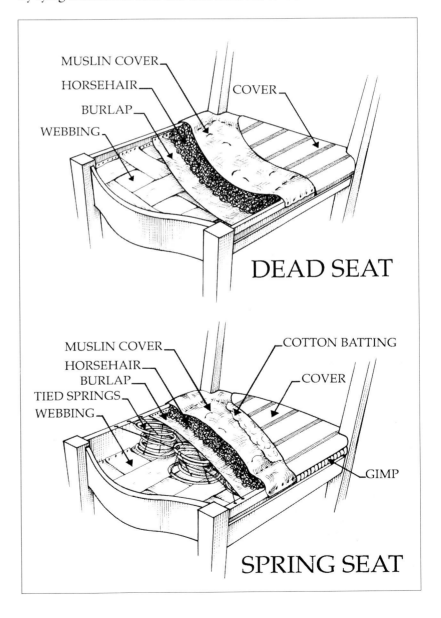

chairs.[34] Upholstered chairs that were adjustable continued to signal the presence of illness as much as the desire for relaxed comfort. In the 1880s, the manufacturers of the Marks adjustable chair still advertised the product both as a chair for invalids and a dandy reclining chair. In early twentieth-century Pittsburgh, the Spencer family's reclining chair was known to children as the "sick chair" (fig. 23).[35]

In the 1830s, advertisements for upholsterers called specific attention to the spring-seat chairs they offered. The first form widely and specifically advertised as such was the "spring-seat rocking chair," which appeared in upholsterers' notices as early as 1829.[36] At first, such "spring seats" appear to have consisted of a spring-filled, stuffed, and covered wooden frame that could rest on a board seat or inside the seat rail (a spring-filled slip seat) in a Boston-type rocking chair. Several of these early rocking chairs survive that bear the labels of Spooner's competitor, the Boston upholsterer and furniture merchant William Hancock. Advertisements for upholsterers in the Boston and Philadelphia city directories as early as 1831 called particular attention to "Patent Spring Seat Rocking Chairs" and "Boston Spring Seat Rocking Chairs."[37] Incorporating spring structures into rocking chairs was a natural development from the early interest in spring structures as aids for invalids; rocking chairs also were associated with the ill or aged members of households in the eighteenth and first half of the nineteenth century and were an inexpensive alternative to wing chairs. Later in the century, rocking chairs still were invalid chairs in special circumstances. In a memoir of growing up in the 1870s near Corning, New York, Jane Williams recalled days spent at a sanatarium called "The Pinewoods" as a guest of the doctor's children. The sanatarium's dining room was furnished with "Boston rockers, instead of straight chairs" for the accommodation of the patients: "When the patients ambled in, they sat down in the rocking chairs and then utterly relaxed, their heads hanging down from limp necks."[38]

Around the same time, however, springs were incorporated into special, personal chairs, such as the singular painted Windsor-type armchair now in the collection of the Metropolitan Museum of Art (figs. 24 and 25). Dating from around 1830, it has a drawer under the seat, a writing arm, and a box-framed, spring-filled cushion seat which rests on top of the board seat. "Spring seat sofas" were another type of such upholstery specifically mentioned in advertisements in the 1830s.[39]

By the mid-1830s, upholstered sofas and chairs containing springs did not always signal illness or age. In the 1840s, upholsterers dropped specific mentions of spring-seat upholstery from their advertisements, probably because the technique was becoming a commonplace for some types of seats. Thus, spring-seat upholstery, like upholstered chairs in general, gradually became a middle-class decency. To this end, an anonymous contributor to Edwin T. Freedley's *Philadelphia and Its Manufactures: A Handbook* (1858) singled out spring-seat upholstery as a particular signal of change and progress in ordinary furniture, noting, "The Cabinet-making business has very much progressed, both in point of taste and extent of production, the last few years. In 1840 there were but few Furniture stores in Philadelphia, and they mostly small ones…A Spring-Seat Sofa was then a luxury—almost a novelty."[40]

There is no single adequate explanation for the larger change in the sense of entitlement of ordinary people to certain kinds of bodily comfort, a change signaled by the rapid acceptance of spring-seat furniture in the second quarter of the nineteenth century. We know very little about what ordinary people thought about this change.

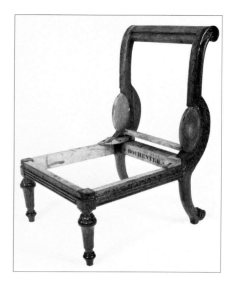

Fig. 21. Chair frame, oak, walnut, and pine, Minges and Shale, Rochester, New York, 1883-1893. High-quality chair frames without upholstery are mostly empty space. Spring-seat structures were nailed, sewed, and tied into such frames in a state of compression that sometimes put such structures under a damaging amount of pressure.

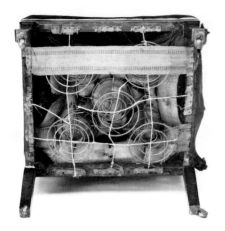

Fig. 22. Viewed upside down, the seat of this damaged upholstered chair reveals the construction sequence in the spring seat. First, coil springs were sewn to the interwoven strips of chair webbing. The light-colored twines at the bottom of the springs were a later addition, an attempt to stabilize an old spring structure. Then the springs were tied together in a state of compression using as many as eight different ties, visible at the top of each spring. The twines also were lashed to the seat frame. Finally, a fabric cover, in this case burlap, was nailed to the chair frame over the tied springs. Stuffing material, in this instance horsehair, then could be added on top of this fabric.

Fig. 23. "Mary, Elizabeth, and Why-Why in the sick chair," photograph by Charles Hart Spencer, Pittsburgh, Pennsylvania, May 1906. Courtesy Elizabeth Ranney.

However, Loudon's 1833 *Encyclopedia* may serve as one early benchmark of a new attitude about bodily comfort. Upholstered furniture, both with and without springs, played a key role in Loudon's discussion of cottage interiors for workers. He devoted considerable space to describing inexpensive sofa beds that could serve for both sitting and sleeping in cottage parlors. Deeming ownership of a sofa in particular "a great source of comfort," Loudon argued that "the cottager ought to have one as well as the rich man."[41] Advertisements and advice literature of the 1830s and 1840s seem to evince a general increased interest in upholstered furniture, particularly with spring seats as an improvement in comfort, when these furnishings were relatively costly and beyond the reach of many consumers. This interest in the mediation of physical sensation in chairs also coincides with other changes in sensory life, such as the possibility of improved domestic heating with the parlor stove and the gradual improvement in domestic lighting culminating in the development of kerosene in the 1850s. Thus upholstery springs may be one more expression of the sensibility of softening that reached its fullest popular expression after 1850.

Yet the presence of spring structures in many chairs produced after 1840 is puzzling because it seems unnecessary in relation to the typical uses of those chairs, and sometimes even detrimental to the structure of the chair itself. This is particularly so with the more formal seats of parlors—reception chairs, small parlor side chairs, and tabourets (upholstered stools). Because these seats were used less frequently than other household chairs and in circumstances requiring strict decorum, certainly sitters had less need for the absorption and distribution of force that springs could provide. If we try to link springs in beds and springs in chairs conceptually, the underlying message of springs is that comfort is linked to relaxation. In this sense, employing springs in reading chairs or furniture for private rooms seems in keeping.

Perhaps in different contexts or at other levels of popular thought, springs in chairs bore other kinds of meanings. In their first decades of use, springs probably were a fashionable novelty as well as another way of putting money "into" chairs, because they increased

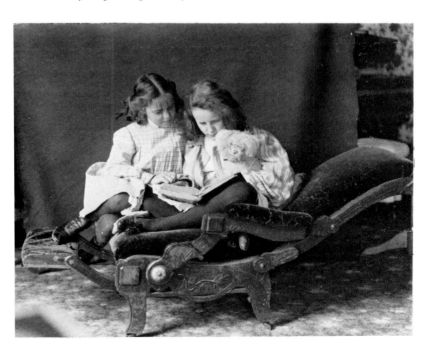

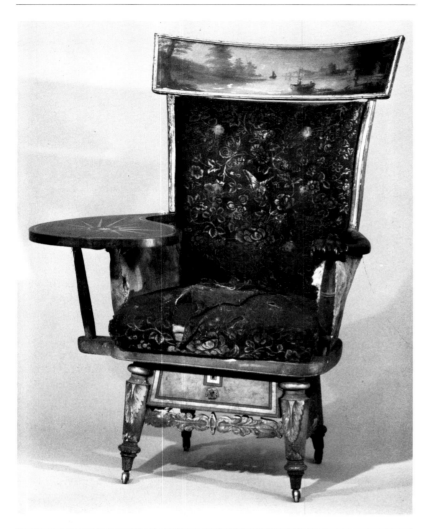

Fig. 24. Armchair, mahogany, wooden inlay and painted decoration, embossed wool plush, probably by Boston, Massachusetts, manufacturer, after 1828. The board seat on this chair is low, suggesting that it was always designed to have a box spring seat. Several rocking chairs with similar boxed spring construction from the shop of William Hancock of Boston, Massachusetts, survive in collections at Old Sturbridge Village and the Essex Institute. Courtesy Metropolitan Museum of Art.

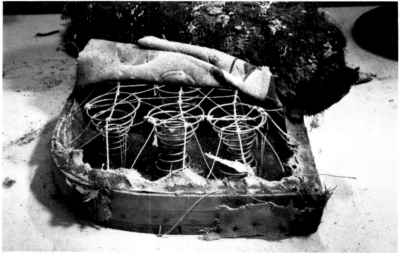

Fig. 25. Detail of fig. 24's box structure during conservation in 1981. Courtesy Metropolitan Museum of Art.

Fig. 26. Advertisement for Gustav E. Sparmann, "Manufacturer of Iron Back Frames," in Improved Commercial Directory and Mercantile Report Combined, of the Furniture, Carpet and Upholstery Trades of the U.S., 1874-5. *Although the finished chairs were expensive, demand for wire or "iron back" chairs was large enough that frame production was a specialty in the furniture trade in a few places such as New York. The spring edge, an innovation of the 1860s, consisted of a row of upholstery springs with a wire or piece of bamboo fastened across the front of an upholstered seat, replacing a rigid "edge roll" of stuffing materials. Both innovations allowed creation of seats that were even more resilient; in fact, wire frames transformed the entire chair into an "elastic" structure. Because of the amount of workmanship involved in constructing a stable seat with so little frame as an anchor, wire frame upholstery and spring-edge seats were more expensive than traditional wooden frames.*

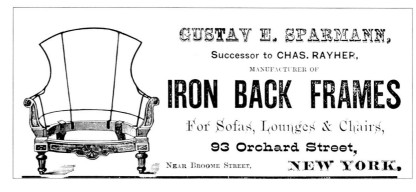

the cost of upholstery. Stiff little armless parlor suite chairs, for example, once had dead "slip seats" that could be removed for easy recovering. They were intended for formal, short-term social use, and thus the presence of springs may have been more a function of the chair's place in a set that "matched" in all respects, including identity of structure, than a significant improvement in their comfort.

Although adjustable furniture was the object of much patent interest, ordinary people seem to have felt that the best chairs were not those that were adjustable, but rather those whose structures were increasingly elastic. Chairs with springs in their backs as well as seats had been introduced by the 1850s and, by the 1860s, the "spring edge" and the wire frame chair appeared, whose entire seat and back structure was, in essence, a large tensile spring (figs. 26-28).

Elasticity may also have served aesthetic functions. Spring seats returned to their original shape when a sitter rose, so chairs maintained a smooth appearance. Further, the inclusion of springs in traditional types of chairs allowed such "improved" seats to be at once modern and traditional, to be stylish at the same time that they expressed their historical origins, which had little to do with bodily comfort but everything to do with serving as long-standing symbols of economic and social power.

Why should increased elasticity, rather than adjustability or scientific design, have set the standard for desirable seating? One possible answer may lie in the conjunction of traditional expectations about the appearance and aesthetic function of chairs, particularly upholstered chairs, with popular interest in new technology as a herald of progress. "Elastic" springs were the objects of deep interest among inventors in several fields of technology, most particularly transportation, where they not only lessened the amount of jouncing that passengers experienced in both carriages and railroad cars but also helped preserve the equipment from damage. *Scientific American* paid particular attention to inventions of this stripe; one article in the issue of July 31, 1847, "New Wagon Springs," praised a new design for "a wagon hung upon invisible spiral springs" which promised "improvement in comfort and economy:" "It is said to be easy and graceful in motion, especially in crossing gullies or rough ground—it having more the motion of a light boat in gliding over the waves, than a vehicle upon wheels." Another praised Thomas Warren's patent spring, meant for use in vehicles and furniture, as a "perfect invention."[42]

The forces harnessed in springs seemed mysterious and exciting to mechanics and inventors in the first half of the nineteenth century, perhaps all the more so for their practical usefulness. Two articles in the *Scientific American*'s ongoing series "Science of Mechanics" that discussed the "Elasticity of Bodies," including metal springs, suggested that elasticity was particularly interesting because it

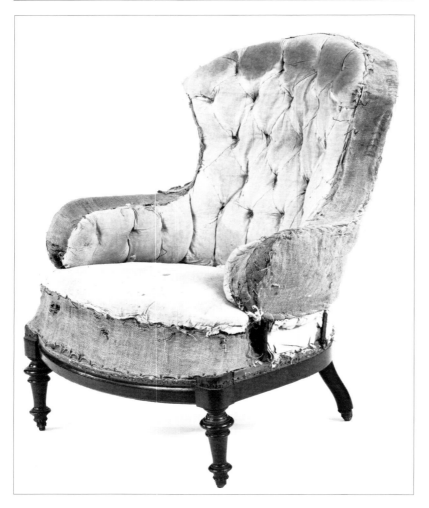

transferred momentum without "perceptible loss of power." "The cause of elasticity, or the philosophical principles of the elasticity of metallic bodies, has never been clearly explained," the magazine pointed out. "It is in fact, difficult to comprehend that the particles composing the distended surface of a tempered steel spring, do not remain in actual contact with each other. Yet there is abundant evidence that such is the fact; that the attraction of cohesion is not sensibly diminished." The elasticity of springs could be turned to the most mundane of uses, from improving the ride of carriages to "Improved Blind Fastenings" for windows and spring door stops.[43]

Thus, springs in seats were one of the few ways in which technological progress could be harnessed inside a particularly traditional artifact, the chair. For someone unacquainted with woodworking, the use of machines for making chair frames was not necessarily apparent. However, springs could be perceived through the act of sitting, even if they were invisible on the surface. And a practiced eye could discern their presence by the depth and shape of chair seats. Thus spring seats made technological progress manifest in furniture.

Further, we may conjecture that elastic structures in seats were congenial to the broad sensibility of refinement because of their responsiveness to the human body as well as their mediation of physical sensation as the chair seat "gave" in the act of sitting down. Adjustability also made chairs responsive, but resilient upholstery was more subtle in its working and, again, maintained the appearance of

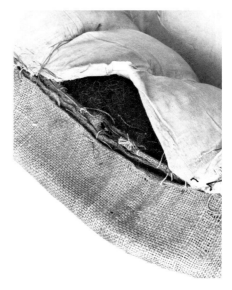

Fig. 29. Simple buttoning and pleated diamond tufting. A number of variations on pleated diamond tufting also were used, including biscuit and bun tufting (which formed rectangles and squares), and star tufting, which consisted of diamond shapes that formed a wheel with a single center button. Drawings by Kenneth H. Townsend.

the traditional chair while avoiding the connotations of illness or total relaxation connoted by adjustability.

Increased padding in chairs, particularly pleated tufting, was another innovation of the nineteenth century. Padded upholstery presents subtle problems of understanding and interpretation similar to those of springs in seats. It mediated bodily contact with chair frames; it also made chairs and couches warmer, mediating the sensations of heat and cold. However, although it is resilient, padding is not necessarily soft, as pleated tufting in most nineteenth-century American furniture demonstrates.

Before tufting developed into a pleated, sewn-in method of anchoring stuffing and of elaborating chair surfaces, it consisted of a simple form of stitching through layers of seat or mattress stuffing (figs. 29 and 30). The large single stitches were spaced evenly through the upholstery and often did not appear through the show cover of a piece of furniture, although in the nineteenth century they were frequently marked with decorative buttons. In the late nineteenth century, lounge catalogs applied the term "tufting" to both buttoning and to pleated tufting. At the level of popular taste, simple buttoning was an acceptable paraphrase for more labor- and material-intensive techniques of pleated tufting.

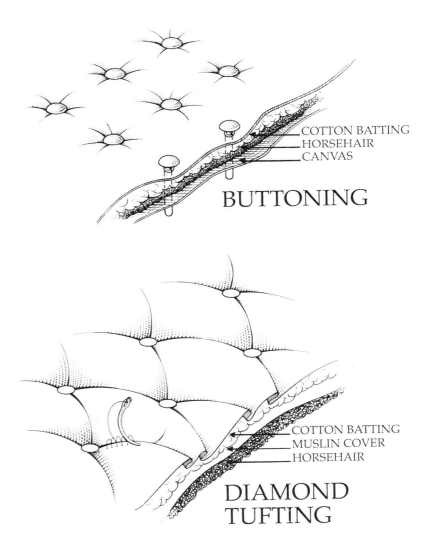

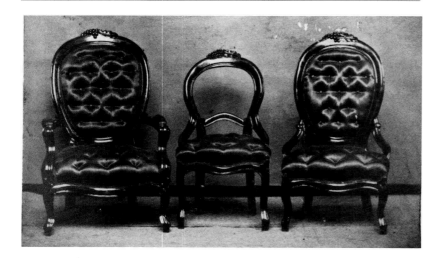

Fig. 30. Chairs from parlor suite with horsehair covers showing simple buttoning, photograph in Descriptive Catalogue of Sofas, Lounges, Tetes, Chairs and Parlor Suits, *Rand and McSherry, Baltimore, Maryland (1872). Courtesy Smithsonian Institution.*

During the first half of the nineteenth century, French upholsterers developed additional methods for building up the padded surfaces of chairs, particularly the vertical ones of seat backs and arms through the use of sewn-in channel and pleated tufting. Pleated tufting contained one final layer of stuffing material, usually cotton, sewn in place in muslin over the stuffing layers above the layer of springs (see fig. 27). The varied forms of pleated tufting broke upholstered surfaces into facets, stuffed and held in place by folding this cotton undercover and buttoning the points of each tuft.

Contrary to its appearance, most pleated tufting was usually not soft, although it contributed to the overall elasticity of a piece of furniture. In America, particularly in the ordinary products of upholstering manufactories, it seems to have been stuffed rigidly full, especially on the vertical surfaces inside chair backs and arms. Thus pleated tufting on many pieces of furniture was as much a contribution to the aesthetic standards that favored complexity as it was a contribution to the physical comfort of a piece of furniture (fig. 31). As late as 1954, the author of one how-to book devoted exclusively to tufted upholstery noted that this was so: "Tufting has a natural tendency to be hard," he wrote, "in spite of the soft appearance it gives."[44] Soft, "sloppy" stuffing was more usually applied to the more expensive upholstered chairs of the 1880s and 1890s and was considered a particularly "French" upholstery characteristic.[45] Unfortunately, it often is difficult to tell how soft or rigid nineteenth-century upholstery was, because the stuffing breaks down over time and springs lose some resiliency.

Judging from the surviving objects and trade catalogs, attitudes about what constituted acceptable parlor seating furniture did change, gradually and unevenly, in the direction of chair types that were traditionally considered informal and comfortable. Parlor rocking chairs became standard components of middle-class parlor suites, and larger-scale, completely upholstered, and less posture-specific furniture, such as the common lounge, became popular. Critics regarded spring-seat furniture, particularly overstuffed "Turkish" pieces, as "dishonest"; the anonymous author of the decorating advice chapters in *How to Build, Furnish and Decorate* (1889), for example, excoriated "luxuriously debilitating puffy sofas and chairs which our ancestors would have scorned." The same author, however, also disliked "stiff, high chairs" and was trying to define some middle ground in furnishing as had the commentators of the previous generation.[46] But the middle ground itself seems to have shifted toward more informal furniture. It is fascinating that this

Fig. 31. Side chair, cherry with carved and gilded decoration, show cover missing, probably United States, about 1875. This chair has lost its decorative cover, but its original structure remains intact, including an example of a stitched edge roll on the back. A pattern of dirt and chalk marks and the button holes on the seat indicate that the chair once had pleated tufting. As a shortcut on cheap furniture, experienced upholsterers sometimes did not sew pleated tufts in muslin before applying the decorative show cover. Rather, they "fingered in" the tufts by sight using the cover material itself. Given the probable use of this chair as a reception or occasional chair, tufting was an aesthetic choice.

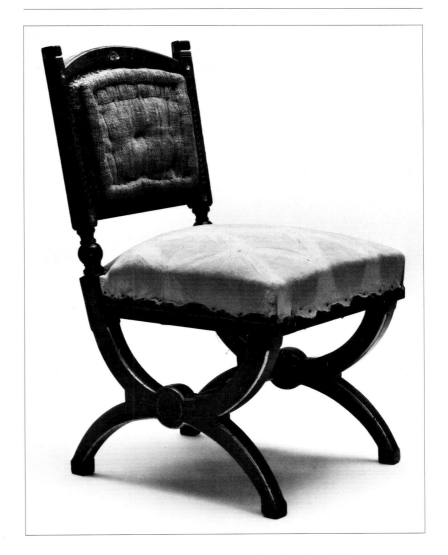

change occurred while the conventions of parlor furnishing and popular thought about the formal social character of parlors, as well as customs of the room's use, seem to have remained unchanged.

In the 1880s, other authors applauded this move toward greater informality and poked fun at traditional standards of deportment. "How to Sit on a Divan" not only offered advice on how to use a new form of household furniture properly, it also offered as an object lesson a proper young woman who attempted to sit perched on the edge of that piece of furniture as her upbringing had suggested she do (and as her clothing probably demanded).[47] In 1883, one commentator even turned the middle-class critique of appropriate domestic comfort on its head by suggesting that furniture, even the beloved rocking chair, had made unfeeling barbarians of our nation's colonial founders:

> The popularity of comfortable furniture, such as this lounge, goes a great deal toward civilizing the people generally. It seems to us impossible for the human race to be good-natured and good tempered if forced to sit in a "bolt upright" position in the extreme corner of a horse-hair covered sofa, with arms and back built on the very straightest and most perpendicular principle... It is not surprising that our forefathers were given to atrocities and

cruelties when they were brought up to endure such tortures as could be inflicted by the furniture of even twenty years ago; it served to deaden the sensibilities.[48]

Throughout the last half of the nineteenth century, the forms of upholstered parlor furniture continued to reflect their jumble of origins—upholstery as a symbol of social and economic power, upholstery as a source of bodily comfort, and the new spring seat as a manifestation of technology's progressive impact on traditional furnishings. Many parlor seats were "elastic," yet their forms did not invite repose. Additionally, some forms of upholstered seating furniture, such as lounges, seemed to invite behavior and deportment that was not acceptable in formal social settings. Even as a slow change in favor of less posture-controlling, larger-scale, and completely upholstered seating furniture occurred, the social restraint of etiquette and the physical restraints of women's full formal dress made "getting comfortable" a complicated proposition.

CHAPTER FIVE
THE QUEST FOR REFINEMENT:
RECONSTRUCTING THE AESTHETICS
OF UPHOLSTERY, 1850-1910

> Our desire is to give some specimens of plain, simple, but substantial furniture, which, by proper and tasteful enrichment of painting, staining or carving, or the addition of hangings, trimmings and embroidery, may be made so rich and elegant in appearance as to stand the test of critical observation and not offend the eye of correct taste.
>
> Henry T. Williams and Mrs. C. S. Jones, *Beautiful Homes* (1878)

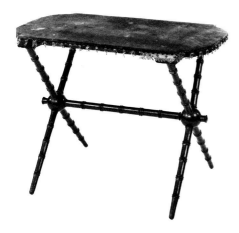

Fig. 1. Upholstered table, walnut, silk plush top with decorative nailing, Charles Drey Polcher, Jr., New York, New York, 1872. According to the surviving bill, the table cost twenty-six dollars. Courtesy Society for the Preservation of New England Antiquities; photograph by J. David Bohl.

Victorians found symbolic meaning in parlor furnishings not only when they displayed an obvious message, as paintings and prints do. They also valued the symbolism of certain formal visual and tactile qualities of objects. The preference for such qualities as intricacy, attributes that even moderately priced upholstery available to middle-class consumers embodied, was linked to real changes in the sensory lives of ordinary people, a new popular appreciation of the act of looking that was itself connected to new technologies of image-making.[1] A mutually reinforcing process of applying meaning to appearances, which in turn strengthened popular preferences for those appearances, took place. This process of meaning-making was self-conscious, time-linked, and cultural, and it can be described and analyzed. It created a constellation of objects, aesthetic preferences, and symbolic meanings centered around the concepts of "refinement" and "cultivation" and reinforced the parlor's role as a ceremonial space.

Even small-scale, "minor" elements of parlor upholstery illustrate what Victorian culture thought was beautiful, and why. Certain kinds of room decorations seem alien to contemporary eyes—fussy, dirty, and useless—yet they were common, clearly were prized, were considered suitable for parlor display, and, finally, were thought to be beautiful. Just as some of the large, important pieces of upholstery typically found in parlors contain levels of elaboration, these small elements also are characterized by a high degree of careful detail. An upholstered table, dating from around 1880, displays attention to detail in both its wooden frame and its upholstery (plate 10). The wood has been turned and carved to imitate the appearance of bamboo, and it has been stained black, or ebonized, to imitate the appearance of ebony. Modern observers would not necessarily understand this double transformation of the wood. Many nineteenth-century observers, however, would have recognized it immediately, because this kind of transforming workmanship was common in the displays of expositions and was much admired.[2] The top of the table seems to have a decorative cover, but the fabric is permanently attached. Cut as a series of lambrequins, it consists of appliquéd layers of silk-pile velvet and wool flannel, with silk stitchery. Tables with fabric tops were sold by fashionable upholsterers in America by the early 1870s; two such tables, one of which can be matched to an 1872 receipt from Charles Drey Polcher, Jr., "late with L. Marcotte and Co.," survive at the Grange in Lincoln, Massachusetts (fig. 1). Instructions for making such tables at home appeared in household art books by the end of that decade, and catalogs offered them as craft "kits" (figs. 2-4).

Sofa cushions, another minor form of room upholstery, also display a high degree of elaboration in their decorative covers. Between 1850 and 1910, they evolved from a state of being stuffed hard (even using materials such as sawdust) to being soft and yielding. Fashions in their covers changed somewhat, but these covers were more notable for being graced by a large amount of devoted and loving needlework elaboration, from Berlin woolwork to embroidery, from appliqué of commercially available fabric "patches" to transfer of photographic images and painting (plate 11). Periodicals that offered decorating advice often suggested novel treatments for cushions, because these could be used to update a room with small expense. Sofa cushions sometimes mirrored upholstery techniques used on parlor seats, as did one sofa cushion design published by *Godey's* in June 1872. The cushion was covered with two tones of blue satin and featured a ruffled border.[3]

A third form of minor upholstery, shelf lambrequins were introduced to American home needleworkers in the early 1850s. Directions published in women's periodicals of the 1850s and 1860s repeatedly introduced such decorated brackets as a European fashion and a popular novelty in Philadelphia and New York; the September 1877 issue of *Peterson's Magazine* informed readers that plain bracket shelves could be "made ornamental" with shelf drapery.[4]

Shelf lambrequins were not a prominent part of a room's

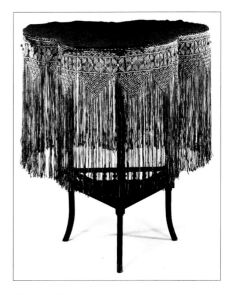

***Fig*. 2.** *Upholstered table, ebonized wood, cotton cloth over wooden top, macramé fringe, United States, 1880-1885. Courtesy Wadsworth Atheneum; gift of Miss Alice and Miss Emma P. Foster.*

***Fig*. 3.** *Upholstered table, engraving in Henry T. Williams and Mrs. C. S. Jones,* Beautiful Homes *(1878). This table was ornamented with a fabric top and lambrequins of cloth "pinked out and ornamented with satin-stitch embroidery," a treatment that made them "very much more elegant."*

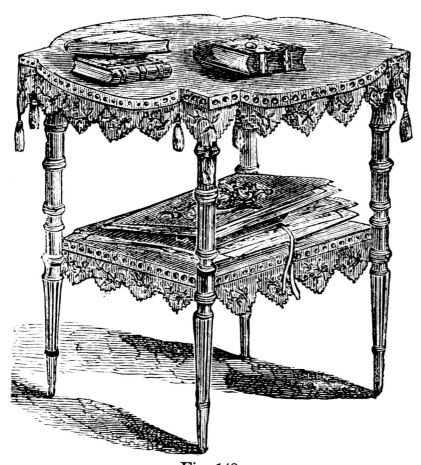

Fig. 142.

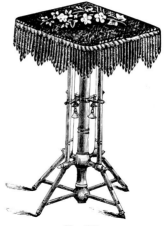

No. 1741.

The above cut, No. 1741, represents a small square Table, covered with plush, and surrounded with a deep tasseled fringe.

The top may be embroidered in plain satin stitch, if intended to hold any heavy object, as a large album, bible, or other book ; but if a more ornamental effect is desired, a branch of sweet briar or cluster of pansies in rococo and chenille will add much to its beauty.   Price for above, all complete, $25.00.

These tables come in round, oval, square, clover leaf, and other shapes.   Prices, in gilt, from $8.00 to 15.00 ; and in black, from $1.50 to 10.00.

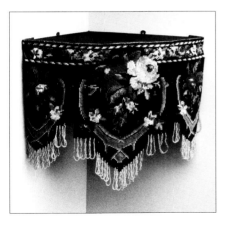

Fig. 5. Bracket shelf with lambrequin, painted wood, Berlin work with glass bead fringe, United States, about 1870. A decorative shelf lambrequin could disguise and embellish a plain or not well-made bracket shelf like this one, making it suitably ornamental for the parlor.

upholstery, yet they were the object of considerable needlework effort and show remarkable complexity (fig. 5). They typically have complex outlines, repeating scallops or small shield shapes.[5] These shapes are like those of window valances (also called lambrequins or pelmets), so shelf drapery was not unrelated to other forms of upholstery.

Shelf lambrequins in needlepoint (Berlin work) often used many colors, which, in combination, created shading and the illusion of three dimensions in the designs. The visual and tactile texture of shelf lambrequins also can be complex, thanks to the combinations of materials and stitching. One otherwise crude-looking lambrequin actually was made with a particularly complicated stitch called the "double Leviathon," which created small textured blocks (fig. 6). The beads and wool and silk yarns in others react to light in different ways (fig. 7; plate 12). Trims finished the edges, added additional contrasting materials, and created complex outlines; fringes of beads or tassels also created interest because they were apt to move, creating variations in light and shadow (see fig. 5). Lambrequins made with other popular needlework techniques such as crochet or macramé offered complex textures and variations of light and shade rendered in one or a few colors (see fig. 7).

Close examination of shelf lambrequins makes it possible to appreciate the amount of detail in a single small lambrequin that appears in a stereograph of a parlor (fig. 8). In the corner above the piano hangs a bracket shelf with a needlework lambrequin, itself only one small component of an extremely complex decorative scheme. A ceramic figure stands on the shelf, and a collection of what appear to be bird feathers is tucked into the space between the shelf and the wall. This small assemblage in "Mrs. L. H. Owen's Room" is an intricate composition in itself, its juxtaposition of elements and materials carefully thought out. The room displays what we might call equivalent levels of detail, because the eye of an onlooker can only take in a finite amount of the detail in the entire room and perceives an equivalent amount of visual information when focusing upon a smaller section of the room. Single objects such as the bracket with lambrequin, the rococo revival chair with needlework

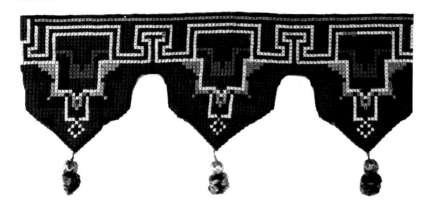

Fig. 6. *Shelf lambrequin, Berlin work with silk tassels, cotton backing, United States, 1870-1880. This lambrequin is embroidered with the "double Leviathon stitch," which was used to create emphatic texture in a geometric grid rather than to follow delicate representational patterns.*

upholstery in the lower left-hand corner, or the "Sleepy Hollow" chair with bun tufting visible in the mirror's reflection offer complex visual experiences for the careful looker. Such objects are arranged in a number of many small, complicated groupings; these are, in turn, orchestrated into one large scheme.

What did the makers and consumers of such visually complex parlor furnishings think about the aesthetic experience such objects provided? How did they describe upholstery, and what did their descriptions signify? What did they *see* when they looked at and selected furnishings for their parlors? Repeatedly, writers of advice books and articles in ladies' magazines, books on the displays at international expositions, and mail-order catalogs employed a particular vocabulary for the appearances of admired examples of "decorative art," including both the large and minor elements of upholstery. Such objects were described as "rich" in appearance, "elaborated," well "finished," "elegant," and "ornamental"; they were praised for their detail, for their "softened" or "softening" effect, and finally for their contribution to the "refinement" of a room.

Both the large and small elements of room upholstery were described with the same vocabulary. In the December 1856 issue of *Peterson's Magazine*, Mrs. Pullen provided instructions for a "whatnot," a hanging half-basket that women could fashion into "one of the most useful and elegant ornaments of the drawing-room" (fig. 9).[6] An 1854 description of the upholstery in the LaPierre Hotel in Philadelphia praised the bridal suite's draperies, "a *rose* red, be it understood, of the most delicate shade, softened still more by the pure transparencies of the lace embroideries falling from the rich canopies above the bed."[7] In 1878, a rustic cornice made from spruce branches and "ornamented with the delicate little spruce

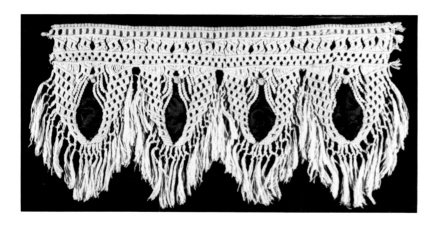

Fig. 7. *Shelf lambrequin, macramé of cotton twine, satin backing, United States, 1870-1890.*

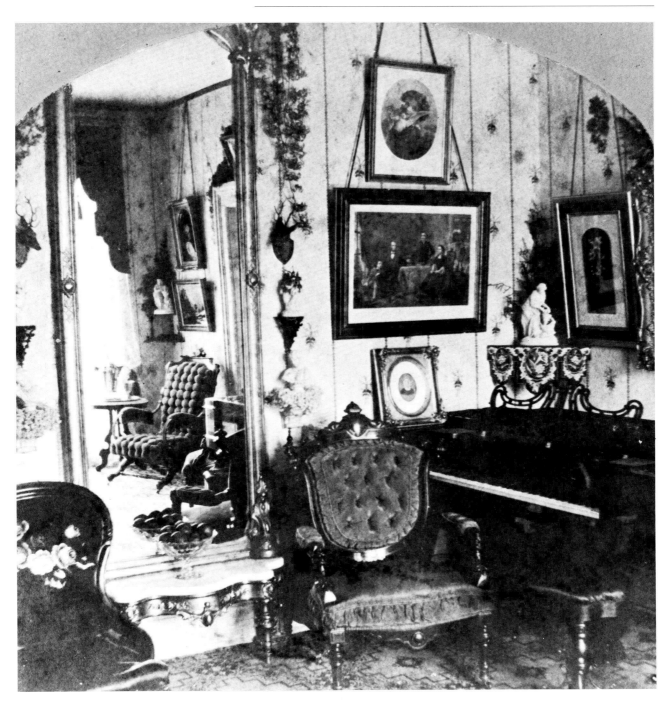

Fig. 8. *"Mrs. L.H. Owen's Room, at Trembley House, Trumansburg,"* stereograph by W.L. Hall, Trumansburg, New York, about 1870. *While the levels of detail visible in this stereograph are remarkable, imagine the additional stimulation of color that is missing in all such views. Courtesy Smithsonian Institution; private collection.*

twigs" was praised for being "complicated in form, and rich in color as some wonderful mosaic" with "the richness and variety of the brown color."[8] The same descriptive vocabulary was still in extensive use after 1900, when the 1908 Sears, Roebuck and Company catalog offered a "Rich Persian Striped Couch Cover," guaranteed "an ornament in any room" for $2.59. Another, available for $3.50, was touted as "one of the heaviest and richest Oriental couch covers ever put on the market."[9]

Even when this specific vocabulary did not appear, a particular technique of description often was employed that implied these qualities. Here each element used in making an object, or each object serving in the composition of a room, was described in careful, realistic detail capable of satisfying the mind's eye of the reader. In such descriptions, the aesthetic standards by which such furnishings were judged are implicit in the levels of detail described and praised. Such descriptions occasionally refer to more than one sensory experience, as the descriptions of hotels and photographers' parlors did: the softening of sound by thick carpets and the visual detail of gorgeous upholstery and gilded wood both were recounted.

By the 1880s, this kind of description reached its apex of elaboration, coincident with the proliferation of upholstery in parlors. The author of "The Best Room. Its Arrangement and Decoration at Moderate Cost," winner of second prize in an 1888 essay competition for amateur decorators who were readers of *The Decorator and Furnisher,* devoted more than fifteen hundred words to a tour of a single room, "a combination of parlor and drawing-room." She offered her readers vivid detail and concluded by employing some of the signal terms applied to prized aesthetic features:

> Diagonally across from the fireplace, the upright piano can stand, pulled out from the wall and covered with a scarf of dark terra-cotta plush…this scarf would be much improved by a design of conventionalized pomegranites and leaves, worked in shades of pink and greens and outlined with gold thread…two small odd-shaped chairs of different designs, one gilded, with a cushion of pale blue plush, the other, with a back of dark wood the cushioned seat in shades of brocaded copper…The windows in the recess should be draped with filmy sash curtains, while from the square frame around them depend heavy rich hangings of dull blue, with a dado of conventionalized flowers and leaves on a ground of old pink…I think now that we have a room which can be fitted up at moderate cost, which is full of soft rich color, and which is pervaded by a general air of comfort, culture and refinement.[10]

Catalog descriptions and images of parlor furniture sold by mail-order firms such as Sears, Roebuck and Company at the turn of the century demonstrate well the popular connection of particular kinds of descriptive language and specific formal qualities in upholstery. Such descriptions frequently call attention to decorative elements in a formulaic, repetitive fashion. Illustrations of every item allow comparison of descriptions with the visual characteristics of pieces in a way that cannot be done in catalogs directed "to the trade" alone; furniture men knew what they were looking at and needed little more than factual information on price lines and decorative options. In comparison, the loaded vocabulary used to sell "refined" furniture to a new group of consumers—newly prosperous rural and small-town Americans—indicates how the process of "educating to ascribe" (teaching people what consumer goods are expressions of desired social and cultural characteristics) proceeded. It also demonstrates how design economics interacted with the preferences of consumers of limited incomes for visual intricacy and with their understanding of "refinement" as manifested in choices about design and materials.[11]

In the 1897 catalog section headed "Princely Parlor Furniture," Sears offered its customers "parlor suits" of from three to six pieces, ranging in price from $18.50 to $47.00, as well as a range of couches, lounges, and "Fancy Stylish Pieces." The upholstery options offered were all factory-made fabrics associated with refinement, machine-woven cotton or silk tapestry, pile fabrics (either "Wilton rug," "crushed plush," or corduroy) or brocaded or damask silks, which

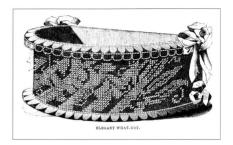

ELEGANT WHAT-NOT.

Fig. 9. "Elegant What-not," engraving in Peterson's Magazine *(December 1856). This whatnot was to be made of cardboard, lined with silk or satin, and decorated with a beaded Berlin work front, cord, tassels, and ribbon. The author of these instructions insisted that increasing the visual intricacy of the piece by quilting the lining was an "elegant improvement."*

represented the top of the line (fig. 10). Most of the suites were free-ranging interpretations of some "Louis" style; several "Turkish" sets represented the design cutting edge of the Sears line. All depended, for their aesthetic effect, on elaborate outlines of their frames, the contrast of fabric and wood profiles, the color and texture of the fabric, and the ways in which the fabric surface was broken up with banding, the use of cords, or tufting. The chair backs of "no. 9505" featured a fantastic design of scrolls, floral ornaments, and a carved crest shaped much like a crown. The shaped back and seat were upholstered "plain," but their shapes were defined by cording and elaborated by the fabric pattern's design. The description vowed that the set was "not only perfect in detail and handsome in outline" but "one of the richest and most stylish appearing parlor suits...of 1897." "No. 9500," a five-piece suit for $11.35, was guaranteed to be "an ornament to any parlor" with its carved back and plain-seat upholstery of tapestry or plush, outlined and broken visually into bands by cording.[12]

Fig. 10. Parlor Suites, engraving in Sears, Roebuck and Co. Catalogue No. 104 *(1897).*

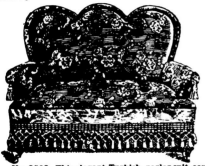 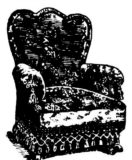 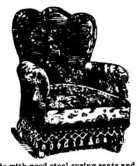 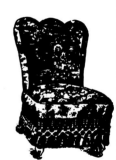
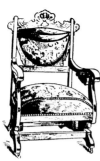 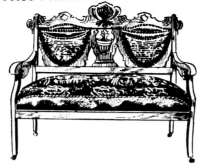 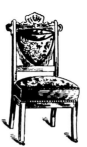

Visual intricacy (attention to detail, ornament, and decoration) signaled cultivation and refinement so much that it supported whole categories of furniture whose function was mostly their contribution to the appearance of the parlor. One such piece was a "Fancy Chair" (the descendant of reception chairs) described in the *Sears, Roebuck and Company Catalogue No. 111* for 1902, "a dainty, odd chair, with neat, graceful lines, made of curly birch, finished a rich mahogany color; back is finely carved and is handsomely covered in silk tapestry, damask or brocatelle. A beautiful parlor decoration " (fig. 11).[13] The caption advertising a five-piece parlor suite (proclaimed to be a $30.00 value available to customers for $15.45) in the same catalog guaranteed that "in every point of appearance attention has been given that no detail shall be overlooked whereby the suite shall be less finished and artistic than it should be… Neither time nor money has been spared in elaborating on the pattern to make it tasty and desirable in every respect." Another suite, "Our Big Five-Piece $20.75 Leader," featured frames that were "beautifully carved, decorated, and ornamented…very highly polished and finished." Guiding the tastes of new consumers, the catalog noted that "the backs of this suite are diamond tufted, as shown in the illustration. This can only be found in the highest grade furniture such as this suite represents."[14]

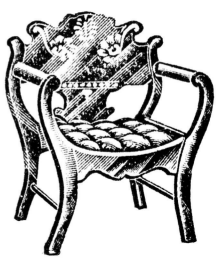

Fig. 11. Fancy chair "No. 1R5455," illustration in Sears, Roebuck and Co. Catalogue No. 111 *(1902).*

Underlying these descriptions of individual pieces of upholstery and of entire parlors are sets of mental constructs resonant in more than one realm of Victorian culture, constructs that are acknowledged in shorthand through this extremely compressed descriptive vocabulary. Some terms applied to evaluate the appearance of things—"refined," "finished," "polished"—are familiar in other kinds of Victorian popular literature that advised readers on other facets of their lives and taught them how to judge the quality of experience—books on etiquette and popular technology, popular histories, didactic sentimental fiction, and the like. Along with the specific terminology, the minuteness of these descriptions is a clue to a set of assumptions about the world—an operating sensibility that valued fine, carefully rendered detail and elaboration of shapes and surfaces. This sensibility also valued a number of other formal characteristics that operated on the senses of hearing and touch but especially upon the dominant sense of sight. These formal features were perceived as expressions of a set of ideals in the world. This sensibility construed these sensory experiences to be analogous to valued processes or activities in a number of other spheres of human action—social behavior and technological change, for example—and therefore applauded their expression wherever it could be found.

What we may call the nineteenth-century "aesthetic of refinement" ("aesthetic" being here defined as the set of guiding constructs for appreciating the world perceived by the senses, rather than the criticism of taste) as it was made manifest in Victorian parlors and in upholstery (and, arguably, in many other kinds of rooms and categories of objects) was not constructed out of thin air. Rather, just as Victorian culture's commercialization of symbols built upon historical precedent, particularly in the commercialization of gentility, some formal qualities of things it valued also emerged from historical traditions. Types of textiles that had once been extremely expensive and rare continued to be prized for upholstery, for example, even though they now could be woven by machine. However, the aesthetic of refinement also ascribed additional meanings to fine things, and it insisted that whole new categories of furnishings, including homemade upholstery, also could be made to demonstrate refinement.

The standards of the aesthetic of refinement employed sets of sophisticated analogies between realms of human activity, as between behavior and the appearance of objects. The "softening of the world" of refined behavior could be symbolically rendered through upholstery and drapery in the parlor. "Refinement" could be rendered visually as attention to and appreciation of detail. Social "polish" was manifested through competence in the use of specialized artifacts and also through ownership of objects that displayed high "finish." "Finish" incorporated the characteristics of smoothness, shine, and ornament, which were expressive of increasing control over materials, just as "finished" or "polished" manners indicated perfect self-control. Finally, all these valued characteristics in the material world and in social behavior were demonstrations of artifice, the techniques of improving natural materials with human skill; thus refinement also implied the treasured and enlightened ideal of progress.

The sensibility that linked these varied aspects of human activity can be reconstructed by analyzing the "semantic taxonomy" of Victorian culture, a language that cut across categories of culture and society not usually directly compared —technology and art, for example, or etiquette and technology.[15] The work of some anthropologists who have examined the relationship of aesthetics to other components of culture provides the model for looking at the Victorian aesthetic in this way. Clifford Geertz has described the work of Robert Faris Thompson among the Yoruba tribe of western Africa, where semantic connections are made between the appearances of things and ideas of the proper nature of all kinds of human action. Yoruba carvers and their audiences consider precise, clean line the foremost aesthetic quality; for the Yoruba culture, Thompson argued, "the vocabulary of linear qualities, which the Yoruba use colloquially and across a range of concerns far broader than sculpture, is nuanced and expressive."

> It is not just their statues, pots, and so on that Yoruba incise with lines, they do the same with their faces. Line, of varying depth, direction, and length, sliced into their cheeks and left to scar over, serves as a means of lineage identification, personal allure, and status expression; and the terminology of the sculptor and of the cicatrix specialist...parallel one another in exact precision. But there is more to it than this. The Yoruba associate line with civilization: "This country has become civilized," literally means, in Yoruba, "this earth has lines upon its face."[16]

The rules applied to the appearance of Victorian decorative arts objects thus arguably have the capacity to express ideas about such "big questions" as the relationship of the human body to the world of the senses (both the "ideal" world and the "real") and the societal constructions of people in that world (again, in both their ideal and real forms). In other words, decorative arts objects as expressions of sensibility may also serve that process of self-measurement and comparison—against other people, a code of morality, a standard of material living—in which people engage more or less consciously, and more or less constantly.

The research of Daniel P. Biebuyck into the arts and rituals of the Lega people of central Africa also links visual qualities and sensibility in another culture and offers a particularly striking demonstration of this connection between the appearance of objects and the way people think about them. Biebuyck deciphers the connections among Lega artistic standards, notions of value in relation to the natural world, conceptions of moral development and ethical value for individuals and whole villages, and a remarkable semantic taxonomy through which the Lega people express the relatedness of these aspects of their culture.[17] Biebuyck's observations center on the importance to Lega culture of *bwami*, a large, many-leveled organization that is a means of teaching the "theory and praxis of a moral philosophy that must produce harmony in social relationships and individual happiness and beatitude."[18]

One fundamental set of concepts that the Lega incorporate in their system of value is the opposition of darkness, ruggedness, and the absence of order versus light, smoothness, and the presence of order and harmony. For example, ivory carvings with a smooth and glossy patina represent the highest level of aesthetic appeal; ceremonial stools are also polished to a high gloss. The highest level of *bwami* initiates is also said to be "smooth." Light-colored and smooth natural objects—white birds, white mushrooms—serve as natural analogs of ivory carving and other such beautiful and pleasing things. New initiates rub themselves with the same oils that are used to polish ivory carvings and thereby express their own developing "smoothness." The semantic taxonomy organizes both significant objects and people in these terms, which refer also to the ideas of unison or harmony in singing (*kukonga*); the related term, *kubongia*, which describes all special objects such as carvings or stools, implies the creation of harmony and unison. Moral, artistic, and natural qualities are thus folded together and expressed in terms that every Lega can "speak" with some degree of competence; *bwami* initiates become more adept than the average Lega over time.

While cultural anthropologists studying the meaning of art forms benefit from the distinct advantage of working with living groups of people, past sensibilities and sensory preferences can be at least partially reconstructed. Art historian Michael Baxandall has recovered some of the cognitive style that Renaissance people brought to bear in their judgments of pictures in the fourteenth century. He does this in two ways—by analyzing some of the practical or social skills that people turned to the purposes of viewing pictures, and by comparing (much as Biebuyck does in reconstructing Lega semantic taxonomy) Renaissance descriptions of the techniques and characteristics of the work of specific artists alongside their surviving works. Thus judgments of quality in pictures were connected to judgments of quality in other areas of life such as hunting or etiquette. In one instance, Baxandall discusses the common use by painters of the Renaissance's highly developed grammar of pious and secular movement and gesture as a means of expressing the mental and spiritual condition of figures in the composition. Orators, popular preachers, and dancers made extensive use of this grammar of motion and gesture to make their points more clear to large crowds. Painters incorporating these gestures into compositions of figures provided the informed members of the public with an additional means of interpreting the meaning of pictures.[19]

As the Renaissance developed language for evaluating the qualities and success of paintings, authors drew upon the descriptive language used to evaluate other aspects of life that were considered worthy of critical judgment: literature, etiquette, the performance of music and dance, and hunting. The same semantic taxonomy described and measured all these things of value. For example, the term *sprezzatura* (which is difficult to translate but was roughly analogous to the ideal of "ease") was associated with favorable judgments of human performance in music, dancing, hunting, etiquette, and painting; laborious displays of skill were to be avoided at all times.[20]

Victorian culture transformed ordinary domestic artifacts into symbols by means of a theory of associations, where a chain of thoughts linked an object, such as a rocking chair, to larger cultural concerns or ideals, such as motherly women and the proper character of family life. The semantic taxonomy organized another level of associations along particular lines. While the rhetoric of middle-class comfort emphasized homey, familial symbolism as appropriate to the formation of character, parlor furnishings were more than simply domestic—they were also worldly. Even while lambrequins, portières, layers of draperies, and fabric-swaddled chairs, tables, mantels, and pianos seemed "cozy," their formal qualities of finish, complexity, and softening could be understood through this taxonomy to express popular understanding of progressing civilization and refinement (fig. 12). Thus they also referred to the world of culture.[21]

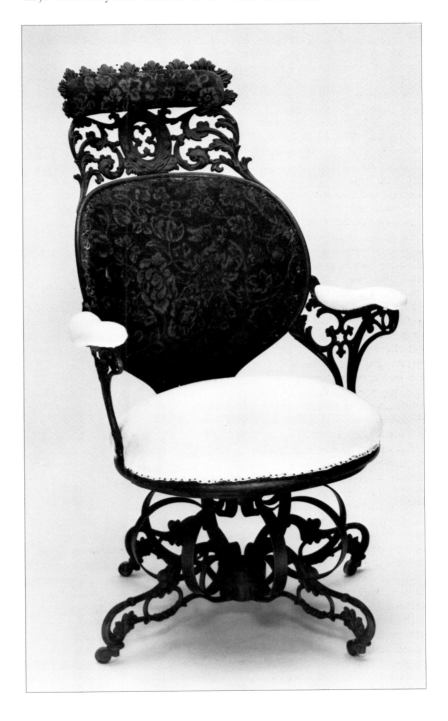

Fig. 12. Centripetal spring chair, cast iron, sheet metal, wood, embossed wool plush, Thomas Warren, American Chair Co., Troy, New York, 1850-1860. An object of admiration at the Crystal Palace, this type of centripetal chair was an example of technological refinement with its patented spring base, molded metal edge to hold the wool plush in place, and ornate cast iron headrest. It also exemplified "refinement" in the elaboration of design elements—the red stamped plush pattern set against the black metal framing and the voids in the cast iron frame.

In concert with a set of related terms—"cultivation," "elegance," "richness," "finish" or "polish," "ornaments" or "ornamental," and others—the concept of "refinement" cut across the boundaries of nineteenth-century thought about individual behavior, the nature of technological and social progress, and the advancement of civilization, which was often conceived in relationship to "progress" in the home. The set of ideas linked together as manifestations of "refinement" seems to have influenced popular aesthetic preferences in household furnishings, because refinement was associated with specific visual and tactile characteristics.

The *Oxford English Dictionary* devotes considerable space to definitions of "refine" and "refinement." Some encompass technological uses such as metallurgy, as in "to free from imperfections or defects; to bring to a more perfect or purer state"; an obsolete French usage of *refin* referred to "fine wool or cloth." Both these uses express the idea of application of technique and labor to the practical arts. By the eighteenth century, the ideas behind "refine" and "refinement" included the concept of progress—"an instance of improvement or advance toward something more refined or perfect," both in the realm of technology and science and in the world of the humanities, as in "to polish or improve (a language, composition, etc.); to make more elegant and cultivated." This concept of improvement and advancement not only encompassed scholarly learning but included a broader notion of personal cultivation—"fineness of feeling, taste, or thought; elegance of manners, culture, polish" (the *Oxford English Dictionary* defines "polish" as being "free from roughness, rudeness, or coarseness"). This grouping of definitions is significant for its conflation of material and social qualities; it also contains the possibility of expressing ideas about moral character in terms of progress. The concept of "refinement" is very much like the association of shine and smoothness in objects and moral perfection in human character that Lega language and culture express. Thus we can think of refinement as suitable for expressing certain key qualities of human action or existence: technical control of materials and resources; control of time for the purposes of improvement; attention to detail; and the development of "fineness of feeling," self-control, and mastery of social forms.

The terms related to "refine" and "refinement" also fold together qualities associated with scientific or technological activities, progress in modes of living, personal development, and the physical characteristics of objects. Of particular interest are the terms "cultivation" and "elegant," or "elegance." "Elegant," which is derived etymologically from the Latin word for 'choosing carefully or skillfully,' refers to both people and artifacts in "refined grace of form; tastefully ornamental," to the broader notion of "modes of life, dwellings and their appointments, refined luxury," as well as to expressions of ingenious technological or scientific problem solving (as in the "elegant solution"). The origin of "cultivate" and "cultivation" is in the Latin *cultivare*, the verb meaning "to till (the ground)." Its primary meanings developed from this Latin source; all refer to the bestowing of "labor and attention" on the land, plants, and animals, with the implied sense of constancy and care in this employment. When "cultivation" was first applied to the notion of "developing, fostering, or improving (of the mind, faculties, etc.) by education and training...refinement," the implication of careful, steady attention to detail remained. Conceptually, although not etymologically, related notions that deserve further explication include "polish," "finish," and "ornament," as well as a handful of other object descriptors. These related terms also express the idea of control, mastery, and what the Victorians might have preferred to call "art" or "artifice" (the display or application of skill).

For ordinary people living in the second half of the nineteenth century, "refinement" was not a matter of reduction to a pure essence but rather a process associated with progress and proliferation. "Refinement" in etiquette was popularly conceived as attention to social detail and the increasing nuances of polite behavior, including competent use of highly specialized domestic artifacts. "Refinement" in the realm of science and the industrial arts was perceived at the popular level as a certain form of progress, the process of perfecting and proliferating the technology and productive activities that increased human comforts and embellished basic needs, especially in the context of the private household (a sort of Victorian version of the *General Electric* appliance advertisements that trumpeted, "Progress is our most important product."). Architecture plan books and "household arts" books of the 1870s and later also expressed the idea that popular interest in the embellishments of domestic interiors generally represented a form of progress. The "Publisher's Preface" to *Our Homes: How to Beautify Them* (1888) noted, "It is not alone the mansions of wealth and luxury which have experienced the results of this decorative advancement, but the humble homes everywhere through the land reveal the beautifying touch of taste and skill."[22]

The question of self-mastery, the personally willed refinement of the individual, is the crux of the conceptions of etiquette and civility over which the Victorians spilled so much ink. No matter how often the authors of etiquette books protested that manners were as much a matter of proper feeling as proper form, the message of the medium of etiquette books was that codifiable form was all.[23] Well into the twentieth century, the real message of most manners books was found in the hundreds of pages of text devoted to renditions of minutely described formal calling rituals, table manners course by course, and the ins and outs of introductions on the street. One author of an inexpensive and popular manual summed up the message of the manners-book medium in this passage, titled "Attention to Small Matters":

> There is nothing, however minute in manners, however insignificant in appearance that does not demand some portion of attention from a well-bred and highly-polished young man or women. An author of no small literary renown, has observed, that several of the minutest habits or acts of some individuals may give sufficient reasons to guess at their temper. The choice of a dress, or even the folding and sealing of a letter, will bespeak the shrew and the scold, the careless and the negligent.[24]

The importance of manners was not simply a question of self-control in the world for the purposes of self-defense and self-presentation. Interest in social polish and the increasing complexity of social relations reflected the nineteenth-century sense that, as one contemporary adviser wrote, "Each successive age, since former periods of barbarity in the dark and feudal times has tended to produce an increased refinement and civilization in this respect."[25]

Complicated manners were an expressive form for individuals to master. They were comparable, in their increasing polish and refinement, to the progress of human civilization, which also was expressed through the increasing complexity and refinement of the material world. In the terms of the prevalent, common-sense belief that the physical environment of the home shaped moral character, refinement in both the appearance of the objects used in the home and in the realm of human relationships also were necessarily linked (fig. 13). Authors arguing for the use of more upholstery in rooms described drapery in the same terms applied to etiquette; center table covers were "a most elegant mode of adornment, giving a sort of grace to what would otherwise appear stiff and awkward."[26]

An enthusiastic sense of American civilization's unstoppable advance through improvements in invention and production methods

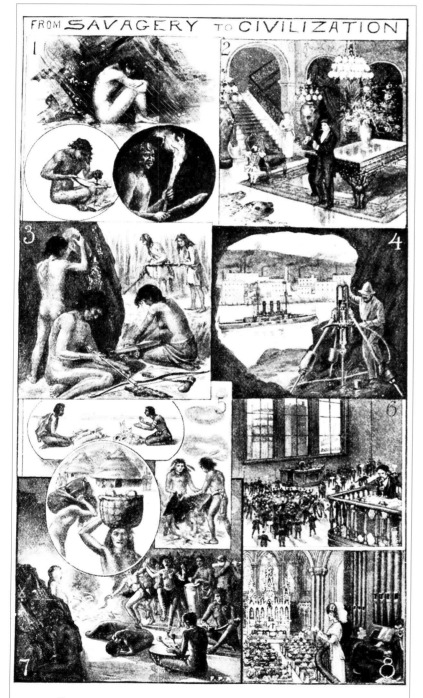

Fig. 13. "*From Savagery to Civilization," frontispiece in William DeHertburn Washington,* Progress and Prosperity *(1911). The frontispiece of Washington's book-length exercise in American boosterism was an ingenious, highly compressed set of visual comparisons with the concept of progressive refinement as its fundamental assumption. In the images of modern life, individuals were more physically comfortable, more expressive, more secure, and capable of a high degree of control over their surroundings. "Progress" also assumed a highly specific tone of greater "refinement" particularly visible in the images of the complex, intricate interiors of the modern home and modern worship.*

and the blessings of economic plenty also led to an equation of "more, and more complicated, things" with refinement in civilization. This belief guided the pen of the "anonymous" author of *Eighty Years' Progress* (published in Hartford, Connecticut, by "L. Stebbins" in 1867), a two-volume compendium and overview of settlement, business, technology, education, art, and "social and domestic life" in the United States between the birth of the republic and 1860. The chapter "Social and Domestic Life" began by documenting the "somewhat uncommonly low average of comfort at the end of the Revolution" and then documented "the general progress of the nation" in the categories of "Domestic Architecture, Furniture, Food, Dress," and "Mental Culture, Intercourse, etc." The general thesis of the chapter was that both the number and ingenuity of new inventions and the proliferation of inexpensive domestic comforts—glass and china, wooden furniture, pianos, less expensive food, and kerosene lighting—all demonstrated "steadfast, and essential, and solid improvement" in the lives of most Americans. The blessings of mechanized weaving technology (the author praised domestic carpet production and the weaving and printing of cotton as a "beautiful" process) were signaled out as improving the quality of life, both in terms of comfort and aesthetic standards.[27]

At about the same time, the author ("An Antiquarian") of a series of eight "lectures" published in the *Household Journal* under the general title, "Our Home: Its History and Progress, with Notices of the Introduction of Domestic Inventions," carried the argument of *Eighty Years' Progress* to its logical extreme. After charting the increasing complexity of and improvements in household architecture, heating and lighting, sanitation, and furnishings, the author declared that "our American home...is the valued result of years of conquest in the realms of commerce and science. It is curious to observe how, in each advancing step, fresh wants were created, which, in their turn, encouraged and accelerated the efforts of science and art as applied to the convenience and embellishments of home."[28] To this author, the progress of civilization led inevitably and suitably to the proliferation and refinement of *things*, especially the objects dedicated to perfecting, through both "convenience and embellishments," the bulwark of republican civilization, the home (figs. 14 and 15).

A related manifestation of refinement in the world of things was a peculiar form of specialization, which had reference both to the world of technology and increasing popular attention to detail in the realm of etiquette. This kind of specialization consisted of creating variations upon common domestic objects with specific, narrowly defined uses. The proliferation of special-use silver flatware and domestic chair types for specific locations and functions (as in "window chairs," "reception chairs," "nursing rockers," "porch rockers," and so on) are only two examples of attempts at analyzing and separating out ("refining") categories of human behavior and providing them with their own supporting artifacts.

In the world of familiar artifacts, the popular understanding of refinement was always progressive and was equated with increasing complexity within each object and with increasing specialization of forms within categories of objects. This set of assumptions figured largely in *The Growth of Industrial Art* (1892), a large government-financed publication arranged and compiled by the Honorable Benjamin Butterworth, U.S. Commissioner of Patents. "Plate 80," "Chairs and Stools," was typical of the book's two hundred full-page plates (fig. 16). The twelve images were arranged chronologically and progressively, from "No. 1," the "Primitive Seat," to the latest patented forms of folding chair. The plate caption, which noted that

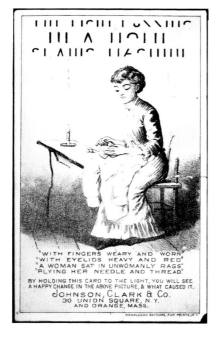 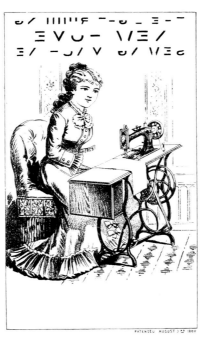

Figs. 14 and 15. Trade card for Johnson, Clark and Co., New York, New York, after August 3, 1880. The seamstress in this puzzle card, whose image appears on both sides, becomes a refined person when the card is held to a light source. Not only does she have less work to do once she owns a Johnson, Clark and Co. sewing machine, but she is materially transformed, dressed in elaborate parlor clothing and seated upon an appropriately softened and finished Turkish-style upholstered chair.

2,596 patents had been granted in the United States for chairs and stools, was also a concise statement of the intellectual assumptions contained in "refinement" as a process naturally associated with all civilizations, even dead ones.

> The Egyptians were among the first to make chairs. On the tombs at Thebes are found representations of almost all the kinds of chairs which modern ingenuity has devised. Thrones, couches, sociables, folding, reclining, lazy back, leather seated, cane seated, split bottomed chairs, with curved backs, sides and legs with claw feet and foot pads, and upholstered with gorgeous coverings. The Egyptians, being an Asiatic race, it is presumable from the squatting posture in their paintings and bas reliefs, that the introduction of the chair came in the progress of refinement.[29]

In upholstery, some of the characteristics that Victorian culture popularly associated with refinement originated with the characteristics of valuable furnishing textiles of the seventeenth and eighteenth centuries.[30] Along with the simple expense of obtaining raw materials such as silk in quantity, the important factor in determining the cost of most fine furnishing fabrics was the skill and amount of labor involved in spinning, dying, and weaving. Tapestry, for example, used readily available woolen yarns, but weaving was extremely time consuming; fine silk damask was more difficult to weave than its woolen counterpart, and the thread cost more. Weaving plain or patterned velvets of wool and silk was also a highly skilled process: the fabric was woven with an extra warp which was raised by means of wires and sheared by hand.

The desirability of the best (and most costly) furnishing textiles, at least those produced in Europe, always involved some calculus of costly and/or finely textured materials and skill in weaving. Expensive textiles for upholstering included one or more of the characteristics of close weaving, complex surfaces (as in brocaded or voided pile fabrics) or very smooth ones (as in silk velvets), elaborate patterns, or additional handwork applied after the weaving process (as in embroidery and other needlework). However, as the terms of

Fig. 16. *"Chairs and Stools," engraving in Benjamin Butterworth,* The Growth of Industrial Art *(1892).*

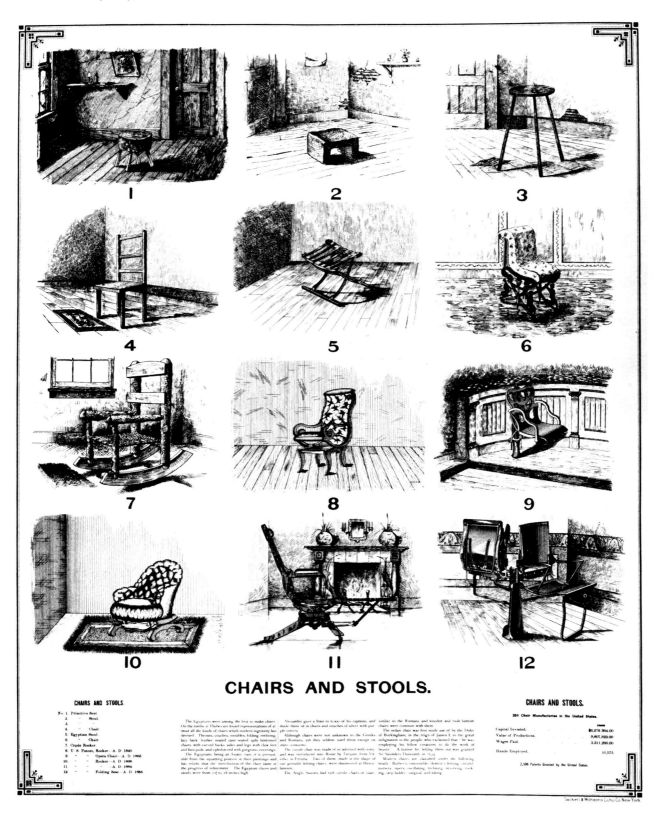

CHAIRS AND STOOLS.

textile production changed in the eighteenth and nineteenth centuries, factory-produced textiles became available that paraphrased the characteristics of what were still expensive, hand-loomed fabrics. For example, nineteenth-century factory-woven mohair pile fabrics such as "Utrecht velvet" or voided cotton velveteens, or "velours," could offer a version of the patterns and pile textures of expensive hand-woven velvets. Factory-made textiles with complicated figures

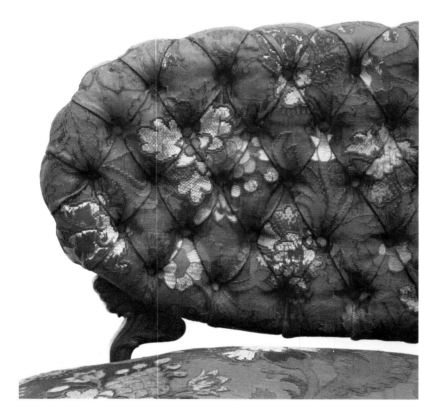

Fig. 17. Detail of fabric on Turkish chair, figured cotton and silk, probably "silk-faced tapestry," 1890-1910. Woven to have a dimensional quality with the figures "embroidered" of silk threads having patterns of their own, this was an inexpensive, "rich" fabric. See chapter 6, fig. 2, for a full view of this chair. Courtesy Grand Rapids Public Museum.

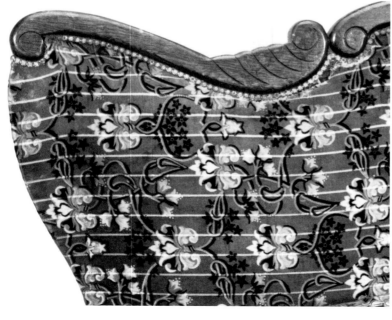

Fig. 18. Detail of voided and printed cotton velvet on Roman divan, 1900-1910. See chapter 7, fig. 20, for a full view of this divan.

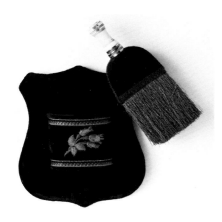

Fig. 19. Upholstered parlor whiskbroom and cover of silk plush and chenille embroidery over cardboard, United States, about 1880. Any object, no matter how utilitarian, could be refined, softened, and introduced to the parlor through the addition of upholstery.

or a high degree of surface texture were still considered as "rich" as their earlier counterparts, but the connection between appearance and cost had been altered (figs. 17 and 18).

The volume of fabrics employed in upholstery was another aesthetic preference with historical roots. The idea of abundance in the use of textiles—the simple ownership and employment of large amounts of yardage—also clearly originated in the historical scarcity of textiles and the association of ownership and display with wealth. Both women's clothing (where dresses might use as much as fifteen yards of fabric) and upholstery, particularly window drapery, demonstrate continuing pleasure in extravagant-looking waterfalls of fabric. Abundance in drapery also meant covering hard surfaces for the purposes of social ceremony and display. In the aesthetic of refinement, abundance and draping developed a new association with "softening," a characteristic associated with civilization's progress.

Along with certain materials, surface characteristics, and the volumes of fabric employed, the best also could be expensive because of the labor-intensiveness of its production and its high degree of workmanship. Workmanship was most visible in the cut of materials, their ornamentation, and elaborate manipulation —the artifice of fine craftsmanship. Many of the new technologies associated with making consumer goods such as upholstery in the nineteenth century partly—but only partly —broke the linkage between elaboration and cost, as when the tufting machine made buttoned surfaces common on cheap furniture. The traditional understanding that elaboration denoted cost was transformed, at the level of popular thought, into an equation between such artifice and expressive value, despite the carping of several generations of domestic and design reformers that cheap artifice was dishonest. Thus, the prized qualities of upholstery were tied into historical traditions, but these associations were elaborated further in ways that reflected the particular preoccupations of Victorian culture, especially its search for evidence of progress in the form of increasing refinement. The more artifice (or elaboration) that existed everywhere in the world, the more progress was manifest (fig. 19).

Covering rough or hard surfaces in association with social ceremony is a furnishing practice with a long history. The medieval noble household was necessarily mobile as the lord kept tabs on large holdings in highly changeable political circumstances. Nobility invested in easily portable forms of furnishing that were also concrete displays of wealth—"plate" (silver and gold vessels and dishes) and other small precious objects, personal garb, and elaborate textiles such as tapestries. These latter formed portable decor and were used to make canopies, cover walls, form platforms and seats or beds of estate, and cover the rough wood of "stepped buffets," shelves that were used to display plate.[31]

The practice of using valuable textiles as loose and temporary furniture covers survived in middle-class households of the seventeenth and eighteenth centuries, when "turkey work" carpets were used as table covers rather than on floors. Even in the nineteenth century, before the arrival of the "Turkish taste" with its use of loose textile covers over couches and other seats, the practice of making rough seats temporarily more ceremonial and refined by covering them with textiles on special occasions may have survived in modest households. In Mrs. C. M. Kirkland's short story "Fashionable and Unfashionable," the rural and untutored (but virtuous) Plummer family prepared its "new frame house" for a homecoming party in honor of the daughter Susan, who had spent the winter with city cousins. In addition to filling spare pitchers with flowers and placing green boughs "here and there,...temporary seats had been formed, the rough material of which was carefully hidden by calico spreads and curtains."[32] Instructions for homemade upholstered furniture that consisted of padded and fully covered wooden boxes and barrels were common in architectural advice books, domestic economy manuals, and instruction guides for household arts beginning in the 1830s.[33]

Furnishing textiles, in their made-up forms, mediated and softened the sensory relationship of the human body to the parlor through the sense of touch, the most fundamental of the "proximate senses."[34] They improved physical comfort when they covered and padded seating surfaces and limited drafts and cold by covering doors, windows, and floors (in the form of carpets). Upholstery also served as a metaphor for the "softening" function of culture. It appealed to the sense of sight and controlled light in the rooms. As

Fig. 20. Cotton tapestry wall covering in dining room of the Voigt House, Grand Rapids, Michigan, about 1907. Courtesy Voigt Collection, Grand Rapids Public Museum.

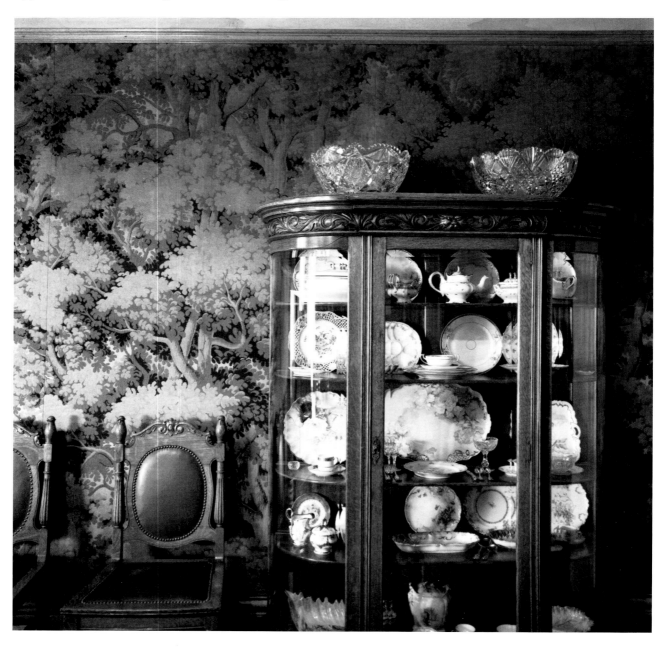

How to Build, Furnish and Decorate advised in 1883, "All that tends to soften too hard and prominent outlines; all that lends distance to effects that would otherwise be harshly and painfully near; all that gives variety and an indescribable charm to the mind and sense, should be cultivated in the fitting up of a drawing-room."[35]

When factory-woven cotton tapestry was moderately priced and readily available from both American and European looms, some houses used it in place of wallpaper. In 1907, the walls of the dining room in the Voigt house in Grand Rapids, Michigan, were hung with such fabric in a pattern of trees in blue, browns, black, and creamy white. Even now, despite subsequent fading, the fabric gives a particular soft quality to light and sound in the room (fig. 20). Upholstery also changed the sensation of space in a room by rounding and blurring the forms of pieces of furniture, by providing contrast to the hard forms of ceramics, metals, glass, and wood. Sometimes textiles were used to create padded walls in high-style rooms or to create "tents" in rooms that reflected exotic "orientalized" taste around the turn of the century. This visual softening seems to have been as important as its tactile counterpart. Softening hard and plain objects by covering them with textiles made them more ceremonial.

Softness also could be more visual than tactile in seating furniture. Upholstery did pad seats, but its softening function was a relative characteristic, especially when the furniture of the 1850s through 1870s is compared to the overstuffed forms of the late nineteenth and early twentieth centuries. The author of *The Practical Upholsterer* (1891) noted that the introduction of "French Work" had led to "a decided revolution…during the past few years," in which parlor furniture was "upholstered very soft" with "very soft 8-inch springs" as well as other stuffing.[36] Never meant to be physically "comfortable," much parlor furniture was instead the highly "controlled" furniture of self-controlled "parlor people," people who understood the refinement of etiquette. Horsehair seating (which could be woven in attractive patterns or dyed in colors and was valued for its sheen, as bright as silk) was hard, springy, and stiff. Mohair plush, one form of "poor man's velvet" of the 1880s and 1890s, had deep pile and held color beautifully, but the pile was quite stiff and could be hot and scratchy.

Drapery that controlled appearances on both sides of windows; table and mantel covers that swaddled and softened furniture outlines that were tactilely and visually harder; and the sophisticated softening of highly controlling seating furniture by means of fabrics having patterns, shine, pile, and rounded profiles or forms of tufting—all these could be read as material analogs to the refinement of civilization (fig. 21). Civilization in turn controlled the world by softening the rough, unrestrained relationships of people through etiquette, especially in the ceremonial realm of the parlor, and by the influences of high culture. "A Greek got his civilization by talking and looking, and in some measure a Parisian may still do it. But we, who live remote from history and monuments, we must read or we must barbarize," one character in William Dean Howells's 1885 novel *The Rise of Silas Lapham* mused. "Once we were softened, if not polished, by religion; but I suspect that the pulpit counts for much less now in civilizing."[37]

Elaboration and visual intricacy were qualities in household furnishings that made manifest refinement and cultivation—fineness of work, ornament, and detail (a high degree of "finish"), visual and tactile richness, and the creation of complex compositions. The visual quality of "finish" incorporated polished smoothness of surface and workmanship that did not reveal itself through any remaining

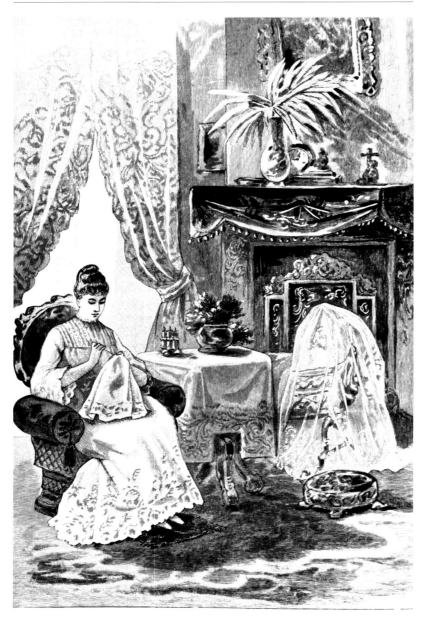

Fig. 21. *Woman sewing in her "softened" parlor, frontispiece of* Art and Needlework *(1889). Because the softening effects of upholstery were gentle influences, rather than demanding and overtly didactic, they also could be read as a particularly "feminine" sensory experience. Textiles already enjoyed an association with the feminine sphere, even if they were the products of professional upholsterers. Courtesy Henry Francis du Pont Winterthur Museum Library; Collection of Printed Books.*

roughness or visible marks left by the craftsman. It was often associated with woodworking, but it could refer to detailing on many kinds of objects. Seamless, effortless-looking but intricate workmanship was the analog of truly refined, polished manners, which were never meant to be awkward or affected.

As a quality associated with furnishing textiles, "richness" had both visual and tactile qualities. Although it could also imply costliness in objects, "richness" was used to describe visual variety and intricacy in many forms. The term was invoked to describe buildings in 1854: "The style of street architecture should be rich rather than classical," declared the editor of *Harper's New Monthly Magazine* in 1854; fifty years later, the term was used in reference to the same qualities in objects such as the "Rich Persian Striped Couch Cover" offered by Sears, Roebuck and Company.[38] In textiles, the typical characteristics of "richness"—physical weight, luxurious surfaces, and deep color—could be reproduced through less expensive means that paraphrased the "rich appearance." *Our Homes: How to Beautify*

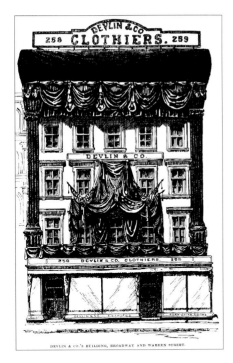

Fig. 22. *"Devlin and Co.'s Building, Broadway and Warren Street" decorated in mourning for Ulysses S. Grant, engraving in* The Decorator and Furnisher *(September 1885). In an article titled "Funeral Decoration," Devlin and Co.'s display was praised for being "beautifully and suitably draped": "A solid, massive band of black concealed the roof line and formed an annex to the frame work of careful and delicate drapery that encompassed the entire structure as if it were a picture." The funeral drapery was praised for its framing and vignetting of the building, in keeping with the aesthetics of window and door draping.*

Them informed its readers that although portières could be made from "rich silks, satins, and damasks, ...a very rich yet cheap material is found in wool blankets dyed any desired color."[39] Richness also described detailed workmanship and visual intricacy no matter how expensive the material, as when Fanny N. Copeland informed the readership of *Peterson's Magazine* that the "effect" of window valances was "made much richer by a fringe, which may be attached to almost every kind of piped valance with a certainty of improvement."[40] The Victor Manufacturing Company of Chicago advertised its "Parlor Suite No. 336" in terms of its richness: "You will observe the rich upholsterings, the back being arranged with bisquit tufting and the front ruffled and buttoned."[41]

Apart from the qualities of the texture or prints on fabrics themselves, furnishing textiles could increase visual complexity through the artifice with which they were cut, sewed, and embellished with fine details. Appreciative observers enjoyed the interplay of folds and shapes and the juxtaposition of drapery with other surfaces below. Even a rapid survey of other decorative uses of textiles—clothing and building draping, for example—indicates an increasing interest in artifice in the employment of fabrics, especially after 1870, and an overarching aesthetic of fabric use that cut across categories (figs. 22-24).

Properly finished ornament, evidence of the progress of craft, was a metaphor for higher levels of civilization. One 1850 *Godey's* article, "A Visit to Henkels' Warerooms," suggested how even a visit to a furniture manufactory could encapsulate the progress of refinement. The author regarded "more florid and ornate" furniture styles "where the *carver* is to decorate and embellish" as "rising higher" than "simple styles of construction." Further developing the connection of "finish" to progress, the anonymous visitor to Henkels' manufactory and warerooms proceeded through the establishment in a sequence that made furniture-making a clear metaphor for civilization's progress and refinement. The visitor passed "hundreds of respectable and temperate artisans, fashioning sumptuous and splendid articles, from their rudest commencement up to the most elaborate decoration and finish." The tour culminated in the arrival at "the saloons, where is displayed the perfected furniture in all its variety of graceful forms, beauty of execution, and delicacy of finish." Having arrived at the "present" in these furniture displays, the author then stopped to admire the fine details of carving in particular, "the hanging foliage, budding flowers and waving scrolls."[42] He showed evidence of his own refinement in his attention to these small niceties.

Increasing accuracy in the rendering of illusionistic, three-dimensional detail on the surfaces of textiles, including carpets, printed fabrics, and needlework, also signaled progressive refinement at the popular level. The author of an article on the "Mosaic Hearth Rug" in *Frank Leslie's Ladies' Gazette of Paris, London, and New York Fashions* remarked, "It is wonderful to what perfection the manufacture of carpets has arrived. First, checks, stripes, and stars were considered wonderful inventions of the loom. Then came flowers trailing over a ground of some positive color...and clusters of fruits were beautifully interwoven in the loom; now we have whole pictures rendered, as with the hand of an artist, perspective foreground, all preserved until one shrinks from treading on anything so perfect" (fig. 25).[43] The trellises, clinging vines, and flower bunches of Victorian wallpapers and printed fabrics probably provided similar pleasures (fig. 26; plates 13 and 14).

Fiction sometimes parodied the taste for naturalistic depiction in carpets and on furniture by making these objects the focus of admiration among characters that were "rubes." *High Life in New*

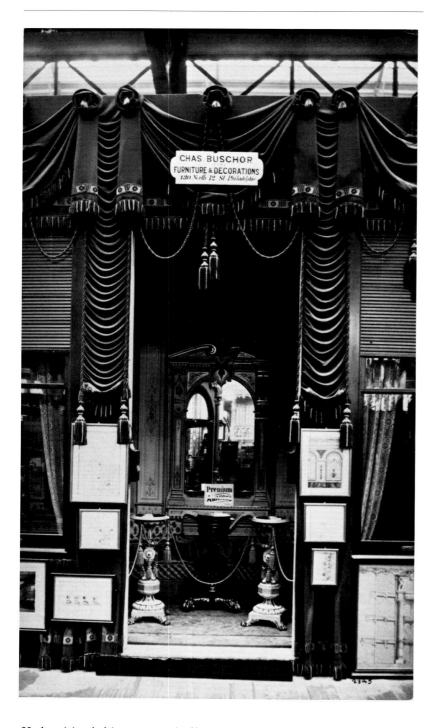

Fig. 23. *Drapery, entrance to exhibit of Charles Buschor, Main Building, Centennial Exhibition, Philadelphia, Pennsylvania, photograph by Centennial Photographic Co., 1876. Buschor was a furniture carver, designer, and decorator who worked in Philadelphia between 1876 and 1886. Courtesy The Free Library of Philadelphia, Print and Picture Department; photograph by Joan Broderick.*

York satirized this presumed affectation when Slick encountered such furnishings as "little square benches,...all kivered over with lambs and rabbits a sleeping among lots of flowers, as nat'ral as life." Slick also admired naturalism in painting. A rooster on a coat of arms was so "Nat'ral, it seems to me, as if I could hear it cockadoodledoo right out."[44]

Design reformers debated whether accurate naturalistic rendering or "conventionalized" (flattened and somewhat abstracted) depiction of design motifs was more advanced and refined. Yet even with the animosity that proponents of the two points of view displayed toward each other, it was simply the terms of progress and refinement that were under debate, not the desirability of increasing progress in design nor the desirability of intricacy itself. Charles Locke Eastlake acknowledged as much when he complained about exactly the kind of popular eye we have been describing. He loved detail as much as any of his peers, but he only approved of certain kinds and believed the characteristics of "elegance" and "richness" were being ascribed to other kinds of details falsely:

> The taste of the public and of the manufacturers has become vitiated from a false notion of what constitutes beauty of form. Every article of upholstery which has a curved outline, no matter of what kind the curve may be, or where it may be applied, is considered "elegant." Complexity of detail, whether in a good or bad style of ornament, is approved as "rich," and with these two conditions of so-styled elegance and richness, the uneducated eye is satisfied.[45]

Ideally, visual complexity was an integral component both of whole rooms and of single objects furnishing those rooms; "Turkish cushions for settees and sofas" were praised for their "rich

Fig. 24. Coffin upholstery, engraving in Illustrated and Descriptive Catalogue of Undertakers' Supplies, *Stolts, Russell and Co., New York, New York (about 1870). As drapery in clothing, building displays, and rooms reached new levels of artifice, so too did the upholstery of coffins. An article in the July 1885* Decorator and Furnisher *entitled "Decoration in Burial" described a display of completely upholstered coffins at the Convention of Undertakers: "A royal purple casket of the heaviest Geneva velvet occupied one side of the apartment and was lined with that delicate shade of cream satin....another of white cashmere, draped in heavy folds, hanging in half moons and caught at every interval with splendid white silk tassels, each draping being trimmed with a narrow silk fringe."*

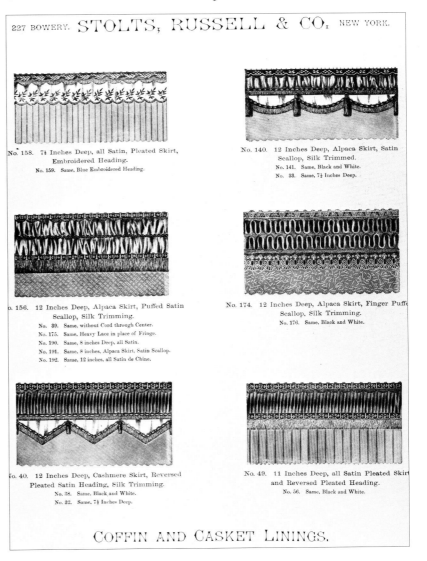

Mosaic Hearth Rug.

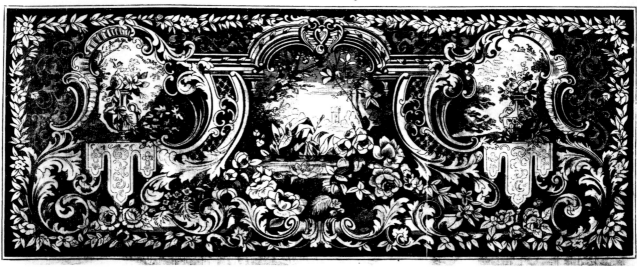

appearance" in an 1891 issue of the *Decorator and Furnisher* because "the details of ornament are very minute."[46] Complex compositions could vary in scale from the entire arrangement of artifacts in a room setting to juxtapositions of materials, techniques, patterns or imagery, and textures within a single artifact, suggesting a general interest in long, careful looking. Consider the exercise of viewing photographs of interiors, from the last quarter of the nineteenth century in particular, as if through a lens of increasing magnification. The same interest in detail and elaboration is expressed in the whole decorative scheme, on the display of a single tabletop, and finally in a single object on that tabletop. "Mrs. L. H. Owen's Room" in Trumansburg, New York, demonstrates such an interest (see fig. 8). Furniture and drapery trimmings and hardware exemplify the level of visual detail given to small components of decorative designs (figs. 27 and 28; plates 15 and 16).

The tenets of the popular aesthetic of refinement implied that a general appreciation of intricate detail was a natural outgrowth of progressive artifice, the mark of the self-controlled and masterful human hand on the rough material of the natural world. If, as the historian Carroll L.V. Meeks suggested in 1956, Victorian picturesque taste laid "consistent emphasis on visual qualities," why might this be so? The character of this set of aesthetic preferences was not, Meeks observed, a simple regurgitation of earlier styles. Through an analysis of the century of American railroad architecture between 1815 and 1914, he argued instead that nineteenth-century art and architecture combined a formal vocabulary of "picturesqueness" with selective restatement of the ornamental vocabulary of past historical styles. The formal qualities of the "special mode of vision" that he christened "picturesque eclecticism" were variations in silhouette and surface treatment; a sense of movement in masses and outline (which often took the form of asymmetry); visual intricacy; and roughness (or emphatic texture). These preferences stood in opposition to the classical preferences of the century before and, to Meeks's mind, were the outgrowth of a larger cultural shift "from reason to sensibility"—that is, the growth of romanticism among intellectuals and artists. At the same time, however, Meeks argued that picturesque eclecticism was so dominant that there was no separate vernacular stream of architecture. "The

Fig. 25. "Mosaic Hearth Rug," engraving in Frank Leslie's Ladies' Gazette of Paris, London, and New York Fashions *(1854).*

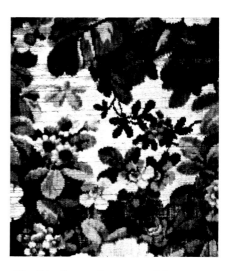

Fig. 26. Carpet fragment with naturalistic design of scattered flowers, wool and cotton, United States, about 1855.

Fig. 27. *"Turkish" fringe, wool, silk, wooden tassel cores, probably United States, 1880-1890.*

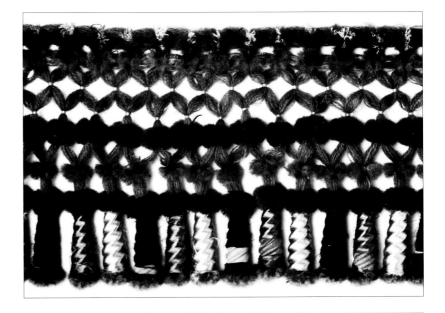

Fig. 28. *"Curtain Poles," engraving in Daniell and Sons Catalogue, Spring and Summer,* New York, New York *(1885).*

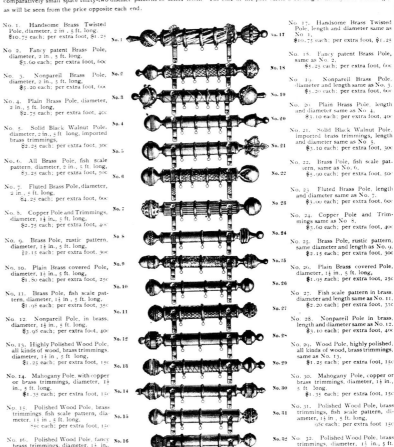

picturesque point of view," he asserted, "dominated all strata of taste and was so universal as to constitute a broadly inclusive system."[47] Meeks's list of the basic characteristics of picturesque eclecticism in architecture can also be applied to analysis of decorative arts objects; the group of shelf lambrequins seems to display some of these five characteristics. Some qualities, asymmetry in particular, can only have a limited application to design of decorative objects that must be balanced in order to function, as a chair or a teapot must. Asymmetry will instead turn up in ornament, for example, or in the design of a chair or lounge back.

Popular enthusiasm for visual detail actually reflected important changes in the sensory life of ordinary people in the nineteenth century. Innovations in the technology of image-making in the nineteenth century introduced people to a new realm of visual detail. Photography showed Victorians how the world "really looked" by rendering enormous detail with apparent impartiality. So did engraving, particularly wood engraving, the inexpensive medium employed by newspapers, periodicals, and trade and mail-order catalogs until the turn of the century. Microscopes, once available only to the wealthy or to dedicated scientific amateurs, became relatively common by 1860. Their revelations of an intricate visual world hitherto unseen were another stimulus to an enthusiasm for detail and ornament.

Mid-nineteenth-century commentators were highly conscious of the proliferation that had occurred in published images, especially in illustrated books and popular periodicals. "A Chapter on Book Illustrations" published in *The Ladies' Repository and Home Magazine* for October 1869 stressed the wonder of this change, which also was a result of the availability of cheaper wood-pulp paper for printing:

> Among the wonders of the day we number the rapidity with which we are favored by the publishers of our own and foreign lands with illustrated works in prose and verse. What a feast for many of us to stroll into one of our large bookstores, just before the Winter holidays, and inspect the choice treasures fresh from the hands of, we might say, the wonder workers! What trophies of the genius, taste, and skill of the nineteenth century—the culmination of ages of patient thought and persevering labor![48]

The lead article in the August 1859 issue of *Godey's* described the technology of engraving for readers and also suggested that the proliferation of images was "the best [method] for diffusing knowledge amongst mankind...the rapidity and cheapness with which an object now can be sketched, engraved, and printed, suggests the possibility of obtaining an instrument for forwarding the improvement of mankind more powerful than the press for printing words."

> Pictures have a great advantage over words, as they convey immediately knowledge to the mind; they are equivalent, in proportion as they approach perfection, to seeing the objects themselves, and are universally comprehended...Not only have the facilities for multiplying designs by means of engraving been instrumental in conveying knowledge through the medium of the eye, but the arts and sciences, in all their varied branches, have been highly indebted thereto.[49]

Wood engraving was the process of choice for most of the popular periodicals and less expensive books because it was easier to execute (therefore cheaper) than steel engraving, and the cut boxwood blocks could easily be added to pages of set type. Its vivid depictions of news events, sentimental or comic illustrations in fiction, and renderings of consumer goods also encouraged the pleasure of looking at detail. Because it is a linear medium, produced by cutting away from a block of boxwood on the end of the grain, wood engraving cannot render tonal variation (as lithography can) except by means of built-up surfaces of lines. Outlines and textures represented by such linear means seem to suggest that the objects depicted are almost "hyper-real," and they invite a certain kind of deep looking. "A Chapter on Book Illustrations" suggested that these qualities were "valuable peculiarities," and that their "brilliancy of effect, a richness and crispness of touch, with gracefulness and freedom of handling [line]" made wood engravings an excellent means of translating the artist's hand into a mass medium, creating a revolution in art for ordinary people.[50]

The second, and ultimately most profound, revolution in seeing in the nineteenth century was the development of photography.[51] Indeed, nineteenth-century photographic images are often astonishing in the amount of detail they render. Daguerreotypes presented what seemed an almost infinite amount of detail, thanks to the slowness of the exposure time, the mirror-like quality of the sensitized plate that received the image, and the fact that the image was not enlarged in developing (in other words, it lost none of its resolution). Stereographic views, especially those from the first few decades of the process, were also cherished for the minuteness of their detail, the worlds contained in their images. Oliver Wendell Holmes's 1859 essay, "The Stereoscope and the Stereograph," articulated the delights of long, thoughtful looking through a stereopticon, a visual form of loitering:

> This is one infinite charm of the photographic delineation. Theoretically, a perfect photograph is absolutely inexhaustible. In a picture you can find nothing which the artist has not seen before you; but in a perfect photograph there will be as many beauties lurking, unobserved, as there are flowers that blush unseen in forest and meadows. It is a mistake to suppose one knows a stereoscopic picture when he has studied it a hundred times by the aid of the best of our common instruments.[52]

Where might evidence be found to support these speculations on increasing visual acuity among common people in the nineteenth century? The diaries and letters of ordinary people living in the nineteenth century say little about their aesthetic preferences. Objects typically provide what Baxandall has described as "complex non-verbal stimulations" that are rarely articulated, much less preserved in letters and journals.[53] Many official accounts of the various expositions provide lengthy descriptions of many decorative arts objects, but their authors tend to be highly trained observers with a distinct aesthetic point of view. Other kinds of descriptions of visual phenomena, those written by popular journalists, are more useful in an effort to reconstruct ordinary seeing. For example, an anonymously authored history of the Brooklyn and Long Island Fair, held to aid the United States Sanitary Commission in February 1864, offered descriptions of some of the textile displays, which found favor because of their great variety and the abundance of visual stimulation they offered (fig. 29). Of the Berlin work (the "worsted department"), the author noted,

This was one of the most interesting, as it was naturally one of the

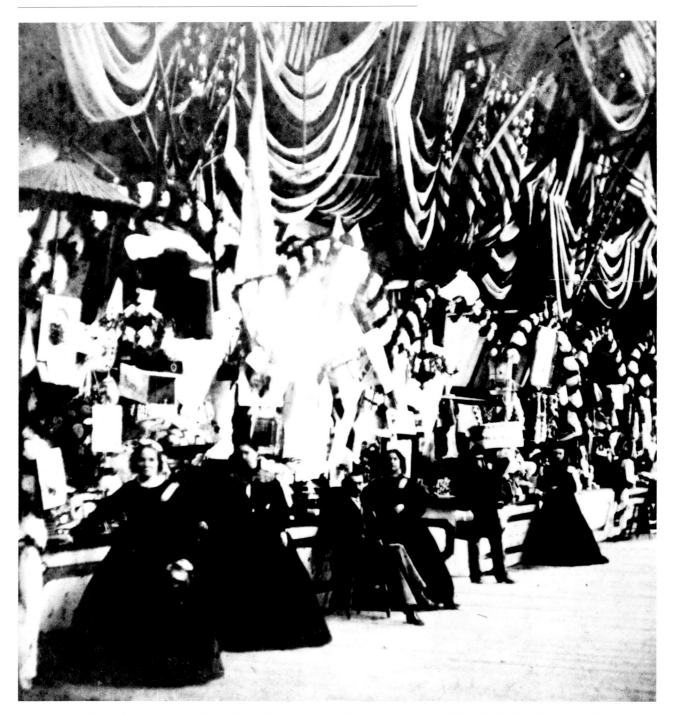

most brilliant departments of the fair…The richness, vividness, and variety of the articles which heaped the tables, fluttered from the pillars, or glowed from the walls, gave one the impression of a bevy of rainbows playing hide and seek in the room.[54]

Fig. 29. Ladies' fancywork, display at the Philadelphia Sanitary Fair, stereograph photographed and published by James Cremer, 1864. Courtesy Smithsonian Institution; private collection.

A hanging display of throws and bedspreads, seen from below, "presented a spectacle of wonderful brilliancy, completely tapestried as it was with afghans, quilts, and spreads, of the most vivid colors."[55]

Decorating advice literature sometimes offers not just deep description of the contents of successful rooms but clues to the ideal experience of looking at them as well. *How to Build, Furnish and Decorate* described the parlor, the room most devoted to culture and the richest in the possibilities it offered for refined looking:

> And now let the reader take a rapid survey of the drawing room here theoretically furnished. The door is flung open, and he crosses the cool Chinese matting, and steps upon the velvety pile or Persian carpet…The walls, mirrors, seats and pictures seem to form one continuous, harmonious, though varied, panorama of pleasing forms and colors, mingling and contrasting. The pieces of furniture are not instantly received on the retina of the eye as so many inky blotches on a white wall; but slowly, and as the eye becomes accustomed to the room, one by one the different parts are unfolded. Bits of color, unobserved at first, starlike appear…the room [is] the more enjoyed the more occupied.[56]

Deciphering the aesthetic of refinement as it applied to upholstery suggests that the consideration of formal aesthetic content is retained properly within broader discussions about how people create meaning. In the case of Victorian culture, we can, through such means as the study of popular texts, find broad areas of cultural concern that shape the forms of association and meaning people bring to those objects they consider important.[57] If the modes in which the ideals of refinement were expressed seem redundant, that is because cultures never communicate important messages once. Whatever important messages Victorian furnishings carry are repeated many times elsewhere, through many vehicles.[58]

All analyses of material culture are plagued to some degree by one question: how are we to know the extent to which makers and users of artifacts themselves understood the levels of meaning that historical analysis now ascribes to what remains of their material culture? How, for example, can we know that a parlor maker who chose to drape every flat surface or opening into a room with elaborately cut, patterned, and embellished textiles *knew*, even if only tacitly, that these furnishing choices were symbolic analogs of parlor etiquette? In truth, we often cannot know such a thing with absolute certainty. What we can do is to map the terrain of plausible meaning, chart what a motivated individual who is not a specialist could know, and speculate how participation in his or her culture's sensibility was possible. Thus the concept of taste in any facet of cultural expression itself is largely a product of a matching process. While one individual may be able to appreciate a visual experience in certain ways, another, having a different degree of formal and informal training, will "see things another way," so to speak.[59] Both individuals are operating within the range of visual cognition of their culture. Not every participant in Victorian culture was equally fluent in, or personally comfortable with, the use of the full range of visual discriminations and their cultural analogs from other spheres of activity. It is clear that popular literature in many forms made a concerted effort to educate its readership in these connections. Such variation among people constitutes levels of competence in making aesthetic discriminations. It is in part a demonstration of artifactual competence, one's ability to employ artifacts for the purposes of communication and to appreciate the levels of information contained in their appearance and use. Some Victorian consumers found rich nuanced levels of meaning in their possessions; others brought less to the experience of owning and using goods.

Objects that present a particular form of play on visual qualities—visual punning—support the notion that visual sophistication was increasing on the part of the public (fig.30). The

CLEVELAND UPHOLSTERING COMPANY,

WHOLESALE MANUFACTURERS OF
~ UPHOLSTERED FURNITURE, ~

LOUNGES, COUCHES, EASY CHAIRS, ROCKERS &C.

130 RIVER STREET,   **CLEVELAND, OHIO.**

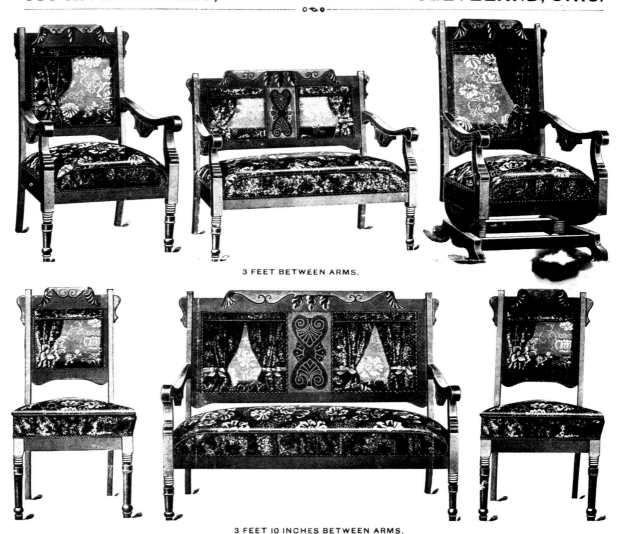

3 FEET BETWEEN ARMS.

3 FEET 10 INCHES BETWEEN ARMS.

═══════ NO. 61 ═══════

JUST OUT—OUR NEW CURTAIN BACK SUIT.

THE BEST Suit on the market for the money. Six Pieces Silk Tapestry, assorted colors, trimmed with fine silk plush, spring edges. Sixteenth Century or Antique Oak, polish finish, workmanship and finish guaranteed first-class. Send for sample of Tapestry. Price $37.50. Terms 2 per cent. 10 days—60 days net.

Fig. 30. "Just Out—Our New Curtain Back Suit," broadside for Cleveland Upholstering Company, Cleveland, Ohio, about 1890.

assumption behind such plays on visual qualities, such as *trompe l'oeil* effects on painted curtain papers, is that the observer understands what relationship the visual pun has to the thing after which it is modeled. It is doubtful that anyone who purchased a set of window shades painted with a design of cornice, draperies, and lace curtains believed that those shades were the real thing. Rather, they constituted a visual pun on that "real thing," an expression of possibilities and participation in the refined aesthetic.[60]

Elaborately decorated domestic objects made of atypical materials—tours de force or "plays" on technological skill—were popular exhibition items at all the expositions beginning with the Crystal Palace—bedsteads of papier-mâché, tables of glass, and the like.[61] Generic household goods that contain sophisticated visual play, as does the ebonized and faux bamboo upholstered table (see plate 10), proliferated in the second half of the nineteenth century and seem to have been appreciated by ordinary people (fig. 31). Some visual play originated with elite taste; the decorators of the French Empire particularly delighted in rooms hung as tents and drapery appearing to be supported by spears. Interpretations of this level of wit in furnishing were made popular by the second half of the nineteenth century. An article on draperies which appeared both in *Godey's Lady's Book* and *Peterson's Magazine* around 1860 introduced one such pun, a "novel and pleasing effect" in which "the drapery appears to be supported by a rope instead of a cornice" (fig. 32).[62] A suggestion for a single sofa cushion appearing in the March 1888 issue of *The Decorator and Furnisher* described another typical visual pun that also reflected the infatuation with intricacy—"a Sofa Cushion covered with wine-colored plush, one side of cover turned back, revealing a gorgeous bit of striped embroidery in gold and silk."[63]

The popular aesthetic of refinement thus received some of its most sophisticated statements in artifacts where the visual message was not strictly formal but also referred to other ordinary objects (always using the aesthetic of refinement) in the form of visual punning or play. If these kinds of upholstery were common, they rarely survive. Perhaps they seemed too extreme in their artificiality and inexplicable to the simplified, "modern" popular eye of the 1930s and later. Understanding the pun behind such objects affirmed their sophistication to adherents of this aesthetic and afforded them a pleasure that is difficult to reconstitute and understand now. Perhaps Marcel Duchamp's statement about the lifespan of his own art is pertinent in trying to understand the aesthetics of objects made in eras other than our own: "No painting has an active life of more than thirty or forty years—that's another little idea of mine. I don't care if it's true, it helps me to make that

Fig. 31. Lounge with cotton chenille cover woven to look like a tigerskin, engraving in 1890 Catalogue for the Buffalo Upholstery Co., Buffalo, New York.

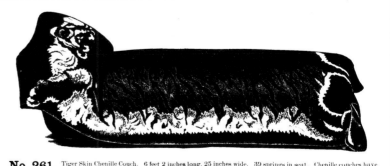

No. 261. Tiger Skin Chenille Couch. 6 feet 2 inches long, 25 inches wide. 39 springs in seat. Chenille couches have spring edges.

distinction between living art and art history. After thirty or forty years the painting dies, loses its aura, its emanation, whatever you want to call it. And then it is either forgotten, or else it enters into the purgatory of art history."[64] The Victorian aesthetic of refinement can never be experienced again as a living idea, but explorations into the language associated with decorative objects such as upholstery can at least partially reconstruct its dimensions and meaning and give us some sense of its power.

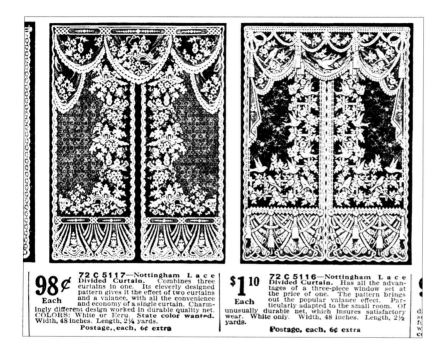

Fig. 32. Panel curtains, illustration in Montgomery Ward and Co. Catalogue No. 97, Fall and Winter *(1922-1923). More than sixty years after Fanny Copeland's drapery pun, and at the level of popular taste, curtains that were "puns" continued to be offered. Panel curtains 72C5117 and 72C5116 were one-piece lace curtains woven to have a "valance effect." The latter had tassels woven into its design.*

CHAPTER SIX
COMFORT AND GLITTER:
POPULAR TASTE FOR FRENCH AND
TURKISH UPHOLSTERY, 1875-1910

Taste, there can be little doubt, depends, in a great measure, upon association. We can account for it often on no other grounds. Our tastes and distastes proceed, for the most part, from the power that objects have to recall other ideas to the mind. And persons of superior cultivation have not only established for themselves a higher standard of grace or excellence, to which they refer, but they have attained to a quicker perception of the relation of things to each other. They trace the connexion immediately, and, as it were, intuitively; and they at once distinguish between what is allied to elegance, and what is, in however remote a degree, connected with everything displeasing or vulgar.

Emily Thornwell, *The Ladies'*
Guide to Perfect Gentility (1856)

"French" and "Turkish" upholstery, the two most popular styles of the waning quarter of the nineteenth century and first decade of the twentieth, demonstrate the "power that objects have to recall other ideas to the mind," as Thornwell put it. They also illustrate the relationship and meaning of form and style in parlor upholstery, as such qualities were popularly understood. The forms of French and Turkish seating furniture are, respectively, emblems of the gala apartment's social facade and the developing understanding of comfort as bodily relaxation (figs. 1 and 2). "Turkish" upholstery, in

Fig. 1. Tête-à-tête, mahogany, brocaded satin, Parkersburg Upholstering Company, Parkersburg, Virginia, about 1900. This settee, typical of moderately priced French-style furniture of the late nineteenth century, interprets the curving shapes and some details of Louis XV (rococo) design (such as the shell in the center of the crest rail), yet it has very little expensive carving on the frame. Confining the upholstery to the seat and a small panel also made the tête relatively inexpensive to produce. Courtesy Smithsonian Institution; photograph by Jeff Tinsley.

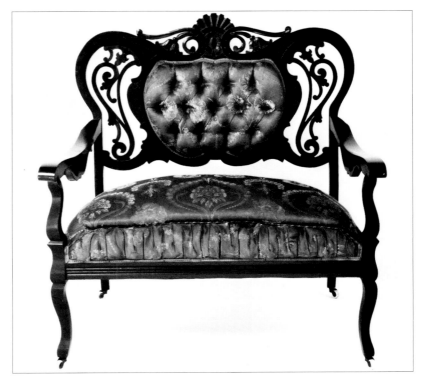

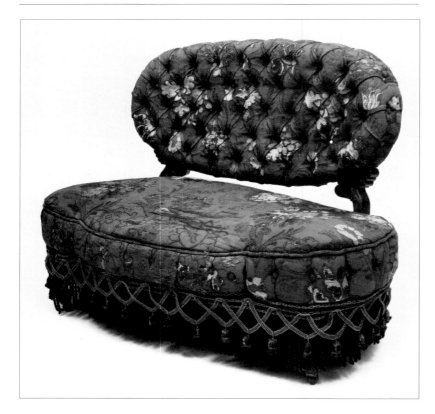

Fig. 2. *"Turkish" tête-à-tête or settee, walnut, cotton and silk tapestry, metallic ("tinsel") threads, cotton, wool, and silk trim with wire core, probably Grand Rapids, Michigan, about 1900. Fig. 17 in chapter 5 is a detail of the fabric covering this settee. Courtesy Grand Rapids Public Museum.*

the form of overstuffed seating furniture, also offers a preview of the typical forms of upholstery found in the living room of the twentieth century.

Victorian decorative objects can be characterized as belonging to the overarching aesthetic that found refinement in detail, finish, and elaboration. However, an examination of Victorian sources indicates that writers of both furnishing advice and of captions in trade and mail-order catalogs assumed readers to be, or to want to be, aware of other sets of visual distinctions (figs. 3 and 4). These constituted "style," a coherent set of options for proportion, arrangements of components, and ornamentation. Not only did proportion and arrangements of elements in architecture and furnishings distinguish styles, but the kinds of ornamentation, mostly derived from historical sources, also expressed them. Popular periodicals freely used the names of the various historical styles that proliferated after 1850, which suggests their assumption that readers knew at least a little about them. In a typical instance, an 1877 newspaper article from the Yonkers *Statesman* described the facade of the new house of John B. Trevor as "French," its library as "Queen Anne," and its dining room as "Gothic in style, Eastlake in character."[1]

The materials used to make upholstered furnishings set distinctive limits on the ways in which style is expressed. In much of the upholstered seating furniture of the period from 1875 to 1910, for example, the wooden frame carried a great deal of information. Historical style also was displayed through the use of appropriate fabrics, or through the colors and pattern (printed, woven, or applied to the fabric surface) of upholstery fabrics (fig. 5). Upholstery that was popularly considered "French" at the end of the nineteenth century consisted of a few specific types of fabric, such as silk damask. It used a palette of pastel colors and was ornamented with a narrow range of images. "French" scrolls, bowknots, and flower garlands, however, could be applied to any type of fabric (fig. 6).

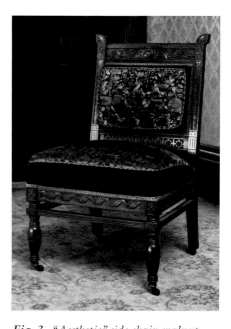

Fig. 3. *"Aesthetic" side chair, walnut, silk damask and silk-pile velvet, wool and silk trim, probably United States, about 1880. This chair was originally part of a suite; four other chairs from the suite still survive. Courtesy Voigt Collection, Grand Rapids Public Museum.*

Fig. 4. *"Colonial" armchair, mahogany and voided cotton plush, United States, about 1910. These chairs (figs. 1-4) would have been understood as belonging to distinct styles—"French," "Turkish," "aesthetic," and "colonial," although this last chair is an interpretation of early nineteenth-century neoclassical furniture. All four chairs are similar, however, in that their upholstery and carved frames create complex compositions of solids and voids, hard and soft surfaces, and smooth and rough textures. All express the interest in elaboration characteristic of the popular aesthetic of refinement.*

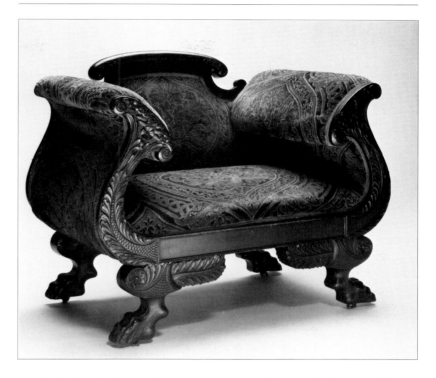

Style in upholstery also can be expressed through the ways fabrics and trims are cut and sewed in drapery and the way fabrics, trims, and stuffing are applied to structures. Sometimes the form upholstery takes on a chair—rounded and curving, stuffed tightly and stitched to have squared edges, having flat planes for surfaces or highly dimensional ones through the use of tufting or binding with cord—seemed to transmit information about "style" regardless of the fabric employed. In the late nineteenth century, overstuffed furniture was "Turkish" no matter what fabrics covered it.

Sometimes upholstery techniques carried loose style cues. Pleated tufting, which had both structural and aesthetic functions, was associated with French upholstery style—rightly so because it was a French innovation. Rococo and Renaissance revival furniture often seemed bald and less finished without the embellishment of tufting, particularly on seat backs. In the late 1860s and 1870s, when English design reformers offered rectilinear furniture as an alternative to curvaceous French chair design, they also turned to flat upholstered surfaces as suitable to such chair frames. Sensing a continued demand for ornament, however, American manufacturers of cheap upholstered furniture made these plain surfaces richer in appearance by adapting other techniques employed on French-style furniture, such as using more than one fabric and contrasting trims (plate 16). Tufting, which could hardly have been thought a "reform," was nonetheless considered more refined and desirable than flat upholstered surfaces. And furniture manufacturers, including shops producing high-quality custom work, almost immediately began to combine "reform" chair frames and "French" upholstery techniques (fig. 7).[2]

Thus the concept of rigorously defined "style" in upholstery is laden with caveats. Still, certain combinations of all these elements—fabric types, colors and designs on fabrics, and specific forms of drapery and upholstered furniture—seemed to signify distinct things to consumers. Most likely, not all consumers understood and employed these elements with equal fluency and

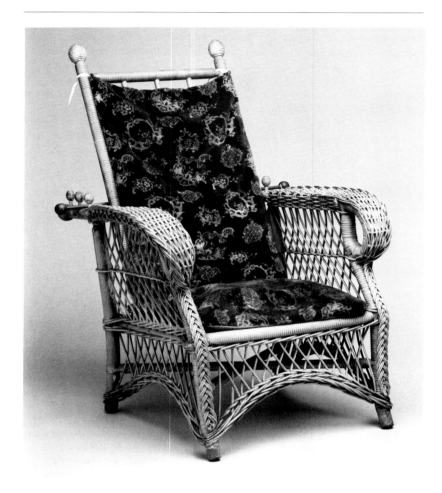

Fig. 5. Child's adjustable ("Morris") chair, wicker and cotton velveteen, Wakefield and Company, Gardner, Massachusetts, about 1900. The cotton velveteen on this chair is printed with flower sprigs interspersed with asymmetrical motifs consisting of c- and s-scrolls; the surrounding fields simulate lace netting.

pleasure, just as many were unconscious of the rich meanings underlying the aesthetic of refinement. But for motivated parlor makers, style in upholstery was yet another way of embellishing statements of social identity through parlor furnishings.

In the first decades of the new republic, the houses of upper middle class mercantile and professional men in America's coastal cities or among the planter elites continued to reflect a genteel, non-domestic conception of the parlor as a setting for the display of personal cultivation, with the "select company" as its appropriate occupants. The spaces such elites created for socializing often reflected their interest in French fashion and culture, partly a consequence of contact with the French fleet's officers between 1780 and 1782. The Swan and Morton families of Boston, for example, surrounded themselves with French books, paintings and "philosophical instruments"; after the French Revolution, they were able to export royal furnishings for their houses. The furnishings particularly of the "saloon" (drawing room) and dining room of the Swan family's country house, built in 1796, demonstrate the early version of the aristocratic parlor ideal. These rooms were "furnished with elegant furniture brought from France, consisting of large armchairs, heavily gilt andirons, beautiful blue and gold vases, while on the walls were rare and valuable French pictures."[3]

The French influence on American furnishings forms a continuous thread in nineteenth- and early twentieth-century decor. Even when various trends in design reform offered attractive and successful alternatives, large groups of consumers continued to gravitate toward parlor furnishings that they understood as "French."

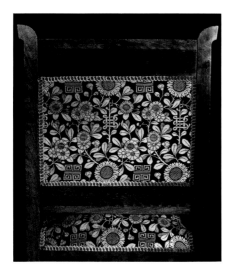

Fig. 6. *Back of side chair in fig. 3 showing black-and-gold silk damask. The seat and back of this chair were covered with fabric featuring conventionalized sunflowers, one of the most characteristic motifs of "aesthetic" design of the 1870s and 1880s. However, the upholsterer had no qualms about breaking up the pattern to the point of illegibility on the back rest, where pleated tufting serves purely aesthetic purposes. Courtesy Voigt Collection, Grand Rapids Public Museum.*

At midcentury, French style provided the most fashionable models for parlor makers with aspirations toward gentility, whether it was called the "French Renaissance," rococo revival, what interior decorators and furniture manufacturers called the "Louis Quatorze," "Louis Quinze" (rococo), or "Louis Seize," or the various hybrids sarcastically labeled by wags as "Louis d-Hotel" (fig. 8).

Information about new French furnishings could be gleaned from a variety of sources, including foreign periodicals of design directed to the furnishing trades; the goods imported by enterprising retailers; and émigré French decorators and craftspeople. According to Kenneth Ames, the French-inspired designs of nineteenth-century Philadelphia furniture manufacturer and dealer George Henkels relied upon French periodicals and other publications about furnishings, particularly those by Desire Guilmard, and upon imported furniture from prominent French manufacturers, which Henkels also offered for sale.[4] An 1850s Henkels ad informed readers that "George J. Henkels, No. 173 Chestnut Street, has just received from Paris, several suits of Splendid Paris Furniture, in Rosewood, for Drawing Rooms. Also a full assortment of the most elegant embroidered brocatelles. The richest goods ever imported into the country."[5]

Well-to-do Americans often received an appropriate dose of French furnishing tastes through contact with French émigré decorators. In 1856, gun manufacturer Samuel Colt commissioned Ringuet-LePrince and Marcotte, a decorating firm with offices and workrooms in both New York and Paris, to provide furnishings for Armsmear, his new Hartford, Connecticut, house. Some of the pieces Colt bought were American in origin; other furnishings were imported directly from Paris. The fabrics used for hangings throughout the house probably were imports as well.[6] Wealthier Americans could also gather ideas on French style and purchase objects for their household in their travels. In France in 1884, the Codman family purchased a quantity of French furniture, including two overstuffed "Turkish" chairs, one scaled for a child (figs. 9-12).

All these contacts had many specific, visible effects on American taste. For example, French émigré decorators seem to have reintroduced American consumers to the decorative slipcover, which could be used to refresh the appearance of a room periodically with less expense than replacing attached covers.[7] Such covers, in cretonne and later in various chintzes and cotton toiles, were a dramatic departure from the ghostly linen or blue-striped ticking covers most housekeepers had employed as a way to protect good upholstery. Until the early twentieth century, most American housekeepers continued to use slipcovers mainly as protective sheaths for valuable upholstery rather than as decoration; at that time, they also gained some currency as a sanitary form of upholstery.[8]

By the 1850s, French design seems to have dominated production of middle class furniture, at least in urban settings, and was the style of choice for what *Godey's* in 1850 had called the "modern" parlor (fig. 13). The commercial parlors of hotels and steamboats, whose French-inspired interiors offered aspiring parlor makers versions of the gala apartments of the best families, encouraged and sustained American fascination with these styles. Consumers with modest budgets could carry the style into their parlors through less expensive American-made knock-offs of French designs available in such warerooms as Henkels' Philadelphia establishment and its less pretentious contemporaries. The era's rococo revival was popular partly because it supported and coincided with the new taste for making parlors that reflected aspirations toward parlor gentility. Design elements understood as "French" could be, and were, incorporated into the products of furniture makers located

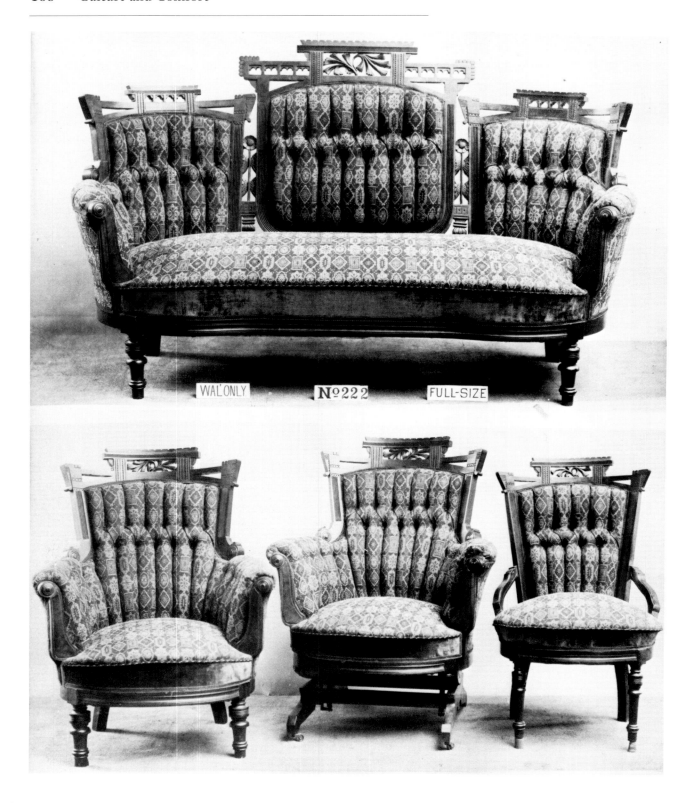

Fig. 7. Parlor suite No. 222, photograph in advertising mailer for H. H. Shrenkeisen and Co., New York, New York, 1880-1885. This parlor suite combines "renaissance revival" curves derived from French-inspired "renaissance revival" furniture with such "Anglo-Japanese" (a modern term) details on the frame as the sunflowers on the triple back of the settee. Anglo-Japanese motifs were associated with the "aesthetic" design reforms of the 1870s and 1880s. The pleated tufting is like that found on French-style suites that would have been labeled "Pompadour" or "Napoleon" ten to twenty years earlier. Courtesy Smithsonian Institution.

Fig. 8. Side chair, walnut, figured wool and silk rep, attributed to Alexander Roux, New York, New York, 1860-1870. The frame of this chair combines elements of the rococo on the crest rail with "French Renaissance" vase-shaped legs and the overall proportions of neoclassical chairs. Courtesy Smithsonian Institution.

far from established centers of fashion. For example, after the expansion of their house in Springfield, Illinois, in 1856, Mary Todd Lincoln purchased for her pair of parlors a locally produced sofa that grafted rococo revival curves and carved clusters of fruit and flowers onto proportions and details from "pillar-and-scroll" (late neoclassical) furniture. The black horsehair upholstery of this piece was not perceived as an expression of French style, but it was long-wearing and offered a handsome sheen resembling silk upholstery fabrics.

Although French furniture design continually reprocessed its eighteenth-century triumphs throughout the nineteenth century (something that commentators noted at the time), one area where

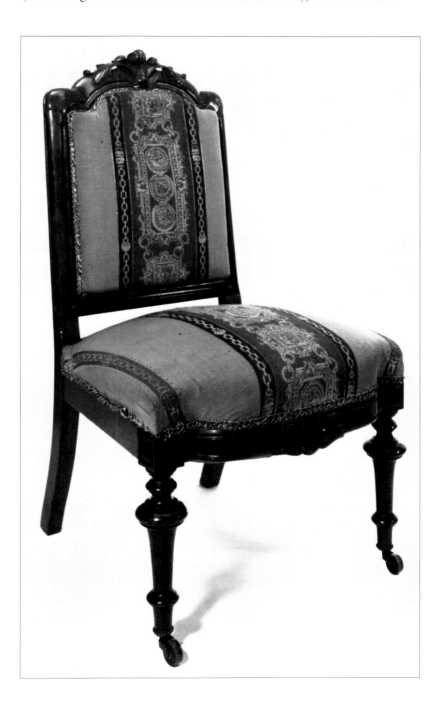

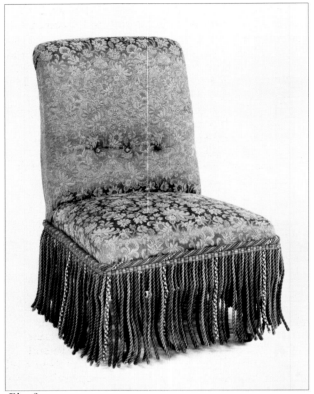

Fig. 9

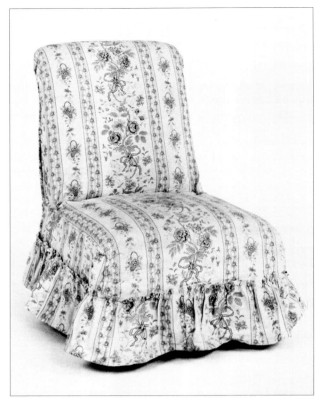

Fig. 10

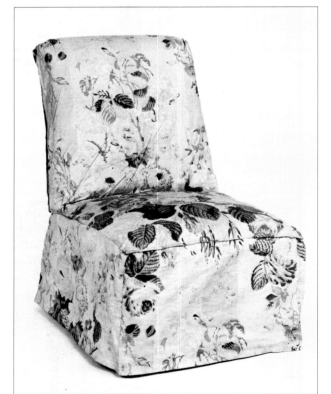

Fig. 11

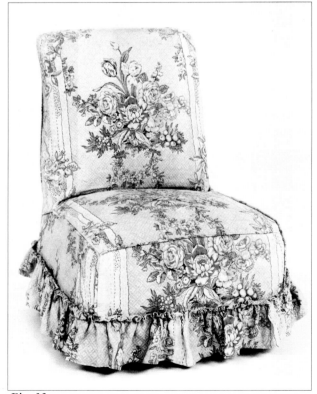

Fig. 12

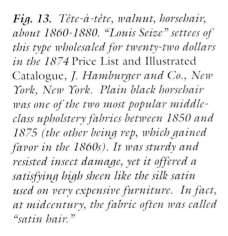

Figs. 9-12. Child's Turkish chair, brocaded silk, silk and wool bullion fringe, France, 1884. Covered with a succession of decorative slipcovers after the practice introduced to the Grange by French émigré decorator Leon Marcotte, this chair was used in the drawing room of the Codman family house. The printed cotton slipcover in fig. 10 dates from 1885; the slipcover in fig. 11, of the same fabric, dates from about 1900. The printed cotton chintz slipcover in fig. 12 was made in about 1930. Courtesy Society for the Preservation of New England Antiquities; photographs by J. David Bohl.

Fig. 13. Tête-à-tête, walnut, horsehair, about 1860-1880. "Louis Seize" settees of this type wholesaled for twenty-two dollars in the 1874 Price List and Illustrated Catalogue, J. Hamburger and Co., New York, New York. Plain black horsehair was one of the two most popular middle-class upholstery fabrics between 1850 and 1875 (the other being rep, which gained favor in the 1860s). It was sturdy and resisted insect damage, yet it offered a satisfying high sheen like the silk satin used on very expensive furniture. In fact, at midcentury, the fabric often was called "satin hair."

innovation did occur was upholstery (figs. 14 and 15). In an 1882 article in *The Decorator and Furnisher*, Theodore Child noted that

> while the cabinet makers remain imitators of the Renaissance and Louis XIV styles, the two styles most in vogue for the moment, the modern upholsterers and decorators have almost created a characteristic Nineteenth Century style in their treatment of hangings and of wholly upholstered furniture. The Parisian *tapissier* gathers up, crumples and rumples plush, broche (brocaded) silks, lampas, satins and scores of rich tissues that Lyons is continually turning out, with an art, a grace, an indescribable *chic* that can only be compared with the *chic* of the Parisians modistes and dressmakers (fig. 16).[9]

Ingenious drapery techniques had marked French upholstery particularly since the Empire (1804-1815), when Napoleon's personal designers Percier and Fontaine experimented with tent rooms and fantastic asymmetrical swag drapery suspended over windows by spears. Similar bravura technique marked French upholstery of the later nineteenth century. Designers mixed many kinds of fabrics and needlework techniques as well as ingenious cutting and "gathering, crumpling, and rumpling" that could be applied to any kind of decorative surface—mantels, tables, chair backs, and pianos. *The Decorator and Furnisher* and upholsterers' cutting books such as *Practical Decorative Upholstery* (1889) and *Cutting and Draping* (1905) published many examples of these kinds of scarf draperies. One "French Arrangement of a Fireplace" consisted of "a combination of dark green plush, set off with old pink silk, which is embroidered with floss silk in delicate shades of green, pink, and gold, edged with long tassels in variegated chenille. Ball fringe in gold gimp around the mantelboard, and the side scarf end."[10] Although skillful effects were more difficult to attain than Child's writing suggests, certain elements of this kind of drapery were easy to paraphrase. Do-it-yourselfers concocted their own renditions in the drapery craze of the 1880s and 1890s, when ordinary consumers blended both the "household art" influences of the aesthetic movement and French-influenced drapery techniques.

While French style enjoyed widespread popularity, authors of popular fiction and essays always expressed ambivalence toward French manners, dress, social habits, and house furnishing.

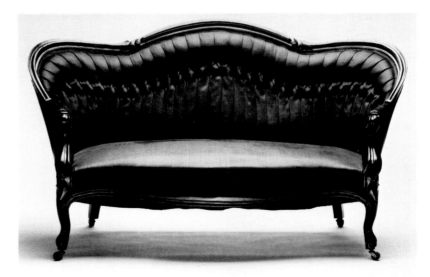

Nonetheless, they understood what surviving artifacts also attest: Americans wanted at least an echo of French cultivation in their parlors. Thus, at the same time that *Godey's Lady's Book* published articles cautioning that the French were not properly domestic people, the magazine took care to introduce its readers to the proper French terminology for modern parlor furnishings in the early 1850s. *Godey's* also published French fashion plates each month.[11]

The manner in which the French lived—Parisians in particular—fascinated middle -class Americans because it seemed so undomestic to their eyes. Author Caroline Kirkland had even insisted that the French had been forced to borrow the Anglo-American concepts of "home" and "comfort" because their own language (and, therefore, their culture) did not contain them.[12] Women's magazines such as *Godey's* offered their readers articles with such titles as "How They Live in Paris" and "The French at Home," taking care in the latter to point out that "the French and Americans differ so entirely in their manner of keeping house and managing the culinary department, that it becomes a matter of interest to compare notes,

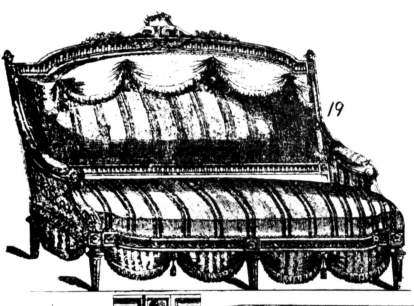

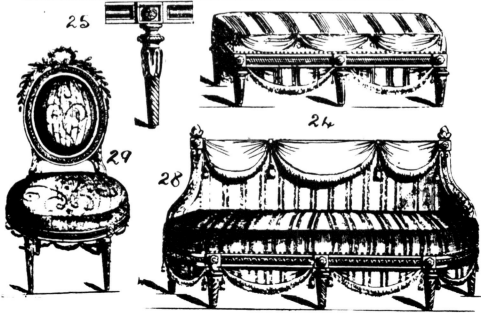

Fig. 14. Eighteenth-century upholstery designs by Richard de LaLonde (active 1780-1790), illustration in Thomas Arthur Strange, An Historical Guide to French Interiors, Furniture, Decoration, Woodwork, and Allied Arts *(1903). These designs probably were reproduced from his* Cahiers d'Ameublement *(about 1780). Certain details in lavish eighteenth-century upholstery, such as the neoclassical swags on these chairs, were reinterpreted on chair backs and seats in late nineteenth-century French upholstery.*

Fig. 15. *Suite No. 97 ("crinoline suite"), illustration in McDonough, Price and Co. catalog, Chicago, Illinois (1876). This firm introduced to midwestern consumers an approach to French suite upholstery also seen at the Centennial in model rooms (see plate 2). Overstuffed, with printed show covers in "coteline" (which seems to have been a printed ribbed fabric), the suite resembled custom furniture offered to well-to-do clients on the East Coast by fashionable decorators in the 1860s and 1870s. Courtesy State Historical Society of Wisconsin.*

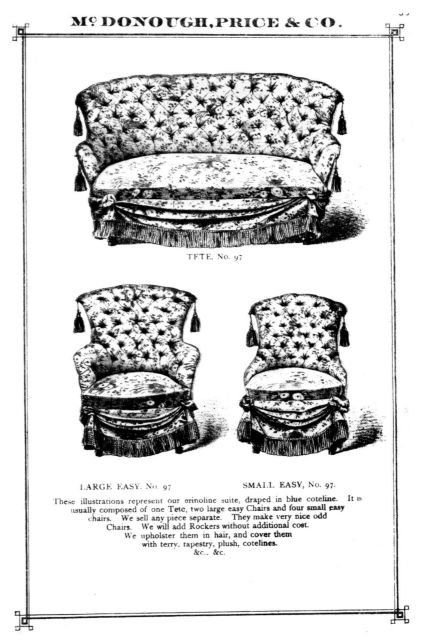

and see which plan is best."[13] While at first reading the tone of such pieces seems simply descriptive, the articles often suggested that the more public character and fashion-consciousness of French family life was strange and discomfiting. The preface to "How They Live in Paris," a translation of an 1847 article from *Le Magasin Pittoresque* reprinted in an 1859 issue of *Godey's,* implied that the "grand-looking palatial house" illustrated was a sham because it actually contained apartments rented to impoverished seamstresses as well as to families of means.[14]

French style in clothing and furnishings also seemed dangerous to domestic commentators because it violated the harmony of means and ends that was, in their view, the prized expression of middle-class, domestic values. "Fashion" was changeable and extravagant, and, because the French were the most fashionable people in the world, French fashion contained the seeds of destruction of the American

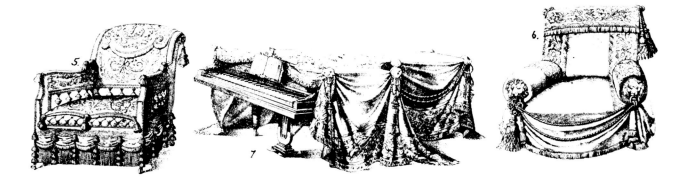

republic. The authors of moral tales about furnishings set up French taste as the epitome of fashion's uncontrolled, irresponsible consumption and of inappropriate middle-class striving after an unnecessary facade.

In Harriet Beecher Stowe's *Pink and White Tyranny* (1871), fascination with French taste and its effects upon domesticity are a constant theme. John Seymour, the steady son and now head of an old New England mill-owning family, marries a shallow fortune-hunting young socialite named Lilly and returns to the ancestral manse with fashionable bride in tow. She finds life apart from the world of fashion in New York and Newport depressing and convinces Seymour to allow a complete redecoration of the house. (John's spinster sister thereupon packs up the treasured family heirlooms and moves across town.) The result is "the transformed Seymour mansion, where literally old things had passed away, and all things become new."

> There was not a relic of the past. The house was furbished and resplendent—it was gilded—it was frescoed—it was *à la* Pompedour, *à la* Louis Quinze and Louis Quatorze, and *à la* every thing Frenchy and pretty, and gay and glistening. For, though the parlors at first were the only apartments contemplated in this *renaissance*, yet it came to pass that...there was no way to produce a sense of artistic unity, peace, and quietness, but to do the whole thing over, which was done triumphantly.[15]

Stowe's discussion of the ability of French fashion to transform the Seymour household suggested that through its embellishments, the transformed house, a product of the highest artifice, was no longer an organic entity and repository for family history. Rather, it was an extreme outcome of the popular sensibility of refinement.

The etiquette of the fine gentleman, not by any means exclusively French but often labeled so, also created ambivalence among both the domestic comfort theorists and the authors of etiquette books at midcentury. The concern about insincerity in etiquette was given a specific national cast as the argument against fashion had been. In another essay in a second collection of domestic tales entitled *Little Foxes* (1866), Harriet Beecher Stowe (in her pseudonym Christopher Crowfield) outlined for the purposes of argument several popular positions on "French politeness." When Bob Stephens, Crowfield's son-in-law, attacked elaborate manners at home as "tedious" and uncomfortable, Crowfield defended them in such a way that still expressed ambivalence about the "races" of people who originated it. His open admiration of "how the element of courtesy pervades every department of [French] life" and "how carefully, people avoid being

Fig. 16. *Details from plate of "Recent French Furnishings" in* The Decorator and Furnisher *(July 1890). Here some of the late eighteenth-century upholstery treatments visible in LaLonde's designs were interpreted by fashionable Parisian upholsterers.*

personally disagreeable in their intercourse" (a view the author confessed was gained largely from literature) was qualified by this precept:

> It is true, as a general rule, that those races of men that are most distinguished for outward urbanity and courtesy are the least distinguished for truth and sincerity; and hence the well-known alliterations, "fair and false," "smooth and slippery." The fair and false Greek, the polished and wily Italian, the courteous and deceitful Frenchman, are associations which, to the strong, downright, courteous Anglo-Saxon, make up-and-down rudeness and blunt discourtesy a type of truth and honesty.[16]

Despite these stereotyped views of "racial" groups, Crowfield remained reluctant to reject what Bob Stephens called "all the delicacies that ever were hatched up in the hot-bed of French sentiment," qualities that Stephens claimed bore the "loathsome, sickly stench of cowardice and distrust."[17] Crowfield countered:

> Now it is the reaction from such a style of life on the truthful Anglo-Saxon nature that leads to an undervaluing of courtesy, as if it were of necessity opposed to sincerity. But it does not follow, because all is not gold that glitters, that nothing that glitters is gold, and because courtesy and delicacy of personal intercourse are often perverted to deceit, that they are not valuable allies of truth. No woman would prefer a slippery, plausible rascal to a rough, unceremonious honest man; but of two men equally truthful and affectionate, every woman would prefer the courteous one.[18]

By the 1870s, the argument about whether French design and fashion were appropriate for Americans had gradually evolved until it was more often about the nature of that intangible quality "good taste" than about the nature of proper moral character expressed through the furnishing of rooms. It is safe to say that Stowe was sincerely worried about the moral state of her readers, but the complaints against popular design tastes proffered by Sir Charles Locke Eastlake, Clarence Cook, and others had a different cast. They debated what refinement really was, who could claim to be refined, and how refinement could properly be manifested through one's possessions. Their writing echoes that of the domestic critics writing decades earlier, but the midcentury question had been rephrased. Rather than arguing about the virtue of consuming fashionable furnishings, the newer critics discussed what *kind* of fashionable consumption was admirable. As they had at midcentury, upholsterers continued to bear the brunt of the blame for the public's bad taste. They were still perceived as milliners for houses, foisting upholstery styles as though they were new spring bonnets.[19] "Good taste" advocate Clarence Cook announced that fashion was trivial and should be beneath proper notice rather than the object of moral anxiety.

> I am not in for a tilt against fashion; fashionable people may do what they like; 't were vain to say them nay. They may buy embossed brass coal scuttles, and put them in front of dummy fireplaces...they may put china cats nursing their kittens on their satin sofas, and enjoy their being taken for real ones by old beaus and maiden ladies...they may do anything that comes into their nonsensical, pretty heads...If you only want to be in the fashion, and to have things either come from Marcotte's, or Herter's, or

Cottier's, or look as if they came from one of these places, you must consent either to pay the round price for the real things, or to put up with such second-rate copies of them as your small means will buy.[20]

However vocal such design reformers' criticisms of "fashionable" —usually French—furnishings were, they always existed in tension with the fact than manufacturers continued to produce French-inspired upholstery for ever-widening circles of consumers. "Reform" styles of upholstered furniture were popular in the mid-1870s and 1880s, but, by the mid-1880s, French style, particularly in upholstery, experienced a renewed burst of popularity (fig. 17).[21] Gothic, Elizabethan, Anglo-Japanese, and Eastlake furniture always was produced side-by-side with pieces of French design, and French upholstery never was out of fashion. Even the furniture forms of the rococo revival of the mid-nineteenth century seem never to have disappeared completely, although they may have been confined for a time to regional markets such as the deep South.

Throughout the second half of the nineteenth century, French styles of both the eighteenth and early nineteenth centuries were subject to periodic scrutiny in the popular press, just as French clothing and manners were. They provoked similarly ambivalent, even parallel, responses. In a series of articles apparently reprinted from *Harper's Bazar, The American Cabinet Maker, Upholsterer and*

Fig. 17. Settee, mahogany, silk satin damask, Berkey and Gay Company, Grand Rapids, Michigan, 1890-1900. Courtesy Grand Rapids Public Museum.

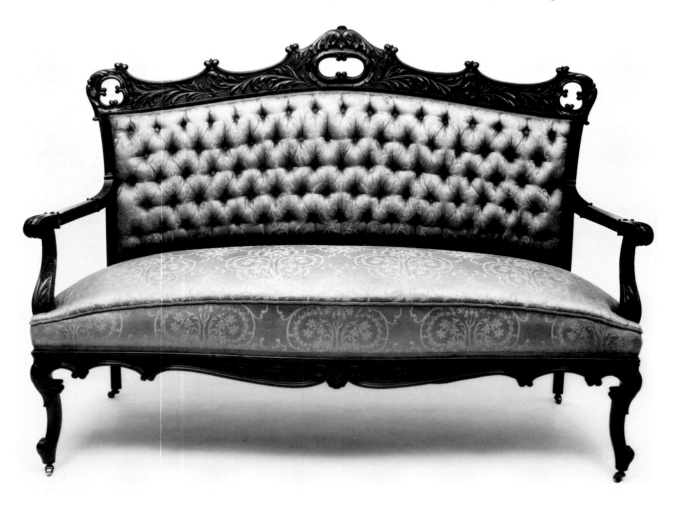

Carpet Reporter noted that, no matter how protected and talented the artists and craftspeople of Louis XV had been, the manufacture of "Louis Quinze" furniture itself was of "no worth" because of flaws in its design and dishonesty in its execution. Veneering, "in its glory in the reign of Rococco," was considered a particular abuse because it masked "the universal face of furniture [with] falsehood." The technique was analogous to elegant yet insincere manners. However, the author's disapproval was qualified. Despite these defects, the Louis Quinze "yet was not altogether without elegance" because of its appeal to bodily comfort.

> Whatever faults it has, it is the only style of all that has ever paid the least attention to comfort. The straight back, the upright lines, the honest and sturdy supports of the Gothic, the perfect grace and beauty of the Renaissance, are nothing at all to be compared, for comfort to the aching, the worn, and the weary, with the deep-seated deliciousness of the Louis Quinze. What comfort has crept into the Gothic and the Renaissance—the properly tilted back, the seat at a healthy angle from it, the elastic support of springs—is there only because the Louis Quinze taught them that such a thing could be.[22]

Perhaps one reason that French style in furniture, particularly in parlor upholstery, was able to maintain its power in the marketplace was because it eventually seemed to mediate the apparently incompatible demands of the cultured facade and bodily comfort. This was especially the case when French upholsterers introduced, and consumers gradually accepted, a range of new overstuffed types of seating furniture called "Turkish" that encouraged relaxed seating posture and began to approach modern-day sensibilities about bodily comfort.

French upholstery also bore a chain of associative possibilities, however, that remained attractive to middle-class Americans. It could be associated with a fragmentary, romanticized understanding of the gracious social life of the eighteenth-century salon. It may also have borne associations to American elite culture of the eighteenth and early nineteenth centuries. Deciphering the symbolism of French upholstery involves outlining the meanings that were possibly ascribed to it and how parlor makers and users linked them in the game of associationism, where ordinary objects became both personal and cultural symbols.

Like Emily Thornwell with her observations about taste and associations, commentators on architecture and decorative arts in the mid-nineteenth century often maintained that the ability to see and appreciate the subtleties of historical detail required a high degree of personal cultivation.[23] However, as the popular understanding of the sensibility of refinement developed, the chains of associations that could be made using parlor furnishings for their wellspring encouraged ordinary people to move from the personal and private realm of domesticity to a form of cosmopolitanism. Refined, rich, and ornamental furnishings made manifest the connection of each consumer to the progress of civilized living. Furnishings contained associative possibilities, which, when fully appreciated, introduced "history" and "progress," making the parlor both a more complete version of the world beyond its walls and the culmination of civilization's presumed continual improvement.

The adaptation of styles—forms, proportions, and ornaments—from one culture by another, later culture for its own purposes was not a new phenomenon in the nineteenth century, but it appears to have gathered substantial momentum after 1825.

Perhaps the most important and well-known example of such reuse occurred in the fourteenth and fifteenth centuries when Europeans rediscovered the arts and learning of the ancient classical world. The Italian Renaissance looked back to "a generalized classical age no more specifically of *one* date than is the scene of Raphael's School of Athens—and aspired to be not merely like that but in fact better: by synthesizing antique and modern knowledge there would come the most truthful philosophy, the best literature, the finest works of art."[24] The historical revivals associated with what has been called the "American Renaissance" in the fine and decorative arts and architecture of the late nineteenth century have been compared to the way in which the earlier Renaissance in Italy employed the past.

This kind of historical associationism, which employed the past in a highly self-conscious and scholarly yet synthetic manner, tended to be adopted by highly educated people in the second half of the nineteenth century and practiced by those tastemakers linked in some way with individuals of wealth.[25] When the E. J. Berwinds (whose fortune was made in coal mining) installed Louis XVI drawing rooms and salons in their Newport, Rhode Island, mansion, The Elms, they not only expressed Mrs. Berwind's preoccupation with Marie Antoinette; they also participated in a spectacular but ultimately not very influential taste culture of economically elite consumers. When they could not find eighteenth-century French furniture to buy, such consumers could own fabulously ornate nineteenth-century copies, because mainstream French decorators and consumers themselves

Fig. 18. Display of modern French furniture at the Columbian Exposition, photomechanical reproduction in The Book of the Fair *(1893). Many French furniture makers of the nineteenth century simply continued to reproduce the designs of the ancien régime in lavish materials for wealthy customers with conservative tastes in both Europe and America.*

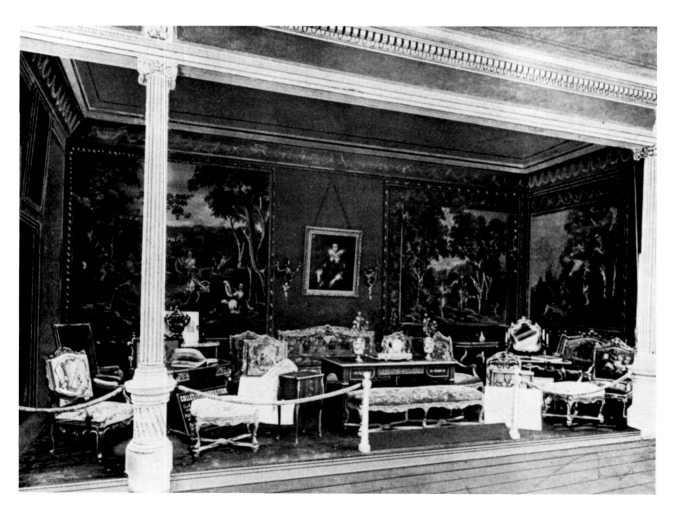

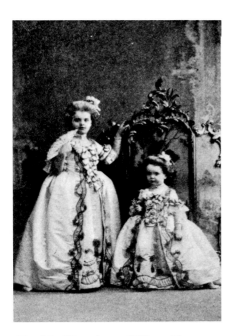

Fig. 19. "Daughters of Elinor Glyn. Margot and Juliette Glyn dressed for a fancy ball as the daughters of Louis XV," photograph in Harper's Bazar *(February 1903). Elinor Glyn was a wealthy author of romantic historical fiction.*

were caught up in reproducing expensive, accurate copies of such forms (fig. 18). By creating such grandiose European settings for themselves, the Berwinds, Morgans, Astors, and their friends were involved in a highly self-conscious modeling process as "princes" of commerce (fig. 19).[26]

For most Americans, however, historical associationism was a somewhat different phenomenon. It was one facet of a heady new sensation enjoyed by consumers—that the world was at their command and could be contained in each individual home, particularly in the parlor. The use of historical design was very impressionistic and, in furnishing, usually was carried out piecemeal. Few people could afford to construct complete historical fantasies, as did the Berwinds and their peers. Advice authors suggested that fragmentary quotations of historical styles had the advantage of making ordinary parlors "cosmopolite."[27]

This kind of late nineteenth-century furnishing advice, in which associationism was praised for its romantic rather than scholarly content, continued the mid-nineteenth-century romanticism that inspired eclectic architecture. In 1854, the editor of *Harper's New Monthly Magazine* compared the associative potential (what he called "romantic suggestion") of Broadway, the "street of palaces," to "such a street in Genoa." The Italian street suggested to sensitive strollers that "plumed and doubleted gentlemen, and ladies with gorgeous stomacher and ample train will issue from the lofty doors and pass on to some princely feast."[28] Juxtapositions of small decorative objects could inspire sets of associations as rich as those inspired by streets of large buildings. An exhibit of vases by French manufacturers at the Crystal Palace was praised because one was "oriental," another "antique," while "a third recalled the breakfast-table of Mesdames Pompadour or DuBarri; a fourth intimated the Majolica of Guid Ubaldo of Urbino; a fifth recalled the tazze of Jean Courtois or Liotard." Further, mixing and matching historical ornament on single objects also evinced "the spread of a popular knowledge of the history of art," enjoying the triple blessing of being romantic, creative, and expressive of progressive refinement.[29] French design seemed exemplary of the "refinement" of specialization that was associated with civilized progress. The royal workshops of France, operating without constraints of money and time, had developed the most varied furniture forms during the eighteenth century, as well as the highest expressions of craft. The specialization of seating forms seen in Victorian furniture—reception chairs, corner chairs, window chairs, invalid chairs, and so on—had been foreshadowed in eighteenth-century French seating. Furniture historian Francis Watson has noted that

> although the principal classes of seat; the stool, the chair, the arm-chair, and the day-bed or sofa, were all established before the end of the reign of Louis XIV, they evolved into a wealth of varied forms and specialized functions throughout the eighteenth century...In the latter part of the century particularly the proliferation of new forms and new names is extraordinary...*sultanes, obligéantes, confortables, tête-à-tête, confident, en confessionale* are only a few of the names current during the late eighteenth century, names which, if their meaning is sometimes baffling...at least emphasize the interest in comfort and social life which was a hall-mark of the period. Chairs, in particular, were created in the most specialized forms such as the various types of *voyeuse* with their padded backs on which the spectator leaned his arms whilst watching others play cards or games of chance.[30]

But the linkage was more profound than a simple genealogical relationship of forms. That such special-use upholstered chairs had historical origins in the cultivated society of the *ancien regime* may have, among some individuals, made even keener that sense of pleasure associated with special-use objects that was so much a part of the popular sensibility of refinement. In an article on the French salon, Theodore Child discussed both the progression of nineteenth-century French furniture styles in terms of their specialization and their evolution toward increased bodily comfort, a trend that was viewed as another manifestation of civilization's progress.

> Now, just as the First Empire reflected the sympathies for Caesar that filled the master's head, so the Second Empire reflected the love of material comfort, which filled the people's heart. The destination of modern furniture is the realization of this comfort, and comfort and glitter are the characteristics of the house furnishing of the time of Napoleon III. To have called for comfort and exact suitableness for special uses in all the utensils that we employ, was a distinct progress.[31]

As widely disparate groups of consumers took up French taste in the late nineteenth century, the rhetorical purposes behind using French furnishing also varied considerably. While members of economic and social elites used French styles as a statement of their role as princes of commerce, a second group of consumers for French upholstery used it in additional ways. Those segments of the middle class who could afford to choose "French" style as a coherent decorating statement for drawing rooms were using it in concert with sets of intriguing conventions that associated particular historical styles with the character of appropriate activity in specific rooms of houses. This form of associationism described, in effect, national character through style. A type of popular history, it contributed to the cosmopolitan character of the self-conscious Victorian middle - class household.

The 1857 parlor of the Tucker family, as well as that of the Lincolns, demonstrate that by 1850 a standard set of conventions had developed in which household parlors were meant to be French. Such conventions not only allowed a certain ease in the execution and planning of interiors but also were a popular code that could be rapidly understood as a visual analogy to the character of the activity designated for that room. "Gothic/library," for example, made a statement about the serious character of learning. In the context of French upholstery, the bundle of conventional associations was "French/parlor/decorum/feminine." Turkish furniture, on the other hand, was associated with the relaxation of decorum in masculine activities of the Orient, such as smoking. These sets of associations were not constant in meaning; the "masculine" and "feminine" cues were subject to considerable change by 1900.

Such conventions were continually reinforced by advice from typical commercial decorators, who abounded by the 1880s but who have been little studied by students of the history of design.[32] The parlor furnished in 1907 by the Voigt family of Grand Rapids, Michigan, epitomizes the turn-of-the-century conventional use of French style in the parlor as a signal of culture (fig. 20). The Voigts had acquired money, thanks to their flourishing dry goods and flour milling businesses. By 1897, they were wealthy enough to build themselves a sizable new house (fig. 21). But they were thrifty enough to retain their older furnishings even as they decorated in the new house. Scattered throughout the house were pieces of an 1870s parlor suite in the Louis Seize mode (much like the settee illustrated

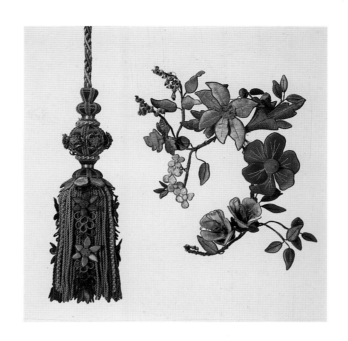

Plate 4. *Drapery trims, silk wrapped over wire, cardboard, wood, and wool, about 1860. Probably of French manufacture, these elaborate trims were used on the drawing room draperies of the Morse-Libby House. They suggest the vivid colors, attention to minute details of design, and theatrical character of the furnishings found in expensive, gala parlors of the mid- and late nineteenth century. Designed and decorated solely for the purposes of entertaining, the Morse-Libby drawing room epitomizes the ideal of the parlor of culture. Courtesy Victoria Society of Maine.*

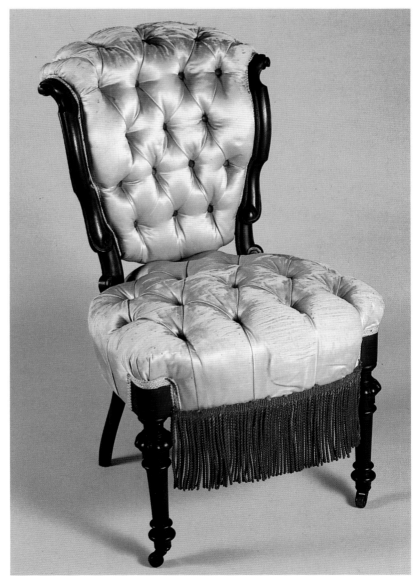

Plate 5. *Side chair, walnut, silk satin, silk and wool bullion fringe, Morse-Libby House, Portland, Maine, about 1860. This chair, which was probably used in an upstairs sitting room, was upholstered in a manner similar to that used on the house's drawing room chairs—satin upholstery, contrasting buttons, and a fringe over the chair rail. About the turn of the century, this chair was probably reupholstered with fabric similar to the original, and it retains the original fringe. Courtesy Victoria Society of Maine.*

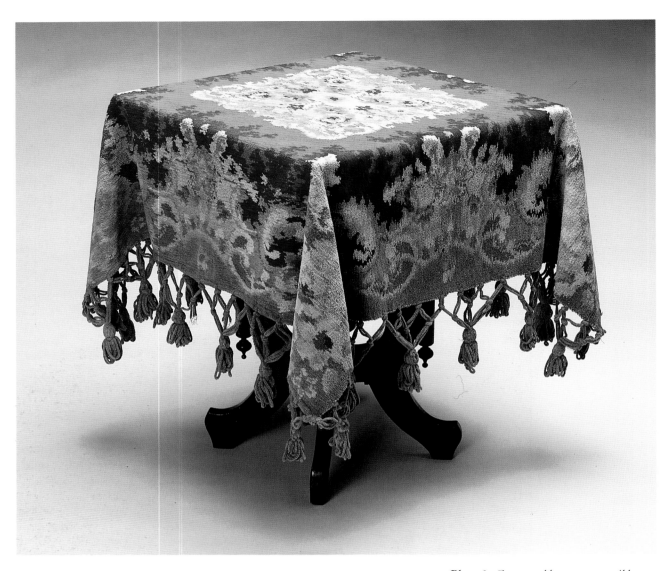

Plate 6. Center table cover, reversible figured cotton chenille, probably United States, 1890-1910. Richly colored and textured chenille table covers sold for as little as one dollar at the turn of the century. In simple parlors, they were important elements of the upholstery.

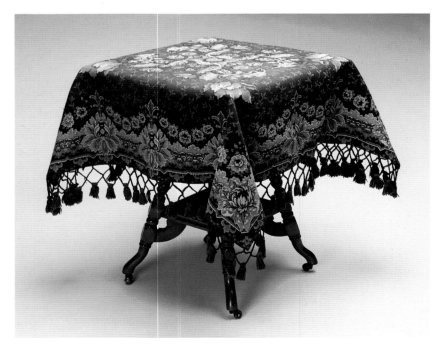

Plate 7. Center table cover, reversible figured cotton, probably United States, 1900-1915.

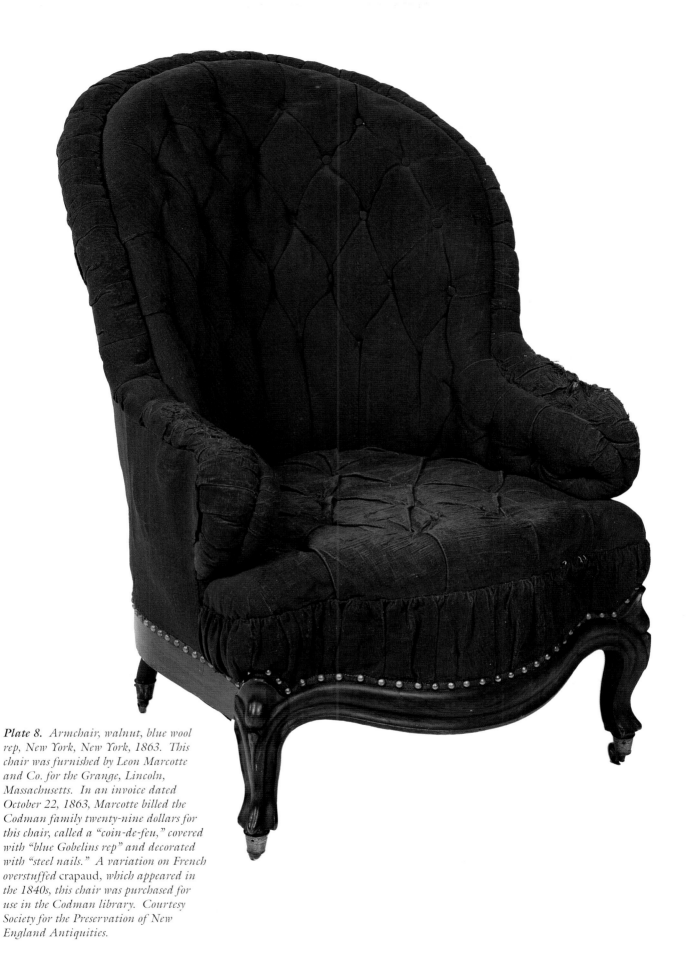

Plate 8. *Armchair, walnut, blue wool rep, New York, New York, 1863. This chair was furnished by Leon Marcotte and Co. for the Grange, Lincoln, Massachusetts. In an invoice dated October 22, 1863, Marcotte billed the Codman family twenty-nine dollars for this chair, called a "coin-de-feu," covered with "blue Gobelins rep" and decorated with "steel nails." A variation on French overstuffed* crapaud, *which appeared in the 1840s, this chair was purchased for use in the Codman library. Courtesy Society for the Preservation of New England Antiquities.*

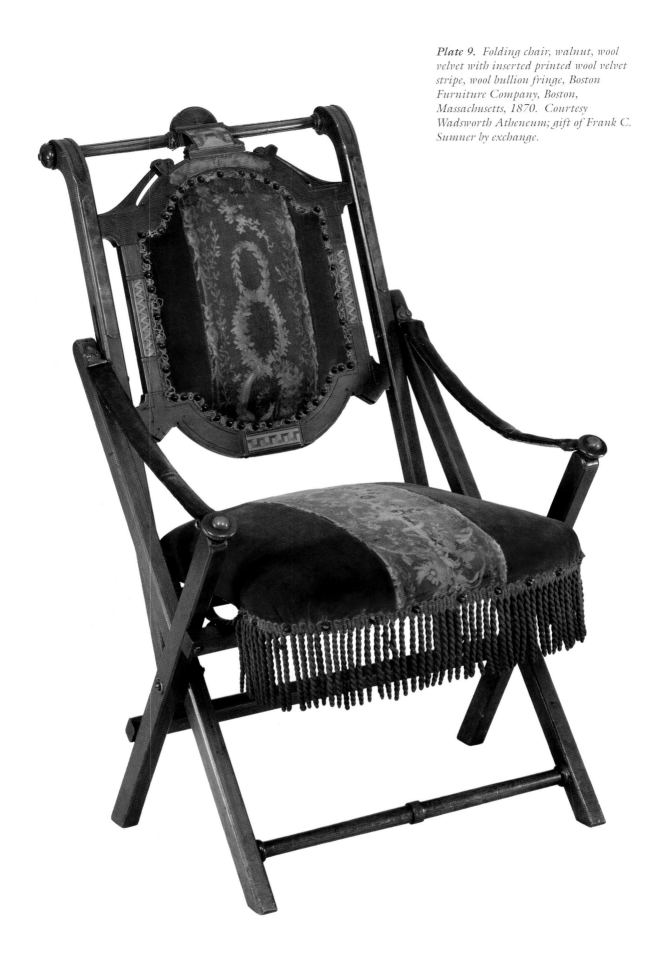

Plate 10. *Table, maple carved to look like bamboo, ebonized finish; upholstered top of silk velvet, wool flannel, and silk embroidery, United States, about 1880.*

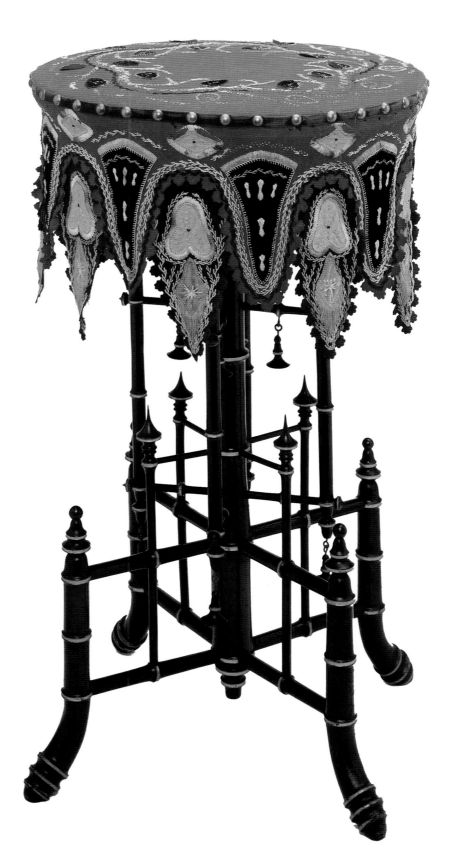

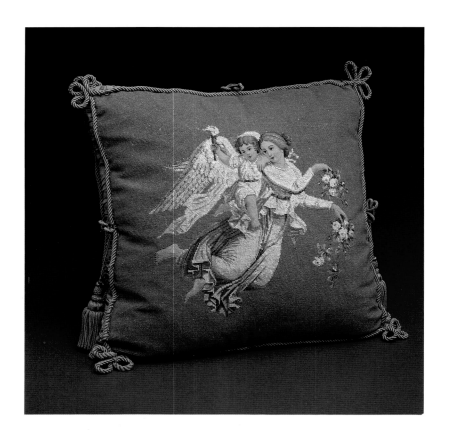

Plate 11. Pillow, beaded Berlin work with silk sides, silk cording, and tassels, probably United States, about 1860. This drawing room pillow depicts in beadwork Bertil Thorwaldsen's bas-relief Day. The reliefs of Thorwaldsen, a Danish sculptor who worked in the neoclassical style, provided a number of patterns for Berlin embroidery.

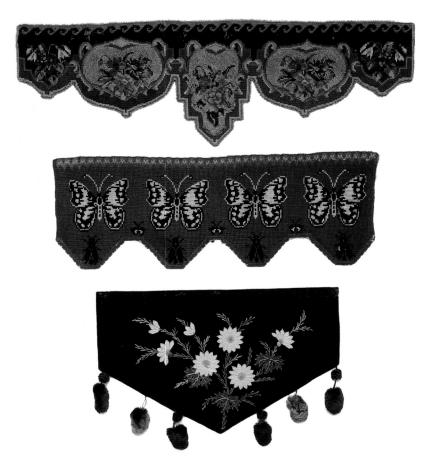

Plate 12. Shelf lambrequins, beaded Berlin work, Berlin work, appliqué, and machine embroidery, United States, 1850-1900. The maker of the top lambrequin emphasized its complex shape by edging it carefully with clear glass beads that would reflect light.

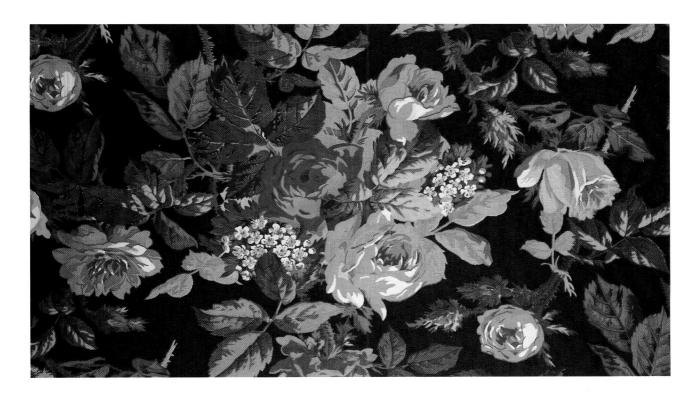

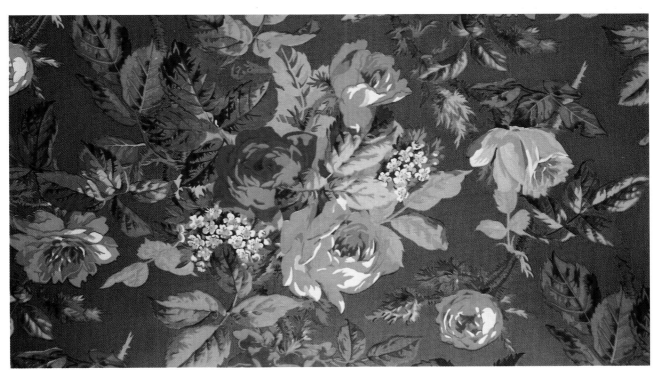

Plates 13 and 14. *Samples from folder of "Furniture twill," Cocheco Manufacturing Company, Dover, New Hampshire, dated October 28, 1886. The mills produced eight colorways of this patterned fabric. Courtesy Museum of American Textile History.*

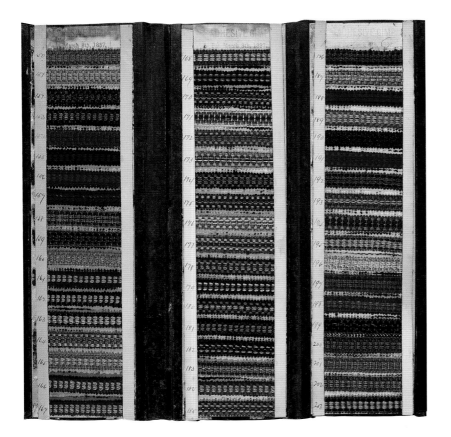

Plate 15. Samples from folder of "Edwards" Adhesive Gimp, patented March 7, 1887. "Edwards" Adhesive Gimp, meant to save money in upholstery workshops, shows how even narrow edgings highlighted the colors in upholstery fabrics. Courtesy Goldie Paley Design Center, Philadelphia College of Textiles and Science.

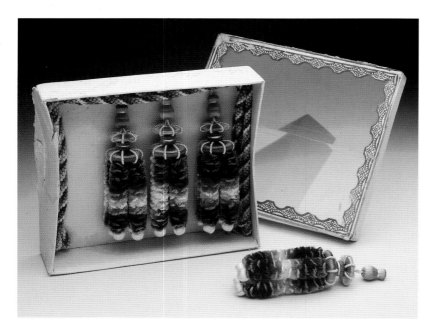

Plate 16. Drapery loops in original packaging, silk, cotton, and wool, France, 1870-1890.

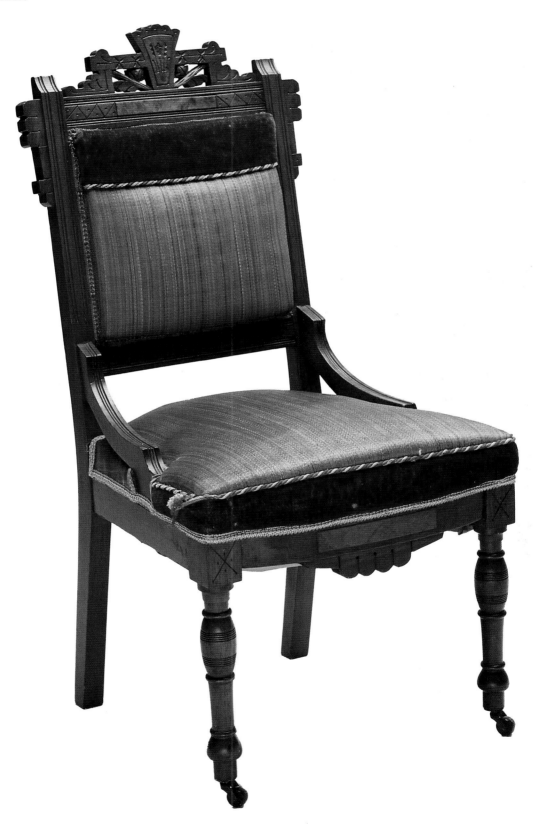

Plate 17. *"Reform" or "Eastlake" side chair, walnut, horsehair, mohair plush, United States, 1875-1885.*

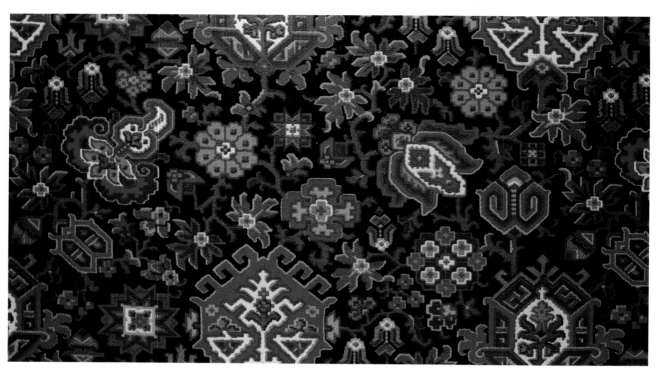

Plate 18. Sample card of cotton cretonne printed in a "Turkish" design, Cocheco Manufacturing Company, Dover, New Hampshire, dated June 16, 1886. Courtesy Museum of American Textile History.

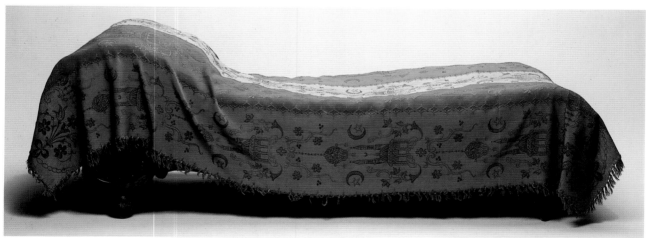

Plate 19. "Turkish" couch cover, cotton, United States, 1900-1915. Woven to look like strips of fabric sewn together and reversible, this inexpensive couch cover is a large-scale cotton rep of the type called "armure" in the early twentieth century.

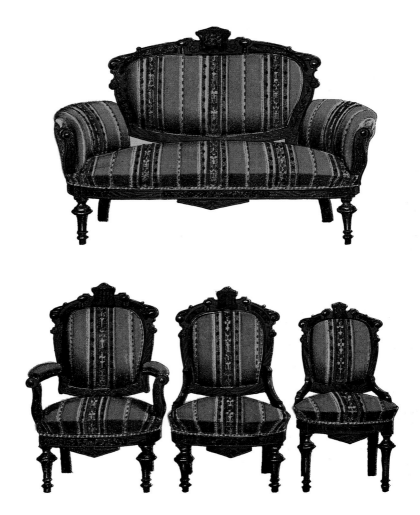

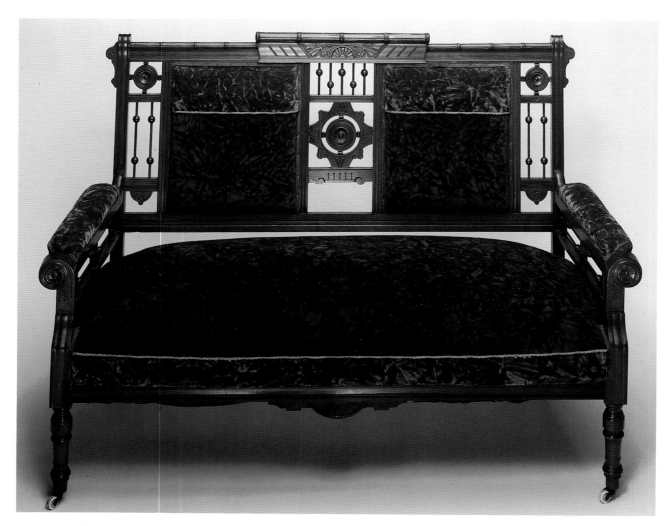

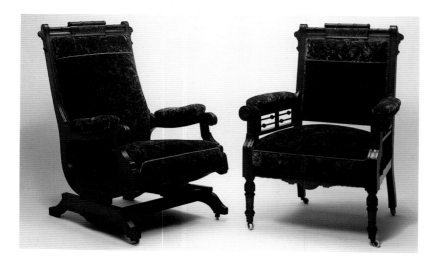

Plates 21 and 22. *Three pieces of a parlor suite, walnut, red and golden-yellow crushed mohair plush, United States, 1885-1890. Typical of moderately priced suites of the 1880s, this grouping suggests formality by its rectilinear, throne-like design, including the crest rail at the top of each piece. Adding platform rocking chairs to parlor suites accommodated the middle-class interest in both comfort and formal furniture.*

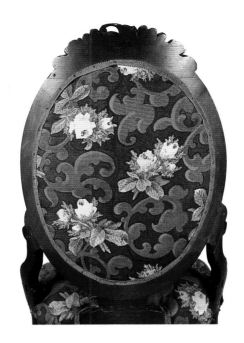

Plate 23. *Detail of side chair. Protected from the sun by its placement in the Tucker family's parlor, the back of this chair is little faded, suggesting the richness of the parlor suite's upholstery when new. (For a full view of this chair, see chapter 7, fig. 12.) Courtesy Castle Tucker.*

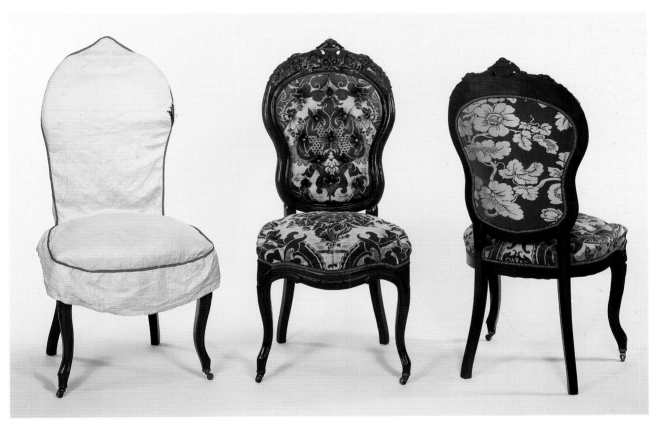

Plate 24. *Side chairs, rosewood, silk damask, silk slipcover with silk piping; probably Boston, Massachusetts, 1863. This fabric would have been called a "satin damask" at the time the suite was produced. Courtesy Wadsworth Atheneum; gift of Mrs. Horace B. Clark by exchange.*

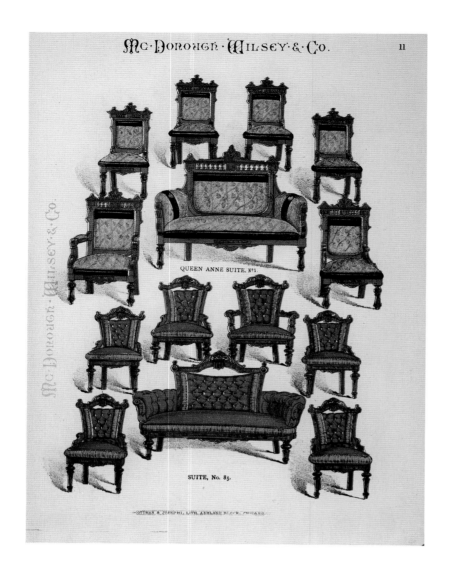

QUEEN ANNE SUITE. Nº1.

SUITE, No. 85.

OTTMAN & JOSEPH, LITH. ASHLAND BLOCK, CHICAGO.

Plate 25. *Page of suites, chromolithograph by Ottman and Joseph in* Catalogue of McDonough, Wilsey and Co., *Chicago, Illinois (1878). This page contrasted a rectilinear "reform" design, called a "Queen Anne" suite, with a suite whose design was a distant cousin to shield-back chairs. Typologically and visually, the suites are more alike than different. They employ the same grouping of seat types and approximately the same scale. The wooden frames of both employ most of their decoration on the crest rail (at the top of the seat back), including a center cartouche and "ears" at each corner. The rectilinear design of the Queen Anne suite has untufted upholstery with a printed or woven design to add interest. It is embellished with flat bands of contrasting fabric, while the other has curvaceous pleated and ruffled surfaces considered appropriate to French-inspired design. Despite these differences, the upholstery on each has roughly the same visual relationship to the wooden frames and employs the same strategy of using contrasting bands of fabric to create visual and tactile contrast. Courtesy State Historical Society of Wisconsin.*

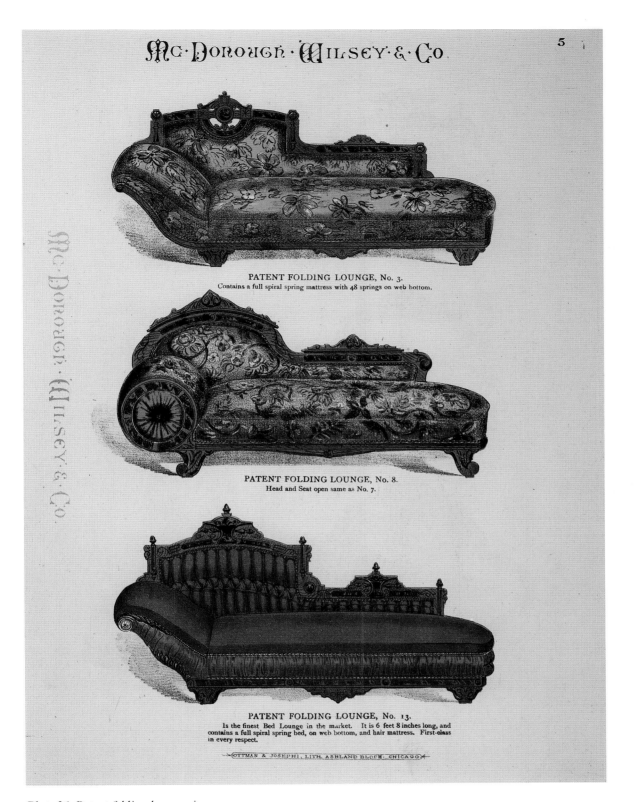

Mc·Donough·Wilsey·&·Co.

PATENT FOLDING LOUNGE, No. 3.
Contains a full spiral spring mattress with 48 springs on web bottom.

PATENT FOLDING LOUNGE, No. 8.
Head and Seat open same as No. 7.

PATENT FOLDING LOUNGE, No. 13.
Is the finest Bed Lounge in the market. It is 6 feet 8 inches long, and contains a full spiral spring bed, on web bottom, and hair mattress. First-class in every respect.

OTTMAN & JOSEPHI, LITH. ASHLAND BLOCK, CHICAGO

Plate 26. Patent folding lounges in Catalogue of McDonough, Wilsey and Co., *Chicago, Illinois (1878). "Bed lounges" were the studio couches of the nineteenth century. Their elaborate, colorful upholstery made them suitable for parlors in modest households. Courtesy State Historical Society of Wisconsin.*

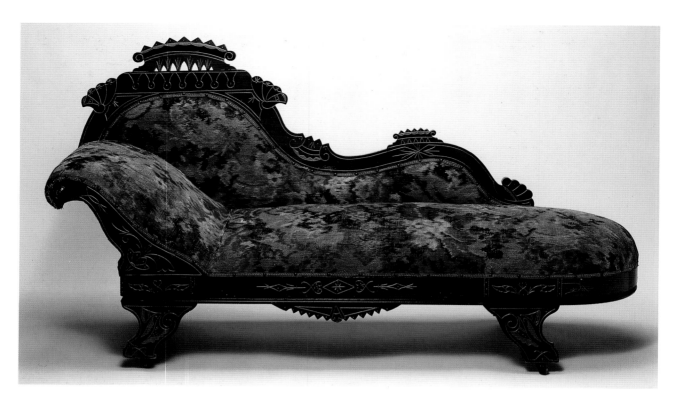

Plate 27. *Lounge, painted oak, tapestry carpet, Martyn Brothers, Jamestown, New York, about 1885. The large enameled nails used with the gimp on this lounge helped to hold the carpet cover in place and provided a decorative element.*

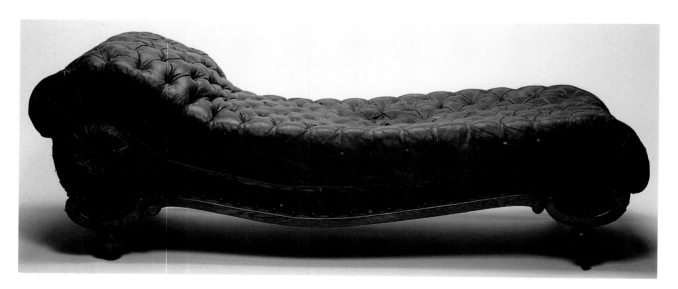

Plate 28. *Turkish couch, oak, leather cloth, about 1905. Leather cloth, also called "American cloth," was oil cloth intended for upholstery use.*

Plate 29. *Detail of chintz drapery panel with matching fabric-covered wooden rod, original hollow brass curtain rings, about 1850. The simply designed panel was probably expensive due to the costliness of the imported fabric and trim used rather than the skill and time required to make it. Women with small furnishing budgets could have easily made copies at home using inexpensive fabrics such as domestic cotton prints.*

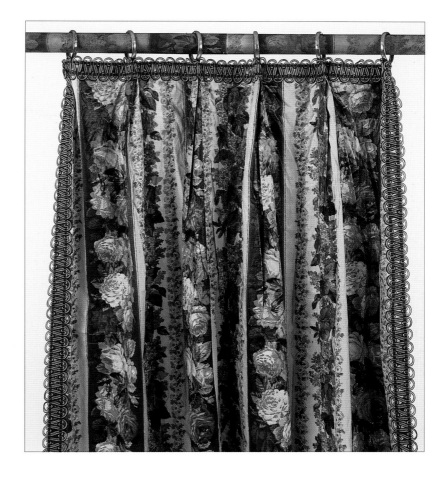

Plate 30. *Valance, silk brocade, about 1860. The rich appearance of this lambrequin (the term often was used to indicate a flat valance) is due to its elaborate figured fabric, trims, and complex shape. However, because the valance is completely flat, the cutting and sewing involved was simple. Courtesy Society for the Preservation of New England Antiquities; gift of Mrs. James Lee.*

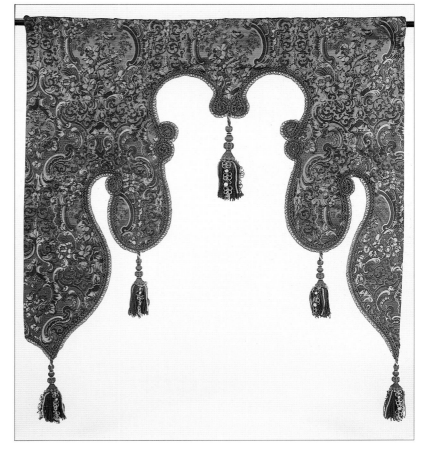

Plate 31. *Stamped metal cornice with valance of green wool damask, hanging in upstairs bedroom in Castle Tucker, Wiscasset, Maine, fabric probably manufactured in England, 1857-1858. Sea captain Richard Holbrook Tucker obtained the window draperies and hardware for his newly purchased Wiscasset house in Boston, Massachusetts. This valance hung in the "Green Room," the family sitting room that eventually became the billiard room. A similar set in red damask, now missing, is believed to have hung in the family's parlor. A heavy paper interlining and lining of brown cotton provided stiffness to the wool damask. Nailed to the wooden backing of the cornice, this valance originally was used with wooden blinds and lace curtains dyed green; no drapery panels were purchased. Courtesy Castle Tucker.*

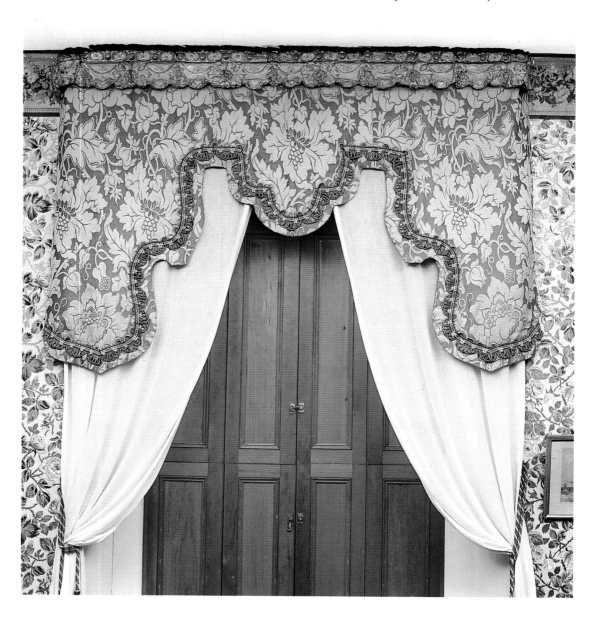

Plate 32. *Window shade, stenciled design on linen, about 1875. Landscapes with appropriately sublime or bucolic subject matter—mountains and lakes, lightning-blasted trees, rushing streams, or rural vistas—were popular subjects for painted shades. By lowering the shade, even windows overlooking muddy, garbage-strewn city streets could be made to express Henry Ward Beecher's "doctrine of windows."*

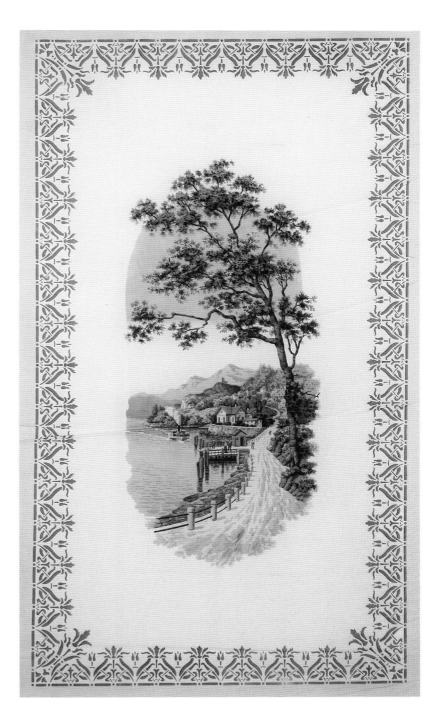

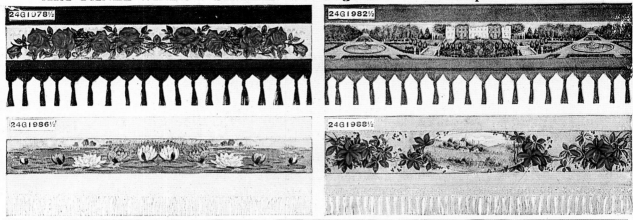

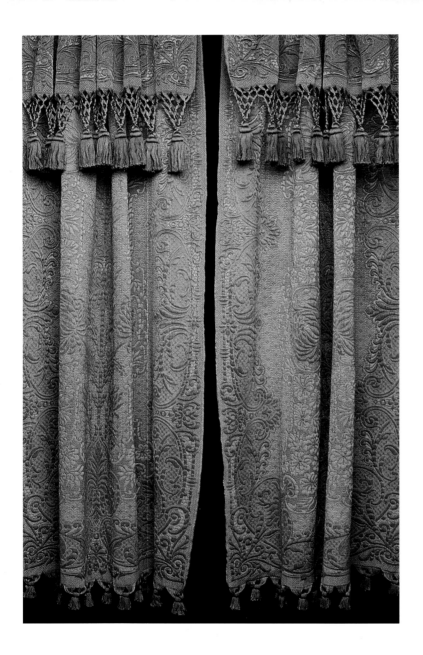

Plate 33. Window shades, engraving in Sears, Roebuck and Co. Catalogue No. 111 *(1908)*. *Sears offered different designs of painted window shades. One design took the form of a decorative "dado"; three showed roses and one a landscape. All could be ordered with fringe for an extra charge.*

Plate 34. Portières, United States, 1890-1911. *Two-color cotton door curtains, woven to be reversible and in a standard length of nine feet, could be adjusted to fit any doorway by folding the tops over rods or catching them at the fold with curtain rings. Knotted fringes and tassels made the excess length a decorative element, and the folded tops mimicked the appearance of a valance.*

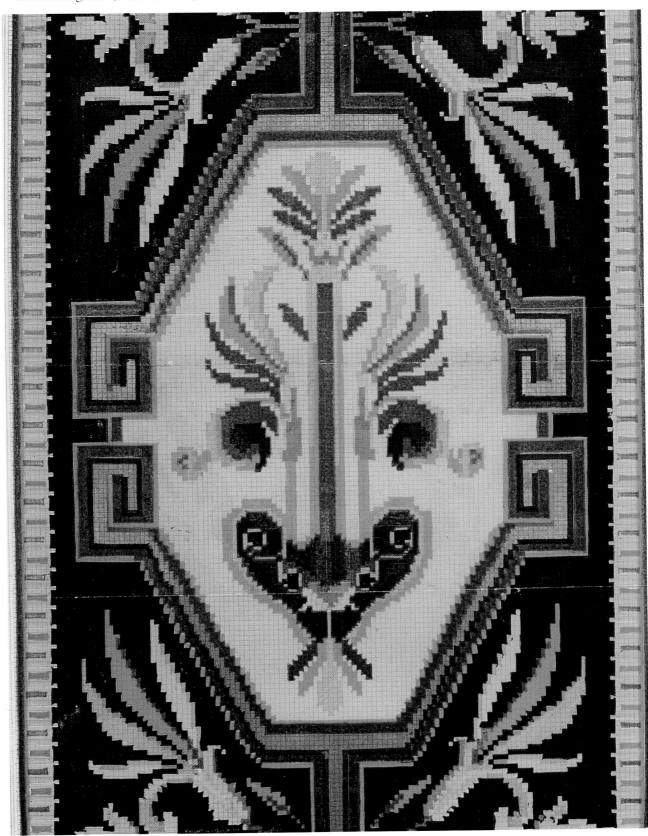

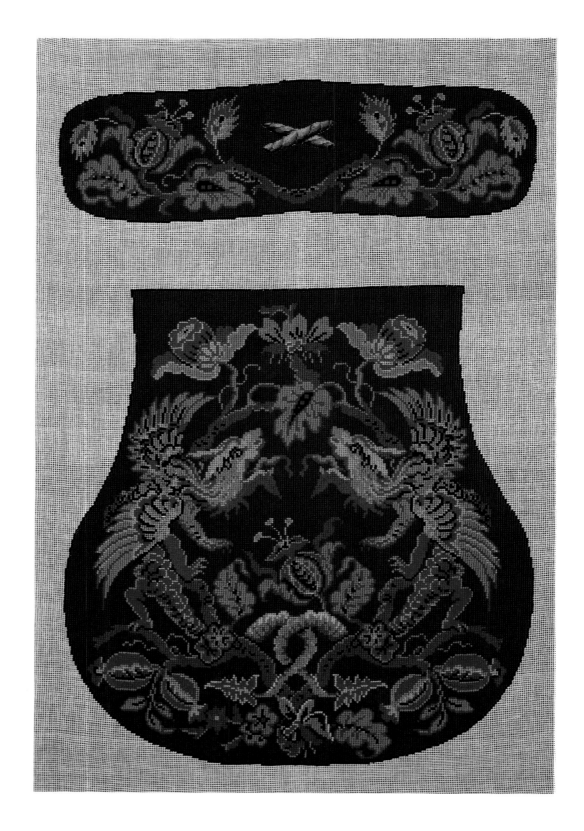

Plate 36. *Unused chair seat and back, Berlin work, United States, 1860-1880. The crossed cigars on the chair back indicate that this canvas embroidery project was intended for use on a "Turkish" smoking chair.*

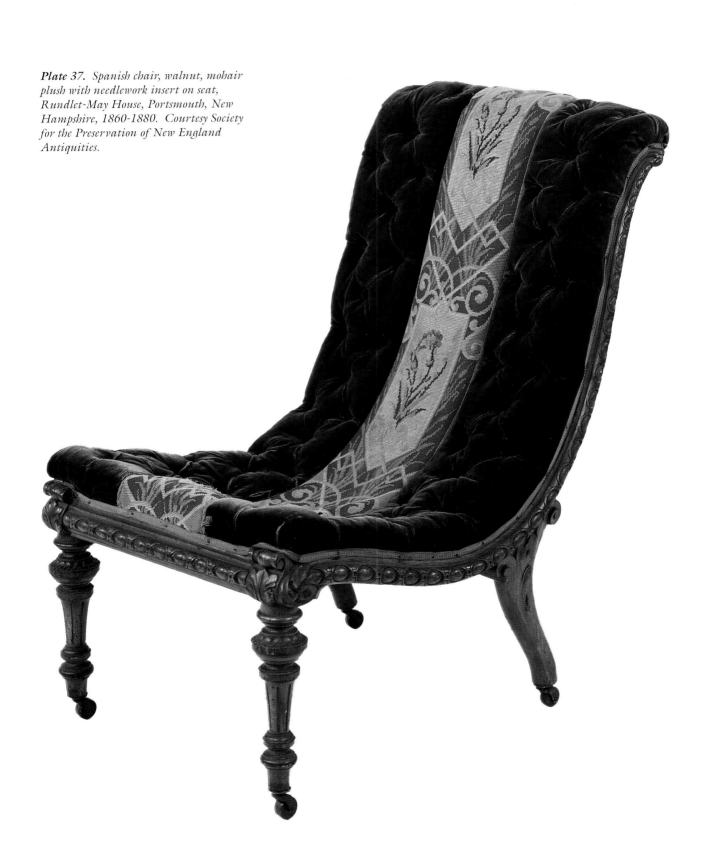

Plate 37. Spanish chair, walnut, mohair plush with needlework insert on seat, Rundlet-May House, Portsmouth, New Hampshire, 1860-1880. Courtesy Society for the Preservation of New England Antiquities.

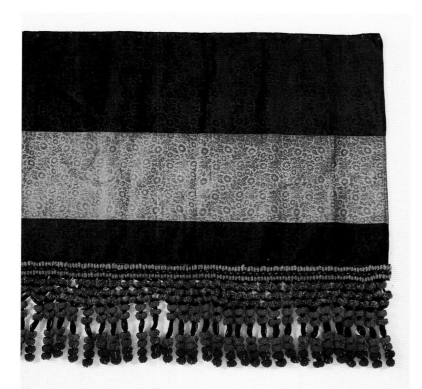

Plate 38. Valance, stamped silk-pile velvet, cotton, wool, and tinsel trim, United States, about 1894. Courtesy Castle Tucker.

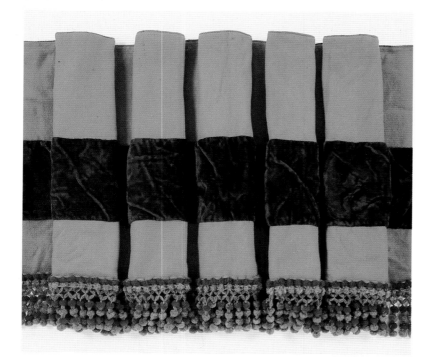

Plate 39. Valance, brushed wool blanket fabric, silk-pile velvet, wool and cotton fringe, made by Jane Armstrong Tucker, Wiscasset, Maine, about 1894. Courtesy Castle Tucker.

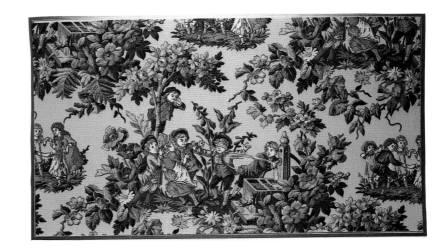

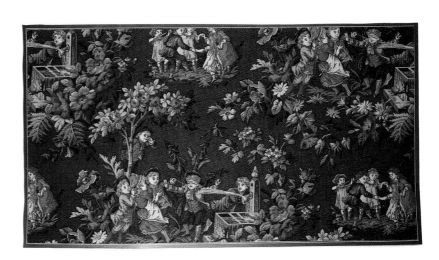

*Plate 40. Sample folder, "3/4 cretonne,"
Cocheco Manufacturing Company,
Dover, New Hampshire, dated October
18, 1886. Courtesy Museum of
American Textile History.*

*Plate 41. Homemade window shade,
linen with cut work and needle lace
inserts, United States, 1870-1880.*

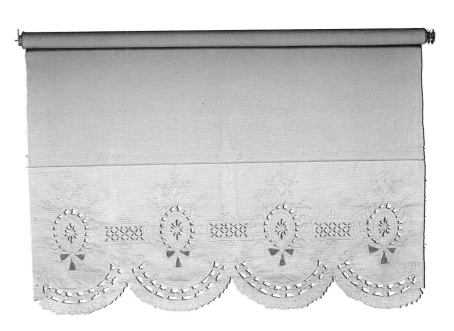

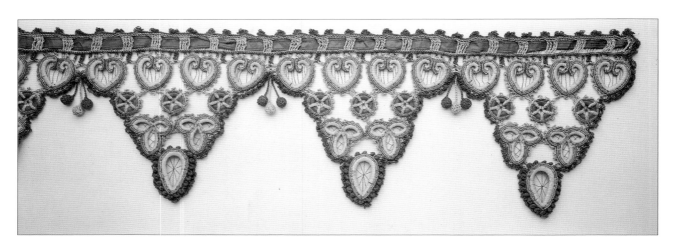

Plate 42. Mantel lambrequin, cotton crocheted, stitched, and wound over cardboard cores, cotton and silk ribbon, United States, 1880-1890.

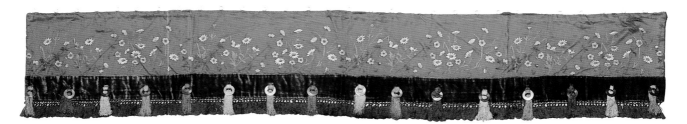

Plate 43. Mantel lambrequin, silk rep, silk velvet, with cotton and silk embroidery, silk fringe, brass rings, 1880-1890. The silk rep used for this lambrequin may have been recycled dress material. Decorative metal rings for home needleworkers were offered for sale in fancy work departments of dry goods stores until about 1910.

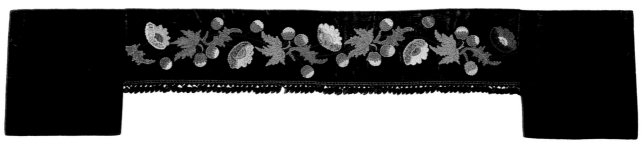

Plate 44. Mantel lambrequin, silk-pile velvet with silk and wool appliqué, couched wool edging and embroidery, cotton and silk "campaign" (bell) fringe, United States, 1880-1900.

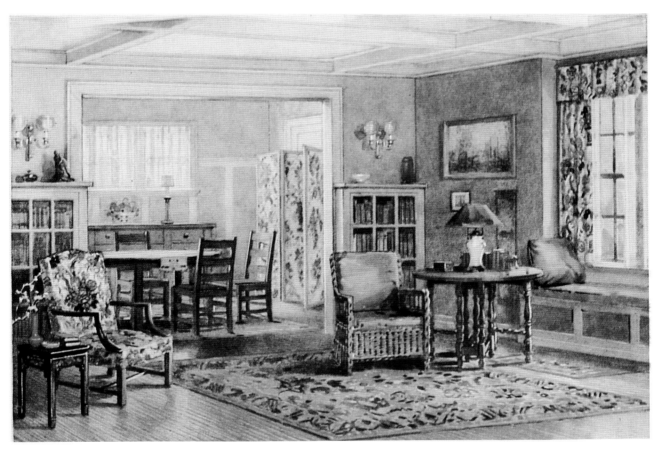

Plate 45. *"A Bungalow Living-Room and Dining-Room with Buff Walls and Floors of Brown Jaspé Linoleum,"* *illustration in Edward Stratton Holloway,* The Practical Book of Furnishing the Small House and Apartment *(1922). In bungalow floor plans, living rooms and dining rooms flowed together through wide doorways as pairs of parlors did in larger houses. Although these doorways have no drapery, portières—often plain velours—still were common in bungalows in the 1910s and the 1920s. Holloway encouraged bungalow owners to use the same fabrics and color schemes "where rooms communicate with a wide opening," which further blurred the distinctions in social life that furnishings suggested. These rooms also reflect the new interest in simplified housekeeping routines and sanitation. All upholstery fabrics here are washable cottons, and the linoleum floor and small area rugs could be kept cleaner than wall-to-wall carpet or larger rugs. The living room curtains, however, still employ both a fabric valance and side curtains.*

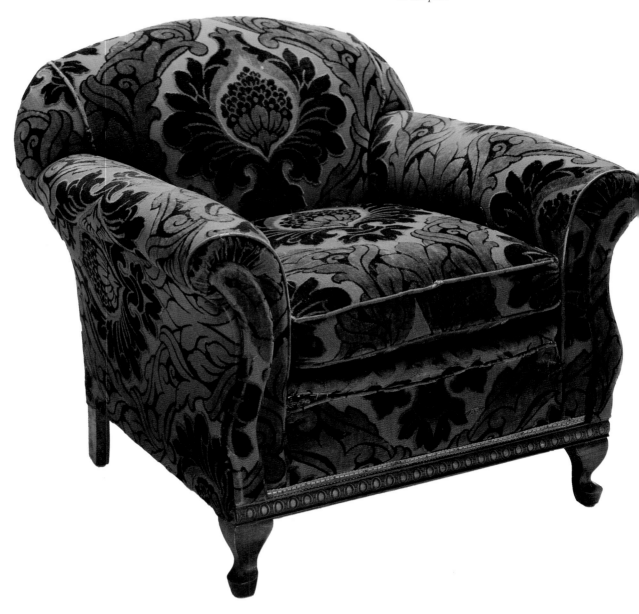

Plate 46. *Club chair, maple, voided printed cotton upholstery velvet, 1920-1930. The velvet used on this chair, part of a three-piece living room set, was printed to give the illusion of dimension to the pile.*

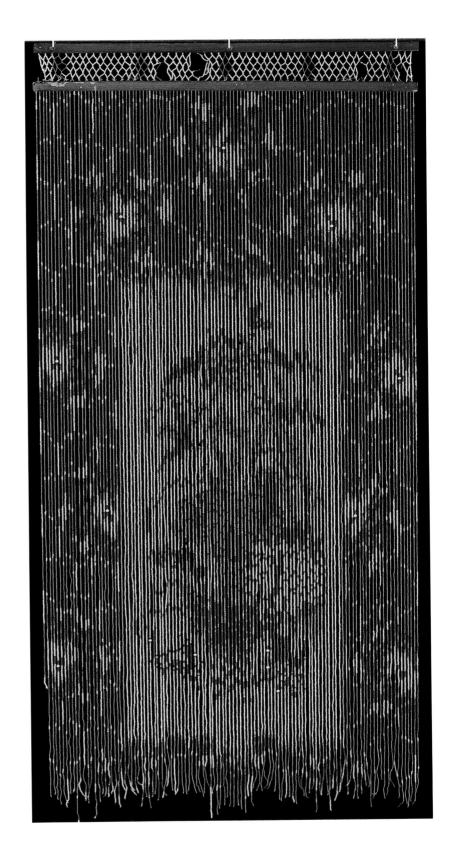

Plate 47. Door curtain, wood slats, cotton string, and glass beads, about 1915. Called "Japanese Portières" in trade catalogs of the period, bead curtains wholesaled for about ten dollars. This example, which has a design of palm trees and hibiscus, strikes a new note in exoticism—popular interest in the Hawaiian Islands.

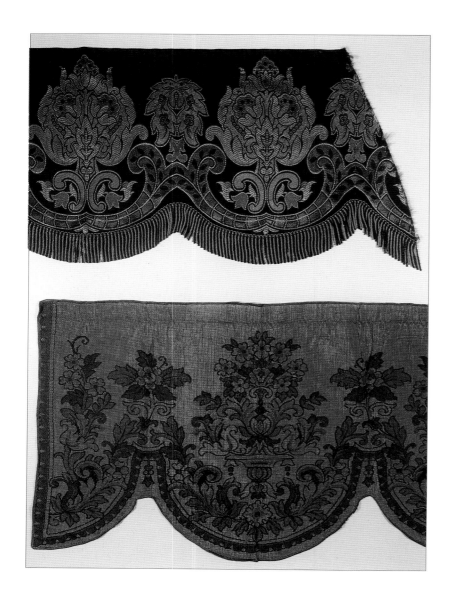

Plate 48. *Valance fabric, figured cotton and rayon, after 1925. By the mid-1920s, valances for windows and mantels could be purchased by the "scallop" in vividly colored and patterned mixtures of cotton and the new fiber rayon.*

Plate 49. *Pillow, rayon satin, about*
1930. Rayon satin was glamorous and
inexpensive, an inviting material for
decorative textiles as well as for clothing.

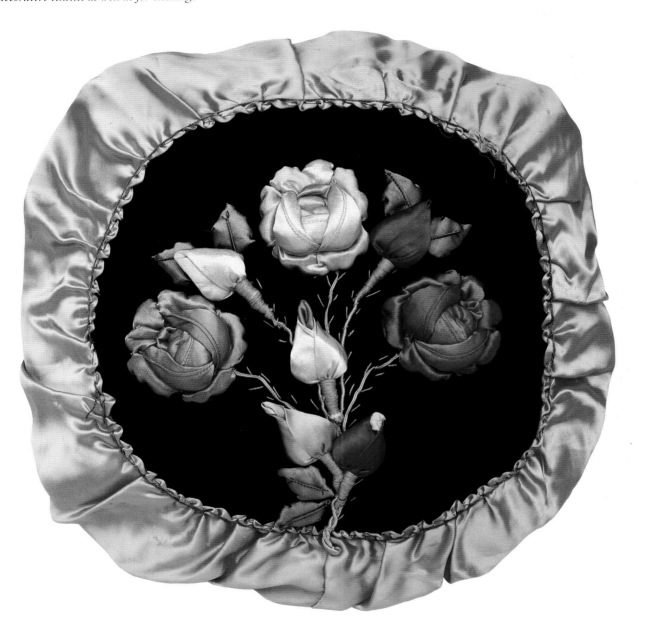

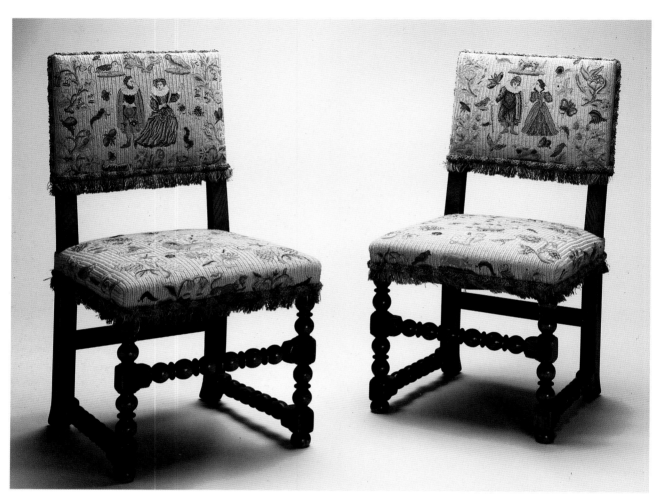

Plate 50. *Armchair and side chair, oak, wool and silk embroidery on canvas, Hayden Company, Rochester, New York, about 1920. Part of a larger set, these chairs have dead seats of horsehair. The animals, people, and plants on the yellow wool ground are finely executed copies of images found on seventeenth-century needlework.*

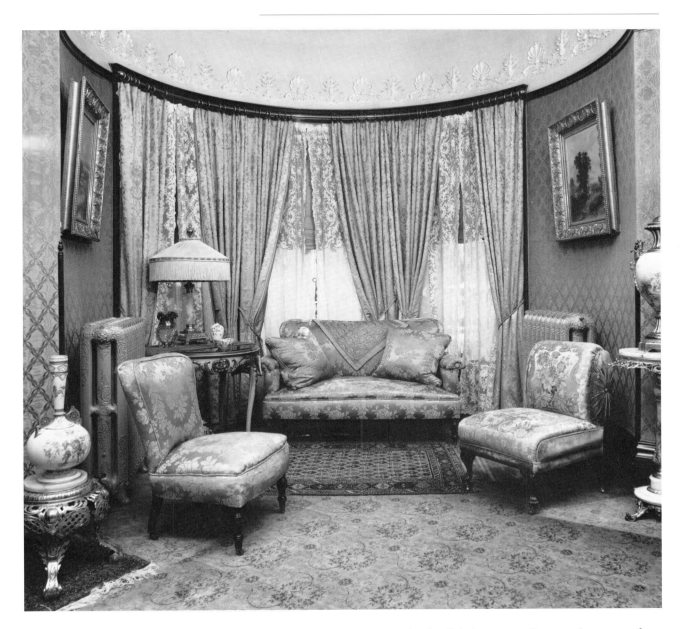

in fig. 13), which attests the family's long-standing employment of the convention of "French" parlors. A surviving suite in the aesthetic taste of the 1880s, now located in the music room of the house, may represent a second stage of parlor decorating in the family's old house, but its location prior to 1897 cannot be documented.

The 1907 furnishings of the Voigt family's parlor also demonstrate the set of cues—fabric types, color choices, and simplified forms of iconography that originated in eighteenth-century French design—that were interpreted as "French" style by the turn of the century. These cues were a paraphrase, a few specific components of eighteenth-century design selected to create "French" style as it was understood by middle-class people. The other public rooms in the house were decorated in dark colors; even the hallway's walls are covered with flocked red and maroon wallpaper, making the space cavelike in its dimness. The parlor, however, was decorated in shades of peach, pale green, and creamy white, with gilt embellishments in the form of pedestals and small tables. The three-piece parlor set and the walls are covered with, respectively, peach silk satin damask and pale green "watered" silk damask. Floral garlands and wreaths appear on many of the room's fabrics, including the wall-to-wall carpet. Plasterwork, the ornament cast into the radiators (which are finished to resemble green-patinated bronze), the picture frames, and the tables and pedestals introduce other "French" motifs, the c- and s-scrolls.[33]

This process of selecting and simplifying an established "style" is how all such decorative formulas are made popular in architecture, in furnishings, even in dress. Selection is done on two levels of each style—form and ornamentation. For example, the typology of forms for parlor suites originally was derived from the typology of social seating types perfected by the French in the eighteenth century. Further, the formulas employed a set of simplified ornamental elements, such as those chosen by the Voigts, that were understood as French. At this level, French style often was severely abbreviated, relying upon simplified festoons and certain trims and repeated use of a few unmistakable iconographic elements, such as the "bow knot" and c-and s-scrolls, that could be applied to any kind of object. (The inexpensive "French" lace curtains shown in chapter 8, fig. 11, employ the bowknot to signify their style.) A few key color schemes, particularly gilt and white or pastels, also were understood as typically French, as were particular fabrics such as damask. The result of this simplifying process can be seen in the French-inspired furnishings that reached entirely new groups of consumers in the last decades of the nineteenth century. These goods included inexpensive price lines of furniture and furnishing textiles, as well as ceramics, popular prints, and other decorative novelties (fig. 22).

How did ordinary consumers know that such objects were French? For those who had little or no contact with French commercial parlors, well-to-do households, and displays at exhibitions, other sources of information could teach interested new consumers—department stores, popular magazines, and mail-order catalogs. When matched to the appearance of the objects themselves,

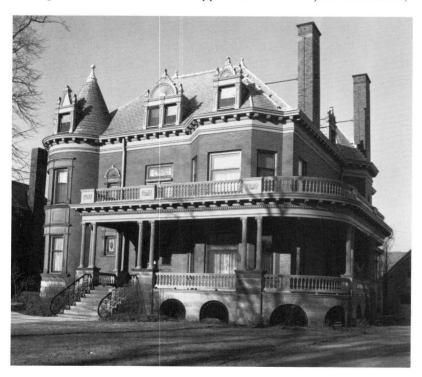

Fig. 21. *Exterior of Voigt House, Grand Rapids, Michigan, 1987. Courtesy Voigt Collection, Grand Rapids Public Museum.*

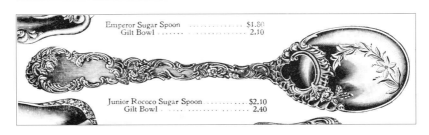

Fig. 22. "Junior Rococo Sugar Spoon," engraving in The Rochelle, *Wendell Manufacturing Co., New York, New York, and Chicago, Illinois (Spring 1898). The spoon handle features c- and s-scrolls, the same design element found in the printed fabric on the chair in fig. 5.*

the descriptors applied to furnishings by such sources in the 1880s and 1890s offered a lesson in the compressed range of design qualities that was considered French. If one was interested and alert, such information was everywhere. Instructions for embroidery in 1895 offered "Pompadour," "La Valiere," "Marie Antoinette," and "Louis XV" designs that featured "bowknots, floating ribbons and baskets" along with "floral groups and festoons." These instructions stated that such designs were considered appropriate for "reception rooms, boudoirs, and music rooms." But because most houses did not have so many separate social spaces, they would be appropriate for parlors.[34] The "Marseilles Shape China" offered by Montgomery Ward in 1895 featured "delicately raised scroll work" on the scalloped edges of each piece.[35] The *Sears, Roebuck and Co. Catalogue No. 110, Fall, 1900* offered a "Rococo couch" and "Rococo Bed Couch" characterized by scrolled skirts and elaborate all-over tufting.[36]

In the late nineteenth century, popular interpretations of French furnishing styles helped promulgate a fragmentary vision of the gala social life of the past and continued to have real charms for ordinary people (fig. 23). Such inexpensive French style represents the final popular ripple of the eighteenth-century ideal of gentility; it was a vision advanced through cheap prints, advertising images, and furnishings that still contained enough style cues to seem gala.

When Theodore Child noted the "comfort and glitter" of French house furnishing of the 1880s, he was, in part, referring to the theatrical character of its upholstery. He was particularly concerned with the appearance of large, overstuffed seating furniture, which was becoming increasingly popular in America. Known as "Turkish" furniture, the descriptor signaled both the presence of objects with design sources or actual origins in North Africa and the Middle East and types of upholstery that had no prototypes in these regions. These chairs were the most recent and most elaborate versions of ideas explored by French upholsterers as early as the late seventeenth century, when they had invented the "sopha" (defined in 1692 as "a form of day-bed like those used by the Turks") and, by the late eighteenth century, the "sultane," another overstuffed lounging couch.[37] Such overstuffed furniture in America originated with designs introduced by the French and interpreted by American makers. This furniture blended upholstery techniques and fabrics popularly understood as French with large-scale, overstuffed forms that were considered "oriental" or "Turkish" in character, although they had no precedent in traditional Turkish furniture. Such forms sent ambiguous messages about appropriate seated posture and were designated "Turkish" in keeping with Western popular ideas about oriental luxury and relaxation (fig. 24).

Between 1850 and 1870, Turkish furnishings in America consisted mainly of versions of the overstuffed "crapaud" armchair, a type introduced by French upholsterers in the 1840s (see chapter 4, fig. 27, and plate 8 for examples of such Turkish chairs). Such chairs sometimes were called "Turkish fauteuils," a term that made the French origins of Turkish chairs evident.[38] What characterized Turkish furnishings as a style group was their elaborate and complete

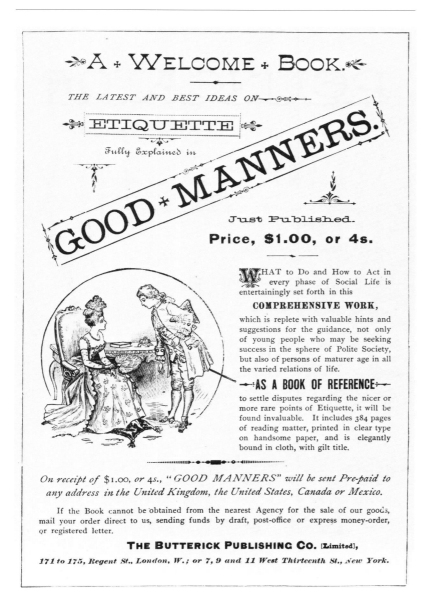

upholstery. Set on low legs that often were covered by fabric or deep fringe, they usually were larger in scale than other chairs. Until the introduction in the 1870s of "saddlebag" upholstery, which paraphrased the carpet-woven bags worn by camels, Turkish upholstery was buttoned or pleated and included an extra roll of stuffing around the top of the arms and back. This extra roll could be manipulated in attractive ways by upholsterers—as an enormous piece of twisted cording, a fan with stitched pleats or cord to mark the channels, or a contrasting pillow attached to the chair back. Turkish upholstery also employed long trimmings that swept the floor; it often had several layers of knotting, applied cords, and fringe.

Another typical French/Turkish form appearing at the turn of the century was a small chair or settee whose overstuffed back almost seemed to float above the seat. It was connected by small supports that were often themselves upholstered. These chairs were structurally fragile and often elaborately decorated, suggesting that they were to function as little-used reception chairs (fig. 25). Many turn-of-the-century forms, such as the pillowback chair with its tapestry upholstery in the Voigt parlor, demonstrate the blending of French and Turkish design elements (fig. 26).

Occasionally, Turkish furniture of the 1850s and 1860s also consisted of "ottomans" (after the Ottoman Empire) and "divans," flat seats or couches. (In the United States, the term ottoman also became a popular designation for hassocks.) Although much Turkish furniture was labor intensive, elaborate, and expensive (some of it employed cut-up Oriental carpets as upholstery), it always had been relatively easy to paraphrase in the characteristic form of the flat couch or ottoman as "do-it-yourself" upholstery projects as early as 1840.[39]

Apart from their complete upholstery, Turkish furnishings were characterized by their invitation to relaxation. In their context in France, ottomans or divans generally appeared in rooms where decorum could be relaxed, as in women's *boudoirs* and smoking rooms for men. By the 1860s, "Turkish" smoking rooms had been transplanted to a few American interiors such as Sylvester Morse's mansion in Portland, Maine, decorated by Gustav Herter in the early 1860s (fig. 27). Morse's smoking room, a small space at the front of the house on the second floor, was decorated in what is clearly a French interpretation of Turkish furnishing textiles. Equipped with a built-in sofa, the facing wall of windows was hung with lambrequins, side curtains embroidered with golden crescents, and tie-backs of red, purple, and black, ornamented with large golden-yellow silk crescents and stars, which were typical elements of Turkish design. Turkish furnishing fabrics of the 1860s and 1870s often were patterned with interpretations of the conventional designs found on rugs and

Fig. 24. Armchair, cotton and wool tapestry, silk-pile velvet, wool, cotton and silk trim, probably United States, 1890-1900. The overstuffed proportions and the multi-layered bullion and netted fringe with bell tassels of this chair made it "Turkish," but the predominantly pale-blue upholstery and the interpretation of eighteenth-century pastoral scenes on its tapestry seat and back also indicated that it was designed to fill a spot in a fashionable French-style room. Courtesy Smithsonian Institution.

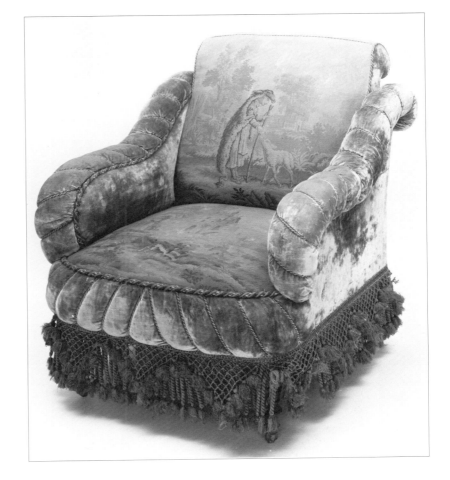

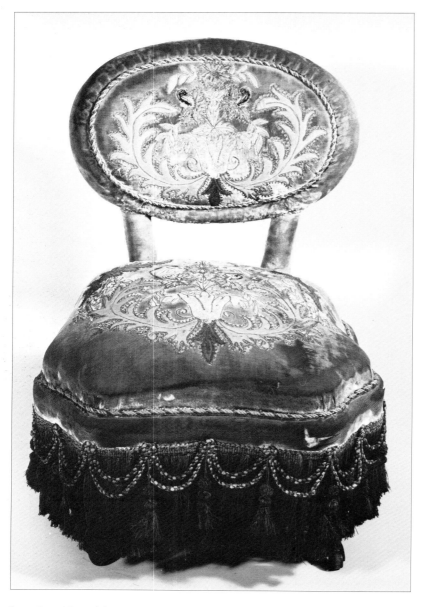

Fig. 25. *Turkish fancy chair, walnut, silk-pile velvet with appliqué, silk, wool, and cotton fringe, about 1885. Courtesy Wadsworth Atheneum; gift of Willie O. Burr by exchange.*

hangings, but, like English-made cashmere shawls, neither the fabric types nor the patterns were exact reproductions (plate 17).

In America, the occasional appearance of such exotic decor in expensive houses was echoed by a few other signs of interest in things "Turkish" about midcentury. Occasional articles in popular periodicals on the houses or dress of the peoples of Turkey, Syria, North Africa, or the Holy Land reflected this curiosity. *Godey's* noted an apparent craze for Turkish proverbs in 1855.[40] "Turkish" fashions, generally small accessory items such as the instructions for a "Turkish Bag in Wool Work" and a beaded "Turkish Purse," also were published by *Godey's* in 1856.[41] American interest in Turkish things was at least partly stimulated by the Empress Eugenie, whose role in fashion may be compared to that of Jacqueline Kennedy in the 1960s. Eugenie socialized with French-educated royalty from Egypt and the Levant, adapted Oriental clothing, and encouraged French decorators to explore types of overstuffed upholstery that were deemed "Oriental."[42]

The imperial adventures of France and England in that sector of

Fig. 26. Detail of pillowback chair (seen at right in fig. 20) in the Voigt House, silk-pile velvet and silk and wool tapestry, United States, 1907. Early photographs of the Voigt parlor indicate that this chair once had deep bullion fringe that swept the rug. Courtesy Voigt Collection, Grand Rapids Public Museum.

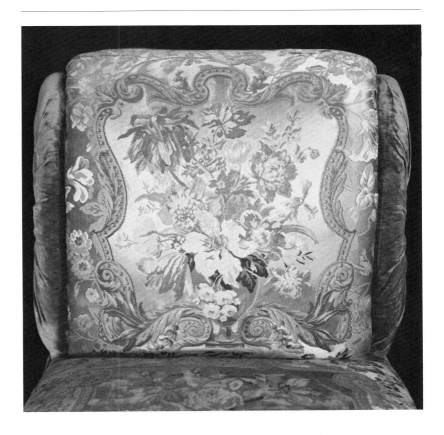

Fig. 27. Smoking room, Morse-Libby House, decorated by Gustav Herter, New York, New York. Courtesy Victoria Society of Maine.

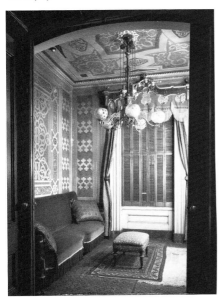

the world had encouraged many forms of artistic expression in Europe depicting oriental scenes. Orientalism was, in fact, a type of romanticism. In painting, it was "a piquant sauce to which clever painters adapted established genres, such as history, the nude, narrative, and even townscapes." Oriental paintings and the settings and themes for plays and operas "satisfied the romantic feeling for the picturesque and for local color" and provided safe outlets for sensuality and expressions of patriotism.[43]

Although American artists rarely took Oriental themes, they created individual studio settings in their studios and households that reflected traveling experiences (fig. 28).[44] Other Americans brought back ideas or a few actual furnishings from eastern tours. Samuel Clemens constructed a carpet-covered divan in the library of his house in Hartford, Connecticut, a recreation of the divans he saw in Turkey. In 1857, Samuel Colt and his bride carried back from Russia embroidered textiles with conventional oriental designs in red, blue, and white that they used to upholster a suite of furniture for an upstairs dressing room.

American interest in the Orient was supported by a simpler set of intellectual structures than the complex Orientalism of imperial Western Europe (fig. 29). While the undercurrent of ideas about the westward course of civilization certainly was popular in the American context, the "feminine" and sexually charged vision of the Orient that motivated artists was much milder and more innocent in mid-nineteenth-century America.[45] When the exotic nature of Oriental womanhood was depicted in American popular imagery, it often had an almost wholesome cast. The illustration published by Frank Leslie of the "scarf dance" offered as an entertainment in the Tunisian Café even showed respectable women in the audience (fig. 30).

Turkish upholstery reached its apex of popularity in America between 1890 and 1915. Popular interest grew from the

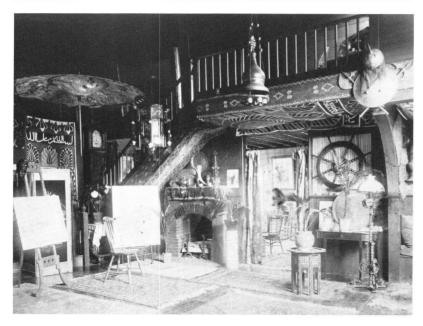

Fig. 28. "*Interior of Kenat's studio, 'The Barnacle,' Kennebunkport, Me.,*" *about 1885. Along with colonial furniture and a Japanese parasol and lantern, this artist's studio featured North African and Middle Eastern lamps, brasswork, a small octagonal stand, and textiles on the walls and under the stairs. Picturesque artists' studios, filled with exotic objects, were popular places for visiting and socializing in the late nineteenth century.*

convergence of several strands of thought and furnishing practice, including the continuing interest in French design (hence French interpretations of Turkish furniture) and changing ideas about what sort of furnishings were appropriate in middle-class homes. This reflected an evolution or reinterpretation of the tension between the cultured parlor and the comfortable parlor. The late nineteenth-century popularity of "Turkish" upholstery also was linked to larger cultural patterns, particularly to the domestication of exotica. The chain of associations inspired by such objects turned back upon itself, blending the "comfort" of domesticity and the relaxed physical comfort that potentially undermined parlor decorum with a popular, not scholarly, sense of the expressive potential of upholstery. When Constance Cary Harrison praised the use of portières for the "whiff" of the Orient they added to the decor of ordinary houses, she implied that they imparted an exotic yet tamed sense to the parlor (fig. 31).[46]

Thousands of ordinary consumers were exposed to the novelties of Turkish furnishings through the North African and Middle Eastern national exhibits at the 1876 Centennial and, more important, through another variation on the model interior, the oriental or Turkish bazaars on the Exhibition grounds (figs. 32 and 33). Books that described and assessed the Centennial, however, tended to illustrate and praise the Japanese national exhibits and the Modern Gothic and "Anglo-Japanese" products of European design reformers at the expense of Near Eastern displays. The author of *Gems of the Centennial Exhibition: Consisting of Illustrated Descriptions of Objects of an Artistic Character...* (1877) contrasted the applied arts of Russia and Turkey in a characteristic manner:

> In the one case [Russia], we see an example of patient progress and self-evolution hardly to be matched; in the other, a fatal and obdurate immovability, a character steeped in Oriental barbarism, from pasha to peasant, in spite of the mask of European polish which slightly veneers life among the upper classes...The Turkish display of those products which represent the artistic phase of national development gave a significant commentary on the place of Turkey in modern history. This people can hardly be said to have any native and organic art of its own.[47]

Nonetheless, the lesser buildings of the Exposition introduced the ordinary visitor to the splendors of the Near East in a most effective and direct way, through a series of small bazaars in the hundreds of outbuildings scattered throughout the fairgrounds. These model interiors were not didactic and overtly "educational," as the exhibits of the large buildings were intended to be. Rather, they were commercial ventures, designed for shopping, eating, and entertainments, a transitional kind of space for fairgoers before the appearance of the sophisticated Midway at the Columbian Exposition of 1893. The authors of a satirical account of a visit to the Centennial suggested the impression these many lesser structures made upon ordinary visitors:

> The foreign display within the Main Building was grand, that outside was grander still. Had our minds been one whit less strong, we should have been bewildered by the conglomeration…Turkish kiosks, Chinese pagodas, Japanese pavilions, Arabian tents, Persian bazaars, Egyptian temples, Mohammedan mosques, Gypsy encampments, and American drinks, enough to confuse anyone. Then monuments, booths, fountains, and cigar stands innumerable.[48]

The Turkish Bazaar received much attention in more popular Victorian periodicals such as *Frank Leslie's Weekly* and in a spate of inexpensive fictionalized accounts of the fair such as *Our Show* and *What Ben Beverly Saw at the Exposition* (1876). The anonymous author of the latter offered for his readers the details of a visit to its coffee room:

> We have all read of the Turkish cafe, where the luxury-loving Turks smoke long pipes and drink the purest mocha. This fanciful looking structure, built in the form of an octagon, with such a queer roof is one, and supposed to be built after the genuine Turkish fashion; suppose we visit it. In the centre of the room are tables and chairs; around the outside are luxuriously cushioned sofas, which have fancifully figured coverings, and have a decidedly hospitable aspect. The curtains are of highly covered, heavy material, and give the room a sort of Oriental air. Behind the counter, on one side, sits a Turkish woman, acting as cashier of the establishment, wearing a gayly embroidered velvet garment—her magnificent black hair, dressed in our modern style…a splendid figure, and a sensitive, refined face, as white as many brunettes of the Anglo-Saxon race. We take a seat on the sofa, and a stalwart young Turk, dressed in a gay, red jacket, immense trousers, and turban, approaches to take our order…In a few moments the smoking mocha appears in a small brass ladle, which holds about three tablespoons full of coffee…We find it to be thick, like cream, the grounds as fine as flour, the flavor delicious…Near us, groups are smoking the famous long Turkish pipes, with stems about six feet long, and seem determined to enjoy a solid comfort from the experiment. Customers come in rapidly…parties and groups are continually looking in, and passing through, to see the novel spectacle, and the lady at the counter, is a continual target for numberless glances from bright eyes; but the Turks are not to be abashed by smiles or laughter, but mind their business, well contented, so long as they can do a flourishing trade.[49]

Hung with "handsomely embroidered curtains," the walls lined with "divans along the sides, covered with blue and strawberry

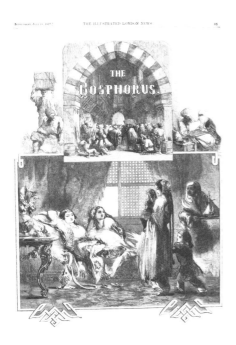

Fig. 29. "*Lights of the Harem,*" *engraving in* Illustrated London News, Supplement *(18 July 1857).*

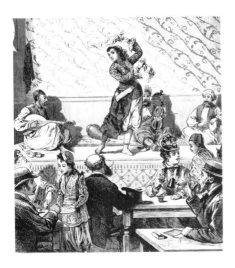

Fig. 30. "*Scene in the Tunisian Cafe—the Scarf Dance,*" *engraving in* Frank Leslie's Historical Register of the Centennial Exposition *(1876).*

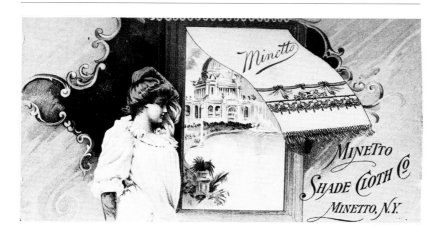

Fig. 31. *Flyer for Minetto Shade Cloth Company, Minetto, New York, about 1895. This vignette (which is outlined by the conventional "French" style cue of c- and s-scrolls) exemplifies the character of popular historical and exotic associationism at the end of the nineteenth century. The windblown shade, with its dado design of French drapery, partly reveals the vista of an exotic oriental building to the dreamy woman at the window. In its composition and the way it uses such cultural references, the advertisement is a precursor to similar twentieth-century advertising techniques.*

covered plush," the reporter for *Frank Leslie's Weekly* pronounced the scene in the Turkish Café and Bazaar "curious and interesting" (fig. 34). For women uncomfortable with the smoke and close company of so many unintroduced strangers, the cafe contained two "waiting-rooms" that were "furnished with lounges and ottomans and hung with Turkish tapestry." These rooms may have introduced many visitors to interiors where most or all of the decorative effect was achieved with textiles. Further, several "bazaars" in the same building sold "rich costumes, carpets, pipes, swords, daggers, hilts, and other articles."[50] The Turkish Café and Bazaar was only one of fifty-six "private exhibition buildings" also run as shops for profit, including the "Jerusalem Palestine Bazaar," the "Bethlehem Bazaar," the "Bosphorus Kiosk Bazaar," the "Oriental Bazaar," the "Persian Bazaar," and the "Tunisian Cafe and Bazaar."[51]

Such accounts of visits to the Turkish bazaar contain clues to popular interest in that country. Although the "refined" young Turkish register girl represented the mysterious orient, her hair in its western style and her delicate features and light skin positioned her on some middle ground between the Eastern and Western worlds. Indeed, an article titled "Turkey: Its Past Condition and Promised Reforms," published in the February 1876 issue of *Frank Leslie's Popular Monthly,* used the homely example of headgear to drive home the point that "on no spot in the world are the customs of the people in all eastern and western countries so blended in proportions as in this city [Constantinople]. Nowhere else are seen the European hat, bonnet and chignon, and the Turkish fez, turban, and yashmach."[52] If the observer was of the appropriate mindset, it was possible to think of Turkey (a location in the orient with blurry outlines at best in popular perception) as both exotic and somewhat familiar.

Even with the constant refrain of the manners book to "sit up straight," the constraints of corsets and bustles, and the use of ordinary parlors for such formal rites of passage as courting and weddings, overstuffed parlor furniture gained in popularity by the 1890s. Cheaper ways of producing such furniture had been developed, but these production innovations themselves must have sprung from the latent demand among some groups of consumers for overstuffed Turkish suites like those advertised by S. C. Small and Co. of Boston, Massachusetts, and the Milwaukee firm Bub and Kipp in their trade catalogs from the mid-1880s.[53]

The most common type of Turkish upholstered furniture in American homes of the late nineteenth century was the overstuffed arm or rocking chair. "Turkish rockers" remained in production in various forms until around 1920 and were a late manifestation of the tradition of introducing upholstered, spring-seat furniture to ordinary

*Fig. 32. "1888. Tunisian
Section—Main Building," photograph by
the Centennial Photographic Co.,
Philadelphia, Pennsylvania, 1876.
Apart from small inlaid tables and
decorative metalwork that could be
appropriated for use as accessories in
domestic interiors, textiles—carpets,
draperies, and fabrics that could be used
as table or furniture covers in western
rooms—were the most influential
domestic furnishings exhibited by Turkey,
Egypt, and Tunisia. Courtesy The Free
Library of Philadelphia, Print and
Picture Department; photograph by Joan
Broderick.*

households through the rocking chair, traditionally the most comfortable kind of chair in houses. In the 1880s, popular enthusiasm for Turkish upholstery also was focused on drapery and carpets, elements that could be incorporated into existing rooms. Between the Centennial and the Columbian Exposition of 1893, factory-organized upholsterers and enterprising American furniture and department stores such as R. H. Macy cashed in on the new interest in Turkish furnishings by setting up "Oriental Departments." They sold a smattering of hammered copper goods, small tables, and other accessories, but the bulk of their business was in upholstery textiles—domestically made and imported draperies, rugs, throws, and pillows ornamented with embroidery and woven with conventional "rug" patterns or stripes. In 1889, the catalog of Jordan, Marsh and Company of Boston offered domestically manufactured "Smyrna Rugs," products of Philadelphia's Bromley upholstery mills, accessibly priced: an 18" x 36" throw rug cost $1.00, 30" x 60" sizes cost from $3.00 to $5.00, and a 12- by 15-foot room-size rug cost $80.00. "Turcoman" portières were available for as little as $1.75 per pair. "Turkish satin" upholstery fabrics cost $1.50 per yard, the same price as black horsehair, which was of better quality. But Turkish satin offered a more satisfying aesthetic experience for consumers interested in the exotic.[54]

By the opening of the Turkish Village at the Columbian

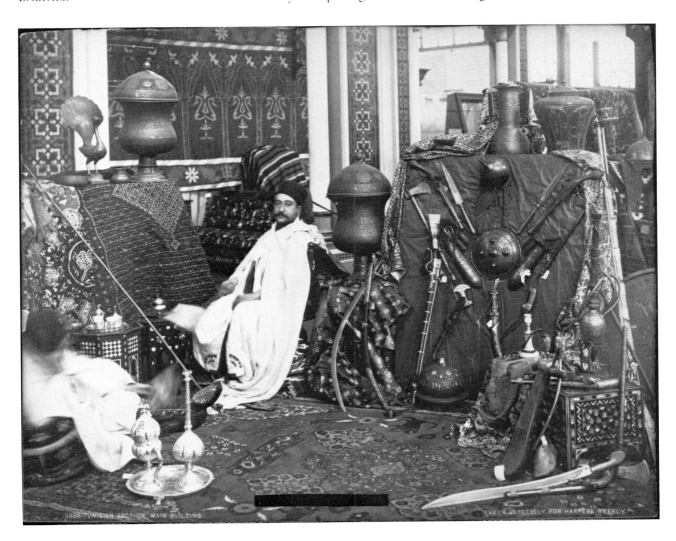

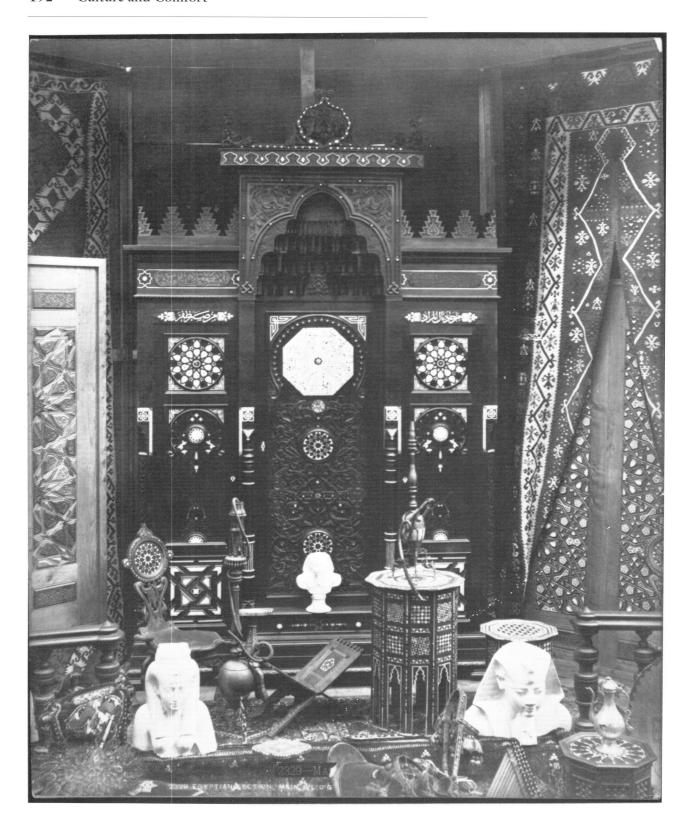

Fig. 33. *"2329. Egyptian Section—Main Building," photograph by the Centennial Photographic Co., Philadelphia, Pennsylvania, 1876. Compare the design of the drapery at the right of the image to the American factory-woven "Turkish" couch cover in plate 19. Courtesy The Free Library of Philadelphia, Print and Picture Department; photograph by Joan Broderick.*

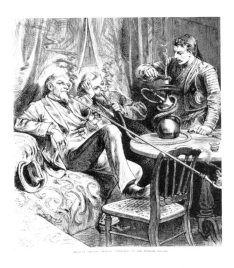

Fig. 34. *"American Visitors Smoking Chibouques in the Turkish Bazaar," engraving in* Frank Leslie's Historical Register of the Centennial Exposition *(1876).*

Exposition in 1893, the range of popular forms of Turkish upholstery was in place. The exhibits marketed Turkish furnishings through model rooms (fig. 35). Juxtaposed beside the "Alpine panorama," the Turkish Village was a concession run for a Constantinople-based importing firm. Intended as a "typical exhibit of the Ottoman Empire," the village was admittedly edited for Western consumption: "Here are no antique castles, no grim weapons or warriers, no peasants or peasants' homes; instead are luxurious pavilions and bazaars, a miniature mosque, a theatre, with Turkish sedan bearers, and costly articles of furniture and decoration, all true to the life of Turkey in Europe and Turkey in Asia."[55] Along with the consecrated mosque, the highlight of the Turkish Village was its refreshment concession and its bazaar, consisting of forty booths that sold Turkish furnishings. These combined recognizable Turkish easy chairs with drapery and other exotic accessories.

A few design writers of the 1890s continued to suggest that Oriental furnishings were laden with associations of barbarism and the harem. The author of one such article on "Draperies and Embroideries in the East" grew overwrought when digressing upon a piece of embroidery from Istanbul, presumably made by "some fair odalisque, of the harem of a Sultan long since gone to his account with Allah." To the potential purchaser, the author suggested that the piece represented "the one poor resource of pleasure in a young life condemned to a thraldom, which was as hateful as its surroundings were mockingly gorgeous…, the spots of the time-tinted surface of the grounding are the tears which fell from the eyes of the patient worker as she nursed over her hopeless activity."[56] However, the settings of the model rooms and bazaar suggest that, by the 1890s, Turkish furnishings had become domesticated exotica. Already sifted through the filter of French design, Turkish upholstery was now reproduced by American looms in the form of "Smyrna art rugs" (reversible chenille rugs woven in oriental designs on American looms in Philadelphia) and striped portières. It also was paraphrased in the form of factory-made divans, ottomans, and "cozy corners" which were often home-upholstery projects.

By the turn of the century, Turkish upholstery was a clue to the changing middle-class formulation of culture and comfort in the parlor. It appealed to the American middle class because it both expressed a cosmopolitan grasp of the world and fitted neatly into new visions of domestic coziness. Turkish furnishings were potentially inexpensive formulations for ordinary households, allowing "culture" to mean the ability to appreciate exotica rather than the cultivation required to meet the rigorous demands of self-presentation. The change in concepts of appropriate parlor furnishing that Turkish furnishings suggest was not uniform, nor did it necessarily reflect the waning force of the idea that comfort was a moral state and the taste for luxury a signal of debilitating weakness in the national (that is, Anglo-Saxon) fiber.[57] This train of popular thought, which worried earnestly about the effects of rooms upon character and the place of room decor as expressions of character, eventually emerged in some decorating literature as the idea of the "living room," which became the room without facade. Until that time, however, some ordinary families, whose small living spaces or typical living patterns set limits on aspirations toward formal parlors, could express culture in the parlor through cozy and iconographically vague Turkish upholstery and related collections of exotic accessories.

Alongside the leather-covered Turkish rocker, lounges were the most popular form of Turkish upholstery by 1900 (see plate 28). They appeared in parlors, family sitting rooms, and libraries. Their typical upholstery fabrics—carpet, or cotton velour—bore traditional

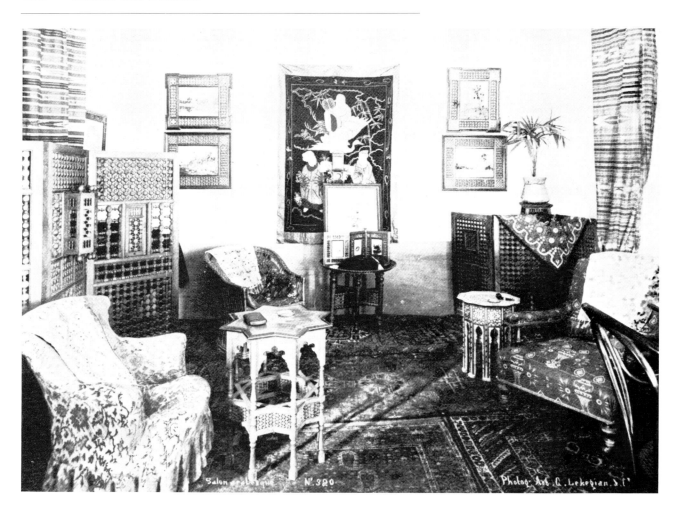

connotations of the richness and luxury of pile fabrics and were woven or printed with conventional designs that loosely approximated oriental rugs. Turkish rocking chairs and lounges with leather covers that suggested the masculine decor of smoking rooms were also popular. Rocking chairs and lounges both continued the connection of Turkish furnishings with situations encouraging relaxation.

Between 1890 and 1920, the fad for creating "cozy corners," which at first often were called "Turkish corners," revived a variation upon the built-in ottoman or divan found in smoking rooms and multi-use rooms in Europe earlier in the century. As parlor furnishing, cozy corners were particularly popular in households where occupants felt a need to complete or update the room but had limited means to furnish it fashionably. These corners often were cited as an excellent do-it-yourself upholstery project, continuing the practice of homemade upholstery for modest rooms.[58] They also were prescribed for small apartments or houses where parlors had to contain convertible beds because they disguised the double function of the room in a fashionable way (fig. 36).

The Turkish corner created about 1895 by the John Curtis family of Dorchester, Massachusetts, seems to have been a solution for a parlor that contained a mixed lot of furniture accumulated gradually (figs. 37 and 38). Before installing the Turkish corner, the Curtis family had been using a dressing case from the 1870s as a parlor étagère. The contrast between the Curtis parlor and ones furnished earlier illustrates how ideas about creating a cultured and comfortable

Fig. 35. Model room ("Salon arabesque") at the Turkish Bazaar, Columbian Exposition, Chicago, Illinois, photomechanical reproduction in The Book of the Fair *(1893). Along with striped curtains and throws, Turkish upholstery was here represented by a* crapaud *with a ruffled skirt, a willow chair with cushion, and an upholstered armchair of the type called a "Cromwell chair" in the 1920s.*

parlor had evolved. The Curtis family displayed on every available surface their broad sense of participation in culture, which included the exotic orient, both the Far East and the Levant as well as Europe. They employed a miscellaneous collection of ceramics, art glass, ironwork candlesticks, and exotica (a Japanese garden lantern, an incense burner), and used oriental rugs (whether real or ersatz it is impossible to tell) as the floor covering. At the same time, the seating used in the parlor, which was doubtless chosen with some care, suggests that this family was particularly interested in comfortable seating. The comfortable exotica of the Turkish corner was a neat summary of both goals. The Turkish corner, with its latticework frame, chenille curtains, pile of pillows, and buttoned upholstery, not only functioned as an overstuffed sofa but contributed to the international eclecticism of the room.

After 1900, cheap factory-woven and printed textiles, simple yardages or finished rectangles of fabrics such as couch covers having conventional oriental-looking patterns, made Turkish style within the

Fig. 36. "A Perfect Bed A Perfect Davenport Combined," advertisement for the D. T. Owen Company, Cleveland, Ohio, in Grand Rapids Furniture Record *(October 1903). Courtesy Grand Rapids Public Library.*

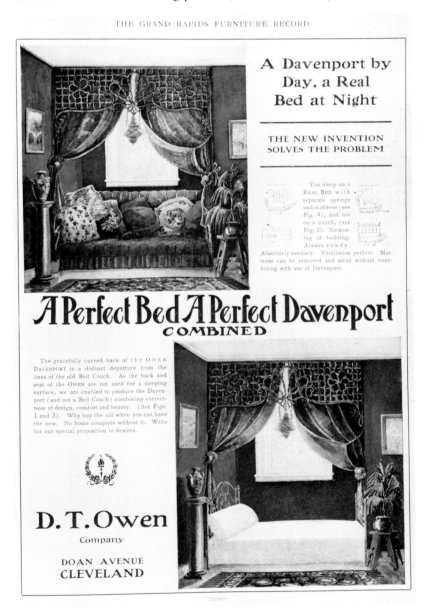

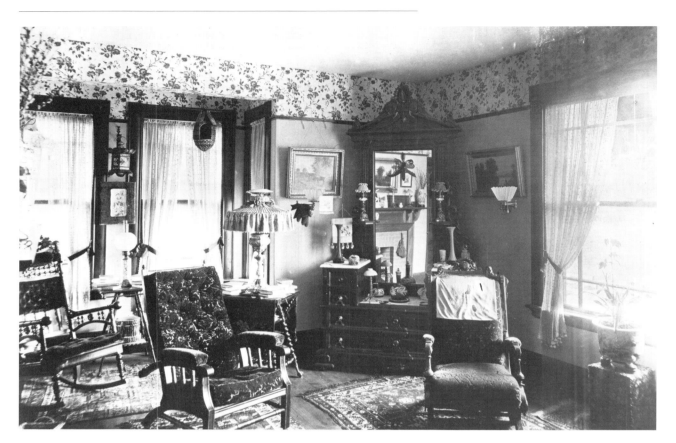

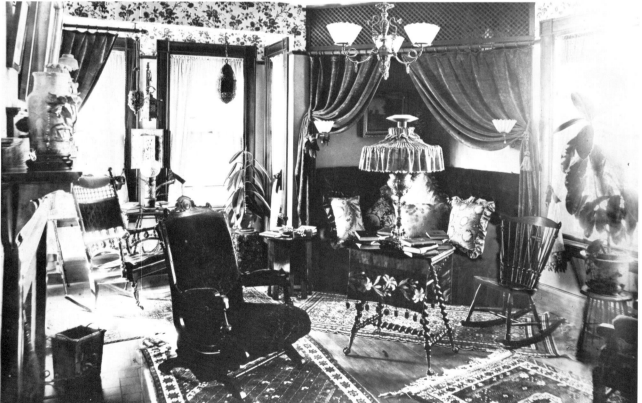

Figs. 37 and 38. *Parlor belonging to the John Curtis family, Dorchester, Massachusetts, before and after the installation of an upholstered "cozy corner," photographs by member of the Curtis family, about 1895. The Curtis family was forced to fill out the contents of its parlor with a bedroom dressing case (serving as an étagère) until it installed its Turkish corner. Courtesy Society for the Preservation of New England Antiquities.*

means of very modest furnishing budgets (plate 18). Readers of some domestic advice manuals were advised that an "Oriental divan" could be had "at the cost of but a few dollars" thanks to "Imitation Baghdad" couch covers (fig. 39; plate 19).

For ordinary parlor makers in the last quarter of the nineteenth century and first decades of the twentieth, Turkish upholstery offered one more set of associative terms that could be employed with a selection of other "styles" to create eclectic settings. The historical elements of Turkish and other styles were simplified in their popular forms and were mixed and matched with increasingly greater freedom, both in room settings and even within individual objects (fig. 40). Within each style, upholstery offered a limited set of formal qualities, and when compared to upholstered furniture of numerous other styles —French, Turkish, aesthetic, and even "colonial" —it is clear that all were unified by their adherence to what might be called a meta-style, an overarching set of formal visual standards. Upholstery generally adhered to this aesthetic of refinement well into the twentieth century.

Throughout the second half of the nineteenth century, then, the work of French upholsterers seems to have defined both the ideal of formal seating for gala rooms, based on eighteenth-century chair types, and new models of informal seating as French upholsterers introduced to Americans their interpretations of Turkish seating furniture. If the aesthetics of upholstery continued to appeal to the sensibility of refinement, the increasing popularity of Turkish overstuffed furniture toward the end of the century also signaled change in ideas about comfort in seating. Comfortable furniture

Fig. 39. *"Plain Couch...without Head or Arms," illustration in* Household Discoveries *(1908). According to author Sidney Morse, "Couches and sofas having a raised headpiece or arms at either end are giving place to plain couches, after the fashion of the Oriental divan, without head or arms, and covered by appropriate couch covers. An ordinary folding canvas cot bed and a common cotton top mattress thick enough to prevent sagging in the middle is really superior to a sofa or davenport costing much more money. Imitation Baghdad or other suitable couch covers in cotton fabrics are inexpensive, and a row of fancy pillows can be readily made of washable material at slight expense. Thus the entire couch and furnishing may be had at the cost of but a few dollars."*

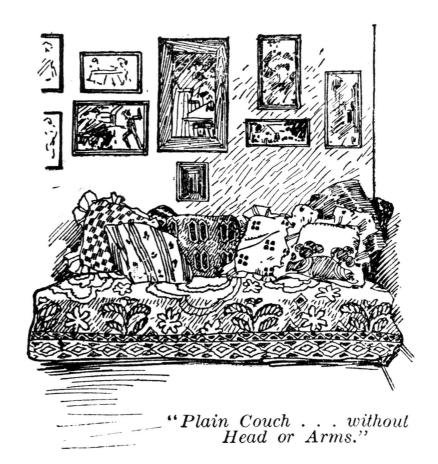

"*Plain Couch . . . without Head or Arms.*"

became overstuffed furniture that did little to control the seated posture of its occupants. At first, such overstuffed furniture appeared in ordinary houses as rocking chairs, a type bearing strong associations with domesticity and with age and infirmity, or as overstuffed chairs and lounges made for use in libraries or sitting rooms. By the mid-1880s, some trade catalogs began to offer factory-made overstuffed parlor sets. Further, the size of Turkish upholstered furniture increased as the turn of the century approached, providing even fewer cues to deportment except perhaps a general invitation to relaxed posture. Trade catalogs from the first decade of the twentieth century that offer a range of overstuffed sofas sometimes acknowledge their products' origins in Turkish furniture; the Bishop Furniture Co., for example, described its overstuffed sofas as Turkish in a catalog from about 1910. (Eventually such sofas came to be called "Chesterfields.")[59] Overstuffed, exotic-looking Turkish furniture survived into the 1930s with "style moderne" interpretations (fig. 41).

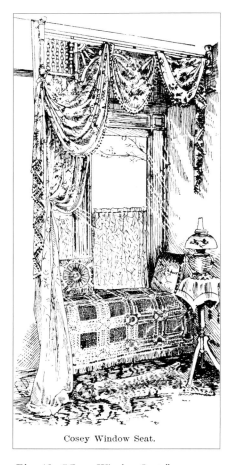

Cosey Window Seat.

Fig. 40. *"Cosey Window Seat," illustration in* The Decorator and Furnisher *(October 1891). This plan for a cozy corner featured fretwork draped in the French manner (scarf drapery, which was not difficult for amateurs to imitate). The seat, however, was covered with a blue-and-white coverlet, an heirloom with family associations and colonial revival overtones. A "leopard rug," praised as "novel and handsome" in the accompanying article, provided the required exotic symbolism.*

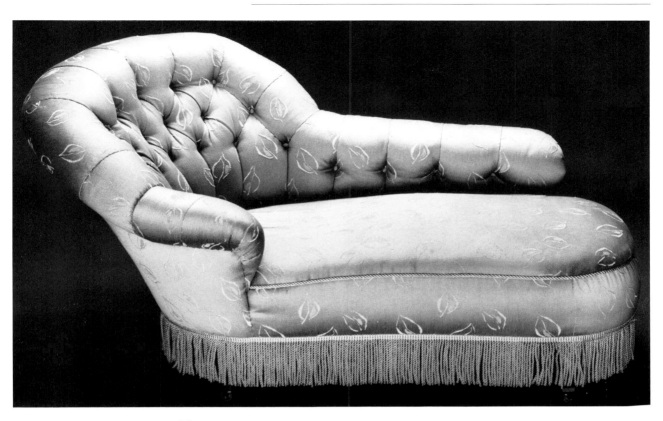

Fig. 41. *Lounge, cotton sateen with brocaded cotton design, United States, about 1930.*

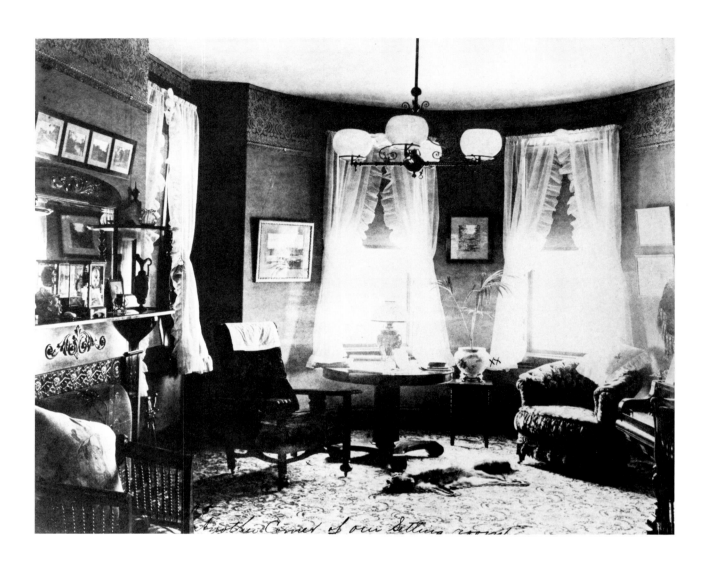

Another Corner of our setting room.

CHAPTER SEVEN
PARLOR SUITES AND LOUNGES:
CULTURE AND COMFORT
IN FACTORY-MADE SEATING FURNITURE

Fig. 1. *"Another Corner of our Sitting room," parlor/sitting room of Mr. and Mrs. William Wilson Carter, by unidentified photographer, 1895-1900. This amateur blueprint photograph, perhaps made by Mr. Carter, is one of a group documenting the first apartment of the newly-wed couple. This modest room combined an overstuffed Turkish chair, an adjustable Morris chair, and a "colonial" fancy chair. Courtesy Society for the Preservation of New England Antiquities.*

A room could be designated a "parlor" by assembling the best seating furniture in the house there, including lounges, easy chairs of various forms, and fancy rocking chairs. Alice Neupert's mother created her front parlor in Buffalo after this fashion in the 1880s; so did newly-weds Mr. and Mrs. William Wilson Carter in 1894 (fig. 1).

However, purchasing a parlor suite (or "suit"—both terms were in use throughout the period) was probably the single easiest way to create a parlor in the second half of the nineteenth century. A parlor was recognizable and could be considered completely furnished, if somewhat bare, when its furnishings included only a parlor suite and a center table, placed in a room containing a carpet, a mantel, and decorative window draperies (fig. 2). This compressed vocabulary of parlor furnishing could also be employed in other spaces, such as the large "parlor" in a family hotel at a camp meeting resort. Each suite, grouped around a center table, represented a separate "parlor" for a single family or party of visitors (fig. 3).

Custom-made sets of drawing-room furniture, which included sofas, chairs, tables, and other cabinetwork, had been available for sale in the United States in the first decades of the nineteenth century for well-to-do clients, but no particular formula existed for the number and kind of pieces of furniture included or ordered in these sets. In 1857, the decorating firm of Ringuet-LePrince and Marcotte invoiced Samuel Colt, the inventor of the revolver, for a matching set of furniture of eleven pieces for the drawing room of his new house, Armsmear, in Hartford, Connecticut. The invoice listed two "Stuffed front sofas, arms & legs in carved Rosewood"; one "Stuffed Corner Divan"; four "Rosewood Medaillon [*sic*] Armchairs"; and four sidechairs to match, all of which were provided with yellow and white satin damask upholstery. The set also included two elaborate rosewood center tables and two card tables made to match. The number of chairs in the set may have been selected for the two card tables purchased for the room. The seating furniture alone cost the substantial sum of $822, which included some discounts to Colt from the firm.[1]

Around this time, more modest yet still up-to-date and prosperous households also contained large sets of matching parlor furniture. A catalog for a New York City house auction in 1853 described the front parlor's furniture as being "EN SUITE"; it included a "Sofa" and a "Tête-à-Tête," a "Sewing Chair," an "Arm Chair," and four "Parlor chairs," all of rosewood and "crimson plush." A marble-topped étagère, "mirror back and doors," and a sofa table completed the set.[2]

Before about 1860, matching sets of seating furniture were commonly incorporated into the parlors of ordinary houses in sets of "fancy chairs," which were decoratively painted. The 1856 inventory for the house of George Clinton Latta (1795-1891), an entrepreneur living in Charlotte, New York (a village on Lake Ontario near Rochester), listed "sets" among the contents of a pair of parlors; these sets were two groups of six "fancy chairs" valued together at eighteen dollars. Latta's parlors represent a transitional type of furnishing

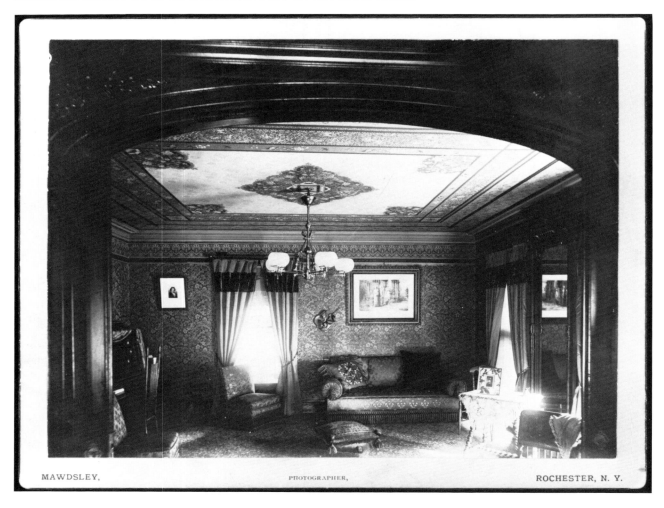

MAWDSLEY,   PHOTOGRAPHER,   ROCHESTER, N. Y.

between the older multi-purpose parlor and the parlor as reception room. They were carpeted, had "damask and lace window curtains and strings" (valued at thirty dollars), and contained two center tables, a piano, a bureau, a bookcase, twelve paintings (family portraits), and a "tête tête" valued at twenty dollars.[3]

By 1856, Latta was an older man, and his family's parlors probably represented a mixture of old and new furnishings. Prosperous middle-class families with money to spend and the opportunity to furnish from scratch could purchase sets of parlor furniture whose size and character anticipated a trend toward the seven-piece set, called "parlor suite," that became a furnishing formula in the 1860s.[4] Captain Richard H. Tucker, who operated a shipping line out of Wiscasset, Maine, and owned his own vessels, sailed to Boston to purchase furniture for his new house. Mrs. Tucker was indisposed, recovering from the birth of their first child, but Captain Tucker knew exactly what to purchase to create a respectable parlor. From A. G. Manning, a furniture dealer located conveniently near Boston's Maine Depot, he bought an eight-piece "parlor sett" for $165 consisting of a sofa, two armchairs, four side chairs, and a matching lounge.

Trade catalogs dating between 1858 and 1870 also suggest the gradual development of a standard formula for sets of parlor seating furniture (fig. 4). The catalog from the firm of George Henkels of Philadelphia, dating from about 1855, offered a range of pieces in a variety of styles and prices but indicated no standard formula for the

Fig. 2. Unidentified interior in Rochester, New York, photograph by Peter Mawdsley (active 1887-1904), Rochester, New York, about 1890. An expensive, fashionable room that reflects the "aesthetic" taste, this parlor nevertheless consisted of little more than a suite, a piano, carpet, and curtains.

number of pieces or types of chairs. Henkels priced out the options for sofas and chairs individually; advertisements and accounts of the appearance of his warerooms do suggest that he also kept sets of parlor furniture on the shop floor, ready to be purchased on the spot. Henkels was locally famous for his imported French furniture. In 1855, a well-to-do customer who chose to make up a seven-piece set (sofa or "tête," ladies' and gentleman's armchairs, and four armless side chairs) of French-made rosewood "Style Antique Drawing Room Furniture" would have spent $760 for the privilege. A less expensive seven-piece group, of carved rosewood in the "Style of Louis XIV" (probably of Henkels' own make), would have cost from $141 to $214 with plush upholstery and $124 to $192 with haircloth (the cheapest and least fashionable furniture cover).[5]

The seven-piece middle-class parlor suite became a formula in the 1860s, although some manufacturers were slow to accept it. An unillustrated *Wholesale Price List of Furniture*, published by P. P. Gustine of Philadelphia on February 1, 1867, offered the owners of retail warerooms a complete range of middle-class furnishings, from sets of simple cane-seat chairs to sideboards. While distributors had the option of making up sets of Gustine's furniture (and the price list offered the proper types of pieces), the firm still did not offer a standard number of pieces for a parlor suite; sofas (called "common," "box," "French," and "medallion back") were offered individually, ungrouped with stylistically similar chairs. "Gentlemen's Parlor Arm Chairs," "Ladies' Parlor Arm Chairs," and spring-seat rocking chairs were sold separately. "French spring seat chairs" with "moulded backs" were offered by the dozen.

By the early 1870s, however, the seven-piece parlor suite had become a staple of furniture manufacture. Almost all such suites included a tête (sofa), an upholstered armchair, an upholstered armless lady's chair, and four small chairs having "brace" (a chair with

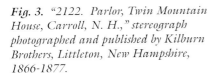

Fig. 3. "2122. Parlor, Twin Mountain House, Carroll, N. H.," stereograph photographed and published by Kilburn Brothers, Littleton, New Hampshire, 1866-1877.

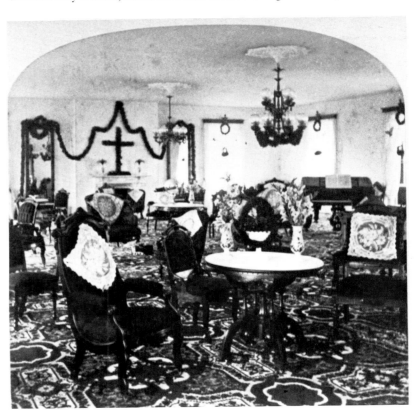

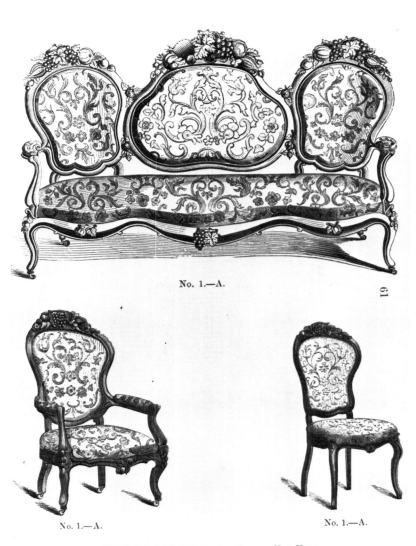

No. 1.—A.

61

No. 1.—A.

No. 1.—A.

FOSTER & LEE. 198 Broóme Street, New York.

Fig. 4. *Suite, engraving in catalog of Foster and Lee, New York, New York, 1858. This company illustrated most of its seating furniture by type, grouping sofas, arm chairs, and other parlor seats on separate pages. However, six pages contained groupings of matched furniture—sofa, arm chair, and side chair—that are plainly meant to be sets. Unusual because it is completely illustrated (most furniture trade catalogs remained unillustrated for another decade), the Foster and Lee catalog is missing its price list; the number of pieces in these sets cannot be ascertained. Courtesy Henry Francis du Pont Winterthur Museum Library; Collection of Printed Books.*

small arms that braces the back to the seat) or "stuffed" backs and an upholstered seat (plate 20). Some catalogs of the 1870s offered consumers as many as fifty choices in wooden frames; wholesale prices typically ranged between forty-eight and two hundred dollars.[6]

That large numbers of trade catalogs offered seven-piece suites in the 1870s suggests the presence of a large audience for new parlor furniture; it also implies that these consumers recognized how ownership of a parlor suite would create a modern parlor. However, none of these suites, even those that wholesaled for as little as fifty dollars, were truly inexpensive or easily accessible to the families of skilled workers, clerks, or other wage earners in the middle decades of the nineteenth century. Two things had to happen before the suite, the consummate emblem of the parlor of culture, could become truly popular: still-lower price lines had to become available, and consumer credit had to be offered to aspiring parlor makers.

Trade and mail-order catalogs do suggest a steady trend in factory production of suites toward lower price lines between 1880 and 1910 as furniture manufacturers became increasingly adept at making compromises in the structure and embellishment of frames and the structure and covers of spring seats. In the 1880s, manufacturers offered expanded lines of parlor suites that would retail for less than one hundred dollars in a range of attractive fabrics. The 1880 catalog of Baxter C. Swan of Philadelphia, a manufacturer who specialized in cheap parlor furniture "For The Trade," offered seven-piece suites in haircloth, printed raw silk, and raw silk embellished with velvet or silk plush bands. Assuming a one hundred per cent markup, Swan's parlor suites ranged between $72 and $225; sixteen would have cost $100 or less.[7] The 1883 catalog of Jordan and Moriarty, a New York City furniture store that targeted its advertising to a clientele with middling incomes, offered "an extensive stock of parlor suites in Hair Cloth, Reps, Brocatelle, Satin, Satin Delaine, Damask, Raw Silk, &c, &c." It illustrated a simple rococo revival grouping with unornamented seats and backs for twenty-five dollars in "haircloth or reps," which were no longer particularly popular or fashionable upholstery fabrics; this suite may have been leftover stock from a failed firm. Still, it must have tempted respectable customers with small furnishing budgets. The firm also offered parlor suites with raw silk upholstery for fifty dollars and higher and with plush covers for seventy-five dollars and higher. To encourage new consumers, Jordan and Moriarty also offered "whatever terms of Installment purchasers may find to be most convenient."[8]

Price lines that were even cheaper developed in the 1890s. In 1895, Montgomery Ward and Co. offered six different five- and six-piece suites costing between $24.70 and $57.79, depending upon their covers. However, the catalog captions indicated particular pride in a five-piece offering, "the greatest bargain ever offered in a parlor suit at $17.50." While the overall quality of such inexpensive suites was probably low, they still paraphrased the popularly desired qualities for parlor furniture: they had spring seats, decorative wooden frames, and showy upholstery in pile or woven figured fabrics, embellished with strips of plush.[9] The cheapness of such catalog suites also was a function of lower markups in the mail-order business.

Figuring out just who purchased parlor suites between 1850 and 1910, an era before scientific marketing surveys, is necessarily a speculative exercise. A pattern of ownership moving down through the economic strata of the middle classes does, however, seem to exist. Secure and prosperous members of the professions, independent merchants, and small entrepreneurs, factory supervisors, and successful freeholding farmers could purchase suites between 1850 and 1880. After 1880, ownership became possible among prosperous sectors of the working classes and small farmers who entered the cash economy. This process of increasing access culminated in the first decade of the twentieth century.

At the turn of the century, suites remained an important furnishing convention for upper middle-class and middle-class people (such as the Voigt family of Grand Rapids, Michigan, self-made German-American dry goods and flour mill owners) whose tastes were conservative, who decorated their homes themselves with the help of local merchants, and whose ideas of appropriate furnishing practices were traditional—at least by the standards of 1910. The other expanding market for suites, especially after 1895, were new consumers such as the modestly prosperous small farmer, who enjoyed a period of relative prosperity and had cash to spend between 1899 and 1920. Mail-order catalogs, Rural Free Delivery (1896), and Parcel Post (1912) offered farmers opportunities to spend that cash. Also among these new consumers were urban, working-class families who had relatively steady, adequate incomes.[10] According to

Louise Bolard More's sample in *Wage Earners' Budgets* (1907), the purchase of decorative furniture became possible when incomes ranged between $800 and $1200; because her sample was from New York City, one assumes the income level and distribution of expenditures reflect the higher cost of living there.[11] Farm families who produced much of their own food probably required less cash to achieve comparable standards of living, as did working-class families in smaller communities.

Installment buying allowed prosperous working-class families in cities and towns to participate in parlor making. More noted that the "installment system" was "almost universal among the working-class" and that pianos, sewing machines, and parlor furniture were the most popular large items purchased in that manner. "The most extravagant tendency is to buy elaborate parlor furniture 'on time'," she observed, "which is far out of keeping with the family's income." The typical cost for parlor furniture was from $75 to $125, which seemed typically to include a "parlor set" and carpet; we know that cheaper suites were available by this time through mail order. By the turn of the century, parlor suites were no longer fashionable in some middle-class eyes, but they had become truly popular. It is impossible to know how much of the vision of parlor gentility that suites had once engendered had been transmitted to working-class clientele; perhaps it had been muted to a general connotation of middle-class respectability. Even as she dubbed it an extravagance, More noted that the purchase of parlor furnishings did indicate "ambition and a higher standard."[12]

The seven-piece parlor suites of the 1870s were, for the most part, of French influence in design, as their predecessor upholstered sets of the 1850s and 1860s had been. Stylistically, many were tied to French nineteenth-century versions of eighteenth-century styles. This was true not only in the case of the furnishings of the "rococo revival," which were produced steadily at least until the end of the 1870s; suites with oval (called "medallion") and shield-shaped backs were also derived from Louis XVI chairs of the 1770s and later.

In addition to stylistic influences, however, the range of forms offered in parlor suites of the 1870s also followed a typology first developed by the French about the levels of social intercourse and the kinds of seating furniture necessary for socializing in the *apartement de société*. This typological order remained intact even when parlor suites in the late 1870s bore "reform" furniture's rectilinear designs, which had been offered by Eastlake and other English designers as an alternative to what they considered bad French taste. Use of the term "tête" to indicate a sofa, for example, derives from the French term *tête-à-tête* ("conversation"; literally, "head-to-head"). In the eighteenth century, the French used *tête* to indicate a small-scale sofa that was really just an armchair doubled in width. The tête was also called a *confidente*. Its name and scale imply that the eighteenth-century tête was meant for conversation (and perhaps also for genteel flirtation).[13]

Of the two large chairs in a suite, one was an armchair, sometimes openly termed a "gentleman's chair," with an upholstered seat and back and upholstered arm rests. The arms were usually open at the sides. The second large chair was, in the 1870s, often called a "lady's chair." It had an upholstered seat and back but was either armless or had recessed, lower arms. The forms of these chairs were derived from French *fauteuils en cabriolet*, armchairs whose curved backs were considered an innovation in seated comfort. (The archetypal "French" chair, *fauteuils en cabriolets* have had many variations of form and use since the eighteenth century and are still in production.) The lady's chair of the seven-piece suite had recessed arms or none at all. Not an arbitrary feature, this design in fact reflected adaptations undertaken to accommodate the encumbrances of women's full formal dress in the eighteenth century. The set-back, small arms of an eighteenth-century *fauteuil* took into account that women wore panniers (introduced in 1717), large padded frames that made formal dresses stand out on either side. (In less formal circumstances, women sometimes folded full skirts up over the arms of chairs.)[14] Parlor chairs of the 1850s and 1860s had to accommodate another form of exaggerated feminine skirt, the ever-expanding crinolines and hoops which required space to spread out around the chair in a large half-circle (fig.5). Thus the original eighteenth-century design could be justifiably recycled. The crinoline had disappeared by 1870 and thus made the lower design of the arms of ladies' chairs unnecessary, but this form survived in parlor suites until the 1880s. It is possible that this survival also was partly associated with doing needlework, because low arms accommodated

Fig. 5. Mrs. Charles Higgins, carte de visite by Wallis Brothers Photograph Gallery, Chicago, Illinois, 1860-1865. Mrs. Higgins's crinolines completely covered the upholstered chair on which she sat for the photographer.

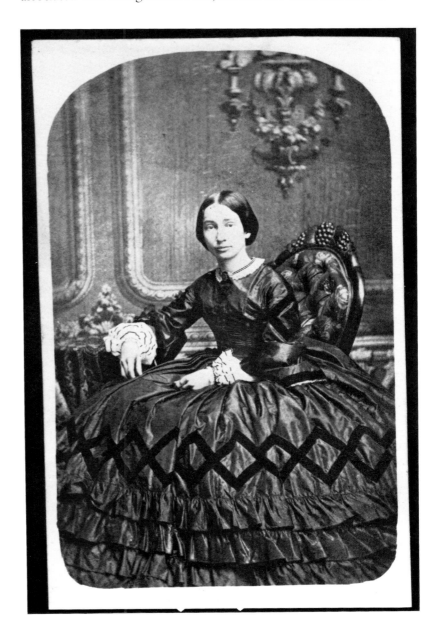

this kind of sewing posture more easily. The disappearance of crinolines did not mean that women were any less encumbered by their formal dress. The form of the obstacles to sitting changed significantly, however—into the bustle and the skirt cage (called the *tournure*).

The rest of the pieces in most parlor suites were small, armless chairs; trade catalogs often referred to them simply as "parlor chairs." They always had an upholstered spring seat, but the chair back sometimes had no upholstered pad. They also were scaled to be smaller than the other chairs of the suite, which meant that they could be moved easily. Small lightweight chairs were an important element in furnishing both gala and private rooms in the eighteenth century, whether to allow individuals to move closer to the fireplace or to form groupings for conversation or card playing. Within the larger, more permanently placed components of a parlor suite, the four small chairs formed a "set" of their own. The 1883 price list of Mackie and Hilton, Philadelphia makers of parlor furniture, lounges, and mattresses, suggested the traditional placement and function of these four armless chairs when it labeled them "Wall Chairs."[15]

The seven-piece parlor suite was a concise catalog of the major types of social seating employed in eighteenth-century French rooms for socializing. The tête suggested relaxed social intimacy, the armchairs promoted the "middle ground" of social conversation with peers, and the movable side chairs (which one author acknowledged were "generally uncomfortable") were meant for short-term sitting at receptions or during social calls.[16] The only notable exception to the typology was the absence of the tabouret or ottoman, an upholstered backless seat that descended from the upholstered stools used in the court of Louis XIV as part of its elaborate system of seating etiquette. Such ottomans occasionally appeared in large, elegant parlors after 1850 and were a graceful seat for women with full skirts (fig. 6). However, they were not incorporated into factory-made suites, perhaps because they echoed the old associations of backless seats with low status.[17]

In parlor suites, the range of sizes and the presence or absence of arms, which made long-term sitting more comfortable by giving arms and hands a natural place to rest, also recalled the etiquette of precedence in seating. For hundreds of years, precedence—the set of formal rules of social status—had been expressed through the use of a hierarchy of seating furniture. In a household where all forms of seating furniture existed, the armchair would stand at the apex of this hierarchy, then the armless chair ("back stool"), high stool, and low stool in descending order. The most honored person in a household would be given the armchair; in fact, the term "chairman" emerged from rules of precedence in seating.[18]

In the etiquette books of the nineteenth century, precedence survived in a gentle form in discussions of the deferential treatment that was to be proffered to guests and aged members of households. A small, inexpensive advice book published in 1857 by the New York City firm of Dick and Fitzgerald described honor in a way that differs little from manners associated with seating today:

> When any one enters, whether announced or not, the master or mistress should rise immediately, advance toward him, and request him to take a seat. If it is a young man, offer him an arm-chair, or a stuffed one; if an elderly man, insist upon his accepting the arm-chair; if a lady, beg her to be seated upon the sofa. If several ladies come in at once, we give the most honorable place to the one who, from age or other considerations, is most entitled to respect. In winter, the most honorable places are at the

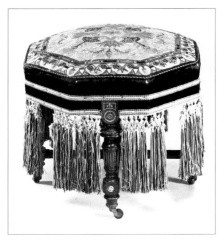

Fig. 6. *Tabouret or ottoman, attributed to Herter Brothers, New York, New York, walnut, silk velvet and silk embroidered needlepoint top, knotted fringe, about 1875. Courtesy Wadsworth Atheneum; gift from the estate of Mrs. James J. Goodwin.*

corners of the fireplace, if you have a fire in it.[19]

Seven-piece suites of the 1870s made a standardized and commercialized, but no less rhetorical, statement about formal social life: they represented the parlor as a gala apartment with French antecedents and the social life within its walls as orderly and hierarchical. The forms not only suggested appropriate use; they also suggested appropriate parlor deportment, which was controlled and dignified.[20] However, when the parlor suite became a codified unit in furniture manufacturing, its market was the expanding group of middle-class parlor makers, people whose houses probably included a single parlor and perhaps a sitting room or a dining room that could double as one. With its gentleman's armchair and lady's chair representing the master and mistress of a household, the seven-piece suite might also, for ordinary people, serve as a symbolic representation of the presence and natural hierarchy of a family in the parlor.

Given the large number of firms offering parlor suites, sales competition was probably intense by the late 1870s and encouraged constant innovation in upholstery, frames, and forms in order to attract and hold consumer attention. Thus, business necessity probably dictated that furniture manufacturers begin altering the seven-piece suite to attract interest, only a decade after its emergence as a standard unit of parlor furnishing. Makers began to include new forms such as corner or window chairs, which also were available separately. With low backs and arms, window chairs were designed to sit beneath a window frame. Such chairs represented a departure from the older typology of parlor suites in that their design was based not upon their place in the choreography of parlor sociability but upon their surface appearance and the novelty of their specialized design and intended placement in rooms (fig. 7). This specialization in chair forms was one manifestation of the popular aesthetic of refinement.[21]

Fig. 7. "Parlor Suit No. 32," engraving in Supplement to Bub and Kipp's Illustrated Catalogue, *Milwaukee, Wisconsin (1885). This suite had once included seven pieces, but the company updated the grouping by reducing the number to six and making all of the pieces different.*

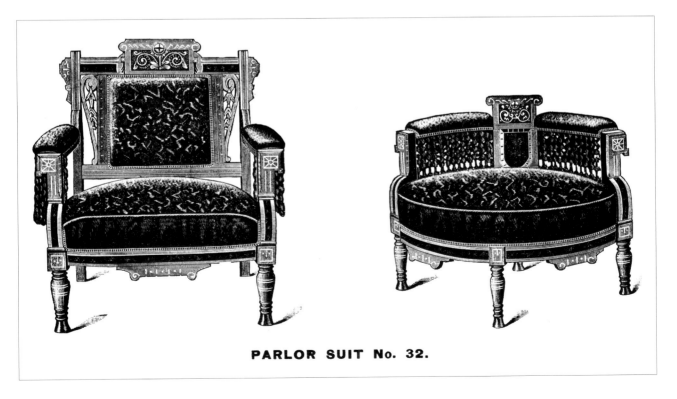

PARLOR SUIT No. 32.

By the 1880s, the number of pieces in suites was commonly reduced to five, which may have reflected the smaller houses of less prosperous consumers. By that time, too, the addition of rocking chairs, the most "domestic" and comfortable of all chairs, further blurred the eighteenth-century typology of gala sociability (plates 21 and 22). In suites of the 1880s, they usually—and appropriately, because they were symbolically associated with women—replaced the lady's chair.

Some evidence suggests that the introduction of rocking chairs into matching parlor decor was an introduction "from the bottom." As middle-class people furnished parlor/sitting rooms for themselves, they selected rocking chairs to accompany their more simple furnishings. Before their incorporation into suites, upholsterers made rocking chairs acceptable for parlor furnishing by gussying up the frames of Boston or Grecian rockers with upholstery. The price list for George J. Henkels City Cabinet Warerooms (about 1855) included "Parlor Rocking Chairs"—with cane seats or spring seats with haircloth covers—only in its cheapest price line of "Plain Style Mahogany or Walnut Parlor Furniture."[22]

The rocking chairs offered with suites of the 1880s were platform models, which could be easily constructed and upholstered to match the rest of the set.[23] In the 1870s, parlor platform rocking chairs with highly ornate upholstery had been sold in large numbers as single chairs. They could be purchased as a matching addition to a suite: the August 17, 1880, price list of Gerrish and O'Brien of Boston offered seven-piece parlor suites and noted that "we furnish a 'Patent Rocker' to match each suite." Or they could be employed as a single chair, ornate enough to be the prize of the parlor, in smaller or more modest households.[24]

The owners of rocking chairs often viewed them as objects of sentimental attachment, and one occasionally finds an example of an older rocking chair, updated for parlor use, in house museums. In the Voigt house in Grand Rapids, which retains its 1897 and 1907 interiors almost intact, a simple armless rocker (the type described as a "nurse rocker" because it accommodated a comfortable lowered-arm position for women holding babies or doing household work) was upholstered in an elaborate silk lampas fabric, woven for a seat and chair back, to make it compatible with new overstuffed "French" parlor furniture (fig. 8).[25] The incorporation of rocking chairs into parlor suites, even in disguise as platform rockers, may be the most decisive statement about middle-class efforts to embrace in one piece both values—domestic comfort and facade of culture—in the parlor.

The reduced size of suites and the incorporation of rocking chairs probably reflected both the furnishing possibilities in smaller parlors and the use of such spaces as both sitting and reception rooms. Still, the frontal and upright nature of the seats in modest parlor suites suggested appropriate deportment and emphasized the parlor's importance as a formal social space. Furniture forms, even when they were large and padded, suggested the desirability of controlled posture and of dignified ease rather than relaxation. It was certainly possible to lounge on a parlor tête or to fling oneself down in a sprawl in an armchair —or even to sit with one or both legs off the floor in some larger pieces—and people probably did. However, the forms taken by most parlor suites suggested that one ought to comport oneself in a gentlemanly or ladylike manner. And, while parlor suites were padded, they generally maintained that "feet on the floor" suggestion. Their upholstery visually softened parlor suites, but until the late 1880s it almost always was stuffed to be tight and hard. Even the fabrics, particularly stiff horsehair and hot, scratchy mohair plush, did not invite repose. The popular introduction of

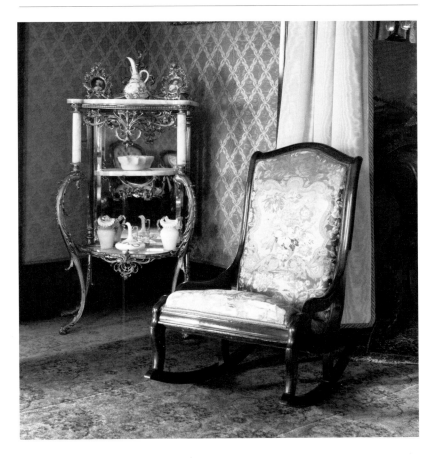

Turkish furniture in the 1880s slowly began to break down these old messages about correct deportment.[26] However, until the 1910s, parlor suites were metaphors of long-standing ideas about parlor etiquette. Their elements were proper seats for the controlled body postures and feelings of "parlor people."

During the 1880s and 1890s, factory-made suites generally included five or six pieces. In its 1895 catalog, however, Montgomery Ward offered a few three-piece suites for small parlors and allowed customers to select a smaller number of pieces from larger sets; in 1908, Sears, Roebuck and Co. still followed this practice (fig. 9). Three-piece sets eventually supplanted larger groupings and became the standard for catalog offerings of overstuffed living-room furniture in the 1910s. Mixed in with various kinds of other seating, the parlor suite at the turn of the century survived as a residual expression of the old vision of parlor sociability, a reflection of the conservatism of some consumers.

Suites not only signaled the nature of appropriate parlor social life; they also allowed ordinary consumers to attain the prized ideal of matched room decor. According to Thornton, unity in interior decoration "became the convention when the concept of *regularité*…came to be accepted as the basis of good taste in architecture…by the 1640s, it must have been a commonplace in grand circles to have the textile furnishings of important rooms matching." *Regularité*, the sense of order and harmony created in rooms by their architecture and decoration, "seems to have been contrived by applying to the interior…the standard precepts of Renaissance architecture" and originally reflected a sense of the proper qualities of intellectual and social life.[27]

Commercial parlors probably played a large role in popularizing

452   SEARS, ROEBUCK & CO., CHICAGO, ILL. CATALOGUE No. 117.   2

NEW DESIGN THREE-PIECE PARLOR SUITE WITH REMOVABLE CUSHIONS, $16.45.

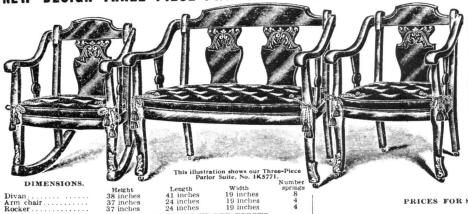

This illustration shows our Three-Piece Parlor Suite, No. 1K5771.

NO. 1K5771 This handsome new design, high grade, Three-Piece Parlor Suite represents exceptional value at the price we ask. We call your special attention to the removable cushion seats. Each piece is fitted with a boxed edge, button tufted cushion, fitted perfectly and securely fastened at the corners by silk cords and tassels. The cushions rest on our all steel indestructible spring construction. They are readily removed for dusting and airing and will wear longer and prove more satisfactory than stationary upholstered seats. The beauty of design, high quality of workmanship and elegance of finish can only be fully appreciated when you see it. The substantial frames are made of specially selected birch, finished in perfect imitation of mahogany. The back is decorated with genuine hand carvings perfectly executed. Furnished in the various high grade coverings by the single piece or full suite as noted below. Shipped direct from factory in Chicago or Eastern Pennsylvania, according to location of customer. Shipping weight, about 100 pounds.

DIMENSIONS.

	Height	Length	Width	Number springs
Divan	38 inches	41 inches	19 inches	8
Arm chair	37 inches	24 inches	19 inches	4
Rocker	37 inches	24 inches	19 inches	4

PRICES FOR COMPLETE SUITE OF THREE PIECES.

The number of this Parlor Suite is No. 1K5771. Always order by number and be sure to state the kind and color of covering desired.

Covering	Fancy Brocaded Velour	Plain Silk Plush	Crushed Plush	Brocaded Silk Plush	Panne Plush
Price	$16.45	$17.95	$18.45	$19.65	$19.95

PRICES FOR SINGLE PIECES.

Covering	Fancy Brocaded Plush	Plain Silk Plush	Crushed Plush	Brocaded Silk Plush	Panne Plush
Divan	$7.15	$7.65	$7.85	$8.35	$8.65
Rocker	5.45	5.95	6.15	6.45	6.65
Arm Chair	4.95	5.45	5.65	5.95	6.15

No. 1K5781 THE STYLE.
The illustration shows one of the newest designs in a high grade Three-Piece Parlor Suite. The graceful curves shown in the top rail, arms and front legs appeal to the taste of those who admire simplicity of outline combined with beauty and strength.

THE FRAME is made of specially selected birch in a perfect imitation mahogany finish, piano polished. The shapely back panels are veneered with genuine mahogany, highly figured. The top rail, arms and front posts are continuous and have rounded edges. The construction is strictly first class in every detail.

THE SPRINGS in the seat are made of the best quality high carbon Bessemer steel, firmly fastened together with corrugated steel bands, interlaced at the top and bottom, and will last a lifetime.

THE CUSHIONS are made of fancy brocaded plush, crushed plush, plain silk plush, brocaded silk plush, or panne plush; either of which coverings you may select can be furnished in plain solid colors of dark olive green or dark red. Read what we say about the different kinds of upholstery materials on page 436. They are made with full box edge and are button tufted. They are securely fastened at the corners by silk cord with silk tassels, and rest on our all steel spring construction, as described above. They are easily detached for airing and cleaning. The added convenience, comfort and wearing qualities will be readily recognized by every housekeeper. Shipped direct from factory in Chicago or Eastern Pennsylvania. Crated to insure safe delivery, shipping weight, 175 lbs.

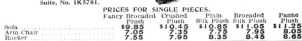

This illustration shows our Three-Piece Parlor Suite, No. 1K5781.

PRICES FOR COMPLETE SUITE OF THREE PIECES.

The number of this Parlor Suite is No. 1K5781. Always order by number and be sure to state the kind and color of covering desired.

	Fancy Brocaded Plush	Crushed Plush	Plain Silk Plush	Brocaded Silk Plush	Panne Plush
Price	$22.75	$24.45	$25.25	$25.95	$26.25

PRICES FOR SINGLE PIECES.

	Fancy Brocaded Plush	Crushed Plush	Plain Silk Plush	Brocaded Silk Plush	Panne Plush
Sofa	$9.85	$10.45	$10.85	$11.05	$11.25
Arm Chair	7.05	7.35	7.75	7.95	8.05
Rocker	7.55	7.95	8.35	8.45	8.65

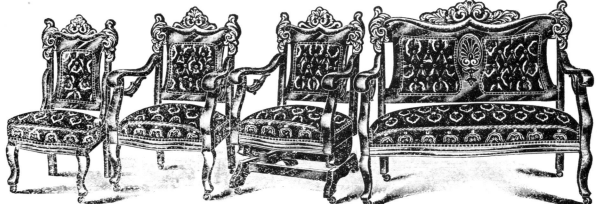

This illustration shows four pieces of our No. 1K5786 Parlor Suite.

No. 1K5786
This beautiful Five-Piece Parlor Suite is a splendid example of up to date workmanship and finish, made of specially selected highly figured birch, in perfect imitation of mahogany. In every detail, workmanship and material is strictly high grade and guaranteed to please. It has deep hand tufted backs, carefully overlaid and fastened securely with metal buttons. The gimp and cord are made to match the coverings. Each piece is upholstered in the very best possible manner with different style of coverings, as noted opposite and described on page 436. Each piece has a full spring seat; springs of the best quality of high carbon Bessemer steel wire with the corrugated steel wire bottom instead of webbing. Our price on this suite represents the actual cost at the factory with but a small margin of profit added. By shipping direct from the factory we save the extra expense of handling, enabling us to quote a very low price. Weight of suite crated, 280 pounds. Shipped direct from factory in Chicago or Eastern Pennsylvania.

The fifth piece is a duplicate of the parlor chair which has no arms.

PRICES FOR COMPLETE SUITE OF FIVE PIECES.

The number of this Parlor Suite is No. 1K5786. Always order by number and send the price which corresponds with the kind of upholstering you select. Be sure to state color desired.

Covering	Figured Velour	Fancy Brocaded Plush	Brocaded Verona Plush	Crushed Plush	Brocaded Silk Plush	Silk Damask
Price	$29.75	$30.95	$31.90	$34.25	$35.45	$36.65

PRICES FOR SINGLE PIECES.

Covering	Figured Velour	Fancy Brocaded Plush	Brocaded Verona Plush	Crushed Plush	Brocaded Silk Plush	Silk Damask
Sofa	$10.55	$10.95	$11.35	$12.15	$12.35	$12.95
Arm Chair	6.65	6.95	7.15	7.75	7.95	8.35
Rocker	7.15	7.45	7.65	8.25	8.45	8.85
Reception Chair	3.55	3.65	3.80	4.10	4.15	4.35

Fig. 9. Three- and five-piece suites offered in Sears, Roebuck and Co., 1908, Catalogue No. 117: The Great Price Maker *(reprint, 1971). As late as 1908, Sears, Roebuck and Co. still accommodated long-standing tastes for the five-piece suite, as well as the old aesthetic preferences for complexity and elaboration in both frames and upholstery. At the same time, the firm offered "colonial" suites that were formal in feeling yet bespoke gradual changes in favor of more simple visual qualities. Courtesy DBI Books, Inc., Northfield, Illinois.*

the ideal of *regularité*, and, by midcentury, middle class consumers wanted rooms that reflected their ability to plan and execute a comprehensive scheme of decoration, no matter how modest. Most had made do with odds and ends of furniture, and the most dramatic antidote to past scarcity and signal of present prosperity was a room that matched from top to bottom. Popular admiration of the matching decor of public parlors suggests why matching remained an important criterion for parlor seating furniture, although suites were criticized as "stiff, and unhomelike" almost from the moment of their commercial introduction.[28] Unified decor was formal and gala; it resonated with gentility. It did not matter whether consumers understood the ideal of gentility and its beau monde imperfectly, nor whether the public's ideals of unified decor were derived from the commercialized gentility of hotel parlors, steamboats, or exposition displays. Parlor suites made manifest their owners' connections with the parlor of culture, even when the suite was embedded in a complex room setting containing many other kinds of furniture.

Although most advice writers advocated "harmonious" rather than matching decor in the 1880s and 1890s, it is clear that popular preferences in room decoration still relied heavily on color matching and the domination of sets of furniture in a furnishing scheme. Advice for homemade upholstery, for example, continued to stress matching throughout the century. Catharine Beecher advised her readers how to make a "green room" with thirty yards of chintz. In the late 1880s, directions for making a room of fabric discussed creating all the furnishings out of a number of yards of one fabric, an inexpensive cretonne (unpolished cotton) print.[29]

The decision to purchase a parlor suite as the centerpiece and starting point of parlor (and, later, living room) furnishing never became unfashionable. Until Victorian furniture was finally displaced by overstuffed living room sets, parlors were repeatedly redecorated around parlor suites purchased years before. In 1882, Augusta Kohrs, wife of a prosperous Montana rancher, purchased her seven-piece cut-plush parlor suite in Chicago for the goodly sum of $300, and the set (which still bears its original figured red plush covers) served as a constant through her parlor redecorating schemes in 1882-1883, 1889-1890 (when the parlor became double parlors), 1900, and 1915.[30]

In the last quarter of the nineteenth century, some innovative manufacturers did try to accommodate advanced tastes for harmonious unmatched furniture with the convenience and guaranteed good taste that parlor suites apparently connoted to ordinary buyers. McDonough, Wilsey and Co. of Chicago offered in its 1878 trade catalog a seven-piece suite with upholstery in several different colors. By the turn of the century, even Sears, Roebuck and Co. offered as one option to select non-matching, "harmonious" suites for its customers.[31] The urgings of furniture advice books aside, evidence from trade catalogs, artifact survivals, and historical photographs suggest that sets of matching furniture continued to be an ideal for many, perhaps most, ordinary consumers.

As styles (manifest in the surface ornament and formal proportions) in average furniture stores today present a somewhat compressed range of the furniture options available from custom producers, factory-made parlor suites generally excluded the most radical furniture designs available from small decorating firms (fig. 10). This was partly due to the calculations of factory owners about what would sell and would therefore merit making new patterns, templates, and jigs for the woodworkers and upholsterers. The fact that most families might own one or two parlor suites throughout their lifespans also encouraged relatively conservative choices.

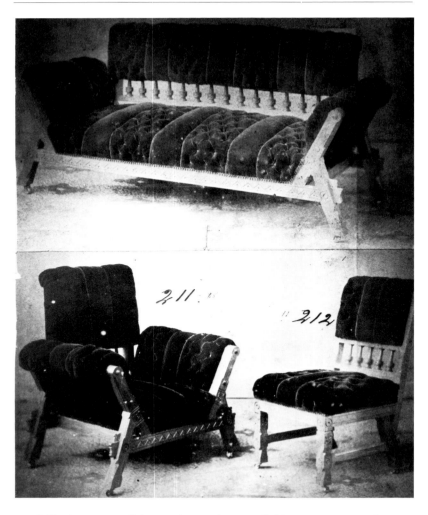

Fig. 10. Modern Gothic sofa and chairs, photograph in scrapbook of Kimbal and Cabus, New York, New York, about 1876. A progressive New York decorating firm in business between 1863 and 1882, Kimbal and Cabus specialized in furniture of the type called "Modern Gothic." The firm did a model room in this style at the Centennial. Although the straight lines of such furniture would have been comparatively easy to paraphrase in factory-made suites, the style may have been too far from the mainstream for manufacturers to gamble on and ordinary consumers to purchase. Courtesy Cooper-Hewitt Museum of Design, Smithsonian Institution.

Still, the range of decorative options available to consumers in factory-made suites was significant. Manufacturers could offer a number of choices in frames by relying upon applied ornament or carving on noticeable places such as the crest rails of chairs at the same time that they used standard legs and seat rails. And frames generally did not constitute the major expense in manufacturing middle-range parlor suites, thanks to sophisticated American woodworking machinery. Depending upon the degree of elaboration in both frames and upholstery, the spring structures and show covers usually accounted for between sixty and eighty per cent of the cost of a suite. The upholstered profile of the individual pieces and the color and contrast of their show covers and trims provided most of a suite's visual impact.

The popular taste for elaboration and visual complexity in objects encouraged great ingenuity in the use of many kinds of materials, including furnishing fabrics. The upholstery of even inexpensive parlor suites could be made "refined" through some combination of many techniques: choice of fabric, including the use of several different fabrics on each piece of furniture; elaboration in the handling of the fabric (buttoning, pleated tufting, ruffling, and puffing); and the use of fine details such as multicolored trims or buttons in contrasting colors and materials. Suites with absolutely plain upholstery were available for less money, but they appear only rarely in photographs. They seemed distressingly bald to consumers, and a purchaser would probably have relieved their plainness with antimacassars, pillows, and throws (fig. 11).

The most popular upholstery fabrics used on factory-made parlor suites tended to have emphatic texture, both visual and tactile. Most fell into a few basic types—satin finishes prized for their sheen, bristly and dimensional pile fabrics, and a few types of woven figured fabrics and printed look-alikes. Middle-class consumers wanted heavy upholstery fabrics both because they implied "richness" and because they were believed to wear better, which was not always the case. Early power-loomed "furniture tapestries," woven with unmercerized cotton yarns, absorbed dirt and grew dingy soon after they were purchased. The wool "rep" popular between 1860 and the early 1880s was relatively inexpensive and sturdy, and it could be dyed deep colors, typically red, green, a sepia brown, and golden yellow. More expensive versions were woven with silk stripes imitating needlework.

With the exception of wool rep (also called "terry"), most suite upholstery fabrics mimicked the aesthetic characteristics of more expensive fabrics. Cotton satine offered the colors and sheen of silk satin, which was used on very expensive furniture. "Satin-de-laine" (satin-woven wool) was sometimes printed to resemble brocaded silks (fig. 12; plate 23), while printed raw silk, which enjoyed a brief span

Fig. 11. *"Suit No. 10" with plain cover (probably rep), photograph in* Descriptive Catalogue of Sofas, Lounges, Tetes, Chairs and Parlor Suits, *Rand and McSherry, Baltimore, Maryland (1872). Courtesy Smithsonian Institution.*

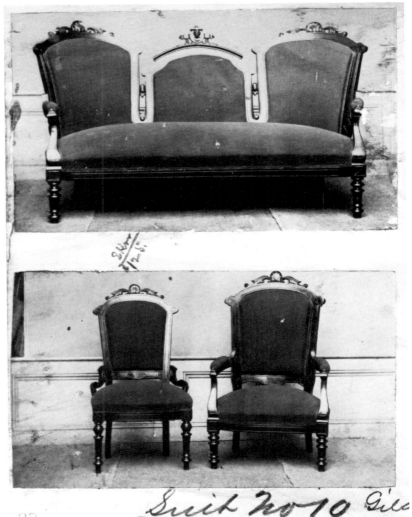

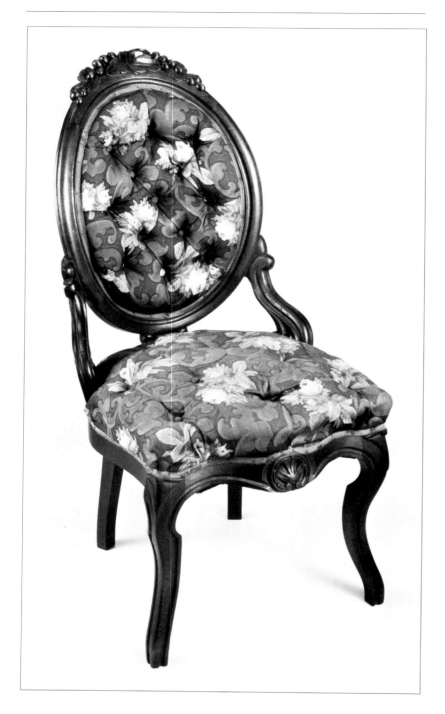

Fig. 12. Side chair, walnut, printed
satin-weave wool (satin-de-laine),
probably Boston, Massachusetts, 1857.
This chair is part of an eight-piece suite
purchased by Richard Holbrook Tucker.
The upholstered fabric was printed to look
like brocaded silk damask. See plate 23
for a color detail of this chair. Courtesy
Castle Tucker.

of popularity in the late 1870s and 1880s, resembled upholstery
tapestry. Mohair plush, which wore better than the wool plush that
also was popular through the 1870s, was used on both mid-quality
and better furniture into the twentieth century (fig. 13), but cotton
velveteens and "furniture velours," as well as heavy corduroy, offered
a cheaper alternative after 1890. Sometimes the cheapest suites were
upholstered with fabrics that paraphrased mid-range upholstery:
"lasting" (a shiny black wool and cotton blend more commonly used
for coat linings and women's shoe tops) was used in the 1870s as a
look-alike for plain, black, power-loomed horsehair.

Advances in weaving technology also made new types of

Fig. 13. Side chair, walnut, wool plush, about 1870. This side chair is part of a seven-piece suite upholstered in dark green wool plush (now largely faded to olive green). Courtesy Castle Tucker.

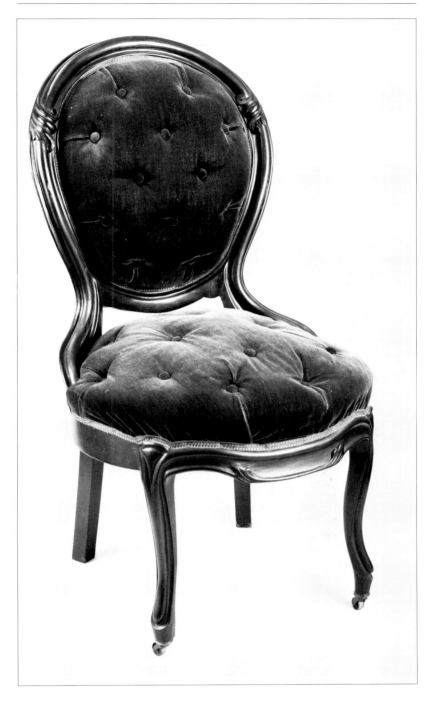

furnishing fabric available to makers of cheap parlor furniture. Imitation tapestry, woven with the jacquard mechanism on the loom, was apparently developed in England as early as the 1830s but does not seem to have been in extensive use in America until the 1880s (fig. 14). By the 1890s, American firms could make it, and the large upholstery weaving industry of Philadelphia made a specialty out of furniture tapestries as well as chenilles and curtain lace.[32] In the mid-1880s, rapid growth occurred in the production and introduction of new mixed-fiber upholstery fabrics, which combined high percentages of sturdy, inexpensive cotton with more valuable fibers such as silk. "Silk-faced tapestry," for example, was mostly made of cotton. Little

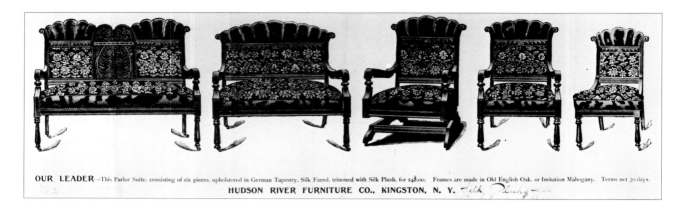

OUR LEADER—This Parlor Suite. consisting of six pieces. upholstered in German Tapestry, Silk Faced. trimmed with Silk Plush. for $45.00.   Frames are made in Old English Oak. or Imitation Mahogany.   Terms net 30 days.
HUDSON RIVER FURNITURE CO., KINGSTON, N. Y.

Fig. 14. Broadside for Hudson River Furniture Co., Kingston, New York, about 1895. This inexpensive six-piece suite was offered in "Silk Faced German Tapestry" with plush trim for $40.00, wholesale. See chapter 5, fig. 17 for an example of this type of fabric.

of this fabric survives, probably because the silk surface wore away and left a very shabby-looking fabric in its wake. The construction of velvets and plushes also changed, so that only the set of warp fibers that produced the pile was made of expensive fibers; the rest was made of cotton, which could withstand the tension of power looms. Velveteens or "velours," popular upholstery fabrics after 1890, were one hundred per cent cotton.

Parlor suites also were elaborated through a variety of techniques for handling fabric and stuffing that were new to the nineteenth century—pleated tufting, ruffling and puffing, and the use of contrasting bands of fabric on the same piece of furniture. Although evidence is fragmentary, it seems that these innovations were transmitted directly to America by emigrating German and French upholsterers (figs. 15 and 16).[33] Sewed, pleated tufting on the backs and arms of chairs and sofas formed dimensional surfaces in a variety of geometric patterns—diamonds, squares, and rectangles. Pleated tufting was freely applied to printed or figured woven fabrics, where it had a kaleidoscopic effect (plate 24). Such tufting was an elaboration upon buttoning layers of stuffing together to prevent its movement on vertical surfaces. Simple buttoning was still in use as a decorative element on seat tops and backs throughout the second half of the nineteenth century, but, by the mid-1870s, trade catalogs offered factory-made suites with "piped, plain, star, tufted or pleated backs." Another technique for increasing the visual impact of tufting was to employ contrasting buttons in the tufts. These were covered with one of the fabrics used on the chair or sometimes were cheaper brown or black enameled buttons.[34]

Applying contrasting bands of fabrics was another way of elaborating the upholstered surfaces of suites. Ruffling or puffing, applying loosely pleated bands of fabric to the fronts of seats or along the sides or the top of the seat back, was a particularly popular decorative option in the 1870s (plate 25). It always cost a few dollars extra. Ruffling was favored on the French/Turkish furniture of the 1880s and 1890s, suggesting that its earlier origins also were French. "Reform" or Eastlake furniture tended to have upholstery with flat surfaces of fabric, considered in keeping with its more rectangular lines, but, to make such surfaces more decoratively complex, manufacturers resorted to a variation on ruffling, offering contrasting bands of fabric, frequently in a pile fabric such as plush, as embellishment for otherwise flat surfaces. Plush not only was pleasing to the touch but also absorbed and reflected light in a pleasing manner.

Finally, the trims of even inexpensive suites offered pleasing visual detail in the cords that covered seams, the gimps that finished raw edges, and the tassels and fringes that became increasingly important

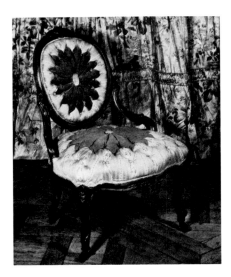

Fig. 15. Side chair, photomechanical reproduction in Colette Lehmann, Mobilier Louis-Philippe Napoléon III *(1977). The upholstery treatment on this chair is a novel variation on pleated tufting, called "star tufting" in the United States. Star tufting is one of many examples of nineteenth-century French novelties in upholstery that were transmitted to America, perhaps firsthand by émigré craftspeople. Trade catalogs and cards show that the technique was used on fancy chairs made by the firm of George Hunzinger in New York and by a few other fashionable upholstery firms. It was undoubtedly expensive because of the sewing skill involved in making multicolored tufts. Courtesy Charles Massin Editions, Paris.*

with the introduction of Turkish furniture. Trims visually tied and mediated the boundaries of multicolored fabrics or more than one color of fabric on a suite. They also provided a visual transition between upholstery and wooden frames.

In their typology of forms, seven-piece parlor suites originally embodied the concept of "refinement" as it was associated with gentility, the eighteenth-century ideal of personal cultivation and self-presentation. Suites were but one component of the commercialization and packaging of gentility, a larger process that included the proliferation of commercial parlors and of etiquette books. Located in the private middle-class parlor, the formula for the number and types of pieces in suites was subject to the ongoing tension between the parlor of culture and the parlor of comfort. Including rocking chairs in suites was an accommodation to domesticity and the comfortable parlor.

If the connection between the seating types in suites and the ideal of gentility became less clear, the elaborated upholstery of parlor suites embodied a peculiarly Victorian conception of refinement. Here, "refinement" motivated consumer preferences in the appearance of suite upholstery, overlaying the skeletal traces of the ideal of gentility embodied in the frames of suite furniture.

In the mid-nineteenth century, families with limited furnishing budgets sometimes purchased only a sofa to serve as their single piece of upholstered seating furniture. By the 1870s, this choice was just as likely to be a lounge, which had become both an important avenue of access to spring-seat upholstery and a cheap piece of upholstered furniture that packed a remarkable amount of aesthetic information into its frame and cover (plate 26). The implications of its name notwithstanding, the parlor lounge usually was a formal-looking, physically stiff piece of furniture whose form contributed to the room's impression of refinement and manifested the tensions between parlor makers' aspirations toward appropriate parlor formality and their desire for domestic comfort.

Even when householders could gradually afford a few other pieces of factory-made upholstery, the lounge was often the most eye-catching and stylish piece of furniture. Its presence informed visitors that the residents of the house were aware of contemporary furnishing trends and tried to follow them. In small houses, the vocabulary of parlor furnishing was paraphrased, necessarily compressed to fewer emblematic objects. With their decorative upholstery, set in embellished wooden frames, lounges could serve the aesthetic functions that entire parlor suites served in larger, more affluent settings (fig. 17). At their cheapest, lounges cost less than the cheapest sofa; in 1878, the Boston firm of Samuel Graves and Son wholesaled "Common Lounges with (12 Springs)" for as little as $3.50 in "enamel cloth" (oilcloth that was used as a substitute for horsehair or leather).[35]

Lounges were descendants of seventeenth-century daybeds and late eighteenth- and early nineteenth-century neoclassical couches. Such couches were often sold in pairs for expensive parlors. Between 1850 and 1870, large sets of parlor furniture still often incorporated a lounge; after 1870, they were no longer offered as part of the formulaic factory-made parlor suite (fig. 31). The Tucker family's parlor suite of 1857 included one as part of the set at the time of purchase, and the double parlors of Southmayd, a Massachusetts summer house that contained furniture by Alexander Roux, also contained an inexpensive lounge completely upholstered with striped rep (fig. 18).

Lounges often appeared in dining rooms, which frequently doubled as family sitting rooms. The Yearick family of Konnarock,

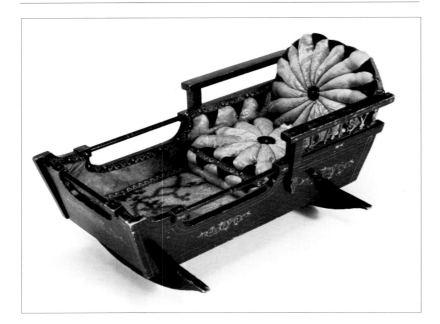

Fig. 16. Doll cradle, ebonized wood with gilded decoration, silk damask and silk velvet, 1860-1900. This cradle, perhaps made by an upholsterer as a gift for his child, demonstrates the use of the novelty "star tufting" technique in the United States. Miniature and toy furniture is often a good source of information on nineteenth-century upholstery because it used the same materials and techniques that appear on full-size furniture.

Virginia, furnished its dining/sitting room with a lounge and rocking chair as well as a table and sideboard.[36] Advice books on furnishing directed to more prosperous consumers suggested that leather-covered lounges be part of dining room furniture. Such a use was associated with upper-class dinner-party etiquette, where men used the dining room as a place to smoke and talk after the meal. Lounges also appeared in libraries and bedrooms; Ella Rodman Church, author of *How to Furnish a Home* (1881), considered lounges "quite a necessary piece of furniture in a bedroom, in order that the bed may be kept in the immaculate condition which is its principal charm, as 'throwing' one's self down on it for an afternoon nap is no improvement to snowy covers, and gives a generally untidy appearance."[37]

A carpet-covered lounge in the collection of the Strong Museum, made by Martyn Brothers of Jamestown, New York, in the mid-1880s, demonstrates where most of the visual information of "style" was typically located on lounges (plate 27). The raised back, which is in essence the back of a parlor suite sofa or tête, has a heavily embellished crest rail that creates a complex outline of voids and solid form. The fanciest upholstery treatment is also located where it can be seen clearly, on the back and across the seat front, which is embellished by ruffling. Typical lounges of the 1870s, 1880s, and early 1890s, having high straight backs and one raised end, contained visual information in the same locations. Backless couches, which became more popular after 1890, often contained most of their visual information across the front, particularly on the raised end.

New lounges contained spring upholstery, but they almost always were stuffed to be rigid and sturdy. Imposing and formal, they exemplified the tension between culture and comfort, seeming to suggest that sitting up straight was most appropriate even as they invited reclining and offered a certain amount of spring-seat resilience. The carpet-covered lounge embodies a formal sofa and a backless reception seat in a single piece of furniture. Folding-bed lounges were, literally, both throne and bed.

Backless couches were found in parlors as well as in more private rooms such as sitting rooms, bedrooms, and libraries (fig. 19). The unidentified Rockland County, New York, family in their modest parlor (see chapter 2, fig. 14) sat across a backless couch as though it were a typical sofa. Such couches did not have to be located against walls because both sides were finished. One particularly popular type of "Turkish" couch, which was relatively expensive in its best quality, often was advertised to be used as library furniture for larger houses.[38] Covered with dark brown or black leather or leather cloth, many versions of these lounges were produced in quantity until at least 1915 (plate 28). Backless couches gave sitters no place to lean, a difficulty parlor makers tried to resolve by piling the surface with cushions.

In trade catalogs issued between 1880 and 1920, the lounge slowly began to be replaced by the overstuffed sofa, which had a symmetrical raised back and two arms. (After 1910, such sofas often had loose seat cushions containing springs.) However, in modest households, the lounge continued to be a centerpiece of parlor furnishing through 1910, at least partly because it did encapsulate so many of the structural and aesthetic characteristics of parlor suites.

About 1900, enterprising manufacturers of inexpensive upholstered furniture introduced a hybrid adjustable lounge called the "Roman divan," which was many times cheaper than its contemporary, the upholstered davenport (figs. 20 and 21). Roman divans offered both "refined" visual qualities and spring-seat structures. They could be adjusted to positions of definite formality with both arms upright; with one or both ends down, they could accommodate reclining postures. Roman divans also served as a transitional form in the move toward cheap overstuffed "davenport" sofas.

Lounges occupied a complicated niche in the burgeoning factory production of upholstered furniture of the second half of the nineteenth century. Through the 1890s, lounge manufacture was related to mattress manufacture. This was partly due to the established popularity of bed lounges, the forerunner of convertible sofas.[39] In the 1870s, the Philadelphia factory of Samuel Cooper produced mattresses as the largest part of its business, which by the mid-1870s occupied a four-story building and employed more than one hundred people. Its annual output was fifteen to twenty thousand mattresses and beds and sixteen thousand lounges; Cooper had another, and surprising, sideline trade in marble-topped tables.[40]

Lounges also were an important part of factory-organized

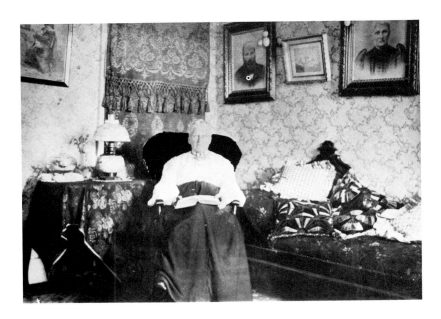

Fig. 17. Parlor in house of John Jay Niles and Hattie Hickok Niles, German, Chenango County, New York, about 1885. A lounge upholstered in carpet and further embellished with homemade patchwork pillows was the colorful centerpiece of this parlor, which also employed other cheap readymade upholstery (the center table cover and portière) to attain a refined appearance. Courtesy Rochester Public Library, Local History Division.

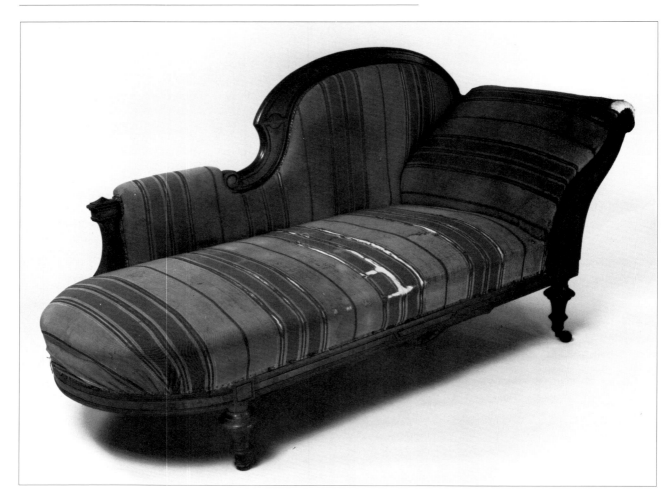

upholstery production among companies that specialized in cheaper furniture lines. In the mid-1870s, J. P. Reifsneider of Philadelphia produced both lounges and parlor furniture in a building that he shared with three other firms. The firms also shared the use of a collection of steam-powered woodworking equipment, including both band and jigsaws, a planer, and a molding machine. Reifsneider produced "about 100 (lounges) every working day," with the upholstering taking place in the "finishing department" over his downtown warerooms.[41] In 1872, the Baltimore firm Rand and McSherry was wholesaling "common lounges," "bed lounges," and "fancy" or "small French" lounges, most of which cost ten to fifteen dollars. The cheapest, the $6.50 common lounge "plain front and back," had no buttoning or other upholstery ornamentation but had a "lasting or fancy cover." ("Lasting" was a cotton and wool blend fabric typically used for women's shoes and coat linings. It had a sheen like horsehair). Rand and McSherry's most expensive bed lounge, having a cover of "lasting," Brussels carpet, or hair cloth, cost twenty-three dollars.[42] The Mueller and Slack Co. of Grand Rapids, Michigan, which billed itself as "Manufacturers of Upholstered Furniture," offered a similar range of goods in the 1890s.[43]

Such a large piece of furniture could be offered for so little money because lounges were subject to a number of ingenious compromises in production. Cost-saving strategies were applied to the frames, the spring structures, the materials used for decorative covers, and the ways those covers were handled to express the aesthetics of

Fig. 18. Lounge, attributed to Alexander Roux, walnut, striped wool rep, about 1870. If a product of Roux's business, this lounge represents a less expensive type of upholstery than is usually associated with his firm. It was used in one of the pair of parlors containing labeled furniture by Roux at Southmayd, a Stockbridge, Massachusetts, summer home. Unlike later factory-made lounges, it has a spring structure resting on webbing. Courtesy Smithsonian Institution.

refinement in ways that still were accessible to families of modest means. In order to reach less affluent markets with upholstered furniture, businessmen whose firms produced and marketed modestly priced upholstery set limits on their choice of materials, on the technologies employed, and on the number and kind of steps involved in fabricating lounges.

Women's "designer" purses and the "knock-offs" that imitate them provide a modern, easily recognizable instance of how this process works. Designer purses are usually canvas bags printed with the logo of a designer and coated to make them waterproof. The designer's initials are themselves recognizable to other women in the know about fashion. However, such bags are also carefully cut out and assembled so that the pattern made by those initials is oriented carefully. The leather seams and handles are rolled, stitched, and finished with welting; the hardware is heavy cast brass. Inexpensive versions of the same bag are made from patterns and materials that, seen in passing or at some distance, resemble the prototype closely. However, seen at close range, the "knock-off" purse has fabric printed with an unknown monogram, designed to look like the expensive one. The binding around the bag edges and handles is synthetic, and the stitching and finishes are much less carefully executed. The hardware is a soft "white metal" of unknown composition, plated with a brass finish.

The owner of the knock-off purse knows well that hers is not an "original." What her cheap purse provides is style, what fashion would call a "status look." Its appearance signals the owner's awareness of and participation in current fashion; she would have the expensive bag if she could. While it could be argued that she is buying a "sham" and should settle for an inexpensive bag that is "honest"—that is, it looks like an inexpensive canvas purse—it also can be argued that she is communicating her up-to-dateness and interest in the fashionable world through this detail. The bag is a rhetorical statement designed to persuade others about her taste and aspirations; it skirts the issue of her means.

Analyzing the economics of furniture design similarly requires comparing and interpreting the processes of production for both

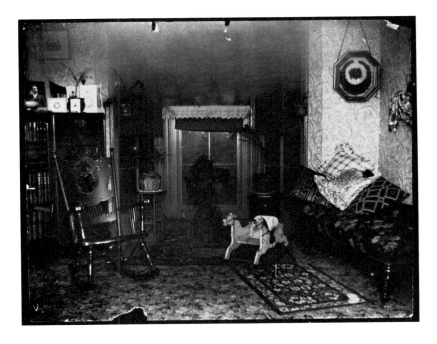

Fig. 19. Parlor-sitting room in unidentified house, United States, about 1885. The carpet-covered lounge piled with homemade pillows appears to be the only upholstered piece of furniture in this modest room; the pillows made upright sitting more comfortable.

expensive and cheap objects rather than rendering judgments about quality.[44] Like manufacturers today, nineteenth-century furniture factories tended to specialize in a price level. One of the major differences between shops that produced cheap furniture and those making expensive items was the amount of handcraftsmanship employed. Firms specializing in upholstery, however, faced problems in cost cutting unfamiliar to companies producing tables or case furniture. The cost of upholstering, always a process involving skilled labor and few specialized tools, could not be lowered readily by the use of machinery in its production (fig. 22). While upholstering could be performed in a large factory setting, little work could be done with the help of machines, and upholsterer's tools changed little in the eighteenth and nineteenth centuries. These tools usually included an assortment of large straight and curved needles, hammers for tacking, "strainers" for pulling welding taut, and "regulators," long, pointed metal tools that permitted rearranging stuffing materials inside chair upholstery as it was built up.

The cost of lounges could be cut, however, by using machinery to make their wooden frames. Power band and jigsaws roughed out frames; jigsaws cut out decorative shapes; planers made straight surfaces and decorative moldings; power lathes turned legs and decorative spindles; routers made simple incised designs, sometimes on more than one piece at a time with the aid of a pantograph; machines bored dowel holes to fit frame parts together. Finishing and decorating lounge frames always required some handwork, but the light and dark areas made by inlay could be mimicked with paint, and carving could be implied in cut-out shapes or incised decoration (see the cover).

In the 1850s through 1870s, the frames of lounges were embellished with curved molding, which could be more or less ornate depending upon the complexity of the molding plane and the

Fig. 20. Adjustable couch (called "Roman divan") oak, pine, printed voided cotton velveteen, stamped metal beaded trim, United States, 1900-1915. See fig. 38 for a detail of the underside of this divan.

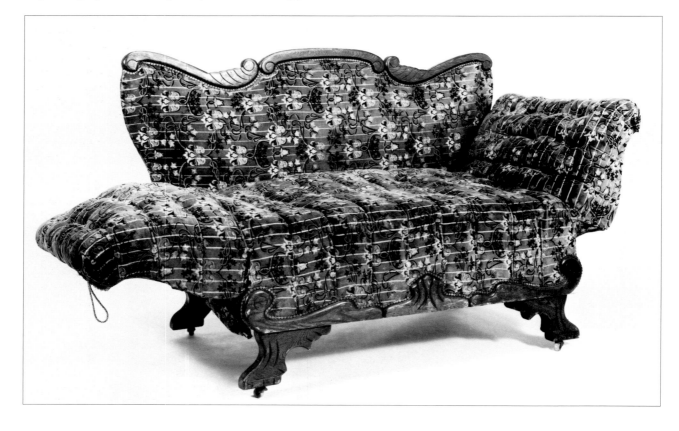

Fig. 21. Roman divans, illustration in Sears, Roebuck and Co. Catalogue No. 111 (1902).

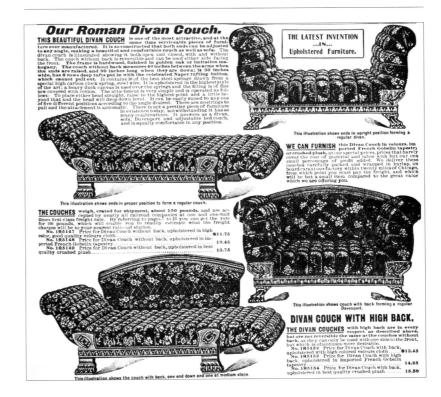

addition of incised or applied carved decorations (fig. 23). In more expensive pieces, the molding was topped off with crests of fruit or flowers like those found on parlor chairs at the same time. In some cheap lounges, the fabric was pulled over the rough wooden frame, requiring no decorative finishing except on the legs, which could be easily turned with a foot- or steam-powered lathe.

When "reform" and "Queen Anne" or "Anglo-Japanese" styles of furniture were introduced to American consumers in the late 1870s, lounge makers were able to take advantage of the rectilinear design of such furniture by using woodworking machines to turn spindles, to cut out complex shapes, and to incise elaborate designs without costly carving. The backs of lounges became complex compositions, the focus of design interest in the relationship of upholstery and decorative frame. Using the same back designs but different seat frames and covers, manufacturers such as the Buffalo Upholstering Company were able to offer customers many choices in lounge design (fig. 24).

During the 1890s, the backless couch became increasingly popular as an expression of the "Turkish taste" in furnishing. Having lost the raised back as a site for embellishment, manufacturers decorated the wooden rail around the couch frame with carving, shaped it and covered it with fabric, embellished it with "Turkish" fringe, and made the raised pillow head more decorative. The raised end often took the guise of a movable pillow even though it was part of the lounge frame. One unidentified maker even used cast metal trim and hairy paw feet (nailed over plain oak stubs), an alternative that may not have saved much money but represented an effort to attract consumer attention with novelty (fig. 25). In couches where little of the frame was decorative, the economics of design were dedicated mostly to reducing the cost of upholstering itself.

Cost cutting in the upholstering process presented makers of cheap furniture with two problems—reducing the costs of creating the structure of the upholstery sandwich and of the decorative or

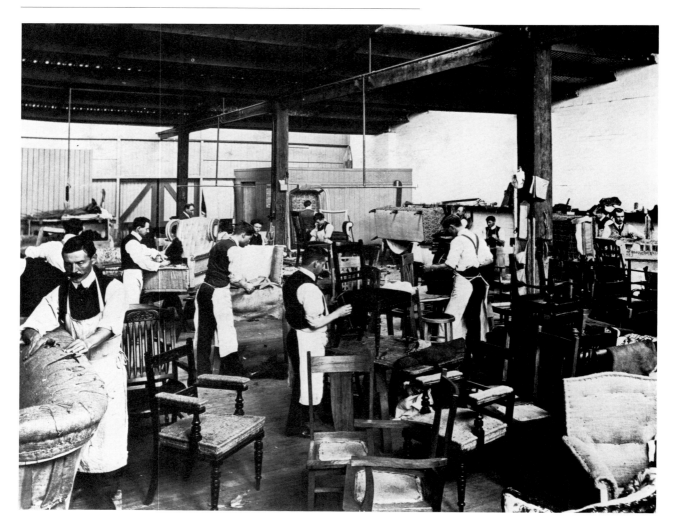

show cover while still offering customers a certain amount of style. By the 1880s, when cheap upholstered furniture proliferated, manufacturers had developed strategies to resolve both difficulties.

Because of its popularity in the furnishing of modest households and the size of the finished product, lounge making is a particularly useful demonstration of the search for shortcuts to reduce the amount of time and skilled labor involved in constructing the internal sandwich of spring-seat upholstery—webbing, springs and twines, fabric, stuffing material, undercover, and show cover. (Cheap parlor suites display some but not all of these shortcuts because of the smaller size of the pieces.) Resilient spring structures could fail in a number of ways—bad spring tying, rotted webbing, improperly tempered springs—and were difficult to repair. However, the public clearly associated resilient seat structures with high-quality upholstery, particularly structures having coil springs. The most expensive springs were the best-tempered and most resilient; the less expensive springs used by makers of cheap furniture always were more stiff, but because they still gave and returned to shape, they were good enough for new consumers. Horsehair was the most resilient stuffing, but it also was the most expensive. Plant materials—tow, moss, wood shavings (called "excelsior")—provided cheaper, although less resilient, alternatives.

The 1890 price list and trade catalog for the Buffalo (New York) Upholstering Company, which billed itself as "the Largest Lounge

Fig. 22. Upholstery workroom, Century Furniture Company, Grand Rapids, Michigan, about 1903. The Century Furniture Company (1900-1940) made high-quality furniture for an upper middle-class and wealthy clientele. In the upholstery workroom, craftsmen began and completed each piece of furniture using a few traditional tools—tack hammers, scissors, curved and straight sewing needles, a long metal "regulator" for moving stuffing around inside each chair, and a "strainer" for stretching webbing. The men's age and dress (white shirts, suit vests, ties, and polished shoes) indicate that they are skilled craftsmen and have come up through an apprentice system. The unfinished furniture on which they work demonstrates their skills —stitched French and English edges, pleated tufting, and spring structures built upon the traditional foundations of interwoven fabric webbing. Courtesy Grand Rapids Public Museum.

Manufactory in the World," demonstrates how differences in frames and seat structures affected price. The cheapest lounge wholesaled for five dollars in tapestry carpet or "Moquette Plush" (a similar carpet with cut pile); it had an "imitation walnut" frame, was upholstered with tow, and contained fifteen springs. The top of the line, with the same fabric cover, wholesaled for nineteen dollars; its frame was oak, and it featured thirty-three springs and a "web bottom."[45]

Cost cutting in production of spring seats evolved along several lines. Producing separately framed, sprung, stuffed, and covered boxes, which sat on blocks in the seat frame like a large slip seat, had been a common strategy for producing upholstered chairs by the 1840s, evolving from the boxes with springs used about 1830 on chairs with board seats. Factory-scale production of box seats appeared in the railroad car-building industry as a way to make seats that were sturdy, easy to remove and replace, and easy to repair and refurbish. Production of spring-filled cushions for chairs and automobiles in the early twentieth century continued this line of problem-solving (fig. 26).

A second method for getting around the problem of constructing web seat bottoms was to close in the bottom of the seat frame itself with a solid board or a series of slats. At least one chair maker experimented with board chair bottoms with metal clasps and hinges in the late 1860s and 1870s (figs. 27 and 28). More commonly, furniture makers employed some kind of box frame as a base for the spring structure, a technique also used in the production of railroad seats. They used a solid wooden bottom or slats rather than webbing for anchoring the springs; the structure then was built up in the traditional manner. This method seems to have been applied first to beds. In August 25, 1831, Josiah French of Ware, Massachusetts, received Patent 6728 for a bed bottom consisting of a box. The end of each spring was seated in a groove in the box bottom and secured with a metal staple hammered in place. A grid of wood was set in place halfway between the box bottom and the top of its frame, with its wooden members running through the springs to hold them in position. By this method, Ware apparently sought to avoid any spring tying at all, as well as attempting to guarantee uniform elasticity in the mattress.[46]

Solid or slatted wooden bottoms, where springs could be fastened in place with staples, became an important design compromise in the seat structure of cheap lounges, as did solid board backs that were often upholstered separately, then attached to the seat frame. Such heavy, large frames gave upholsterers a lot of solid material for anchoring upholstery, which required less skill than building structures over minimal frames hung with webbing. The finished

Fig. 23. *"Lounge 104," photograph in* Descriptive Catalogue of Sofas, Lounges, Tetes, Chairs and Parlor Suits, *Rand and McSherry, Baltimore, Maryland (1872). Courtesy Smithsonian Institution.*

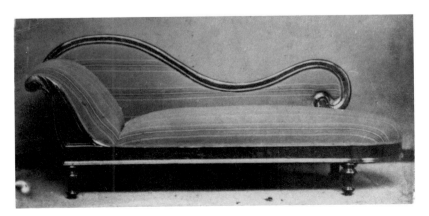

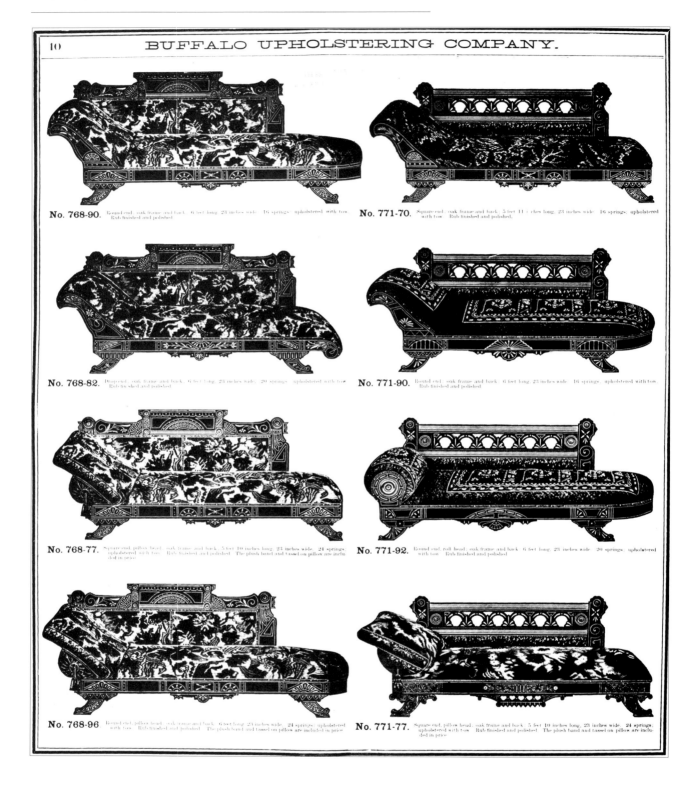

No. 768-90. Round end, oak frame and back, 6 feet long, 23 inches wide, 16 springs, upholstered with tow. Rub finished and polished.

No. 771-70. Square end, oak frame and back, 5 feet 11 inches long, 23 inches wide, 16 springs, upholstered with tow. Rub finished and polished.

No. 768-82. Draped end, oak frame and back, 6 feet long, 23 inches wide, 20 springs, upholstered with tow. Rub finished and polished.

No. 771-90. Round end, oak frame and back, 6 feet long, 23 inches wide, 16 springs, upholstered with tow. Rub finished and polished.

No. 768-77. Square end, pillow head, oak frame and back, 5 feet 10 inches long, 23 inches wide, 24 springs, upholstered with tow. Rub finished and polished. The plush band and tassel on pillow are included in price.

No. 771-92. Round end, roll head, oak frame and back, 6 feet long, 23 inches wide, 20 springs, upholstered with tow. Rub finished and polished.

No. 768-96. Round end, pillow head, oak frame and back, 6 feet long, 23 inches wide, 24 springs, upholstered with tow. Rub finished and polished. The plush band and tassel on pillow are included in price.

No. 771-77. Square end, pillow head, oak frame and back, 5 feet 10 inches long, 23 inches wide, 24 springs, upholstered with tow. Rub finished and polished. The plush band and tassel on pillow are included in price.

product was a much heavier and less resilient piece of furniture (figs. 29 and 30).

In the 1890s, inventors also experimented with the use of metal wires or strips and with wire grids, another development originating in bed production. Wire or mesh could be used as a means of anchoring springs instead of sewing them to a webbing base. Wire did not rot as jute webbing was apt to, and it was more resilient than a wooden bottom. In 1908, Sears, Roebuck and Co. advertised that all its couches and suites with spring seats were sold with "all steel construction," including "corrugated steel wire bottoms" which, the company asserted, was sturdier than webbing. Wire bottoms on furniture also found favor because they were open, available for inspection and therefore more sanitary than traditional structures (fig. 31).

As they experimented with methods of producing economical, if rather stiff, spring structures in lounges, manufacturers also tried to attain desirable visual qualities in their upholstery. Upholstery fabrics always had to be cut by hand from patterns, but the relatively simple shapes of lounges did not require much sewing of covers nor the fabrication of separate cushions before they were applied.

The covers of lounges were typically showy, but the fabrics often were relatively inexpensive. Simple decorative buttoning all over the surface or one row of pleated tufts on a raised back made the upholstery more complex in appearance, but lounges were typically covered with fabrics that imparted visual detail and tactile richness through their pattern and texture—striped rep, printed raw silk, crushed or embossed mohair plush, or "tapestry brussels" carpet (figs. 32 and 33). Small labor and materials savings also could be realized in the process of trimming out lounges by using gimps with adhesive backs or metal stripping as trim.

Furniture manufacturers began experimenting with using the cheaper grades of carpet for chair upholstery in the 1850s.[47] Tapestry carpet (an innovation of the 1830s), where the warp of the carpet was printed with a stretched-out version of the desired pattern and then woven so that it was looped into a pile and the design made visible, was the cheapest and most popular form of carpet upholstery. Patent folding chairs such as those manufactured by the New Haven Folding Chair Company and the Worcester, Massachusetts, firm of Edward W. Vaill frequently had custom-woven carpet with patented designs on their unpadded seats and backs. Carpet upholstery sometimes was

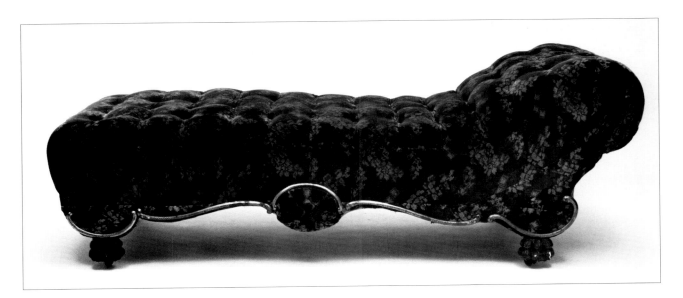

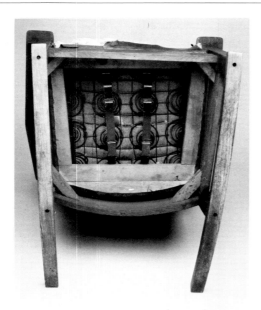

Fig. 26. This chair seat, made with iron bands and wire mesh, was constructed in much the same way as an automobile or railroad car seat.

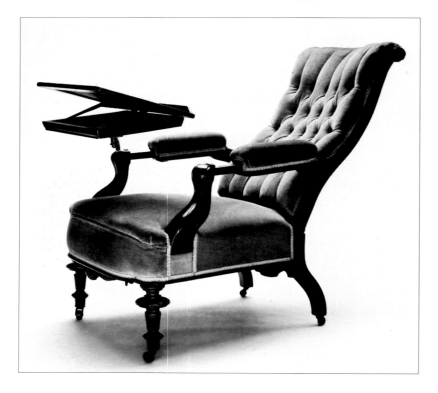

Fig. 27. Reading chair, walnut, brass, modern cotton velvet, P. J. Hardy, New York, New York, 1866-1878.

offered in all of the popular kinds of looped or cut-pile carpet. Vaill's catalog for 1882-1883 offered carpet-seat folding chairs with a rosewood or walnut finish in "Pattern Tapestry" carpet for forty-two dollars a dozen, "Pattern Brussels" or "Pattern Velvet" (cut-pile tapestry) for forty-eight dollars, and "Pattern Wilton" for sixty dollars a dozen.[48]

The apotheosis of carpet upholstery could be found in the factory-made lounge, however. Consumers valued fabrics that looked "rich"—heavy, colorful, and often with pile surfaces. In addition, detail was frequently labeled "rich" because of the historical connotations of work that it bore. Refined upholstery was rich in

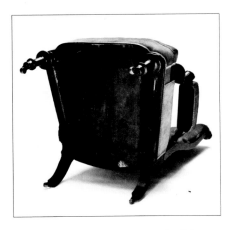

Fig. 28. Bottom view of fig. 27 with board bottom in place. The nature of the original spring structure of this chair cannot be determined because it has been replaced. The hinged board bottom allowed access to the spring structure and anchored the springs.

Fig. 29. Box bottom of Martyn Brothers lounge (see plate 27). Trade catalogs dating between 1880 and 1890 issued by the Buffalo Upholstering Company of Buffalo, New York, offered frames with similar board bottoms and solid board backs wholesale to upholsterers.

Fig. 30. Back of plate 27. Board backs made cheap lounges heavier than backs with webbing, and, because board backs provided a sturdier base, these lounges required less skill of upholsterers.

color and intricate, and it was even better if it bore particular kinds of pattern, naturalistic renderings of floral bunches or garlands.

Carpet upholstery had all these qualities. Because it was so heavy and stiff, carpet upholstery could not be tufted. Therefore, less skill was required to apply it to the lounge frame. It was sturdier than many other inexpensive upholstery fabrics offered in the 1880s and 1890s, such as mixed cotton and wool ("union") rep and printed jute. It also was considerably more visually pleasing than the common inexpensive machine-woven black or gray plain horsehair, which disappeared from catalog offerings in the 1880s. It seemed more appropriate to parlors than did artificial leather, called "American cloth." Consumers who had limited means for furnishing seem to have loved it, and it was not replaced as the fabric of choice until after 1895, when cotton corduroy and velveteen printed in bright patterns became popular.

Tufting signaled both high-quality production and an important component of the aesthetics of refinement to ordinary consumers shopping for factory-made upholstery, just as it did to the clientele of custom upholstery shops. Pleated tufting added to the cost of furniture because it required both skilled labor and twenty to thirty per cent more of the show cover material.[49]

Companies making cheap lounges and mattresses, which also required buttoning to hold stuffing in place, could reduce the amount of skill and labor involved in tufting by availing themselves of devices invented after 1893. These tufting forms and tufting machines produced a mat of backing fabric, stuffing, and cover fastened together by decorative buttons with shafts that clinched. This mat could then be wrapped around a couch form like a large quilt, cut to size and fastened down with tacks (fig. 34).

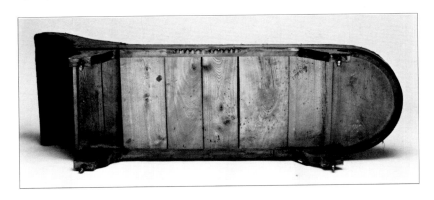

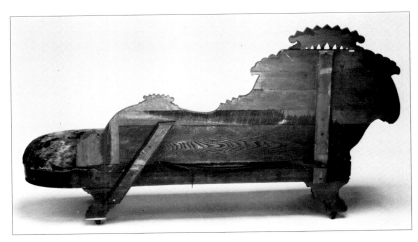

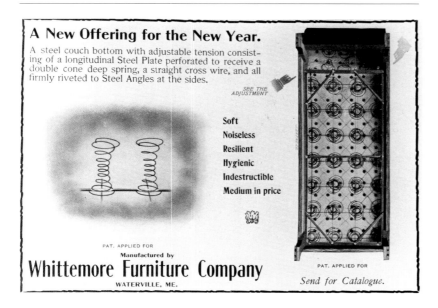

A New Offering for the New Year.

A steel couch bottom with adjustable tension consisting of a longitudinal Steel Plate perforated to receive a double cone deep spring, a straight cross wire, and all firmly riveted to Steel Angles at the sides.

SEE THE ADJUSTMENT

Soft
Noiseless
Resilient
Hygienic
Indestructible
Medium in price

PAT. APPLIED FOR

Manufactured by
Whittemore Furniture Company
WATERVILLE, ME.

PAT. APPLIED FOR

Send for Catalogue.

Fig. 31. Advertisement for the Whittemore Furniture Company, Waterville, Maine, in The Grand Rapids Furniture Record *(February 1903). The steel couch bottom introduced in this advertisement worked very much like the wooden mattress frame patented by Issac Ware more than seventy years earlier. Here the springs were fastened into perforations in a steel frame that could then be fitted into a wooden couch frame and adjusted to fit tightly. The springs were steadied at the top by fastening them with another grid of wires running diagonally across the couch frame. The pattern of buttoning, with clenched button shafts barely visible over a round fabric anchor, suggests that this couch's cover was tufted by machine. Courtesy Grand Rapids Public Library.*

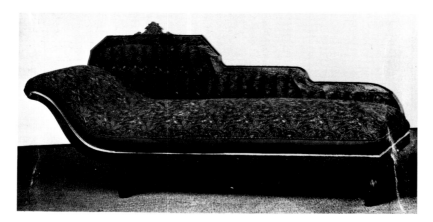

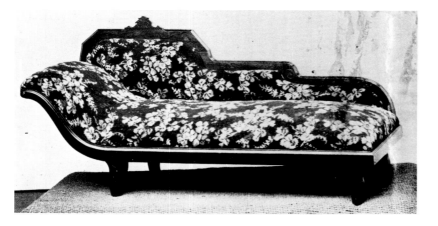

Figs. 32 and 33. "#8 Raw Silk, $12.00" and "#8 Carpet," photographs in James Boyd Co. catalog, Boston, Massachusetts, 1875-1880. Boyd offered his customers a typical range of middle-class upholstery choices on simple frames. The cheapest version was upholstered in striped rep, its surface varied by unnecessary but decorative buttoning. The version in printed raw silk was the most expensive, and the channel and pleated tufting on its back involved the most work of all versions. Tapestry carpet upholstery, featuring a floral design that was probably brightly colored, required the least upholstering workmanship to create a lively effect. The lounge was also offered in wool terry, a finely patterned ribbed fabric, and gained stylishness not only through its fabric but through its shiny enameled buttons, a contrasting band of raw silk, and cording as well.

The tufting machine was responsible for the introduction of "section work" in large-scale upholstery shops. Before then, even in factory settings, the upholstery of a single piece of furniture was the product of one upholsterer, a situation that still exists in better workrooms today. Craftsmen used a price book to determine payment on a piecework basis. In New York, for example, the 1870

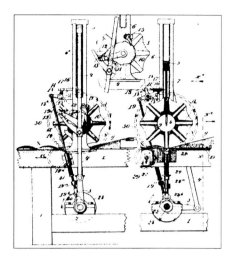

Fig. 34. Patent No. 622,901, illustration in Official Gazette of the U.S. Patent Office *(11 April 1899). The text underneath this illustration calls this invention a "machine for making tufted fabrics." Christian S. E. Spoerl of Scranton, Pennsylvania, filed for this patent on October 22, 1898.*

rate for a parlor suite (probably of seven pieces) was five dollars. As late as the 1890s, custom upholstery work paid quite well, and skilled upholsterers in some cities were protected by unions. When work was steady, the members of the New York Custom Upholstery Local earned between sixteen and twenty-one dollars a week, wages on par with those of other skilled workmen.[50]

At the lower end of the upholstered furniture price spectrum, competition was keen; upholsterers were a skilled labor cost for which manufacturers were eager to find a partial substitute in tufting machines. Upholsterers were equally eager to resist such attempts. In one instance, on May 28, 1898, the craftsmen in the upholstering room of the Paine Bedding Company of Grand Rapids walked out because the company introduced a tufting machine and section work on backless lounges (couches). An article on the strike, which lasted at least until July 3 when Charles Paine was able to obtain an injunction against twenty-one members of the upholsterer's local, described the conflict and the nature of the work:

> Last Saturday the Paine company served notice on its upholsterers that thereafter they would require their work to be done in "section." "Section" means that a part of the work is done in one room by cheap labor and finished by skilled labor in another room. The workmen objected to this division of their work and a meeting of the Upholsterers' union was called Sunday morning. At that time, it was voted to agree to cut off from 25 to 35 cents per couch, but not to accept the divided labor. Monday morning they submitted their proposal, it was not accepted and eight of them walked out.[51]

Paine tried to hire boys as tufting machine operators, but harassment by the striking upholsterers led management to resort to hiring seven girls to operate the machines. At least one other strike was called on account of the introduction of tufting machines, an unsuccessful walkout in 1899 by unionized upholsterers in New York City against the National Parlor Suite Company.[52] Factories that employed this kind of section work required fewer skilled workers and reduced production costs. Cheap couches continued to be produced by less skilled labor, using similar kinds of upholstery section work such as pre-stuffed edge rolls (visible at the back of the workroom in fig. 35).

The "tufting machine" that led to the Grand Rapids strike was probably a form of power press that employed a presser plate and a flat panel or form with either indentations or a set of raised pins to mark the position of buttons. The first such device was patented in 1895.[53] The tufting machine produced a mat of fabric, stuffing, and backing material, punctuated and held together with buttons at regular intervals. Sometimes the buttons were fastened with string, but a number of patents were taken out after 1898 for buttons with metal clinchers that could be bent apart with pressure from the presser plate after insertion into the pad of fabric. Because the tufts themselves were not pleated and sewn into place, machine tufting required less fabric than pleated tufts, and the results could be applied to any plain upholstered surface. Workers soon gave this type of tufting power press the nickname of "hay baler."[54] This type of continuous action power press became the typical tufting machine, such as the one illustrated in a 1903 advertisement for the Novelty Tufting Machine Company (fig. 36).

Machine tufting seems to have provided a satisfactory paraphrase of hand-tufting upholstery to new consumers, although its

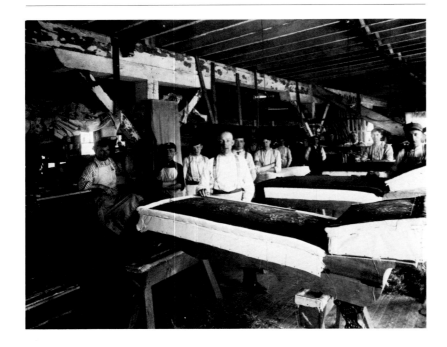

Fig. 35. *Couch upholstery workroom,*
Mueller and Slack Company, Grand
Rapids, Michigan, 1903. This
workroom, where inexpensive couches were
upholstered, shows the different kind of
labor employed for cheap lounges and
section work. Courtesy Grand Rapids
Public Museum.

appearance was much different than handwork. One box or
wardrobe couch, used in an upstairs room at the Voigt house in
Grand Rapids, Michigan (fig. 37), appears to have been tufted by
machine, as does the Roman divan (fig. 38). The couch, which
features a storage unit lined with cedar, was upholstered with forest
green cotton voided velveteen. The raised top is a complete spring
seat structure, featuring wire used as a shortcut for fastening in the
coil springs from the bottom, topped by a mat of velveteen, stuffing,
and cotton duck buttoned together and fastened over the top's frame.
This construction, where the solid wooden sides of a lounge, couch,
or, somewhat later, davenport sofa, disguise a hollow interior
arrangement with a thin spring structure mounted across the top, was
one of the important shortcuts that made cheap "overstuffed"
furniture available to average consumers in the 1910s and 1920s.

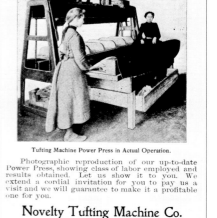

Tufting Machine Power Press in Actual Operation.

Photographic reproduction of our up-to-date
Power Press, showing class of labor employed and
results obtained. Let us show it to you. We
extend a cordial invitation for you to pay us a
visit and we will guarantee to make it a profitable
one for you.

Novelty Tufting Machine Co.
A. FRESCHL, Manager
263 Dearborn Street,   CHICAGO, U. S. A.

Fig. 36. Advertisement for Novelty
Tufting Machine, illustration in
Directory of Wholesale Furniture
Manufacturers of the United States
1903-4.

Fig. 37. Box couch in sewing room of the Voigt House, Grand Rapids, Michigan, 1901-1915. Courtesy Voigt Collection, Grand Rapids Public Museum.

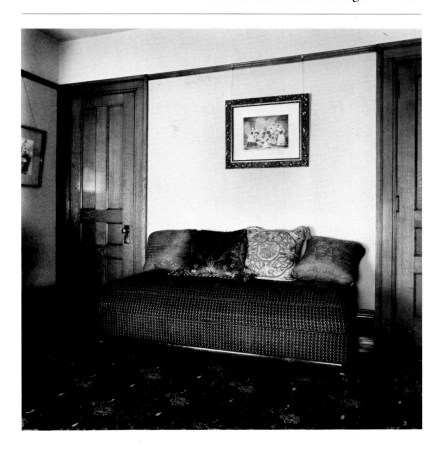

Fig. 38. Detail of fig. 20. Viewed from the underside, the Roman divan reveals the complete range of shortcuts taken by manufacturers of cheap upholstered furniture by the turn of the century. The springs are stapled to pine boards (which are themselves braced with blocks) and are not tied; they are instead braced at the top by thick wire bands. The regular pattern of buttons clenched with metal shanks through round anchors (visible as black circles here) indicates that a tufting machine was used. The board back was upholstered separately, then fastened to the divan with two wooden braces after the piece had been shipped to a retail store or its new owner.

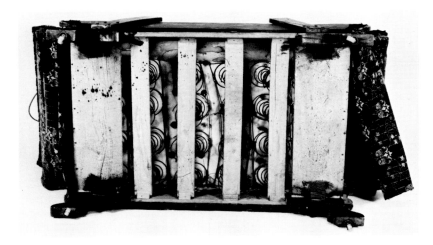

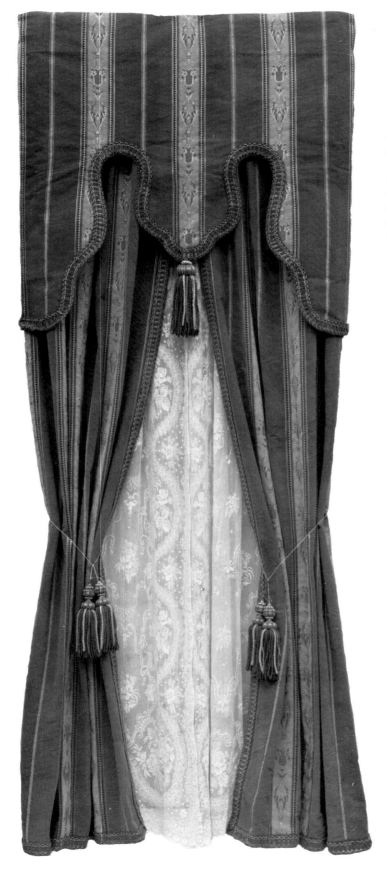

Fig. 1. *Valance and draperies, wool and silk figured rep, 1860-1870. Tambour lace curtains, England or France, 1870-1880. This complete window treatment has a history of use in the New York City residence of John Moore, an importer of agricultural products, at 35 West 49th Street. Courtesy Metropolitan Museum of Art; gift of Mrs. Fred Thompson, 1976.*

CHAPTER EIGHT
WINDOW AND DOOR DRAPERY:
CREATING THE COMFORTABLE THEATER

So many delightful possibilities are concealed by a curtain; not to mention the skillful hiding of defects made feasible with such means, or the softening of angles and happy obliteration of corners.

Janet E. Ruutz-Rees, *Home Decoration* (1881)

Between 1850 and 1900, decorative window draperies became an increasingly important element of parlor decor in ordinary homes (fig. 1). By the 1880s, the largest, most impressive expanses of heavy drapery in many ordinary parlors were the door curtains, or portières. It is tempting to assume that the increasing popularity of window and door curtains was always associated with the desire to make rooms less drafty and cold. However, draperies made their own special contributions to parlor sensibilities, and individual choices in parlor window draping were actually motivated by a variety of goals. Along with the practical impulses to control temperature (including heat in the South) and limit light to preserve other upholstery, control of light for aesthetic purposes, the desire to have privacy or to block out unpleasant views or other "defects," and the "framing" effect of draperies on windows and doorways were also valued for their contribution to the aesthetics of refinement. Further, decorative window shades and lace or sheer curtains signaled respectability to the street and passersby; they were in fact the only element of parlor decor that could do so.

At midcentury, some families who had the means to purchase heavy window curtains still often chose not to do so. In 1857, Caroline Cowles Richards of Canandaigua, New York, noted that her grandmother refused to have curtains or shades at the parlor windows "because Grandfather says, 'light is sweet and a pleasant thing it is to behold the sun.'"[1] Authors of midcentury advice books also argued that draperies were unnecessary, in part because furnishing fabrics were still expensive. The authors of the 1856 volume *Village and Farm Cottages* noted that window curtains were "not, like some articles of furniture, absolutely necessary, and very many dispense with them wholly," although they qualified this statement by observing that curtains could "almost rival the bright fireside in giving to our apartments a warm, cheerful, homelike aspect."[2] In 1860, Fanny Copeland still believed that curtains were "comparatively expensive, and, therefore, will never come into such general use as blinds."[3]

Parlor draperies in particular represented a large investment in households of the 1850s. One 1854 article in *Godey's Lady's Book* stated that parlor curtains ordered through the mail from a local business establishment cost $15 to $150.[4] The fabrics most frequently cited in this kind of advice were invariably expensive—silk and wool damasks, the earlier form of "brocatelle," brocades, and, the most modest of the group, "satin-de-laine," wool woven to have a satin surface (fig. 2). Wealthy consumers sometimes spent astonishing sums of money on ostentatious window drapery. The yellow-and-white silk drawing room curtains created in 1856 for Samuel Colt's house Armsmear, similar in design and ornamentation

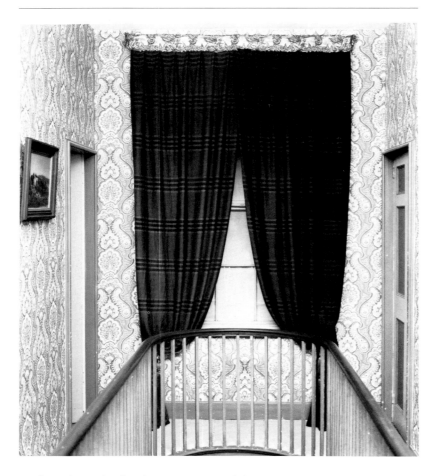

Fig. 2. Curtains, satin-weave wool (satin-de-laine), once used in Castle Tucker, Wiscasset, Maine, 1858-1860. In "Decorated Parlor Windows," an article appearing in the February 1854 issue of Godey's Lady's Book, *the author praised "curtains of Paris stripe" in* "satin laine" *employed in the bedrooms of the La Pierre, a Philadelphia hotel that had opened the year before. The article implied that such curtains were appropriate for use in private houses. Where these curtains were originally used in the Tucker house is not known. Courtesy Castle Tucker.*

to those hung in the drawing room of the Morse-Libby Mansion, cost $568 for two windows, a sum equal to a year's wages for many skilled workers (see chapter 1, figs. 9 and 10).[5]   Such expenditures were atypical, but they are indicative of the kind of resources wealthy families poured into creating opulent facades for their social lives. In 1858 and 1860, the Tucker family spent $28.50 and $30.00 per window on drapery (and, probably, hardware) for its best rooms, a figure which may be taken as a representative expense for middle-class families with ample but not lavish incomes.[6]

Families with limited money to spend on furnishings could, and did, create parlors for themselves without decorative window coverings. However, such window treatments became increasingly important as an expressive term in creating appropriately refined and softened parlor decor. The desirability of ample expanses of drapery, which framed windows and helped create unified decor, had been introduced to many people through commercial parlors and periodicals such as *Godey's*, which occasionally reproduced engravings of draped windows.[7] While many draperies associated with "design reform" of the 1870s still were made of expensive materials, Eastlake himself advocated a number of cheap, washable fabrics, including "the new *cretonne*," as suitable for curtains and practical because they could be washed.[8] This kind of thinking signaled new possibilities for inexpensive "artistic" draperies that could be made at home. By 1877, *Peterson's Magazine* was publishing instructions for "Oriental curtains" made from inexpensive muslin and colorful flannel (fig. 3; plate 29).[9] By the 1880s, a veritable drapery craze was in full swing, which not only increased the amount of fabric employed in parlor decor generally but also encouraged the use of less expensive novelty

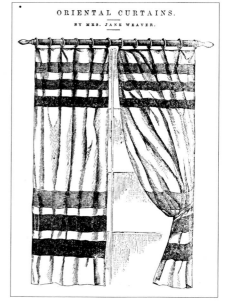

ORIENTAL CURTAINS.
BY MRS. JANE WEAVER.

Fig. 3. "Oriental Curtains," engraving in Peterson's Magazine *(May 1877). The instructions that accompanied this illustration informed readers that these curtains cost only $3.40 to make and suggested that their simple cut and materials liberated housekeepers from dependency upon expensive upholsterers for their parlor draperies.*

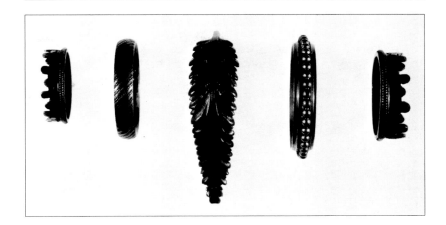

Fig. 4. Curtain rings, stamped and cast brass, 1840-1880. The rings that held most window curtains usually were plain wool or brass. Decorative brass rings, probably imported from Europe, could be used as parts of window decor, along with curtain pins or tiebacks that had fancy heads of metal and glass. People seem typically to have recycled decorative drapery hardware through several generations of curtains.

fabrics for parlor draperies, including fabrics that once were acceptable only for utilitarian purposes or were new to the market. The 1881 catalog for Lord and Taylor, for example, offered ready-made full-length curtains in "printed jute" (burlap) for between nine and twenty-five dollars per window.[10]

Changes in production costs of cotton or cotton-blend drapery fabrics played a large role in encouraging the proliferation of window drapery, particularly lace, the lighter-weight cottons, and linens for shades. Machine-made lace curtains, most of them imported from England, dropped in price dramatically between 1850 and 1890. American production of upholstery goods, centered in Philadelphia, and of cotton prints suitable for furnishing use accelerated after 1880 and were produced largely for the middle-class market.[11] While the 1880 Census found no American upholstery production that incorporated silk, by 1890 the *Census of Manufactures* documented the production of $471,324 worth of curtains, $1,330,287 of furniture tapestries, and $1,910,721 of other upholstery broad goods. "Curtains largely made of silk, but with some admixture of cotton, are now offered to consumers at less price than were 'all cotton' goods ten years ago...," the 1890 Census reported, "equally in 'Other upholstery broad goods', such as brocatelles, light silk damasks for draperies, silk chenilles, etc., the improvement has been exceedingly rapid." In 1890, American weaving of pairs of cotton curtains, finished in the factory for sale, totaled $1,225,364 (676,032 pairs). By the mid-1890s, American production of the cheaper grades of lace curtains was also established, although 1,679,659 square yards ($752,775) of lace were still imported from England in 1898, along with quantities from France, Scotland, and Switzerland.[12] American production of printed cotton furnishing fabrics, especially cretonne (which eventually garnered the name "drapery print"), was also well established by the 1880s.

Thus production capabilities evidently began to meet the requirements of consumer demand already in place, waiting for drapery fabrics to become more accessible. By 1889, Frank A. Moreland could assert that "the modern house is very dependent upon its upholstery decorations for the necessary finish...there is always an uncomfortable sense of bareness when no drapery is furnished, no matter how generously the apartment has been supplied with furniture and other appointments."[13] And women whose families lived on modest incomes could look around their parlors at the long panels of machine-made lace and the curtains or valances of Canton flannel and brightly printed cottons and agree with him.

Actually, the "fully dressed" window between 1850 and 1910 varied little in the elements it employed—shades or blinds (better houses sometimes had built-in shutters); underdraperies of muslin, lawn (at this time, a fine linen fabric), "scrim" or "grenadine" (fine cottons), net, and lace; a valance or lambrequin that could be nailed to a cornice or hung from a decorative pole; and overdraperies at the sides of the window frame. Often these panels could not be closed but hung only as a fabric frame. One factor that did vary was the degree of elaboration involved in each element (plate 30). Elaborate draperies always were money on the wall, so to speak. Their fabrics were expensive; their trims could be more expensive than the fabric; and if they were draperies in the French taste, their cutting almost always required substantial expertise.

The hardware associated with curtains could also be costly. In the 1850s, the fully dressed window often included imported stamped metal cornices, fancy brass curtain rings, and brass "curtain bands" that held back drapery.[14] In the 1850s, even the plainest curtains could be made more ornamental with American-made decorative "curtain pins" (now called "tie-backs") with pressed glass, mercury glass, or ceramic heads. These tended to be treated as permanent elements of window frames by some families and remained in use for decades (fig. 4).[15] The wooden cornices popular in the late 1860s through the early 1880s and the decorative wooden or brass poles popular through the end of the century could cost as much as the curtains below them (fig. 5). Once purchased, however, they often remained in use through repeated redecorations (plate 31).

Most parlor makers usually made a selection of some of these components as a matter both of household economy and other considerations such as seasonal variation, because many housekeepers continued to remove heavy window draperies in summer. One of the most popular ways of draping a window in middle-class households was to use a valance or lambrequin with lace curtains and a shade or blinds, without heavy side curtains. The parlors of Castle Tucker in Wiscasset, Maine, where new curtains and valances were installed in 1858, and the Osborne house of Victor, New York, where similar materials were put in place around 1870, displayed this kind of window treatment (fig. 6).

For families who chose not to use curtains or could not afford them, decorated window shades provided an attractive alternative to draping parlor windows (plate 32). Painted window shades were sold in the United States in the eighteenth century, but shades of fabric and paper seem to have become popular in the 1830s. Making fabric window shades, which involved freehand painting, stenciling, and block printing, was a trade often associated with ornamental carriage and sign painting, especially in small communities where no single type of painting would support an entire business (fig. 7).[16]

Window shades made from painted paper—called "paper curtains"—also were a secondary product of the wallpaper trade and were produced by stenciling and block printing in smaller shops (fig. 8). A broadside for Strout and Bradford of Haymarket Square in Boston, dated September 1856, advertised that its business consisted of (fabric) window shades and oil cloths for tables and floors as well as "GREEN AND BLUE CURTAIN PAPER AND PAPER

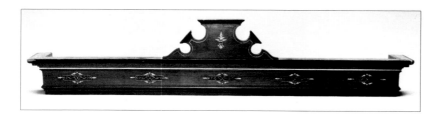

Fig. 5. Cornice, walnut with gilded and ebonized decoration, United States, about 1875. Valances and drapery panels were nailed into cornices. Lace sheers hung over wire rods strung inside cornices like these so that they could be removed and laundered.

Fig. 6. Valance, tabby-weave silk, chintz, silk and wool tassels with wire and wooden cores, about 1870. The top of this valance from the Osborne house in Victor, New York, is unfinished. It is simply overstitched to hold the layers together because the valance was permanently attached to a wooded cornice with small tacks. To stiffen the valance, made of a light, dress-weight silk fabric, it was interlined with thin cardboard cut just as the valance was, including the pleats. Unfortunately, by the time this drapery was made, cardboard was made with wood pulp rather than rags, so both the cotton backing fabric and the silk are disintegrating from acids in the brittle interlining. The deterioration of the silk tassels is typical, given that they are composed of a wooden core wound with fiber. Three of these valances are still used.

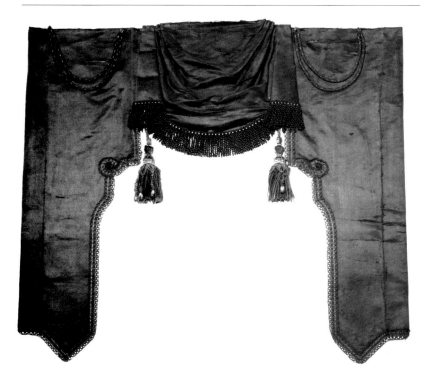

CURTAINS." In this instance, "curtain paper" may have designated simple painted paper available by the yard for shades, while "paper curtains" were pre-cut and printed with designs. Sawyer and Company of Cincinnati sometimes used the term "green curtains" and "blue curtains" to designate shades having a painted design of a complete window with curtains and a landscape seen through the glass.[17]

In the 1850s, architectural and decorating advice writers began to criticize fancy painted shades. The authors of *Village and Farm Cottages* wrote, "At all events, good friends, when you are about to furnish your windows, do spare yourself the expense of getting, and those who pass by, the pain of seeing, those intolerable daubs called 'painted shades,' with their preposterous attempts at landscape and architecture, which are so common at cottage windows."[18] Painted shades were associated with rural taste in sentimental fiction; Mrs. C. M. Kirkland described the decor of a frame farmhouse in 1853 as featuring "a multitude of windows, which were adorned with paper curtains, although the best room had white ones, with netting and fringe half a yard deep."[19] Indeed, in the 1860s, businesses catering to rural clients, such as W. A. Currier's "Kitchen, House Furnishing, and Stove Warehouse" of Haverhill, Massachusetts, offered its rural customers many types of decorated shades, still calling them "paper curtains," "gilt curtains," "landscape curtains," and "velvet curtains" (shades with flocking).[20] By the 1860s, furnishing advice for urbane, middle-class consumers no longer took note of painted shades; such books recommended instead that plain shades in white, buff, green, red, and blue holland linen be employed at windows, and that one color be selected for all windows in order to present a uniform exterior.

Even so, decorative shades continued to be offered for sale because they were more modestly priced than fabric for most curtains. In the 1850s, factory-made painted shades ranged in price from sixty cents to several dollars; by contrast, *Godey's* offered a low estimate of fifteen dollars for parlor curtains.[21] The 1881 Lord and

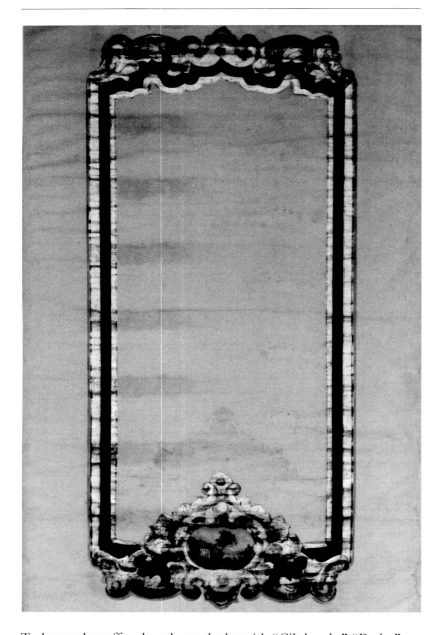

Fig. 7. Window shade, paint, flocking and gilding on unidentified sized fabric, United States, about 1860. This shade employs a variety of painting techniques associated with decorative painting for wagons and signs, including a vignette painted freehand. Flocking also was employed on factory-printed decorative shades as late as 1895 when Montgomery Ward and Co. Catalogue No. 57 *(1895) offered "dado" shades printed with a fence of wild roses and a sparrow chasing a butterfly in "flock and gold" for forty-two cents apiece.*

Taylor catalog offered made-up shades with "Gilt bands," "Dado," and "Painted shading" at twenty-five to thirty cents per yard; custom painting was still available at a cost of seven cents per square foot.[22] In the 1890s, customers who preferred plain colored shades could choose to buy them embellished with fringe and other fancy edgings; materials for embellishing old shades also were readily available for sale by the yard. The 1895 catalog of Montgomery Ward offered decorated shades for as little as thirty-one cents apiece.[23]

Machine-printed paper and linen shades remained an element of window decor into the 1920s, their patterns keeping step with popular tastes in furnishing (plate 33). The borders of some surviving shades reflect the influence of the rococo revival and Eastlake design even if the shades are otherwise undatable. Shades of the 1890s featured dado designs like those found on common chenille portières, suggesting that they could serve as another inexpensive means of attaining unified decor. The market for these decorated shades may have consisted of conservative or less

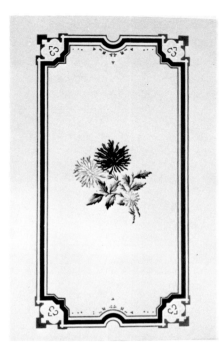

Fig. 8. Window shade, stenciled design on paper, United States, about 1880. "Wallpaper" shades were less expensive than those of painted linen. However, they were less sturdy (because they were ruined by rainstorms) and even less translucent, particularly when painted in deep colors.

sophisticated consumers; their sale through mail-order catalogs well into the twentieth century suggests that the market existed largely in small communities by the 1890s.

Another option for modest parlors was to use shades with lace inserts, sheer curtains with fancy edging and insertions, or curtains made entirely of lace. At midcentury, sheer curtains of muslin ("mull") still served as physical barriers against insects and street dust and were elements of the "summer dress" of important rooms such as parlors. Advice literature rarely discussed sheer curtains as barriers to insects, probably because it was as commonly understood as using bags made from sheer cotton to protect paintings, gilt surfaces, chandeliers, and mirrors from fly specks.[24]

Commentators viewed machine-loomed lace as one of the miracles of burgeoning textile technology throughout the nineteenth century (fig. 9). An article on the history of lace published in the November 1881 issue of *The Household* marveled that "the jacquard system has during the present century so perfected the lace loom that it is no easy task even for a practiced eye to detect the difference between the fabrications of machinery and those by hand…Compare a pillow-worker, making five or six meshes per minute, with a thousand meshes per minute by machine! The modern machine produces 30,000 meshes per minute. In 1800 a square yard of plain net was worth $5; the price constantly fell, till in 1862 it was six cents."[25] Machine production of lace gave ordinary people access to textiles for clothing and home use which, in their handmade forms, were extremely expensive and difficult to produce in wide yardages. Some machine-made lace was so good that it was almost impossible to tell from handmade counterparts, as in the kind known as "valenciennes." Among all domestic furnishing textiles, lace represented the most successful approximation of high-quality and expensive consumer goods through the application of technology. Coarser cotton was universally substituted for fine linen thread in factory production because it was cheaper and withstood the stresses of machine production. However, in their complexity and in the fineness of their design, jacquard-woven Brussels-type lace and other types were just as good as their handmade counterparts.

Fig. 9. Exhibit of Alfred Bailey and Co., Centennial Exhibition, Philadelphia, Pennsylvania, photograph by Centennial Photographic Co., Philadelphia, Pennsylvania, 1876. Alfred Bailey and Co. was one of a number of French lace manufacturing firms founded by English immigrants in the mid-nineteenth century. Its display featured edgings for clothing, doilies and table covers, window shades, and drapery panels, including a lace curtain memorial to George Washington. Courtesy The Free Library of Pennsylvania Print and Picture Department; photograph by Joan Broderick.

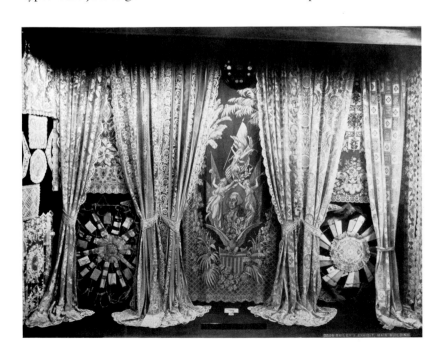

The development of mechanical processes for making lace in stages began in England with production of knitted net in the 1760s. Looms that could produce bobbin-net (also called Nottingham and Brussels net) were developed beginning in 1809; by the 1860s, looms produced net three and one-half yards wide.[26] At first, the designs on machine-made bobbin-net were still "hand run"; professional lace workers and women at home embroidered them with a simple running or darning type stitch or tamboured (chain-stitched) them by hand with a crochet hook (fig. 10). By 1875, a sewing machine that could apply tambour-work to lace net reduced the cost of these curtains. Expensive and delicate "Brussels lace" curtains were made throughout the century by applying handmade bobbin-lace motifs to machine-made netting, but, by the 1870s, completely machine-made imitation Brussels lace was possible. The Jacquard loom apparatus allowed the production of complicated patterns in textiles through use of a series of punched cards (very much like 1950s-style data processing punched cards) that cued the harnesses of the loom to move. The mechanism was adapted to lace machinery beginning in the 1830s (fig. 11). By the 1850s, a number of specialized lace machines produced versions of established lace types as well as imitation crocheted lace and clever "combination laces," blending the appearance and characteristics of several traditional lace types in a way that defies easy identification or description (fig. 12).

Until the 1890s, when English machinery was imported to America, all machine-made lace curtains were European imports. Even so, their prices were startlingly low by the 1870s. The 1875 Montgomery Ward catalog (which, unfortunately, has no illustrations) offered its rural customers three varieties of "German Lace Curtains" ranging in price from $1.00 to $2.75 a pair.[27] By the 1890s, "Nottingham lace" curtains were available by the pair for as little as fifty-nine cents a pair for two yard-wide panels, each three yards in length, having scalloped edges hand sewn with cotton tape. The term "Nottingham lace" was applied in several ways to machine-made lace. Sometimes it signaled the use of the "lace curtain machine" (also called the Nottingham lace machine). It also was applied to curtains that bore certain kinds of designs, particularly large ferns and flowers. In both instances the name referred to England's largest lacemaking center.

By the 1880s, the parlors of ordinary people commonly had lace curtains, hanging by a rod or a recycled cornice without additional drapery, year-round. The spring and summer 1885 catalog of Daniell and Sons, a New York City dry goods firm, offered machine-made lace curtains in "the largest variety ever shown," including "Brussels Point, Tamboured, Irish Point, Cluny, Antique, Guipure d'Art, French Guipure, Scotch and Nottingham," in lengths of three, three and one half, and four yards, with taped and plain edges, for prices as low as seventy-five cents "per window" (fig. 13).[28] The firm advertised that it had "Seven Buildings Devoted to Importing and Retailing of General and High Grade Dry Goods Millinery Fancy Articles Etc." By the early twentieth century, lace curtains were commonly found in working-class households; they provided a backdrop for one Lewis Hine photograph published in *Homestead*, Margaret Byington's study of working-class standards of living (see chapter 2, fig. 13).[29]

Understanding the meaning and uses of window drapery requires one to look at them from both sides of the window glass. Because of their linings, which protected expensive fabrics as well as improved their drape and increased their light-proofing qualities, heavy parlor draperies were not visible from the street. Seen from indoors, they were something else entirely. They contributed to the aesthetic of

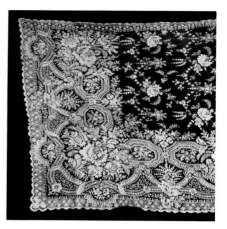

Fig. 10. *Lace curtain, cotton chain-stitch design ("tambouring") on cotton machine-made net ("bobbinet") ground. The machines that made this kind of net were patented as early as 1809. By the 1830s, thousands of English women were employed to chain stitch or darn designs on this net, mostly for clothing. In the second half of the nineteenth century, tamboured lace curtains were one of the luxury items within the factory lace-curtain trade because they involved more hand labor than other types, even after the introduction of chain-stitching sewing machines in the 1870s. In the 1888 catalog of New York dry goods firm John Daniell and Sons, "Handsome Tambour Lace Curtains" with similarly heavy stitching in a pattern of ferns and daisies cost $11.75 a pair. A few curtains of this type were produced in the United States in the 1880s, but most were imported from England, France, and Switzerland. (See chapter 3, figs. 5 and 6, for lace curtains similar to these in use in the Rochester, New York, parlor of the McGonegal family.)*

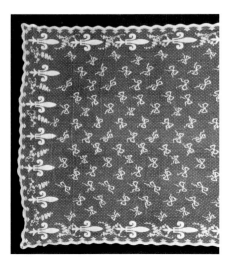

Fig. 11. Lace curtain, cotton, United States, England, or Scotland, 1900. These curtains have a history of use in the Sibley family of Rochester, co-founders of a successful department store that is still in existence. Looking like a darned lace on a square mesh ground, they were produced on the "lace curtain machine," also called the Nottingham curtain machine after the lacemaking center where it was developed in the 1840s.

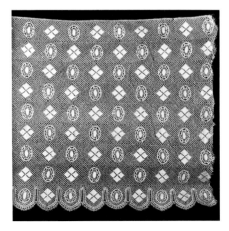

Fig. 12. Uncut length of curtain lace, cotton, probably England or Scotland, 1870-1900. Machine-made lace in this kind of uncut yardage could be used for half-curtains. This particular furnishing lace, made on a Leavers lace machine, imitates handmade bobbin lace.

"matching" by being coordinated with other upholstery. Their detail, including trims, special hardware, and layering, contributed to the visual intricacy of the room setting. In their abundance and intricacy, draperies, especially long, sweeping curtains or multi-layered window treatments, were also an economic statement. This was as true for middle-class families who had curtains made of woolen furniture rep as it was for households that could afford twelve-foot curtains of imported silk damask.

An increasing need for privacy in urban settings was another motivation for curtaining windows. The authors of *Beautiful Homes* (1878) noted that curtaining windows should be "the first thing to be attended to in house furnishing" to protect inhabitants from "prying eyes, or…the feeling of fear at imagining some outside spectator gazing into our apartments during the evening hours." Another author noted tactfully, "If the outer world does not happen to be agreeable in that particular locality, it is well to employ ingenious devices for shutting it out."[30]

Draperies also functioned as frames for the world outdoors. In more attractive rural or suburban settings, draperies created a more ornamental frame for the outdoors than did the plain window frame. In gardening as in room arrangement, the Victorians were highly conscious of "framing" or "vignetting" views through curtains as well as through doorways. The aesthetics of framing and vignetting probably were encouraged by a general heightening of visual awareness that marked the second half of the nineteenth century. Henry Ward Beecher considered this framing quality in his special "doctrine of windows." Beecher wrote, "They are designed to let light in, and equally to let the sight out; and this function is, in the country, of prime importance. For, a window is but another name for a stately picture. There are no such landscapes on canvas as those which you see through glass."[31]

The desire to control the amount of light entering parlors through the use of curtains, shutters, and shades had motivations both practical and aesthetic. Limiting direct sun helped to preserve other elements of parlor upholstery from fading, and parlor windows were often kept darkened when the rooms were not in use. The excellent state of preservation of the 1857 parlor upholstery at Castle Tucker in Wiscasset, Maine, is a function both of the care with which the suite was used and the fact that the parlor shutters were always kept closed when the room was unoccupied.

Heavy parlor draperies also served as a barrier and mediator of the world beyond the parlor's walls by muffling sound and changing the qualities of light. Softened by draperies, light spread unevenly over objects and, broken into patches of light and dark, was the light of the refined parlor sensibility. It revealed tantalizing glimpses of the parlors' contents and added, in effect, another level of complexity to visual experience. Sheer or lace curtains did not make rooms as dark as did heavy curtains; rather, they preserved privacy while admitting a filtered daylight appropriate to sensibilities that found it "unpleasant to have the full glare of sunlight streaming through an apartment."[32] Bright natural light was valued in the uncurtained rooms of the early nineteenth century; it helped to conserve expensive artificial lighting. However, the objections voiced by the grandparents of Caroline Cowles Richards to curtains may also have expressed a Georgian sensibility that preferred light to be even, "rational," and classical in character.[33] Picturesque light also was colored light. It could be provided by both stained glass windows and expanses of colored curtains. For example, the draperies of beautiful rooms described in popular fiction often cast "floods" of colored light into rooms.[34] Harriet Beecher Stowe described parlor curtains that created

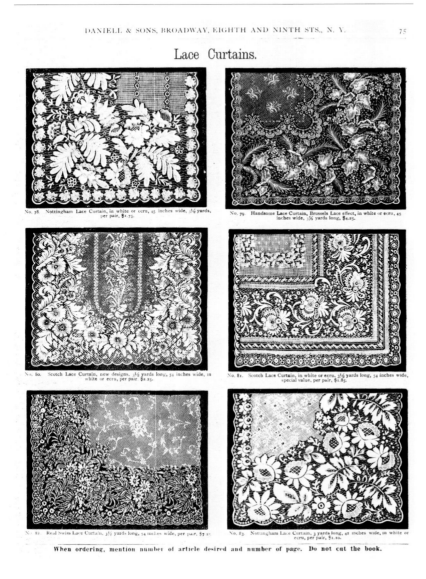

DANIELL & SONS, BROADWAY, EIGHTH AND NINTH STS., N. Y.   75

Lace Curtains.

When ordering, mention number of article desired and number of page. Do not cut the book.

Fig. 13. "*Lace Curtains,*" *engraving in* Daniell and Sons Catalogue, *New York, New York (1888). This plate showed customers a selection of machine-made and handmade lace curtains ranging in price from $1.10 to $7.25 per pair.* Real Swiss Lace" *required much handwork, making these curtains the most expensive. By the 1880s, even the cheaper "Nottingham" and "Scotch" lace curtains (here referring to the places of manufacture) mimicked more than one lace-making technique on the same length of fabric.*

picturesque light in the short story "How Do We Know?" "It was a splendid room. Rich curtains swept down to the floor in graceful folds, half excluding the light, and shedding it in soft hues over the fine old paintings on the walls, and over the broad mirrors that reflect all that taste can accomplish by the hand of wealth."[35]

While the elegant frames of draperies were invisible to passersby, lace curtains and decorative shades could be plainly seen. Especially in large communities, the houses of respectable people were private places, open only to the social circle of the occupants. Thus the content and quality of parlor furnishings —and, by implication, the quality of the person who owned the parlor—were unknown to passersby and people who were outside one's social circle. In an urban setting, where the architectural elements of the facades of houses were often very much alike, one of the only ways that a house could make a statement to the street was through whatever decorative components were visible at its windows (fig. 14).

Made of a textile associated with women's dress, lace curtains and lace-insert shades also connoted the feminine presence in households (fig. 15). Lace was used in complete, layered window treatments as a translucent element, offering pattern and contrast to heavier

Fig. 14. Detail of "Packer Street" by unidentified photographer, United States, about 1885. In this urban setting, the presence of lace curtains is the only clue to the character of the residents of these row houses or apartments.

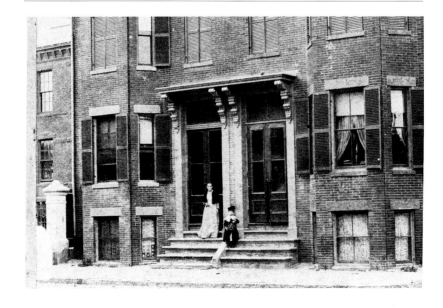

Fig. 15. Interior of unidentified house in Pittsburgh, Pennsylvania, by unidentified photographer, about 1895. Such vast expanses of lace drapery imparted a feminine feel to parlors and softened daylight. One commentator in the 1870s noted that lace curtains refreshed the eyes by providing a contrast to heavier fabrics in rooms. Author's collection.

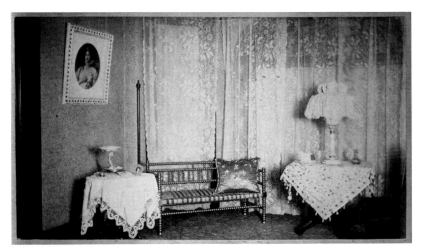

draperies; this usage was analogous to the ways lace was employed in women's dressy clothing. Visible to the street, the cleanliness of shades and lace curtains also suggested the quality of housekeeping inside. The role of lace curtains in signaling the presence of a properly feminine domestic influence may have been more important for modest houses, where women did most or all of their own work including laundering soot- and dust-covered lace curtains (fig. 16).

Many parlor makers seem to have been highly aware of the visual effects created by those parts of window treatments visible from the street. For example, pull-down shades stenciled with designs of flowers or landscapes were often mounted with their decoration toward the street side or were trimmed with decorative pulls and fringes which made them more refined and ornamental (fig. 17). Transparent shades were painted on thin sized muslin so that they admitted light which illuminated the design (fig. 18).[36] They not only presented "art" to the street but can be thought of as a visual play upon Beecher's concept of the window as a "frame" to the landscape, in this instance the window literally doing service as a "frame" for a painting of an ideal landscape. Lace or sheer curtains, private yet translucent, hinted at the "possibilities" behind the curtain

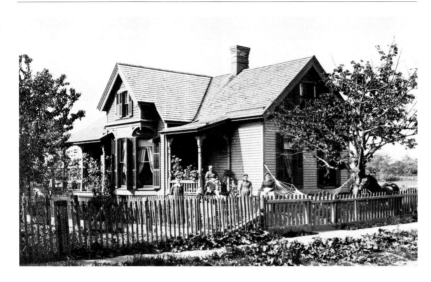

Fig. 16. *House of Catherine Walter, 215 Flint Street, Rochester, New York, by unidentified photographer, 1885-1890. The fringed window shades and neat sheer cotton and lace curtains visible in the windows of this small house suggested to passersby that a conscientious housekeeper resided within.*

and suggested that the owners had, on some level, nothing to hide. Lace curtains in modest households also were indicators of social aspirations. This symbolic use of lace curtains was so common by 1897 that Edith Wharton and Ogden Codman, Jr., declared it vulgar for their well-to-do audience to use them. Charging that "the use of elaborate lace-figured curtains, besides obstructing the view, seems an attempt to protrude the luxury of the interior upon the street," they criticized a practice that had long been in place and was clearly understood.[37] Employed as a frame, as a means of achieving a refined parlor through softened, picturesque light, and as a means of increasing visual and tactile complexity in the composition of the parlor, draperies expressed the presence of a parlor of culture. In their role as barrier to the outside world and signal of a woman's presence in a household, parlor draperies also could mark the presence of the comfortable, homey parlor of a properly domestic household.

Outside a house, visitors received clues to the domestic character of a household from the lace curtains or fancy shades at its windows; upon entering, they also were cued to the theatrical character of even modest parlors by the drapery that framed the room's doorways (plate 34). In the 1880s, embellishing doorways with great sweeps of floor-length fabric was a furnishing innovation to most Americans, but it had long precedent in large houses in Europe. By the seventeenth century, portières were common in European interiors, where they played a role in preserving warmth. In keeping with developing concepts of regularity in decor, door curtains matched the other hangings of important rooms and were made of valuable fabrics such as tapestry, although accounts survive of worn tapestries and coverlets being pressed into service in this manner.[38] In the grand salons of the European houses in the eighteenth and early nineteenth centuries, doors were often draped to match the window hangings, functioning purely as an addition to the decorative plan. Draping doorways continued in France as part of mid-nineteenth-century reinterpretations of the Louis styles.

At this time, door drapery still was rarely used in America, even in grand houses. It does not seem to have been part of the decor of the showy French-inspired interiors in the Morse-Libby Mansion, nor of the Lockwood-Mathews Mansion of Norwalk, Connecticut (decorated by French émigré Leon Marcotte).[39] Still, Harriet Spofford's *Art Decoration Applied to Furniture* (1877) illustrated, without particular comment, a "Louis Quatorze" drawing room in which the doors were draped as fully as the windows. Their uninterrupted usage in France may account for the general usage of the French term *portière* in both England and America during the last quarter of the nineteenth century.[40]

The portière probably achieved its first widespread introduction in America as an aspect of "design reform" (fig. 19). In 1872, in *Hints on Household Taste*, Charles Locke Eastlake praised "some very beautiful specimens of portière curtains...composed of velvet and other stuffs, embroidered by hand and decorated with deep borders, consisting of alternate strips of velvet and common horse girths."[41] Authors of advice books, particularly those writing for do-it-yourselfers, repeated many variations of Eastlake's suggestion that such common, cheap materials could be used to create elegant drapery. In 1878, the authors of *Beautiful Homes* noted, "As regards heavy hangings nothing can be more elegant in appearance than some plain woolen material...embellished with bands of the woolen strips used for saddle-girths. We learned this little secret years ago, and what was our delight on reading Mr. Eastlake's 'Household Taste' to

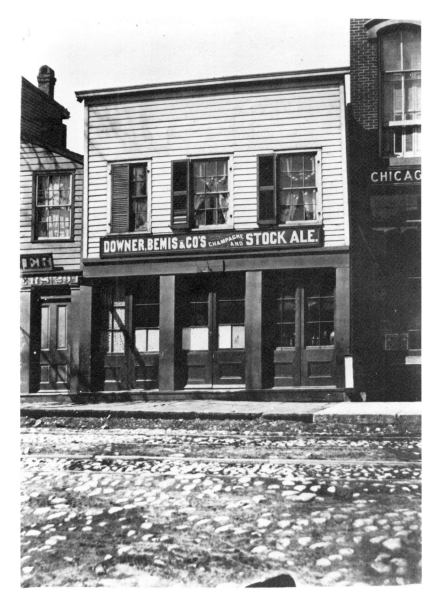

Fig. 17. 292 State Street (now 414), Chicago, Illinois, in Potter Palmer Real Estate Album, about 1870. Curtain and decorated window shades are visible in the building's second-floor windows, which may be in an apartment. Courtesy Chicago Historical Society.

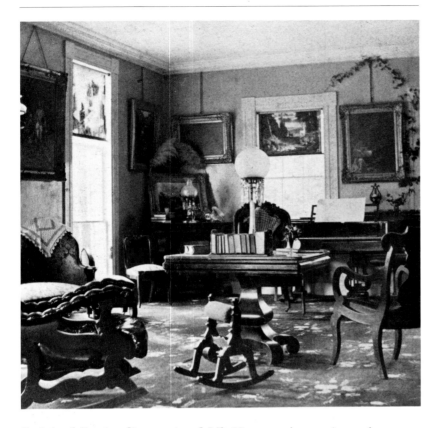

Fig. 18. Parlor in Dewey house, Barre, Massachusetts, stereograph by unidentified photographer, about 1870. Translucent shades painted with landscapes were the only window covering used in the parlor of this house; there is no visible evidence of other hardware on the window frames. Courtesy Society for the Preservation of New England Antiquities.

find the following [instructions]."[42] Homemade curtains and portières that had stripes of contrasting fabrics and embroidery for decoration were commonly offered as projects in advice books of the 1880s, such as Constance Cary Harrison's *Woman's Handiwork in Modern Homes* (1881).

The interest of English and American design reformers in draping doorways grew partly out of the medieval revival associated with John Ruskin, William Morris, Eastlake, and others. In his 1876 report on the industrial arts of the centennial, Professor Walter Smith devoted almost a full page to a wood engraving of a set of "valance and side-curtains, or *portières*" produced by the Royal School of Art Needlework at Kensington, England. Made of deep red mohair plush ("Utrecht velvet") with velvet appliqué and gold embroidery, Smith praised the curtains as "gorgeous in the extreme" and compared them favorably with the work of English embroiderers three centuries earlier, when "England had the reputation of making the finest ecclesiastical vestments in the world" (fig. 20).[43] That women were supposed to execute this kind of pseudo-ecclesiastical needlework for domestic purposes further emphasized the connections between household art and the house as domestic sanctuary.

The overtones of medievalism that made portières so attractive to such elite consumers as Walter Smith did not apparently influence their rapid acceptance as a new convention of parlor furnishing. Rather, ordinary consumers seem to have associated door curtains with "oriental" (commonly called "Turkish") furnishing styles. Exhibits from North Africa and the Levant and commercial "bazaars" at the Centennial Exhibition introduced thousands of visitors to the idea of draping doorways. When *Frank Leslie's Illustrated Weekly Newspaper* covered the fair in Philadelphia, it devoted a number of illustrations to the Turkish Bazaar and Tunisian Cafe, both of which were heavily draped. The paper illustrated both window and door

Fig. 19. *Detail of length of drapery of portière fabric, wool and cotton with metallic threads, 1875-1885. With its "modern Gothic" design of trefoils and arches in shades of brown, sage green, and red, this fabric panel was woven to be reversible, suggesting its suitability for portières that would have been seen from both sides.*

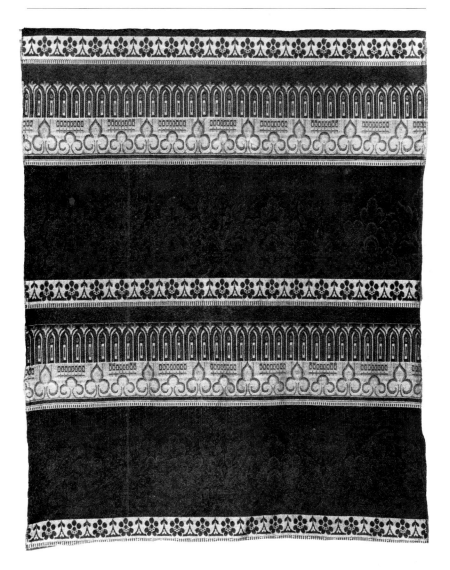

curtains exhibited by Egypt in the Main Building, with the door curtain singled out as "truly magnificent" (fig. 21).[44]

When portières became a furnishing convention in the 1880s, they also reflected the continuing interest ordinary consumers had in maintaining some sense of the theatrical, cultured facade of the parlor. Apparently plucked from the furnishing practices of exotic Eastern cultures, portières made ordinary parlors cosmopolitan. In *Woman's Handiwork in Modern Homes*, Harrison gushed, "There is something thoroughly Eastern in the conception of a portière. The stirring of its stately drapery seems to bring to the senses a waft from 'far Cathay.'"[45]

By the late 1870s, furnishing advice books began urging their readers to remove their parlor doors, including built-in pocket doors, and replace them with sweeping double-sided curtains, which almost always were flat panels hung on a rod and rings or folded over a curtain rod. For these authors, preserving the warmth of rooms was no longer an issue, even though most houses still had no central heat. F. A. Moreland, author of *Practical Decorative Upholstery*, informed his readers that door curtains allowed "more even temperatures" in houses, on the assumption that their houses were warm enough that more solid barriers were unnecessary.[46] Still, in some houses

superb set of door-hangings, decorated after designs furnished by the last-

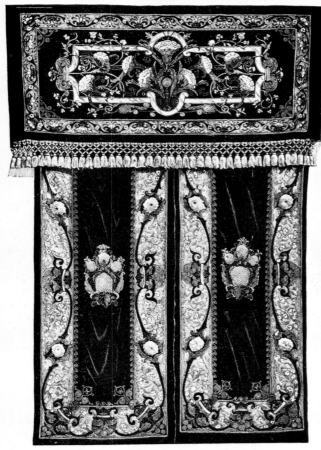

Designs for Door-hangings: Royal School of Art Needle-work.

Fig. 20. *"Designs for Door-hangings: Royal School of Art Needle-work,"* *engraving in Walter Smith,* Masterpieces of the Centennial Exhibition *(1876).*

Fig. 21. *"Egyptian Door-Curtain,"* *engraving in* Frank Leslie's Historical Register of the Centennial Exposition *(1876).*

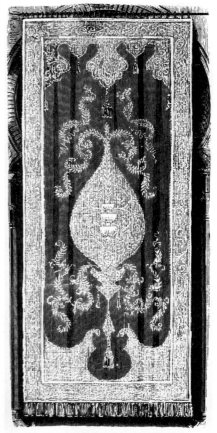

EGYPTIAN DOOR-CURTAIN.

portières were used to preserve warmth in rooms that had wooden doors. Ethel Spencer recalled that, when winter arrived in Pittsburgh, "heavy velour curtains" were hung at the doors of the downstairs rooms that saw steady use (the dining room and the library) as "protection against drafts." The rooms were also equipped with sliding pocket doors.[47] Portières also changed sound, as did heavy window draperies. Spencer remembered that the library and dining room portières in her family's Pittsburgh house "made the family rooms vaguely mysterious. Outside noises were hushed by their heavy folds, and our own voices were strangely muffled. When I think of the winters of my childhood, they have the muffled sound and camphory smell that came with the velour curtains."[48]

However, sets of portières most often hung where they could have done little to make rooms warmer or more quiet. Fade marks on some surviving door curtains suggest that they were rarely, if ever, closed. Rather, their attraction for most consumers was aesthetic. Ample, thick, richly colored and textured, portières concealed the frames of doorways with long sweeps of fabric and blurred the transitions between rooms. When they were made from double-faced fabrics or two different fabrics sewn back to back, they complemented the color scheme of the interior space on each side. The facing fabrics were sometimes very different in their weight and texture, as in the Gibson House in Boston (whose decorations were augmented and updated several times in the late nineteenth century) and the Voigt House of Grand Rapids, Michigan (decorated in 1897 and 1907). In the Voigt House, portières still hang in every first-floor doorway (fig. 22). Each doorway has two sets of portières on brass rods, with sliding pocket doors between, but each set is decorative on both sides. Two-sided door draperies often were bordered with a thick braided cording that contained colors from both facing fabrics. For houses equipped with sliding pocket doors, special portière rods could be fitted easily inside the door frame. The Fowler House (1890) in Moodus, Connecticut, the Gibson House in Boston, and the Voigt House in Grand Rapids, Michigan, all have original oak portière rods in place, mounted with thin brass caps screwed into the door frames at each end. If an ambitious parlor maker was forced to improvise portière rods, however, all that was required was the simple purchase of a pair of brackets and a curtain rod, to be mounted on one side of the door frame.

A little behind the most fashionable interior decorators, department store and dry goods catalogs introduced portières to their customers around 1880 (fig. 23). The 1881 catalog from Lord and Taylor in New York City informed its clientele rather tersely that "folding doors are not used between parlors and the space is draped with curtains. All doors are done away with on the parlor floor, and graceful *portières* are substituted." It offered printed raw silks, tapestries of worsted wool and silk, damask woven wool and jute fabrics, terries (reps), momie cloth (a linen and cotton fabric with a puckered surface), and flannels for making both window and door draperies.[49] Because almost all portières were flat pieces of fabric, caught with drapery pins and rings at the top, they were not difficult to sew and hang.

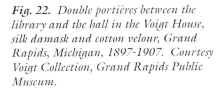

Fig. 22. Double portières between the library and the hall in the Voigt House, silk damask and cotton velour, Grand Rapids, Michigan, 1897-1907. Courtesy Voigt Collection, Grand Rapids Public Museum.

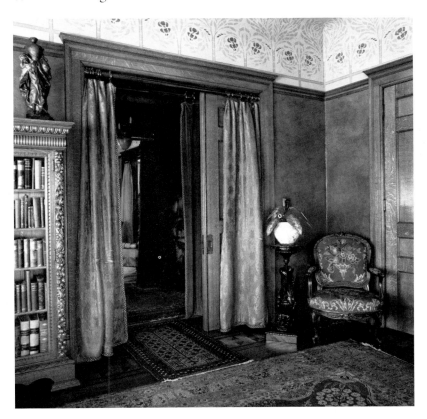

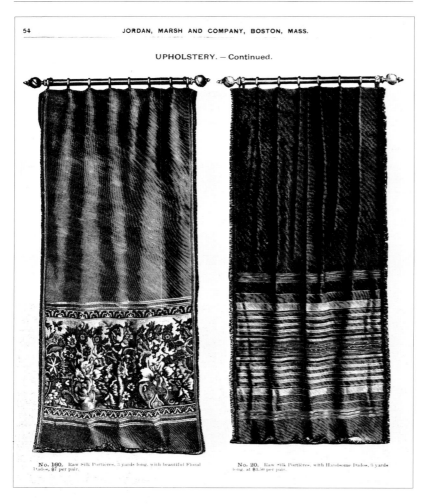

Fig. 23. *Portières,* Catalogue of Jordan Marsh and Company, Summer, *Boston, Massachusetts (1887). The upholstery department offered six grades of imported portières in "Raw Silk," "Silk Turcoman," "Silk Chenille," and "Figured Chenille," typically in patterns with stripes or "dado" designs like those found on wallpaper and window shades, for four to twelve dollars a pair.*

The simple shape of portières also made them easy to prefabricate, and dry goods firms began to offer ready-made versions by the mid-1880s. The 1885 catalog of Daniell and Sons sold "Heavy Curtains and Hangings, suitable for Portières, in all Silk, Shela, French Velours, Turcoman, Egyptian and Roman draperies" for $3.60 to $25.00 a pair (fig. 24).[50] A few years later, weaving mills in both Europe and America were producing ready-made portières on looms with Jacquard attachments. These were usually woven as a reversible double fabric, much like a coverlet or ingrain carpet, which was called "armure" or "tapestry" (although it differed from "tapestry cloth" for furniture covers). Such prefabricated portières typically fell into a few design types. One had a multicolored "dado" pattern on a plain or small repeat-patterned ground. Another variation featured large border designs, while a third bore extremely large, nonrepeating patterns that were variations on rococo or baroque scroll designs. A nine-foot portière might have only one or no repeats of rococo scrolls or "baroque" cartouches. By offering a standard length of nine feet and designing the portière to fold over a rod with a "self fringe" that could be pinned decoratively over a rod, manufacturers could both accommodate the vagaries of individual doorways and allow consumers to paraphrase more elaborate door curtains with separate valances.

Commercially woven door curtains also provide some indication of the long-standing color preferences of ordinary consumers. They were almost always woven in combinations of maroon and red, red or brick-color and green, and brown or tan and green. Brown, green, maroon, and red had been popular colors in upholstery since the 1850s, used in both seating furniture and drapery. "Reform" designers continued to employ them, both in clear colors and new shades that were muted, such as olive greens.[51] Such color combinations still found favor at the turn of the century. The Sears catalog for 1897 offered its tapestry and chenille curtains in such colors as "cardinal," "terra-cotta," olive and nile green, "bronze," tan, and "slate" or "steel" gray.[52] The color names made red, green, brown, and gray more glamorous.

Because they were offered in a limited range of popular colors and patterns, factory-woven portières also may have contributed to the gradual popular acceptance of "harmonizing" rather than "matching" as the ideal use of color in a room. Advice on hanging portières usually informed amateur decorators that they were not to be identical to the curtains in a room. One author noted, "By doing so, you lose a great opportunity for telling colors…But be sure that the coloring is controlled by the other decorations of the room, with

Fig. 24. Portière, voided cotton plush, 1890-1910. Identical on both sides, this door curtain was woven with dimensional "carved" pile, almost one-half inch thick in shades of maroon, red, and pink (now faded to brown). This portière may be an example of the "Figured Double-faced Velour" door curtains offered in the 1891 Price List and Fashion Book of Jordan Marsh and Company, Boston, Massachusetts, for forty dollars a pair. Someone considered this portière too good to throw away after door curtains were no longer in fashion; it was cut down at the top and used as a window curtain even though the fabric was extremely heavy.

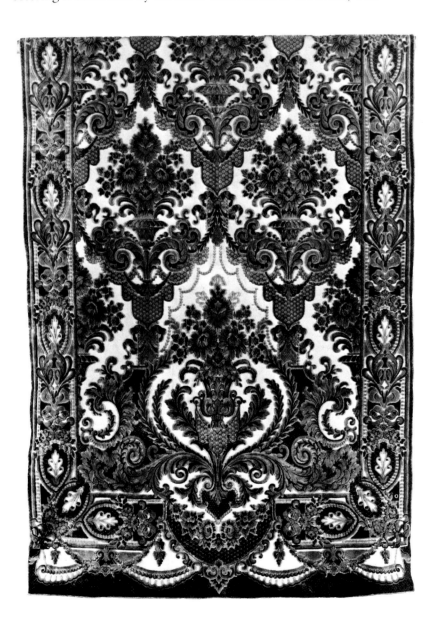

which it must accord."[53] Complex compositions of different fabrics presented a challenge to parlor makers, however. Just as mail-order catalogs were obliged to explain "harmonizing" in relation to suites of the 1890s, dry goods and department store catalogs of the 1880s tried to interpret this departure from the old standards of regularity as an easily followed formula: "These artistic hangings [portières] should harmonize with the furniture, though to avoid sameness they are generally in different designs," the 1881 Lord and Taylor catalog advised. "The curtains may be crossed by stripes, while the furniture covering is figured."[54]

Between 1880 and 1930, textile factories making novelty upholstery goods, such as the Philadelphia mills, produced sets of jacquard-woven portières in the same manner that they produced rugs called "art squares," or "piece-woven" with designs on all four borders. Philadelphians pioneered the power-loom weaving of cotton chenille yarn, which made an especially popular portière fabric, at the end of the 1880s. Production of this particular yarn required a two-stage weaving process: loose fabric was made on a power loom and cut up; these strips were then rewoven on power and hand looms as fuzzy chenille yarn (fig. 25).[55] By 1891, *Dockham's American Report and Directory of the Textile Manufacture and Dry Goods Trade* listed thirteen firms engaged specifically in both production and finished weaving of chenille.[56] Used as door curtains, table covers, and small area rugs, woven chenille was a particularly rich-looking fabric. In most of the heavy prefabricated portières, whether tapestry (both terms were used for the same ingrain-type fabric) or chenille, the left-over lengths of warp thread were knotted off in a "self-fringe" (a hand-finishing operation), or tassels were sometimes applied as ornaments to fold-over tops.

Given the large volume of heavy, rich-looking fabric they provided, prefabricated portières were a bargain, although they still represented a significant investment for families at the poorer margins of the middle classes. A pair of the cheapest chenille portières offered by Montgomery Ward and Co.'s 1895 spring and summer catalog cost two dollars, approximately a day's wages for journeymen in skilled occupations at that time.[57] Ward's "extra heavy" best chenille portières cost five dollars a pair. ("Nottingham lace" curtains, three yards long and one yard wide, sold for as little as fifty-nine cents a pair in the same catalog.) This price range did not change significantly through the first decade of the twentieth century. *Sears, Roebuck and Co. Catalog No. 123, 1911* offered tapestry and chenille portières at a price range of $1.98 to $5.25 a pair. Sales volume was still so significant that Sears devoted four full pages in the 1911 catalog to portières in these fabrics, leather ("Mission Draperies"), and "Tapestry and Rope."[58]

If they did not contribute materially to warmth or to privacy in

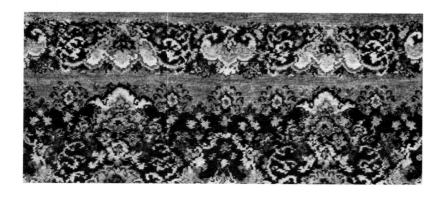

Fig. 25. Detail of portière, cotton chenille, 1890-1910. Cotton chenille door curtains were less expensive and sturdier versions of imported French silk chenille portières offered for sale by department stores in the 1880s and 1890s.

Fig. 26. "*Interior Residence, Fifth Avenue, N.Y.,*" *stereograph from a series titled* "*American Scenery*" *by unidentified photographer and publisher, 115 Washington Street, Boston, Massachusetts, about 1880. The genteel titillation provided by views taken through curtained doorways is suggested by another stereograph with the same view published by Bierstadt Brothers of New Bedford, Massachusetts. Theirs was titled* "*In the Boudoir, Fifth Avenue, New York.*" *Courtesy Society for the Preservation of New England Antiquities.*

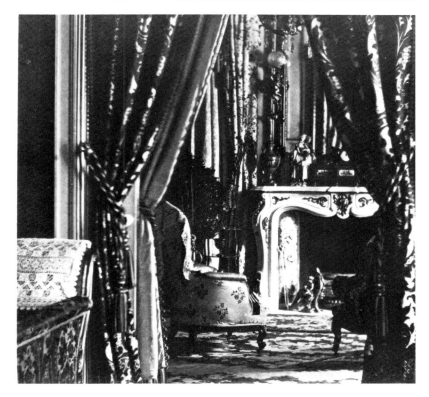

rooms, why were portières so popular? Visiting historic houses such as the Voigt and Gibson Houses, which retain their portières, is perhaps the best way to understand the effect they had on the visual qualities of rooms and on the sensibilities of ordinary people. Through the portière, a theatrical curtain, every entrance became an occasion. Every room also seemed cozier and more intimate because the rectangular architecture of room openings was blurred with long folds of fabric.

Indeed, portières seem always to have been discussed in terms of their visual qualities rather than their contribution to greater physical warmth. "The Portière is preferred to any door at all, and it is certainly very graceful," an untitled note in *The Decorator and Furnisher* stated in 1883. "It may be elegantly embroidered so as to be really a work of art, or it may be of simple curtain material, owing its beauty to its appropriate coloring and the soft folds in which it falls."[59] Articles on door curtains made this aesthetic preference clear well into the twentieth century, as when the author of "Portières for the Country House," published in *Country Life in America* in January 1906, declared, "Doors are ugly things at best; draperies possess lines of beauty…most doorways are greatly improved by their use."[60]

Furthermore, as Constance Cary Harrison's rhapsodic commentary on their exotic qualities suggests, portières were particularly valued as the curtains of the domestic theatre of the parlor (fig. 26). Sitting in one room and looking through to the parlor made it a stage and a vignette, a space framed with curtains where social action could take place, as in the framed vignettes of fashionable rooms offered by some of the model rooms at the Centennial Exhibition. Evidence of room use by the Yearick and Hughes families has suggested that people sometimes sat in a back parlor or dining/sitting room and looked into the adjoining parlor, which was pristine and unused. Their own parlors became vignettes or theatrical sets that could be studied and reexamined with pleasure as a concrete manifestation of that family's refinement, taste, and ability to set aside a parlor.[61]

In painting and photography, the term "vignette" designates an unbordered portrait, a partial view shaded off around the edges of the figure. In commercial photography, vignetting became popular in the 1880s, when the experience of a photographic portrait was common enough that consumers did not expect to have their entire figure rendered. However, the term "vignette" also was applied to other situations where a partial or fragmentary view was revealed through a natural "frame"—a gap between mountains or an ancient wall with a break in it, for example.[62] The fabric of portières created the blurred edges for a vignetted view of the parlor's landscape; the partially revealed contents of the room beyond provided a sense of dramatic anticipation and pleasure to viewers. One author noted, "To one who considers at all the picturesque qualities of an apartment, hangings require no recommendation, for even ordinary furnishing seen through the prettily drawn portière has a deceptive attractiveness given it all out of proportion to its real qualities when seen without the aid of tapestry or Turcoman."[63]

The view through a door curtain became a common convention of room photography as well as commercial imagery in the last quarter of the nineteenth century (fig. 27). It capitalized upon an older artistic convention of the curtain that is partly pushed aside to reveal dramatic action, a convention that emphasized the artifice of the painting. There, the painted curtain also reminded viewers that the world was a theatrical stage, inviting them to look in on the action beyond. The curtain framing Henry Sargent's *Tea Party*, for example, makes viewers feel as though they are omniscient observers of the theater of elite parlor social life. In other instances, curtains partially pulled aside tantalize viewers, encouraging them to enter the space, as they do in Charles Willson Peale's famous self-portrait *The Artist in His Museum* (1822).

Other variations on the drapery of doors also emphasized its visual and theatrical qualities. Bay windows frequently were curtained, across the front as well as on each window. This kind of drapery arrangement had originally been employed as a way to preserve heat, but bays provided an opportunity to create a vignette within a room, arranged with tables, fancy chairs, and pedestals displaying plants or statuary (see chapter 3, figs. 5 and 6). The occasional use of lace curtains as portières and the popularity of rope and bead portières and door valances also emphasized their symbolic character (figs. 28 and 29). Short window valances of bullion fringe appeared in upholstery trim catalogs as early as 1878, but doorway valances of rope or bands of trim became common fifteen or twenty years later, appearing in mail-order catalogs until the late 1920s. The visual effect created by rope portières also resembled that of decorative wooden grilles in doorways, popular at the same time; both were frames rather than barriers (figs. 30 and 31).

As an element of popular aesthetics in parlor drapery, using fabric as frames evolved between 1850 and the 1880s from making windows into framed pictures to creating interior views between rooms. Thus portières made ordinary rooms theatrical, contributing to the already well-developed sense of the parlor as a stage, and they moved the pictorial and theatrical vignette into the real space of the parlor. Popular interest in vignetting and framing, in the suggestive fragmentary view rather than the whole vista, suggests an increasing visual sophistication among ordinary people in the second half of the nineteenth century. As increasing amounts of visual information were

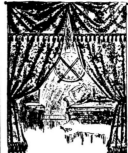

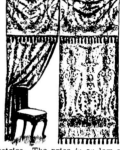

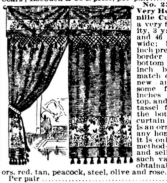

Fig. 27. Portières, illustration in Sears, Roebuck and Co. Catalogue No. 104 *(1897). The small depictions included beside each description not only demonstrated how to hang door curtains, but they also suggested their allure with vignettes of half-revealed rooms beyond the doorway.*

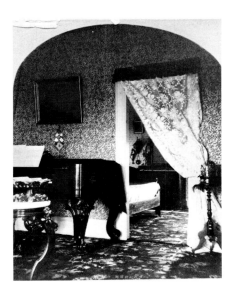

Fig. 28. Lace curtain as portière in unidentified interior, stereograph by W. A. Prescott and Co., about 1880. Courtesy Smithsonian Institution; private collection.

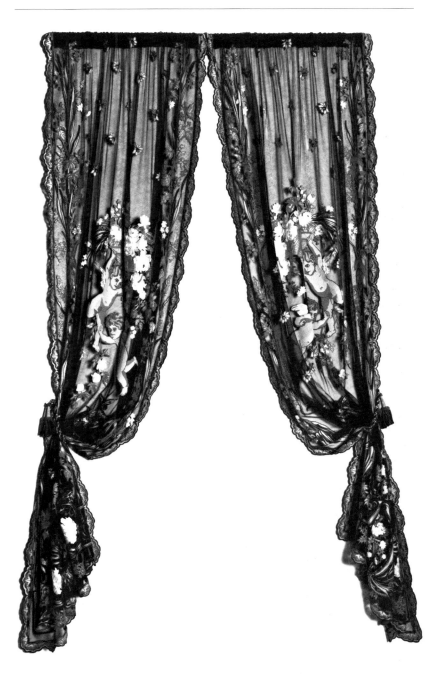

Fig. 29. Curtains, cotton tambour (chain) stitching on cotton bobbinet lace ground with cotton appliqué, about 1900. These multicolored curtains consist of a black net ground with appliqués of cherubs, baskets of flowers, flower sprigs, and a border of iris made from cotton with a close loop pile in natural, shaded colors. They have a history of use as portières between a parlor and music room in the Hot Springs, Arkansas, home of a doctor at the turn of the century. Courtesy Smithsonian Institution.

available through cheap sources—stereographs, illustrated books, popular prints, and advertising trade cards—consumers became conversant in a range of such visual conventions and enjoyed their playful qualities. Inexpensive portières allowed them to make the sophisticated visual convention part of their daily visual experience (fig. 32).

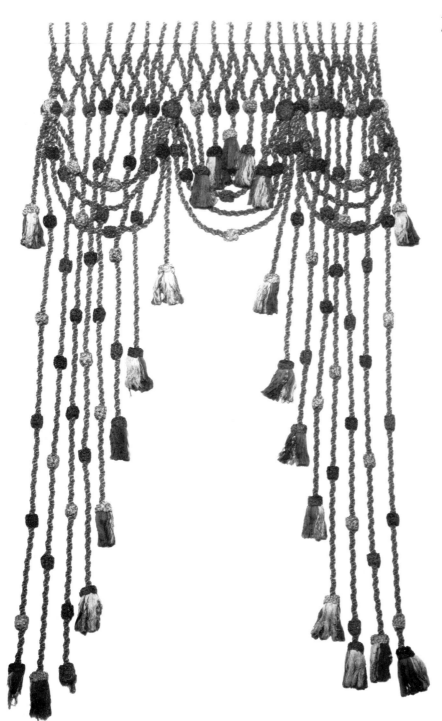

Fig. 30. Rope portières, wool, cotton, and metallic "tinsel," about 1900.

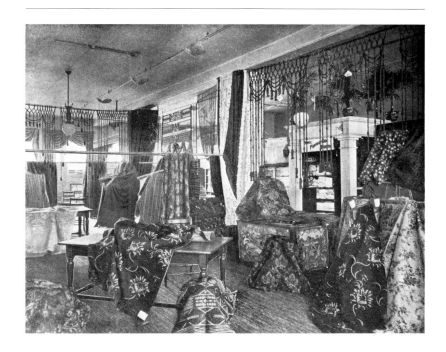

Fig. 31. *"Upholstery Department of William Hengerer Company, Buffalo, N.Y.," photograph in* Grand Rapids Furniture Record *(May 1901). Rope portières reached the height of their popularity between 1900 and 1910. This department store displayed rope portières costing four and six dollars, as well as bead curtains and wooden grilles for doorways. Courtesy Grand Rapids Public Library.*

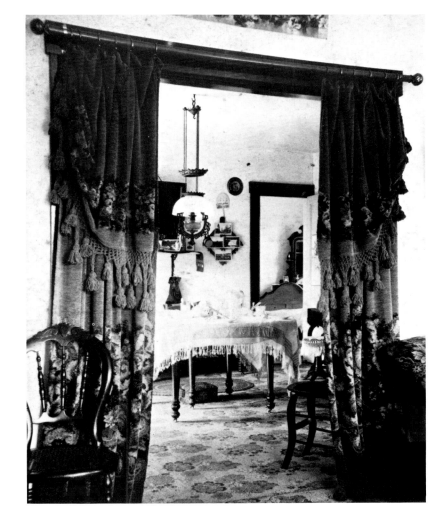

Fig. 32. *Unidentified interior, stereograph published by H. F. Preston, Athol Center, Massachusetts, 1890-1900. The doorway between the parlor and dining room of this modest household is hung with chenille portières, with the fringe caught up to make swags. The photograph features the curtained frame of the doorway itself and a vignette of the dining room table set for a meal. Courtesy Society for the Preservation of New England Antiquities.*

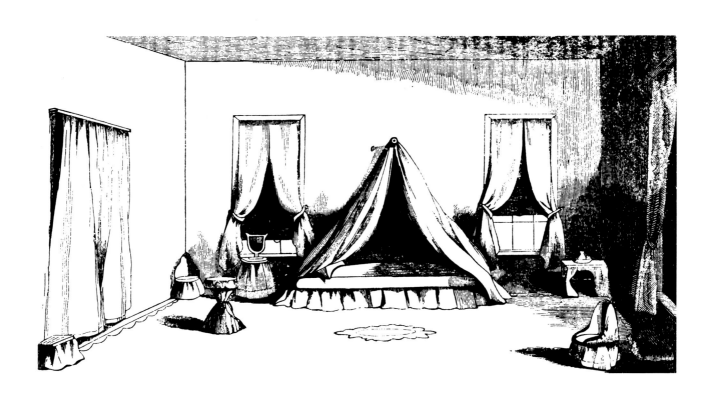

CHAPTER NINE
MAKING DO:
HOMEMADE AND RECYCLED
UPHOLSTERY

Fig. 1. *"Appearance of Room When Finished," engraving in "The Unexpected Visitor,"* Godey's Lady's Book *(January 1859). This quasi-fictional* Godey's *article published instructions for a bedroom containing furniture made from packing boxes, barrels, and fabric. The protagonists, a family about to receive an extended visit from an aunt, are unable to furnish an empty bedroom to accommodate her until another visitor, a thrifty "New England lady" known as Aunt Lorrie, teaches them how to make the furniture, including four chairs fabricated from small oak barrels.*

"Now for chairs," said Aunt Lorrie. "Walter, did you soak those six barrels in the creek to season them, as I asked you to?"

"Yes, auntie, I think they are highly seasoned by this time; I took them out two or three days ago, and dried them in the sun."

"Well, bring them in; they are for chairs."

"Oh, auntie!" cried Pet, "you are not going to make Aunt Fannie sit perched up on the top of an old flour barrel, are you?"

The barrels were taken into the workshop, and under Aunt Lorrie's direction some of the front boards were sawed in halves, and taken out; the staves were then secured at the end, and also sawed away, leaving a back to her chair; Harry Wilson, catching her idea, cut them away in a very pretty shape. When four were so cut, they were taken into the room for the girls to finish. A seat was made by fastening webbing across the large hole in the barrel; then the back and arms were covered with coarse bagging, put on loose, leaving the top of the back open. The bagging was then stuffed with bran, and closed at the top, and there stood a stuffed easy-chair. When covered with the pretty chintz, with a full flounce from the seat, down, and a cushion, nobody would have suspected that the foundation was a barrel (fig. 1).[1]

Upholstery made at home probably was more common than the contemporary rate of survival of its forms suggests. Like most ordinary things, it was used until it was used up, and then it was discarded. It often consisted of recycled materials in the first place. Amateur upholstery reflected a range of motives among its makers. Some kinds, such as Berlin work upholstery, represented a continuation of the long-standing tradition of women's accomplishments, where impressive needlework projects using expensive materials were expressions of the schooling upper-class young women received. Middle-class women who were enthusiasts of the aesthetic or arts and crafts movements used certain kinds of homemade upholstery as vehicles for "reformed" design, expressions of their participation in this particular facet of elite culture. For parlor makers with limited incomes, homemade upholstery was a means of access both to additional bodily comfort and to parlor culture itself.

Published instructions and advice for homemade upholstery in a wide range of forms, from mantel drapery to large, fully covered pieces of seating furniture, appeared with increasing frequency during the second half of the nineteenth century and peaked with what might be called the "drapery craze" between 1880 and 1910. To accommodate the limited skills and purses of prospective amateur upholsterers, do-it-yourself instructions tended to offer simplified versions of upholstery; no one would have mistaken a set of homemade curtains for the products of a professional drapery maker who knew trade secrets of cutting and construction. At the same time, however, such instructions attempted, in a variety of creative ways, to satisfy the aesthetic visual preferences of home upholsterers for visual intricacy, a high degree of finish, and both visual and tactile softness. The authors of instructions for homemade upholstery understood the association of upholstery with domestic ceremony and "softening" the world, and they instructed their readers (in a manner that sometimes reveals the expectation that seekers of advice were newly aspiring consumers) how to make a set of inventive compromises that could yet express the aesthetic standards of this world.

Instructions in books and magazines for novel forms of homemade upholstery associated loosely with the "aesthetic movement" and its tenets of self-expression through household art proliferated in the 1880s and 1890s. Women could use these directions to guide them in the fabrication of mantel lambrequins, table covers, small decorative textile accessories, and some window and door drapery. While some of these "art needlework" projects used expensive materials or even were the products of early crafts kits, others reflect thrifty recycling, into forms other than quilts, of fabrics too good to throw away. Recovering worn furniture and rotating old draperies and furniture to lesser rooms was a common strategy for extending the life of upholstery, but second-hand stores and auctions also were common and important avenues of access to usable upholstery and furniture fabrics for modest households.

The authors of domestic economy and decorating advice books described ideas for upholstering at home in ways that reflect their assumptions about the composition of their readership. At midcentury, homemade upholstery was frequently cited in conjunction with the ideal of appropriate "middle-class comfort" and consumption (fig. 2). Catharine Beecher provided as a model an exemplary middle class "Christian family": it was young, growing, possessed some education, and was, as young families still often are, house-poor—"having spent more than they could afford on the building itself, and yet feeling the necessity of getting some furniture."[2] Using a portion of her parlor furnishing budget of eighty dollars (representing more than one month's wages for a skilled carpenter at the time), the clever wife was enabled to upholster the room by making a lounge (a sofa six feet in length consisting of a covered box base with a mattress-like stuffed pad and cushions for the back), producing a set of lambrequins from thirty yards of "green English chintz," stitching muslin curtains for three windows, and purchasing a voluminous center-table cloth. Here, homemade upholstery was depicted as one method of improving family comfort through the skills of thrifty housewifery.[3] A. J. Downing's sections on cottage furnishing in *The Architecture of Country Houses* also connected homemade upholstery to appropriate levels of domestic comfort.[4]

As store-bought furniture and curtains became available to more families of modest incomes, domestic critics continued to suggest that choosing homemade parlor upholstery was a signal of familial thrift and demonstrated an understanding of true comfort. The 1856 advice book *Village and Farm Cottages: The Requirements of American Village Homes Considered and Suggested...* urged "the young wife or matron" to remember that "for cottages of small expense, all that is needed in the way of couches and easy chairs, may be almost wholly of domestic manufacture. The frames, simply but solidly made of some common hard wood, and of convenient form, might be cushioned and covered by the family themselves." The authors argued that homemade furniture was not only more comfortable, but it was also more respectable (the implication being that it was more honest) than the furniture offered by cheap warerooms, which was "neither comfortable, nor handsome, nor durable." Family production also was the recommended way of acquiring curtains, to be hung from locally made wooden cornices rather than "flimsy gilt" ones from the city.[5]

Such home decorating also was one method of gaining immediate access to consumer goods that expressed important assumptions linking the formation of character to the influence of domestic settings. John Claudius Loudon's recommendations for the furnishing of cottagers' small houses set this precedent with instructions for a "sofa" constructed of a platform of wood with a "mattress" stuffed with hair, wool, or plant material and covered with fabric. These instructions, published thirty-six years before *The American Woman's Home*, were rooted in his belief that "right habits of thinking go hand in hand with comfortable dwellings and convenient, neat, and elegant forms of furniture."[6]

The proliferation of household art books in the decades following the publication of Eastlake's *Hints on Household Taste* in 1868 encouraged women to make draperies, portières, and other embellishments to express themselves in artistic ways (fig. 3). Their authors encouraged women to make their rooms more individually distinctive and artistic as antidotes to a world of ugly consumer goods. Influenced by the revival of "art needlework" in England and the subsequent exhibition of outstanding examples at the Centennial, Clarence Cook encouraged the prosperous readership of *Scribner's*

Fig. 2. *"Plate 23," engraving in the* Workwoman's Guide *(1840).*

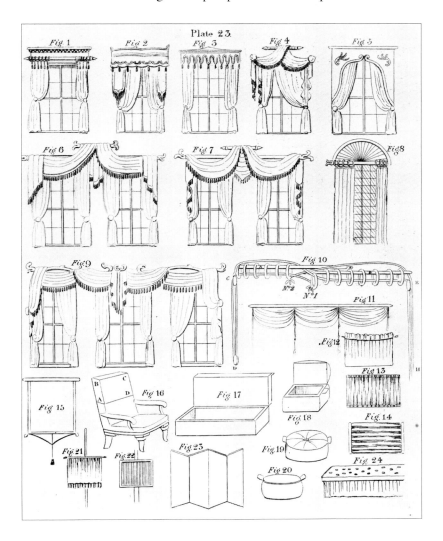

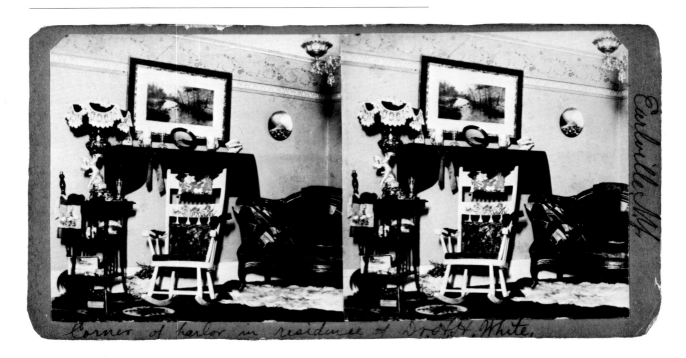

Monthly and readers of his popular 1878 book *The House Beautiful* to take up "serious works" in embroidery — "coverings for furniture, hangings for doors or walls, and the like." The projects advocated by Cook and advisers such as Constance Cary Harrison, author of *Woman's Handiwork in Modern Homes* (1881), were often expensive to make, consisting of materials such as silk plush. Cook allowed that they were "out of the reach of most purses; but many, especially the English things [fabrics], are not costlier than is reasonable in the beginning," and, he argued, their appearance mellowed with age.[7]

Appearing after the 1870s, a third type of advice writing on homemade furnishings abandoned the didactic tone of earlier advice books while it continued to assume that readers must rely upon their own domestic skills as the avenue of access to refined parlor furnishings. It also adapted the rhetoric and design tenets of household art to more popular ends. These sources were often, but not always, directed to rural audiences. *Our Homes: How to Beautify Them* (1888) devoted an entire chapter to "Hand-Made Decorative Furniture," guaranteeing "all the requisites of beauty and convenience" through recycling "such unconsidered trifles as old barrels, boxes, etc." or old furniture, all in "the labor of odd moments." *Our Homes* appeared under the imprint of O. Judd Co., "Publishers and Importers of All Works Pertaining to Rural Life," who published S. B. Reed's *House-Plans for Everybody* and the widely circulated *American Agriculturalist.* The unidentified author described his aspiring home decorator as having "limited means, but refined taste," which reveals his assumption that his audience was cash-poor and probably rural, yet not isolated from the influence of new ideas in room decoration, particularly the "esthetic craze."[8]

Articles having a similar tone and offering instructions on a wide variety of homemade furnishings composed largely of textiles also appeared monthly in cheap magazines such as *The Household*, which was directed to rural housewives.[9] Also, many inexpensive "domestic encyclopedias" often included sections on house furnishing in a chapter or two generally targeted to audiences with limited incomes. All these sources combined both the older motive of simple access to

Fig. 3. Corner of parlor in residence of Dr. H. H. White, stereograph by unknown photographer, Earlville, New York, about 1895. In this parlor, a Boston rocking chair has been converted to acceptable parlor seating through a new coat of decorative paint (including a spray of iris across the backrest), a crushed velvet or plush seat and back cushion, and a padded headrest tied on with three bows. Although the parlor has no fireplace, a mantel shelf decorated with an asymmetrical lambrequin gives the parlor a decorative axis. Courtesy Smithsonian Institution; private collection.

the means to furnish with that of self-expression through the creation of handsome rooms. *Our Homes and Their Adornments*, a product of the People's Publishing Company of Chicago and Philadelphia in 1885, offered thrifty advice on "How to Use the Odds and Ends in Rendering the House More Beautiful," a title that recalled the tone of early domestic economy books. However, it also provided a basic, if somewhat anecdotal, introduction to the vocabulary and principles of interior decoration and suggested that homemade interior decorations not only improved comfort but expressed the "enchantment" of art:

> By interior decoration is meant the addition to the interiors of our homes...such features as will add to the attractiveness of the rooms and lend an enchantment not felt or attained where *habitation* is the only object desired in a house... The addition of furniture of the humblest kind to a room relieves the monotony and gives it an air of comfort; the presence of other articles not strictly in the kind of necessities still further adds to its comfort... *Harmony* is another vital consideration in the matter of decoration.[10]

While it introduced its readership to self-expression through household art, *Our Homes and Their Adornments* also suggested that the goals of household art were not incompatible with limited means and domestic thrift. It demonstrated this under the heading "Use Up The Pieces," which presented the example of a woman for whom purchasing a length of felt was a luxury:

> A friend indulged not long ago in some crimson felt for a screen. There were some pieces left. With the largest, she made the center of a scarf table-cloth, putting some striped stuff on each end; and then there were some long ribbons of the felt left. She feather-stitched them in old-gold, and threaded them into a willow chair, where they did much better than ribbons, not fading, and looking more like use. A little piece still remained. She lined it with pasteboard, first having worked the motto, "Fast Bind, Fast Find," upon it, and made an excellent brush-broom holder for the hat rack.[11]

Until household art books introduced a dizzying spectrum of needle arts techniques and novelties in materials to their audiences, decorative needlework for upholstery purposes included a range of techniques and materials with strong ties to the needle arts of the past and the skills required for making clothing at home. Crochet, for example, could be adapted to the production of chair covers. *Godey's Lady's Book* provided its readers with many such patterns at midcentury, using knitting or netting for homemade tidies and curtains, patchwork for window shades, and braiding to decorate pillows and stools (fig. 4).

In the eighteenth and early nineteenth centuries, homemade upholstery in the form of bed "furniture" (sets of hangings and covers) and show covers for chairs were part of the long tradition of "feminine accomplishments" in the needle arts. Such projects had a strong association because only the daughters of prosperous families had been able to expend the time and materials required for making needlepoint chair covers or an entire set of crewel bed hangings. The objects women made were valuable parts of a family's estate and sometimes constituted part of a dowry.[12] One important type of homemade upholstery, canvas work (petit point or needlepoint), was used to create chair seats, easy chair upholstery, fire screens, and rugs.

NET TIDY.

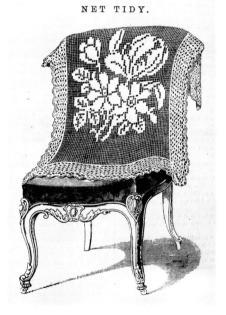

Fig. 4. "*Net Tidy,*" *engraving in* Godey's Lady's Book *(1848).*

Canvas work upholstery never disappeared, but, in the 1820s and 1830s, it evolved into Berlin work, which was also called "worsted embroidery" and "modern embroidery." Berlin work was the first completely commercialized form of needlework — the forerunner of today's crafts kits — and perhaps the first widely practiced form of homemade seating upholstery. The basis of the Berlin work craze was its printed and colored paper patterns, much cheaper than designs painted upon canvas, in which the design was rendered on a grid representing canvas threads. The needleworker could enlarge or reduce the size of the design by using different sizes of canvas and wools because she transferred the design to canvas by counting squares, as practitioners of "counted cross-stitch" do today. The patterns also could be reused.

The invention of a German print seller, Berlin "prints" or patterns were commercially produced after 1810, but their first decade of widespread popularity in England and the United States was the 1830s. Mrs. Henry Owen, author of several books on needlework in the 1840s, estimated that "no less than fourteen thousand copper-plate designs" had been published, and "upwards of twelve hundred" persons, "chiefly women," were employed to color the patterns.[13] Women's magazines on both sides of the Atlantic also published vividly colored patterns for chair covers, decorative stripes and seat bands, and window or sofa cushions in Berlin work. Such patterns appeared in significant numbers in the 1850s in magazines such as *Peterson's* and *Godey's Lady's Book* and continued to be published through the 1870s (plate 35).

Berlin yarns, called "zephyr," were soft, woolen (as opposed to worsted) four- or eight-ply threads dyed in bright colors. Berlin work became especially vivid after the German development of coal-tar dyes in the 1850s. Silk was also used, often as an accent to wool yarns, and beading became common by midcentury. Such materials were not inexpensive, and because Berlin work covered the canvas with stitching it used more yarn than did regular embroidery. A variety of canvases were also used, including types woven with colored threads that marked out a "graph" pattern. These eased the difficulty of counting threads under poor home lighting conditions. For women of greater means, designs continued to be offered that were painted directly on the canvas; for women with means and less ambition, merchants offered partially completed Berlin work panels (the product of sweated labor), requiring only that the background be filled in.

By the 1840s, Berlin work for furnishing use appeared frequently in the United States, both to embellish and update existing furniture and to cover new pieces. The stitchery often incorporated beading and "tufted work," which could not have withstood constant wear from sitters, and it seems likely that Berlin work upholstery survives in disproportionate quantity compared to other kinds of upholstery because the objects it covered were not subject to hard use. Berlin work usually embellished a limited number of pieces in a room, providing an accent or contrast to the larger decorative scheme. "Reception chairs," which seem to have been largely decorative in character, piano stools, footstools, and screens were the most common recipients of needlework (plate 36). For her elaborate Montana parlor, Augusta Kohrs worked a footstool cover with the classical theme of a Thracian slaying a lion; it was mounted on a stool that had horn feet and was embellished with ball fringe.[14] Berlin work strips stitched onto chairs lengthwise seem also to have been popular and common, so much so that manufacturers of upholstered furniture introduced machine-woven fabrics with "center stripes."

Despite the better survival odds of Victorian furniture covered

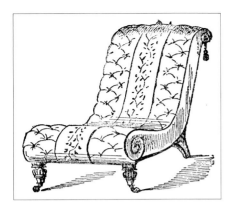

Fig. 5. "Spanish chair," engraving in [John Phin], The Practical Upholsterer (1891).

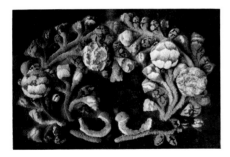

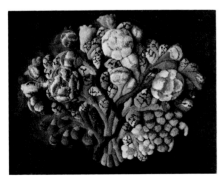

Figs. 6 and 7. Chair seats, wool tufted work on horsehair, United States, 1870-1890.

with needlework, there is good, even amusing, evidence that such furniture actually was common by midcentury. The judges of Class XIX, "Embroidery and Worsteds," at the 1853 fair of the Metropolitan Mechanics' Institute in Washington, D.C., awarded prizes to sixteen chairs, two ottomans, four stools, three fire screens and a number of rugs and table or piano covers — apart from the usual large number of meticulously rendered needlework "paintings" on such subjects as "The War of the Pets."[15]

Berlin woolwork upholstery was not a route to improved access to upholstered furniture but rather a traditional form of feminine self-expression commercialized for middle-class needleworkers. Indeed, women usually were unable to complete their projects alone; they relied upon professional upholsterers to mount their finished products on commercially produced furniture frames. This created special problems as well as opportunities for new sales among upholsterers. In 1845, the English cabinetmaker Henry Wood even published *A Useful and Modern Work on Cheval and Pole Screens, Ottomans, Chairs and Settees for Mounting Berlin Needlework*, a book especially for furniture shops faced with the problem of producing suitable mounts for needlework masterpieces.[16] In 1891, *The Practical Upholsterer* devoted two pages of its chapter on parlor furniture to suggestions for handling puckered and "out of the square" needlework and for selecting fabrics and colors that could form attractive backgrounds for woolwork and crewel work. The author suggested that the "Spanish chair," a sling type descending from the leather-covered campeche chair, was especially "suitable for the display of strips of needlework" because its sling form made mounting long sections simple (fig. 5; plate 37). It was also relatively "inexpensive" because it was "entirely stuffed over," meaning that it did not require upholsterers to work carefully around a decorative wooden framework of seat rails and back.[17]

In the 1870s and 1880s, two variations on Berlin tufted work enjoyed a popular revival. One produced geometric designs in pile cut to various heights; its use seems to have been confined largely to pillows and footstools. The second revived typical closely tufted designs of such subjects as flowers, birds, and blooming branches resembling 1850s Berlin work patterns, the principal difference being that the ground fabric was not canvas. In this technique, the needlework canvas and base fabric (often horsehair) were first fastened together on a frame. When the design was completed, each loop was trimmed and the canvas drawn out one thread at a time, leaving the design on the heavy ground fabric.[18]

Two chair seats in tufted work by an unidentified needleworker, mounted on a pair of small Grecian-style chairs as a later addition to their upholstery, exhibit little wear except where the volume of the wool tufting has distorted the horsehair ground fabric (figs. 6 and 7). The unusual designs of seaweed-like plant garlands and birds would seem to have been the creation of a talented amateur rather than to have resulted from professionally prepared patterns. These chair seats saw little use, understandably so as the lumpy tufting would have been uncomfortable and could have been easily damaged by a sitter's weight.

Why would a home needleworker devote so much attention and time to such a project (fig. 8)? Like the reception chairs, stools, and fire screens of several decades earlier, these chair seats represent a tour de force of women's craftsmanship: their utility is secondary to the display of the needlework skill, and sometimes the wit, of their makers.[19] In this regard, they may be compared to another kind of needlework that has a specific ethnic past and folk character, the Pennsylvania-German *Handtuch* or show towel (a modern term), a

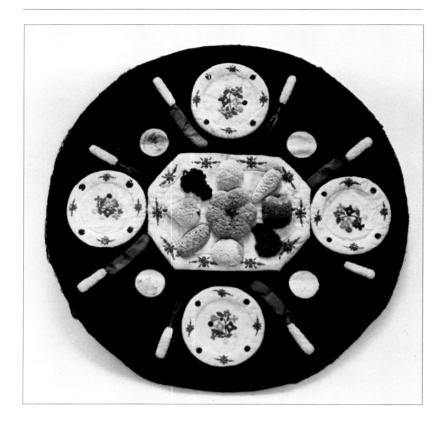

Fig. 8. *Table cover, wool tufted work, appliqué and embroidery on wool, Pennsylvania, about 1860. This table cover is a striking, playful variation on the needlework tours de force of tufted work and beaded Berlin work normally used on reception chairs and fire screens meant for display rather than use. Courtesy Schwenkfelder Library, Pennsburg, Pennsylvania.*

linen towel decorated with drawn work and counted cross stitch and free embroidery. Made well into the twentieth century, show towels were the work of young unmarried women and never were intended to serve utilitarian purposes. Rather, they hung on the painted doors that were kept closed between rooms and presented the quality of their mature stitchery techniques (some years after these women had completed samplers) for the inspection of guests.[20] These tufted work projects were single examples of women's needle skills—a later nineteenth-century version of the canvaswork upholstery of earlier decades—but, like show towels, these "functional" objects were set aside from everyday use and reserved for contexts of display, such as the parlor.

Most advice for making upholstered seating furniture at home focused upon the needs of consumers who could not afford commercial upholstery. These instructions concentrated on a small range of forms that used recycled materials, mostly variations on couches or chairs made with bases of wooden packing boxes or pads and covers that could be applied to existing furniture either as structural or removable elements. As Beecher and Stowe suggested, "If you have in the house any broken-down arm chair, reposing in the oblivion of the garret, draw it out —drive a nail here and there to hold it firm — stuff and pad, and stitch the padding through with a long upholsterer's needle, and cover it with the chintz like your other furniture. Presto —you create an easy chair."[21]

Advice writers often emphasized that such decorative work was possible even in households such as small family farms where all hands were occupied with hard daily labor. Instructions appeared repeatedly for upholstered furniture to be made from barrels, a form worthy of special note not only because it seems emblematic of do-it-yourself upholstery in its transformation of a rough utilitarian object to a softened parlor denizen. As it was depicted in advice books over

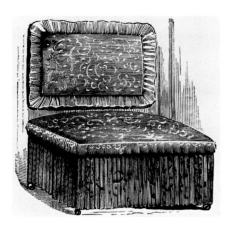

Fig. 9. "A Box Chair," engraving in [George A. Martin], Household Conveniences *(1884).*

time, the barrel arm chair also reflected the popular spread of the aesthetic of refinement.

Homemade couches, sometimes called "box couches," "box lounges," and "box ottomans" (this last term was used to apply both to hassocks and larger seats) were the modest descendants of a form of "ottoman," a built-in seat with a mattress-type cushion and padded back that appeared occasionally in images of European interiors in the first quarter of the nineteenth century.[22] Downing illustrated this type of "ottoman" or "divan" as an appropriate kind of country parlor furniture, probably borrowing the idea from Loudon, but books on home sewing such as *Household Conveniences* and *The Workwoman's Guide* of 1840 also included such box seats as one of the few kinds of upholstered furniture that could be made at home.[23] In small interiors, such couches may have opened up to provide additional storage, and instructions for box couches between 1833 and the 1890s described them as useful for linens, fabric scraps, and clothing (fig. 9).[24]

Instructions for homemade seating furniture rarely recommended that amateur upholsterers tackle spring seating, although Catharine Beecher suggested to her prospective couch makers that they provide an "elastic" base for seat cushions by using flexible wooden slats rather than a solid board top on the couch's box base.[25] Instead, they described a variety of dead and cushion seats filled with straw, moss, husks, cotton, horsehair, or feathers. Some instructions for converting a wooden packing box into a chair suggested just how limited the means of readers aspiring to upholstered comfort were expected to be: "In stuffing such chairs, any coarse fabric will answer; bagging that has been used for packing goods, quite as serviceable as new, may often be had at stores for a trifle."[26] Another advocated "newspapers torn into the tiniest fragments" as acceptable stuffing.[27]

Do-it-yourself upholsterers frequently received advice to recycle carpet scraps, worn clothing, and bedding as chair padding or covers. *Beautiful Homes* instructed its readers to "take any old quilt or 'comfort,' or, in lieu of these, parts of old worn garments, cotton batting, soft pieces of carpet, or indeed, any material that will serve to make a soft foundation. Tack this covering over the entire chair, from top of back down to the seat, putting on layer after layer until a soft foundation is secured." Additional padding was achieved by cutting a layer of wool or cotton "sufficiently thick to form a comfortable pad." Home upholsterers could then make use of their quilting skills to secure this pad under the cover fabric.[28] A pine-framed settee added to the collection of the Farmers' Museum of the New York State Historical Association in 1953 (now deaccessioned) was padded with ten alternating layers of straw and quilts or coverlets. The original show cover was quilted green linsey woolsey. Old clothing, particularly the wide expanses of women's skirts, could also be used for the show covers. For its box chairs, *Household Conveniences* recommended the use of chintz or rep (probably the ribbed, printed cotton furnishing fabric commonly available at that time rather than the woolen rep popular through the 1870s) for the cover; failing that, recycling old dress fabric was considered acceptable. Some homemade upholstered chairs incorporated dress-weight fabrics in their covers, although it is impossible to say with certainty that the fabrics were recycled from clothing.

Padding existing chairs was associated with providing bodily comfort for the aged or ill members of a household. Ladder-back chairs with arms, some with rockers, were a natural object for such improvements because they already were considered relatively comfortable. The rungs of their ladder backs could be augmented with woven slats to form a solid surface for amateur upholsterers to

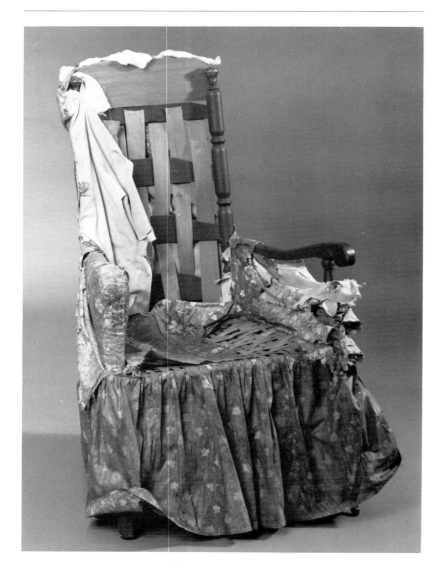

Fig. 10. Homemade upholstered rocking chair, made from ladder-back chair with woven strips of pine to support upholstery, walnut, pine, cotton batting, printed cotton, Massachusetts, after 1840. This chair is one of two such homemade upholstered chairs found in the Emerson Bixby House in Barre, Massachusetts. The ladder-back chair beneath the layers of quilts and padding dates from around 1800. The fabrics covering the chair suggest that it was upholstered after 1840, perhaps coincident with the enlarging and redecorating of the Bixby House in the mid-1840s. The splints woven through the chair's back were meant to support the addition of upholstery; the rockers probably were added at that time. When it was new, the red printed fabric that covers this chair must have added a cheerful note to the room in which it sat. *Courtesy Old Sturbridge Village; photograph by Henry E. Peach.*

work against. In an October 1879 issue of *The Household*, an article titled "Lath and Lambrequins" informed readers that pine lath was a cheap and easy-to-use material to fix "bottomless, backless, or roundless" chairs prior to upholstering them with recycled dress fabric.[29] A skirt could be easily made to disguise their legs (fig. 10). Upholstered ladder-back chairs may have been relatively common; in any event, they were common enough to enjoy such a clear association with old-fashioned rural family life that the American genre painter Thomas Hovenden showed one as the comfortable, supportive chair offered to a wounded soldier in the parlor of a farmhouse (fig. 11).

Americans made over old ladder-backs into upholstered easy chairs well into the twentieth century. In the 1920s, Jane Armstrong Tucker engineered one such transformation as part of redecorating some of Castle Tucker's rooms for the accommodation of summer guests. Wishing to have a pair of matching wing chairs in a particularly large bedroom that was going to be "colonial," she recovered one that the family already owned. She then removed the rockers, built up the arms, and constructed wings on the back of another chair before covering it with padding and the same fabric that she had used on the first chair. Floor-length cretonne skirts effectively disguised the chairs' mismatched legs and feet (fig. 12).

The upholstered easy chair made from a cut-down barrel was repeatedly cited by authors of furnishing advice as an example of the potential transformations of commonly available utilitarian objects into upholstered furniture. A. J. Downing offered three illustrations of "barrel-chairs" that he considered appropriate for simple cottage furnishing, and other architecture advice books soon followed suit: *Village and Farm Cottages* observed in 1856, "We have seen good-looking, home-made chairs, with easy seats and backs, which had been quickly and cheaply manufactured, and with no other frame than a common flour-barrel supplied" (fig. 13).[30]

Many of the instructions for making barrel chairs were so sketchy that a reader unfamiliar with the form would have had difficulty reproducing one. Julia McNair Wright, for example, simply advised her readers that a comfortable sewing chair could be produced from a barrel "sawn into shape, and covered with chintz, over stuffing."[31] Other instructions promised startling transformations of barrels into Turkish-style overstuffed chairs, a metamorphosis certainly beyond the skill and means of the amateur home upholsterer. In fact, the barrel chair seems to have become a symbol for all homemade upholstery. Perhaps it was a particularly attractive example because it seemed to be an emblem of Yankee domestic ingenuity and thrift. Perhaps the transformation of a coarse storage vessel also symbolized the possibilities of self-transformation contained within the activity of making refined furnishings for modest households (fig. 14).

It is impossible to know how many families actually produced homemade upholstered furniture for themselves. Pieces that were not worn out, as most upholstered furniture eventually is, probably succumbed to changing tastes or to their owners' improving financial circumstances and were discarded. At least two barrel chairs dating from the mid-nineteenth century survive in museum collections, both padded with cut-up quilts and upholstered in printed cotton and linen (figs. 15 and 16). The supposition that barrel chairs were relatively common in the nineteenth century may be further supported by the revival of popularity enjoyed by commercially produced barrel chairs around the turn of the century, when they were a small element of the colonial revival. A commercially made example, covered with a turn-of-the-century, factory-woven dark

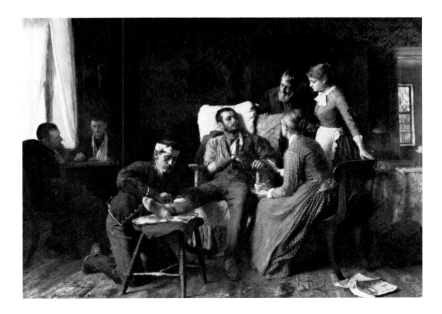

Fig. 11. In the Hands of the Enemy, *oil on canvas by Thomas Hovenden, 1889. The wounded soldier has been seated in a homemade upholstered rocking chair like that in fig. 10. Courtesy Ellen Battell Stoekel Trust; photograph by Joseph Szaszfai, Yale University Art Gallery.*

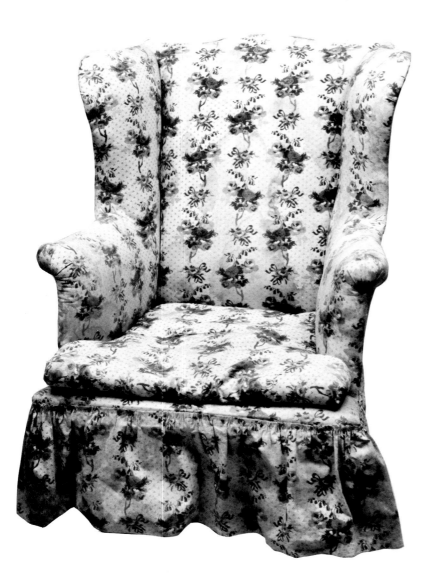

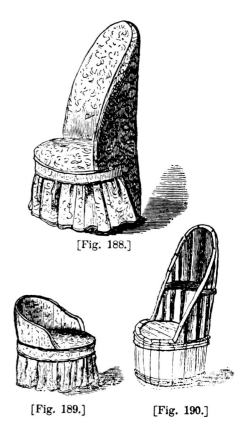

Fig. 12. Homemade wing chair, stuffed with horsehair from an old mattress, covered with unpolished printed cotton (cretonne or drapery print), 1920-1930. The deck upon which the loose seat cushion rests is supported by strips of mattress ticking. Courtesy Castle Tucker.

[Fig. 188.]

[Fig. 189.]   [Fig. 190.]

Fig. 13. Barrel chairs, engraving in A. J. Downing, The Architecture of Country Houses *(1850). In* Beautiful Homes *(1878), Henry T. Williams and Mrs. C. S. Jones wrote, "For children nothing can be more cunning and really comfortable than kegs or small barrels made and upholstered as described previously. When covered with gay cloth, with some name or monogram wrought on the back and seat, these little chairs always afford infinite satisfaction to the little folks."*

green tapestry and featuring a "potty seat" cover under its cushion, survives in the collection of the Codman House in Lincoln, Massachusetts (fig. 17), where it was used as a bedroom chair. Thus the barrel chair, which once signaled aspirations toward increased bodily comfort and the creation of self-consciously decorated rooms, was transformed into an emblem of colonial thrift.

By the 1870s, engravings of upholstered chairs made from boxes and barrels or recycled plain, wooden chairs had subtly made the requirements for success in homemade upholstery more exact. They depicted the finished products as elaborately decorated chairs with ruffled fronts, tassels, and tufting or common wooden chairs with fancy needlework cushions and covers decorated with bows and thick fringe. These transformations were in keeping with the spread of the popular aesthetic of refinement. Descriptions of homemade chairs contained the same implications, urging a high degree of detail and finish in even homemade upholstered chairs and equating the finished product with the progress of refinement in the domestic lives of their makers. When the authors of *Beautiful Homes* (1878) offered instructions for upholstering and embellishing two-dollar rocking

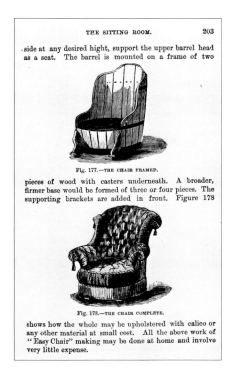

-side at any desired hight, support the upper barrel head as a seat. The barrel is mounted on a frame of two

Fig. 177.—THE CHAIR FRAMED.

pieces of wood with casters underneath. A broader, firmer base would be formed of three or four pieces. The supporting brackets are added in front. Figure 178

Fig. 178.—THE CHAIR COMPLETE.

shows how the whole may be upholstered with calico or any other material at small cost. All the above work of " Easy Chair " making may be done at home and involve very little expense.

Fig. 14. "The Chair Framed" and "The Chair Complete," illustrations in [George A. Martin], Household Conveniences *(1884). By the time these instructions were published, the simple barrel frame "easy chair" had evolved into a "Turkish fauteuil" with button tufting on the head and back, decorative ruffling, and tassels. Projects for furniture from barrels and boxes became more elaborate by the 1870s, so much so that the bases were transformed beyond recognition. Simply building a frame from scratch would have been more sensible than engineering the changes depicted here. However, the central importance of the project was the act of transformation itself, from rough and only utilitarian to refined, both symbolically and functionally useful as a parlor object.*

chairs, they noted, "We really know of no more comfortable chair than the homely 'splint-bottom rocker' that accompanies the farmhouse chair of the western prairies. These quaint-looking but substantial affairs would suit Mr. Eastlake exactly, but as we cannot admire them in their rude state, it has become a subject of some importance to make them as tasteful as possible by means of padding and covering" (fig. 18).[32]

In the eyes of these authors, simply improving physical comfort through upholstery was no longer enough, and the interest in household art, the popular offshoot of the aesthetic movement in the 1880s and 1890s, led to instructions for transforming many mundane domestic objects—broomsticks, milking stools, and rocking chairs—into refined furniture through the application of homemade upholstery (figs. 19 and 20). Such instructions raised recycling from a necessity to an art. Feeding on this new interest in artistic decor, at least one fancy-goods firm, belonging to Mrs. T. G. Farnham of New York City, offered craft kits for "aesthetic" wicker chairs. The kit even included one chair with work partially completed for prosperous amateur decorators who did not need to recycle.

Transforming the mundane into the artistic was no longer exemplary of thrift alone but an expression of advancing civilization, where individual refinement contributed to the progress of all. Williams and Jones articulated this sensibility in *Beautiful Homes*:

> If we can make pretty things that will give pleasure to our selves and others, and that will save expense, (where need be to economize,) then it is wise to surround ourselves with them, and though it is just and right that the wealthy should enjoy all the luxury that money can procure, there is no reason why those less favored, and who perhaps enjoy beautiful objects just as fully, should not be allowed to make for themselves objects as nearly resembling the costly ones as may be, for as Mr. Conway justly observes, "take away all that has been added to our homes by art, and we all become naked savages, living in mud or log huts."[33]

Advice for making this kind of "aesthetic" homemade upholstery largely supplanted instructions for basic upholstered box furniture by the 1890s. The disappearance of the latter type of advice reflected changes in access: the booming factory production of a certain quality of upholstered furniture offered style for little money, and systematic installment buying in towns and mail-order buying in rural communities increased. Barrel chairs or upholstered ladder-backs no longer were necessary avenues to ownership of upholstered furniture for consumers with limited incomes. Homemade upholstery continued to flourish in other ways, through homemade forms of drapery and instructions for smaller objects such as table covers and for renovating the new cheap upholstered furniture itself. Inexpensive decorating advice books showed readers how to support the sagging webbing of their furniture and how to make decorative slipcovers. The anonymous author of the *Modern Priscilla Home Furnishing Book* (1925) advised, "A seat that is beginning to sag should be attended to at once, if we wish to do it at home; otherwise the springs will become crooked, the stuffing will lose its shape, and the expertness of a professional upholsterer will be necessary." The chapter on reupholstering and slipcovering included a picture and instructions for a "home-made stretcher" for tightening webbing and also described how to make and use a "regulator," the long needle used for rearranging stuffing inside a chair.[34]

Many kinds of fashionable French-inspired draperies enjoyed seasons of popularity throughout the nineteenth century, especially

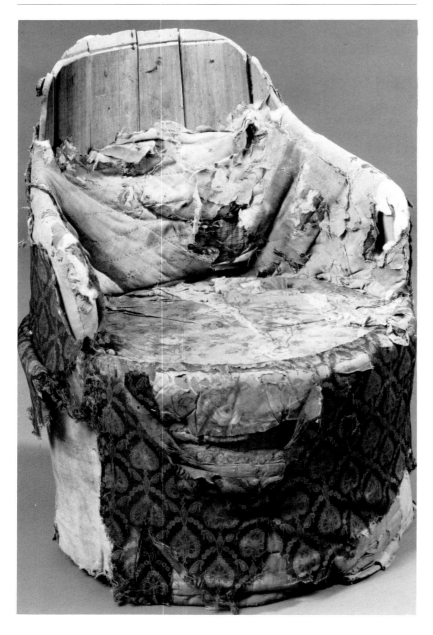

Fig. 15. Barrel chair, chestnut, padded with cut-up patchwork quilt, printed linen cover, about 1850. The upholstery on this chair, for which no history of making or ownership survives, incorporates cut-up quilts as padding on the inside arms and back. Its loose cushion covers a different print than the red-and-black printed linen which is its show cover, an apparent effort to piece out a limited quantity of fabric. Courtesy Old Sturbridge Village; photograph by Henry E. Peach.

those forms that were hung in swags or festoons. Their complicated construction required special skills in handling and cutting fabrics that were often expensive. For these reasons, guides to domestic economy from the first half of the nineteenth century often cautioned women against tackling complex draperies at home, no matter how accomplished they were at household and fancy sewing. The author of *The Workwoman's Guide* of 1840 noted that while "some knowledge of upholstery is of importance to the head of every establishment...It is strongly recommended to those who can afford the expense, to employ an experienced upholsterer, as the patterns will not only be more in fashion, but more tastefully and regularly put up, than they could possibly be by any one not accustomed to the business" (see fig. 2).[35]

Such notes of caution continued to appear in articles and books of decorating advice in the years between 1850 to 1930, particularly in relation to the more complicated styles of upholstery in the "French

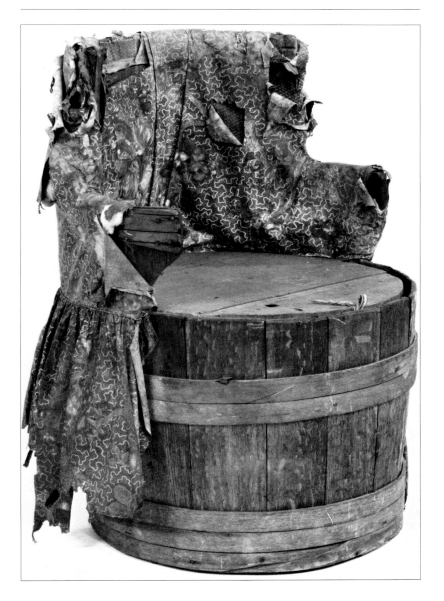

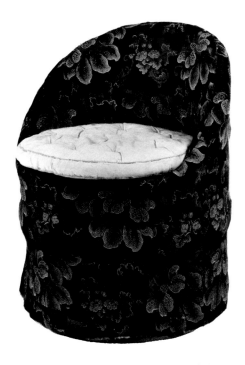

Fig. 16. *Barrel chair, oak, cotton batting, printed cotton, used in Stetson House, Hanover, Massachusetts, 1840-1850. Courtesy Society for the Preservation of New England Antiquities; gift of Dr. L. Vernon Briggs, Boston; photograph by J. David Bohl.*

Fig. 17. *"Colonial revival" barrel chair, chestnut, cotton and wool tapestry, Codman house, Lincoln, Massachusetts, 1900-1930. Courtesy Society for the Preservation of New England Antiquities; photograph by J. David Bohl.*

taste" of the 1880s and 1890s (fig. 21). Helen Anderson, author of a number of articles directed to ambitious amateur decorators in *The Decorator and Furnisher*, urged her readers to "avoid elaborate draperies," especially those that gave the illusion of being "draped carelessly over a pole." "Many of the hangings that are in the style of Louis XVI are a snare and a delusion to the unwary," she warned, and she suggested that those with a hankering for French window treatments instead try a less graceful but cheaper and easier-to-make variant called "scarf drapery" (fig. 22).[36]

Although women's magazines published wood engravings of extremely elaborate window treatments that represented the height of expense and fashion in the 1850s, 1860s, and 1870s, homemade window treatments were probably, as a rule, simply executed affairs. (These images were recycled several times; *Godey's* cuts from the early 1870s reappeared in the advice book *Beautiful Houses* in 1878.) The difficulty in making draperies of swags and festoons lay in the cutting rather than in the sewing. Paper patterns were unavailable (patterns were not available at the time for clothing, either), and the limited instructions contained in articles on draperies do not seem helpful.

An 1860 article in *Peterson's Magazine*, which purported to provide directions "by the aid of which any lady, with ordinary skill, can make and arrange her own curtains, or other window or bed draperies," pictured a selection of valances either pleated or festooned over ornamental rods and discussed the required hardware, but it issued no instructions on how to cut them. Author Fanny N. Copeland coyly noted, "There are almost as many ways of arranging the curtains as of folding napkins for the dinner-table, and they may all be found out by a little ingenuity."[37] Thus, elaborately cut draperies, requiring the skilled work of cutters trained in the craft, always contained the echoes of money spent for skill as well as for cloth and trims.

The execution of straight draperies and valances could be deciphered nonetheless from otherwise vague instructions if a picture for copying them was included. Flat valances, also called lambrequins, could be made from simple cottons, required no special skill to make them drape properly and could be stiffened and hung so that no expensive cornice was needed (fig. 23). Homemade cornices may also have been relatively common, however, and advice books mentioned them as a possible contribution to furnishing from the men of a household (fig. 24). Draperies that consisted of straight panels of fabric, hung with rings of brass or wood from an ornamental rod made of the same materials, also could be reproduced by any housewife who could get her hands on that volume of fabric.

When forms of drapery were easy to cut, both style and expense became functions of the materials and surface decoration they featured. Amateur decorators with limited budgets employed a variety of clever strategies for attaining similar richness and visual variety in their creations. After purchasing a set of window valances made from stamped plush and decorated with Turkish trims, Jane Armstrong Tucker, a woman with an enthusiasm for household art in many forms, produced a similar set of valances for the family parlor. She achieved variety and richness by recycling a heavy, napped wool blanket fabric that probably first saw use in a blanket and by adding strips of purple cotton velveteen and a deep ball fringe of cotton and wool as trim across the bottom of each (plate 38 and 39). This set hung in loose pleats which were achieved by nailing the valances in gathers from the 1857 cornices in the parlor (see chapter 2, fig. 10).

Although women had been sewing their own window curtains throughout the nineteenth century, an increased range of drapery characterized ordinary parlors after 1875, reaching its popular peak in what one advice book called the "esthetic craze" of the 1880s and 1890s.[38] The author of "Artistic Draperies" in the June 1890 issue of *The Decorator and Furnisher* enthusiastically noted that "in no respect has there been a greater change in house furnishing than in the increased use of draperies."[39] Along with window treatments, home decorators turned their attention to draping doorways, as well as mantels, pianos, tables, and bookcases. They swaddled furniture with throws; they refined wastebaskets, "gypsy tables," and umbrella stands with wrappings of fabric. Small forms of drapery, requiring less time to execute, allowed the homegrown aesthetic impulse to display itself in newly popular art needlework techniques— "Kensington embroidery," painting on fabric, appliqué, drawn work, and stitchery with chenille and other novelty yarns.

By the 1880s, the continuing decline in price and improved appearance of American domestic cottons encouraged the proliferation of home drapery. Some directions for homemade upholstered rooms, whose appearance depended entirely upon the fabric covering boxes or the plain wooden frames of furniture, recall the medieval practice of creating formal furniture by draping simple

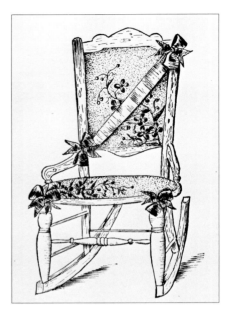

Fig. 18. "*Fig. 39.—Renovated Rocking Chair,*" illustration in [George A. Martin], Our Homes: How to Beautify Them *(1887). The directions accompanying this figure informed readers that "a very cheap old-fashioned rocking-chair" could be "tastefully trimmed up and transformed into a fancy chair for the parlor" by making cushions from "an old comfortable," embroidering their covers with silk or applying an appliqué cut from cretonne, and adding ribbon and bows to increase the "decorative effect."*

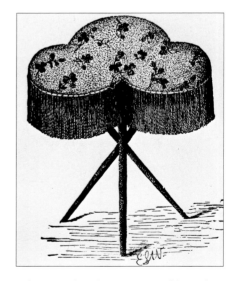

Fig. 19. Cloverleaf or gypsy table made from three broomsticks and fabric-covered board top, engraving in [George A. Martin], Our Homes: How to Beautify Them *(1887).*

THE HOUSE ORNAMENTAL.

The Magic Barrel.– VI.

From a single apple or flour barrel it is possible to make a perfectly lovely couch, much superior to anything that can be bought in the furniture shops.

First, get a carpenter to make you a stout frame of mahogany or walnut, with an ebony leg at each corner. The rest you may do for yourself.

Lay the barrel staves one upon the other, as shown in the illustration, and fasten to the frame with brass tacks and fine copper wire. This gives you an ideal spring, neither too hard nor too soft, and a spring that will last as long as you will. The barrel heads should then be sawed in twain, and fastened to each end of the frame, as shown in the illustration. All you have to do now is to upholster the couch with embossed Spanish leather, and trim with Oriental stuffs, and you have a piece of furniture that is a thing of beauty and a joy forever.

As I have previously remarked, the peculiar value of barrel furniture is its individuality, its exclusiveness. The machine made stuff is uninteresting because it lacks character.

PATIENCE TINKER.

Fig. 20. "The Magic Barrel.- VI.,"
illustration in Patience Tinker, "The
House Ornamental," Grand Rapids
Furniture Record *(December 1909). By*
the turn of the century, do-it-yourself
upholstery in the "household art" vein was
the object of satire, in this instance from
furniture manufacturers in one of their
trade publications. "The Magic Barrel,"
a collection of six sets of instructions for
converting "the lowly flour barrel into the
Barrel Beautiful," ostensibly was
reprinted from The House Ornamental:
A Periodical of Putter. *"Patience*
Tinker," editor of the ersatz magazine,
informed her readers that "with the lowly
barrel, or rather with a number of lowly
barrels, you can furnish your entire house.
To begin with, suppose you buy a barrel of
apples. You won't need the apples; those
you can give away. But you save the
barrel." Courtesy Grand Rapids Public
Library.

wooden furniture with fabric (fig. 25). They also were, in essence, homemade paraphrases of the stylish "tent rooms" that first appeared in France during the Empire period (fig. 26).[40]

Although calico was not typically a furnishing fabric, advice on homemade upholstery encouraged its use, and bright-colored domestic prints were available for between seven and ten cents a yard in the mid-1870s. English chintz, a traditional furnishing fabric that featured a polished or "calendared" surface finish, was by 1880 largely supplanted by both foreign and domestic cretonne, "furniture twill," and "drapery print" (plate 40). Most patterns offered in these inexpensive furnishing fabrics continued the tradition of using large-scale floral designs for furnishing purposes, however. Using both traditional and newer analine dyes, printing mills typically offered consumers from five to nine vivid colors in each print. Dark backgrounds were particularly popular, probably in part because they did not show the effects of coal dust and lamp soot as soon as light colors were apt to. Although a few timely novelties were added each season, reflecting interest in Japanese or Egyptian designs, many furnishing prints typically remained in production for years. The rollers for each design were expensive to produce, which encouraged reprinting, but this continuity also reflected the long-standing fondness of American housekeepers for floral prints, particularly fully opened roses, even if they were rendered in shades of blue or orange.[41]

The costs of such fabrics, while outside the reach of the poorest families, made them accessible to many ordinary households. Cretonne in thirty-two-inch widths cost anywhere from fifteen to fifty cents a yard in the early 1880s; similar floral drapery prints were offered for as low as six cents a yard fifteen years later.[42]

Although machine-woven lace curtains were cheap by the 1870s, several forms of homemade tape lace, called "Battenburg lace," "guipure d'-art," "guipure renaissance," and needle lace experienced a revival for furnishing purposes in the 1870s and 1880s (plate 41). Both required few specialized materials, and they provided one form of lace-making where satisfying results could be obtained quickly with the aid of commercially produced tapes and "Battenburg rings."

Mantel drapery seems to have been particularly popular for parlor embellishment and may be taken as a good index of how the sensibility of refinement encompassed utilitarian objects and turned them to its own purposes. It also provides a case study of the kinds of decorative strategies employed by ambitious parlor makers. Mantel lambrequins originated with simple fabric or leather strips that were fastened across the large openings of Dutch fireplaces, where mantel shelves protruded into the room, as early as the seventeenth century. In wealthy households, they were made to match the other hangings in the room.[43] Decorative or simple, such "chimney cloths" functioned as a screen to keep some of the fire's smoke out of the room.[44]

Nineteenth-century mantel upholstery itself appears to have been a French innovation. In 1841, Sydney George Fisher of Philadelphia admired an upholstered mantelpiece, "covered with a cushion of crimson velvet with a rich fringe of gold hanging from its edge & heavy gold tassels from the corners," in the elegant French-style parlors of Mrs. Israel Pemberton Hutchinson.[45] Mantel draping was such a rarity that Fisher called it a "novelty." Unfortunately, no more detailed description of this mantel cover survives, nor does a description of the "upholstered mantel-piece" displayed by Lewis F. Dennis (praised as a "good specimen of upholstery") at the first Exhibition of the Metropolitan Mechanics' Institute, held in Washington, D.C., in 1853.[46]

By the late 1870s, a simple form of popular mantel drapery consisted of a fabric-covered board with a short valance of fringe or other trimmings, nailed or screwed into the mantelpiece. Clarence Cook described this type of mantel valance as a way of disguising ugly, outdated marble mantels; the Gibson House in Boston, Massachusetts, features an example of this type of mantel upholstery dating probably from the early 1870s (fig. 27).[47]

Popular audiences took mantel drapery to their hearts in the 1880s, however, and used it as another means of making ceremonial and refined the increasingly superfluous fireplace. Until heating stoves became common, hearths and their mantelpieces were the functional axes of rooms. They also were a natural focal point for decoration, both in their architecture and the objects displayed on and around them. In the United States, middle-class households of the late eighteenth and early nineteenth centuries decorated the unused hearths in summer with painted fireboards as well as arrangements of natural materials set into them. Even when houses were equipped with heating stoves or furnaces, architects supplied rooms with full but non-functional fireplaces (vents for hot air) or, in small houses, mantel shelves. S. B. Reed's *House-Plans for Everybody* (1878) offered one plan where the parlor had a marble mantel shelf but was heated with a stove or "radiator" that drew heat from a stove in an adjoining room.[48] Clarence Cook noted and commented upon the customary expectations of people regarding mantels: "However willing people have been to give up fireplaces, they have not been willing to give up mantelpieces, and, indeed, I suppose the keeping up even of a show of fireplaces has been partly owing to the liking for the shelf that has so long been suspended over them."[49]

The symbolic meaning attached to fireplaces as "the center of family life, the spiritual and intellectual center" also encouraged mantel draping.[50] Draping typically was used to emphasize the ceremonial aspects of other significant pieces of furniture such as center tables and upright pianos, those hard-won and installment-bought symbols of family culture. Judging from the number that survive from the 1880s and later, mantel covers and lambrequins seem to have been a typical choice for homemade drapery, guaranteed for examination and praise when suspended from the decorative center of the parlor.

Decorative needlework shelf lambrequins had been popular as a parlor embellishment since the 1850s, and flat lambrequins for windows since the 1860s, but the form reached its height of

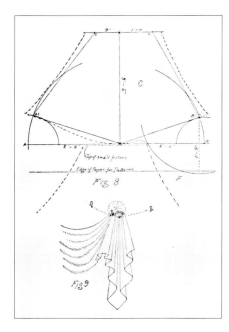

Fig. 21. *Detail of "irregular festoon drapery," engraving in John W. Stephenson,* Cutting and Draping *(1905).*

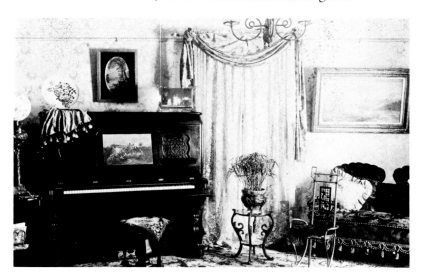

Fig. 22. *Unidentified interior with scarf drapery" of light cotton or printed silk at parlor window, Rochester, New York, about 1900. Scarf drapery achieved its effects by the way the fabric was hung rather than cut and sewed. The author of* Cutting and Draping *(1905) considered it "at best but an imitation of the cut festoon drapery" only suited for temporary purposes.*

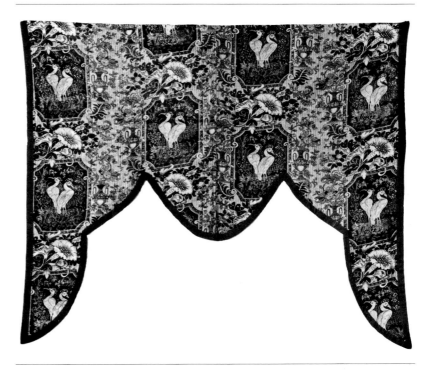

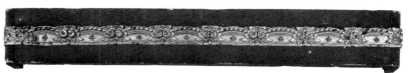

Fig. 24. Cornice, wood, flocked wallpaper, and stamped tin, used in Merrill Tavern in South Lee, Massachusetts, 1850-1870. The maker of this cornice recycled a length of stamped metal cornice to make this homemade piece more decorative. Courtesy Society for the Preservation of New England Antiquities.

popularity after 1880. In an item in the July 1881 issue of *The Household*, Mrs. H. Emmons noted both the range of forms and increased interest among farm women in trying them out:

> So many of the sisters, this past year, have asked questions about lambrequins of different kinds, that I wish I could explain so that you could all see, as I do, some patterns I have, forming a set that can be used for any room, chamber, library, or parlor, and can be cut from any material. There are patterns for window, mantle [*sic*], and bracket lambrequins, and besides a pattern marked out for silk or worsted embroidery about a finger wide goes with them…If any of the sisters would like the patterns, and will send to my address, enclosing eighteen cents in new postage stamps, I will have them cut, marked and sent to them.[51]

Making mantel covers or lambrequins usually followed a set of simple compositional strategies for getting the requisite effect of complexity and richness. The first was to use simple cut-out shapes that required little or no tailoring. Many mantel lambrequins were flat; others used shield shapes that could be repeated many times over when a long expanse was to be covered. Decorating the fabric surface provided interest and detail. When crochet or macramé was used to make a mantel lambrequin, repetition of single decorative shield shapes accomplished the same end (plate 42). Decorating fabric lambrequins could be accomplished through the use of trims such as homemade tassels and ball fringes or, by the 1870s, through embroidery and appliqué (plates 43 and 44). A technique for stretching expensive fabrics, endorsed by the Beechers as well as by

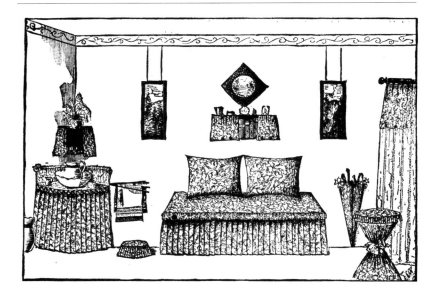

Fig. 25. *"A Room Furnished in Cretonne,"* engraving in *[George A. Martin]*, Our Homes: How to Beautify Them *(1887).*

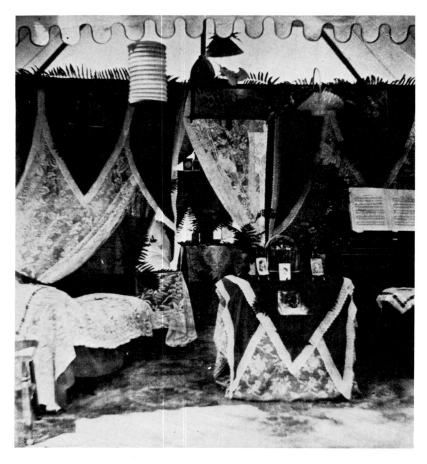

Fig. 26. *An unidentified family's tent at "Lake Pleasant Camp Meeting," stereograph, about 1875. This temporary summer housing suggests how fabrics, including inexpensive lace curtains, could be used to create a cozy and refined room.*

later household art advisers, was to incorporate bands of the more expensive material, prints, or pile fabrics.

Layering many kinds of drapery and home upholstery was another strategy for attaining intricacy with homemade objects, one easily employed by women who were forced to assemble their room decor gradually rather than as a planned scheme completed at once. Along with fancy pillows and throws, tidies on plain furniture both relieved

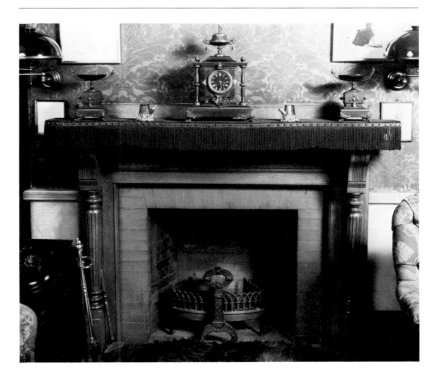

Fig. 27. *Mantel lambrequin, wool bullion fringe, wool baize top, Gibson House, 34 Beacon Street, Boston, Massachusetts, 1870-1880. This mantel upholstery was attached to a board which was then fastened to the fireplace. "Mantel fringe" like this was offered for sale in the 1878 catalog of New York City trim makers Charles A. Schmidt and probably was available elsewhere. Courtesy Gibson House Society.*

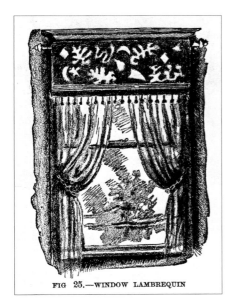

FIG 25.—WINDOW LAMBREQUIN

Fig. 28. *"Fig. 25.— Window Lambrequin," engraving in [George A. Martin] Our Homes: How to Beautify Them (1887). The instructions for this parlor window treatment demonstrate how layering felt and other inexpensive fabrics and decorating their surfaces could create visual complexity. The lambrequin was created from a twenty-inch width of maroon-colored felt, having irregular-shaped fancy designs cut out all over its surface. The felt was then lined with pale blue silesia (a plain-woven cotton lining fabric). Tinsel cord outlined the cut-outs and ornamented the bottom, along with ball fringe. The directions guaranteed that the finished product would give a "beautiful and rich finish to the window and room."*

dull surfaces and updated old furniture too good to throw away or recover. Layering was most successful when there was substantial variation between the types of materials employed, and home decorators freely combined homemade and store-bought elements to create domesticated vignettes, soul-satisfying in their complexity. As the cost of furnishing textiles declined in the 1880s and 1890s, a wide variety of commercially produced items — table covers, portières, couch covers, and lace curtains — became available at prices lower than the cost of similar items made at home.

This proliferation was encouraged by popular household art manuals that applauded the use of inexpensive fabrics that once would have been considered unsuitable for the purposes of household decoration. In the October 1880 issue of *The Household*, "Lenaria" spread this news: "I wonder if the sisters know that you can get cotton flannel in all widths and shades, bronze, old gold, and seal brown, to use wrong side out for table covers, lambrequins, tidies, etc." She advised the use of appliqués of other fabric scraps for decorating them and offered patterns through the mail. Another article in the same issue described how to make "coarse burlap curtains," fringed by raveling and decorated with a stripe of cretonne for the "sitting room." Perhaps because its farm audience had burlap around the premises, *The Household* recommended its use for decoration periodically.[52]

Felt was another popular choice for making lambrequins and table covers, both in homemade and inexpensive commercial forms (fig. 28). Its double width (seventy-two inches) alone made it a bargain, but it also looked "rich." Felt came in a wide range of deep colors and saved sewing because it required no hemming and could even be glued together. In the 1880s, it cost around a dollar and a half per yard, but it dropped in price by one-third by 1895.[53] As in their instructions for seating furniture, authors of advice on homemade upholstery directed to aspiring parlor makers with very limited means encouraged recycling dress fabrics, particularly the expanses of skirt material, for making drapery. Dress fabrics often were recommended for drapery purposes in conjunction with other recycled drapery fabrics, as when the authors of *Beautiful Homes* recommended that "half-worn Turkey-red chintz curtains" be used to line a lambrequin of "Tycoon reps," a dress fabric with long vertical ribs formed by a heavy cotton warp and fine wool weft that was popular in the 1870s.[54] It was printed with "gay-colored patterns...imitations of those of Eastern fabrics, such as cashmere, which it resembles."[55]

Intact sets of draperies were themselves often recycled by re-cutting along newer, more fashionable lines (as dresses often were) or simply by cutting down their length to accommodate such changes as the introduction of radiators into domestic interiors. Most surviving lace curtains have been cut down from their original three-yard length to six feet or less, probably for this very reason. Portières also were subject to this kind of remodeling as door draping went out of style. A set of heavy voided cotton plush portières woven with the raised design on both sides and with a border and center motif design of foliage and scrolls is an example of this recycling (see chapter 8, fig. 24). Perhaps when door curtains were no longer in fashion, the tops were cut off and hemmed roughly so that the fabric panels could be used as window draperies. The safety-pin type of drapery hooks pinned to the new top hem made additional sewing unnecessary (fig. 29). Exposure to strong light from outdoors faded one side of the recycled portières, while the other has retained most of its deep maroon color. Scraps of clothing fabric could be employed for many of the smaller forms of room upholstery, such as lamp mats or table runners. Ultimately, even the colonial revival intersected with the "aesthetic" drapery craze in some kinds of fabric recycling, particularly those forms associated, if apocryphally, with housewifely thrift, such as rag and hooked rugs. Just as quilts of silk scraps were a play on the quilt as an emblem of both female craft and thrift, so too silk "rag rug" portières and table covers were a refined "take" on striped rag carpeting (figs. 30 and 31).

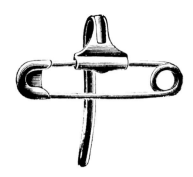

Fig. 29. Safety-pin drapery hook, illustration in Andrew Dutton Co. catalog, Boston, Massachusetts, after 1912. Easily purchased hardware made drapery re-dos easy. Safety-pin drapery hooks were available through mail-order catalogs as early as the 1880s.

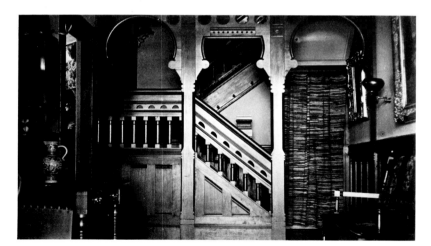

Fig. 30. Hallway in unidentified house probably in Arlington, Massachusetts (near Spot Pond), about 1890. One doorway off this "reform"-style hallway was draped with silk portières woven as rag rugs. In Woman's Handiwork in Modern Homes, *Constance Cary Harrison urged her readers to "collect every scrap of silk, whether new or old, to be found about the house, and to cut and sew it into long strips." She recommended that the strips be sent to a weaver, who would charge twenty-eight cents a yard for weaving. This was, she said, "certainly an inexpensive method of securing an excellent result in curtains or portière."*

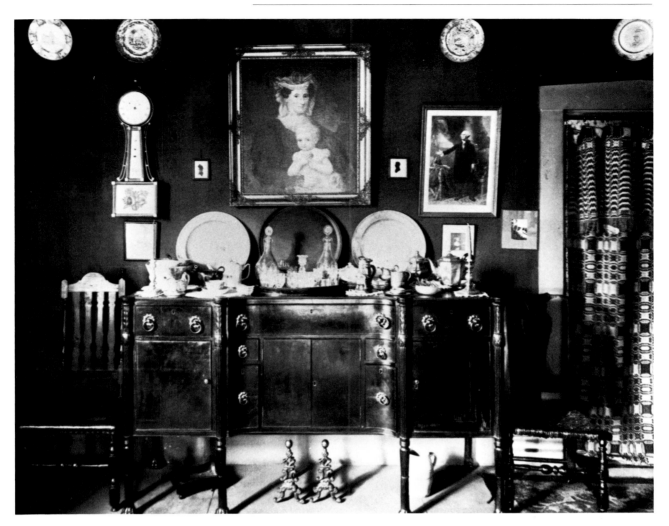

Fig. 31. Blue-and-white coverlet recycled as a portière, probably Colonel Jeremiah Page House, Danvers, Massachusetts, photograph in Mary H. Northend, Colonial Homes and Their Furnishings *(1917). Courtesy Henry Francis du Pont Winterthur Museum Library; Collection of Printed Books.*

CHAPTER TEN
VICTORIANISM IN THE MODERN ERA:
AT HOME IN THE LIVING ROOM,
1910-1930

The old custom of setting apart a "best room" or parlor to be used only on special occasions, as for weddings, funerals, or the entertainment of company, is happily passing away. Only very wealthy people now have drawing-rooms reserved for state occasions. The present tendency is to call all the lower rooms of the house "living rooms," and to have all the members of the family use them freely. A room set apart from ordinary use, and hence shut up much of the time from sun and air, is not good for the physical or moral health of the household. Hygiene demands that sun and air should be admitted freely to all parts of the house. The furnishings themselves, if good care is given them, will be improved rather than injured by ordinary wear, and guests will receive a far pleasanter impression from the easy and graceful atmosphere imparted to a room by daily use, than from the stiff and formal restraints imposed by the old-fashioned parlor.

> Sidney Morse, *Household Discoveries: An Encyclopedia of Practical Recipes and Processes* (1909)

The "modern" parlor had been the target of criticism virtually from the moment that it became a possibility among the middle class in the mid-nineteenth century. In fiction, essays, and books of advice, authors argued that the parlor was "sacrificial" because it wasted family resources, confined family life to fewer rooms in houses, and expressed the middle-class ideal of comfort inappropriately. This was the case not only because parlors were the rooms most subject to the whims of fashion but also because they were unbecoming and artificial—"the apotheosis of all refined discomfort," one writer called them—and hence unnecessary facades.[1]

Such criticism never stopped ordinary families from creating parlors for themselves and furnishing them; in fact, as lower price lines of furniture and furnishing textiles appeared on the market and consumer credit became available, more families became parlor makers. These new consumers almost always furnished according to a set of conventions that communicated information about middle-class identity, favoring decorative objects that adhered to popular standards of refinement, including French-influenced upholstery. Whether by necessity or preference, they created rooms that usually occupied some middle ground, that were both gala and homey.

How ideas about culture and comfort were themselves understood also changed by the end of the nineteenth century. "Comfort," for example, seems not only to have included the long-standing middle-class ideal of the domestic haven and a harmony between economic means and values. Toward the end of the century, as parlor makers opted for large-scale overstuffed furniture that was less posture-specific than earlier parlor suites, the term comfort also increasingly implied some relaxation in the traditional requirements for self-presentation in the parlor, standards that had seemed meaningful since 1850. Particularly after 1915, advice authors began to regard these strictures as "old-fashioned pomposity."[2] Mary Chambers, author of *Table Etiquette, Menus and Much Besides* (1929) announced that a "revolution" in etiquette had occurred, a "happy tendency to naturalness and simplicity in social intercourse." The formal call, the *raison d'être* of so many parlor rituals, was replaced by visits without cards, "sometimes announced previously by telephone, sometimes unpremeditated, and on the spur of the moment."[3] Deportment—the "easy manner" of gentility—was completely neglected in such books.

By the early twentieth century, most authors of furnishing advice, with the exception of those whose readership was well-to-do and able to continue the practice of having both a drawing room and a sitting room, chose the idea of the "living room" in preference to the parlor. The term living room once had signified a multi-purpose room in small, very modest households, a room one had on the way to economic success and future parlor making. Now it began to be defined as the space that served both as the principal family room and public room in middle-class houses and apartment buildings.

The new middle-class "living room" evolved in part from the fact that living space, both in new apartment buildings and in newly built single-family houses, tended to become smaller in the 1910s and 1920s. Not only were houses often smaller than their counterparts of the 1890s; some, such as bungalows, also featured open floor plans where the public spaces of houses flowed together (plate 45). This trend arose in part because people now opted for expensive domestic systems—heating, full plumbing including heated hot water, and electricity and cooking gas—over larger living area. S. B. Reed's revised *Modern House-Plans for Everybody* (1900) suggested that in the last quarter of the nineteenth century, when domestic systems were being refined, families who could only afford houses costing about two thousand dollars or less would obviously opt for ceremony over systems—parlors and formal dining rooms over bathrooms and furnaces. These houses were not planned with any systems other than a kitchen sink.[4] The twentieth-century change in priority from ceremony to systems itself suggests a larger shift in family ideals away from the self-contained Victorian household.

By the 1910s, thousands of ordinary families also redirected a large part of their discretionary income to the purchase of an automobile. Automobiles were the largest single domestic expenditure for many families, exceeded only by the cost of a house itself. In 1913, the Ford Model T dropped in price from $950 to $600, but even the lower figure was equivalent to the average annual earnings of employees in American businesses.[5] Until the advent of the General Motors Acceptance Corporation in the mid-1920s, consumer credit for auto purchases was limited. Still, the Lynds' pioneering sociological study of Muncie, Indiana, found that by 1923 there were two passenger cars for every three Muncie families. It has been estimated that as many as half of the thirty million households in the United States owned or had access to a car by 1930.[6]

By the 1920s, the automobile clearly served as a portable facade, so much so that the family car became the target of criticism because of the resources it diverted from furniture purchases. "So long as our judgment of others revolves largely around what makes of cars they drive, rather than the sorts of homes they live in," *The Modern Priscilla Home Furnishing Book* warned in 1925, "good furniture will wait until the car in the garage is paid for. And then, likely enough, we shall have our eye on a better car and continue to complain because good furniture is not to be had on the bargain counter."[7] By the 1920s, automobiles, not parlor furnishings, were the dangerous, fashionable consumer goods that threatened to upset the middle-class

Fig. 1. "Living Room in home of Rev. Dr. and Mrs. William R. Taylor, at 13 Prince Street, Rochester, N.Y. 1923." By the 1920s, printed cotton slipcovers had become a common decorating solution in many middle-class living rooms. They were "sanitary" as well as decorative; further, some housekeepers used them in summer over mohair and tapestry upholstery because they were "cooler." Although French decorators had provided printed cotton slipcovers to some fashionable clients in the nineteenth century, advice writers informed readers that their use was consistent with English country-house decor. Courtesy Rochester Public Library, Local History Division.

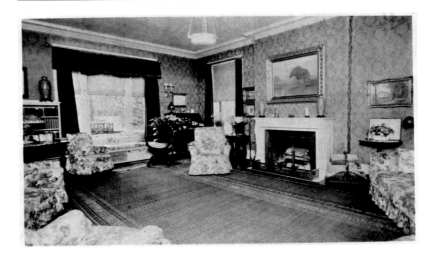

symmetry of means and ends.

The decor of modern living rooms described and illustrated in decorating advice books of the 1910s and 1920s contained many fewer things than the properly refined parlor had at the turn of the century (fig. 1). Deliberate simplification was another harbinger of change in priorities, at least among the authors of such advice and, presumably, among self-consciously up-to-date housekeepers. Changing ideas about domestic sanitation increasingly made some kinds of upholstery seem dirty; rich-looking but dust-catching chenille, for example, disappeared as a fabric for portières and table covers. Charlotte Calkins urged home economics teachers to instruct students to avoid "fringes and tassels...as they serve only to catch dust" (fig. 2).[8]

In those decades, the lives of women became more public as they entered the world of modern shopping and, aided by the automobile, participated in new forms of commercialized leisure. Because fewer servants were available, women who had once been able to rely upon the help of at least a part-time laundress took over all housework.[9] Parlors—even shut-up, rarely used "sacrificial parlors"—required more maintenance than some women were willing to supply. The authors of *The Modern Priscilla Home Furnishing Book* announced to readers, "We have discovered that the world is full of a number of things beside the routine of housekeeping."[10]

Smaller living spaces, changes in housewives' work patterns and priorities, and new, compelling outlets for spending discretionary income were accompanied by the decreasing power of the idea of the parlor as a world within a room, the emblem of family living, and the memory palace of culture. Parlors that were deliberately simplified did appear as early as the 1890s, but they still contained some objects that functioned to support these earlier notions about the room (fig. 3). Displays of mementoes on the desk or mantel and the "art group" of ceramics and glass atop the center table remained common through the 1890s. In decorating advice books of the 1910s and 1920s, the living room was discussed and illustrated as a room carefully stripped of many of the objects that Victorian culture enjoyed displaying and contemplating — emblems of personal cultivation, from fancy needlework to appropriately didactic books, and the eclectic mix of furnishings that carried historical or exotic associations. Helen Adler, the author of *The New Interior: Modern Decorations for the Modern Home* (1916), instructed her readers that "objects of sentimental associations, of affected culture, together with

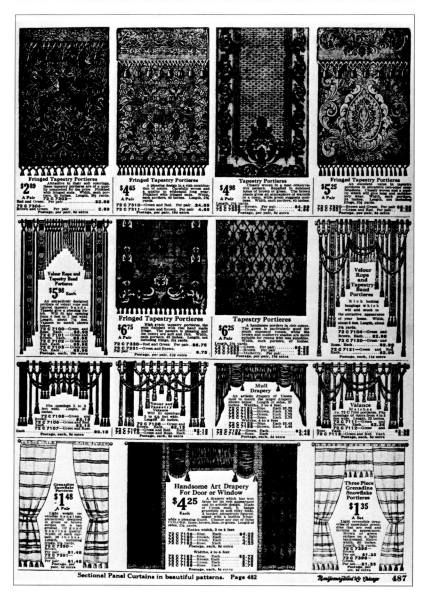

Fig. 2. Door drapery, illustration in Montgomery Ward and Co. Catalogue No. 97, Fall and Winter *(1922-1923).* When progressive house furnisher Charlotte Wait Calkins argued that "portières made of ropes, cords, beads, bamboo, or shells serve no real purpose," she missed one point in favor of their use—creating vignettes through doorways for aesthetic pleasure. Although the use of such upholstery was waning, Montgomery Ward still saw fit to offer an entire page of rope, tapestry, and lighter cotton portières and door valances in 1922.

certain heirlooms and souvenirs which the scheme of decoration refuses to assimilate, should find a happy end in a memory chest where the viewing of them at intervals provides a source of interest and amusement."[11]

Like advice authors describing successful parlor decor fifty years earlier, authors offering guides to living room furnishings suggested that such rooms were successful when they reflected the attributes and aspirations of their owners. However, the nature of those reflections had changed. Helen Koues, author of a number of decorating books and articles for the magazine *Good Housekeeping*, instructed her readers that expressing "individuality" was one of the most important principles that could guide furnishing living rooms. Desirable rooms were "sympathetic," as were desirable personalities.[12] Their furnishings had "charm," another attribute of the modern personality.[13] One of the most influential volumes promoting the cult of "personality" in interiors was Emily Post's *The Personality of a House*; first published in 1930, it was reprinted a number of times through the 1940s.[14]

Fig. 3. Parlor of "Home owned by Constance Winsor Noyes, 71 Sparks St., Cambridge," Massachusetts, photograph by Pack Brothers, January 1895. This dramatically simplified interior probably was meant to be "colonial," but it contained such characteristically Victorian upholstery as a reception chair and a Morris chair covered with a lace tidy. Courtesy Society for the Preservation of New England Antiquities.

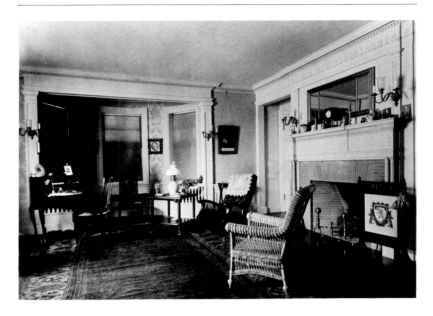

The argument that living rooms properly revealed the personality of a family employed a twentieth-century understanding of the nature of the individual to restate the earlier argument that a parlor should reveal a family's true character rather than its social facade. Occasionally the old rhetoric of "sincere" furnishing appeared again, as when Helen Adler wrote that "homes which cannot free themselves from the clutter of trivial and futile objects are mute declarations of the insincerity of their creator's pretensions to good taste and refinement in other directions."[15]

The early twentieth-century design reformers often were progressives with ties to the Arts and Crafts movement, manual arts training, and social work; they offered a critique of the parlor and its contents that was based upon a narrow, proto-modernist definition of "function." When function was defined as "physical use," it excluded the Victorian conception that parlor furnishings could be used symbolically to make statements about the personal domestic world of family and friends and the world of culture outside the parlor's walls. Charlotte Calkins's *A Course in House Planning and Furnishing* (1916), a book intended as a guide to high school teachers, analyzed common household furnishings in categories related to their appearance and appropriate function. Her notes on selecting furniture urged students to ask such questions as, "Will this article be consistent with its surroundings? For what purpose is it to be used? Will it serve this purpose in a simple, honest, straight-forward manner?"[16] Calkins too demanded sincerity in furnishing, a state that could only be attained through rigorously editing both the design and quantity of personal possessions. Middle-class people were supposed to be functional rather than showy or aspiring; so were middle-class furnishings.

Calkins was one of many reformers who attacked the continuing preferences of ordinary consumers for the old aesthetic of refinement, with its emphasis on rich pattern, visually complex design, naturalistic ornament, and room compositions whose multiple layers had equivalent levels of visual detail. A series of compare-and-contrast exercises with lecture notes composed this critique. A plate comparing "good" and "bad" sofa pillows was accompanied by the statement, "Pictures on sofa pillows and all other objects are out of place. No one should want to rest his head on anything that resembles real rose thorns, tennis rackets, pipes, flags, Indian heads

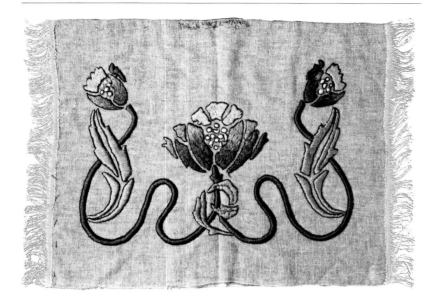

Fig. 4. Pillow sham, mercerized cotton embroidery on linen, 1900-1910. Charlotte Calkins would have approved of the design of this "arts and crafts" pillow sham, which bears an abstracted, conventional design of poppies embroidered on a coarse linen ground with a simple cut fringe for trim. The debate over the relative merits of "naturalistic" versus "conventional" design had been taking place since the publication of Eastlake's Hints on Household Taste *(1868), but designs like this one remained popular through the 1920s.*

and the like. Any of these ideas may be taken as a motif and treated in a flat conventional way, which will be appropriate for a flat surface and will conform to the shape and purpose of a pillow, but the designs will then be far from realistic. Avoid sofa pillows with elaborate ruffles, tassels, or other disconcerting details" (fig. 4).[17]

Edward Stratton Holloway, author of the popular book *The Practical Book of Furnishing the Small House and Apartment* (1922) argued that the taste for naturalism was "vulgar" because of the poor quality of products expressing it; he singled out for criticism the "rose-bedecked carpet" and "mats containing lifelike portraits of huge dogs."[18] These were the sort of naturalistic designs that Victorian Americans found so thrilling in their realism. The author of *Household Discoveries* (1909) also described the "modern tendency" for simplicity, pointing out that the most beloved of parlor upholstery —"flounces, valances, and other superfluous articles," as well as "stuffed plush and other upholstered articles of furniture in bright colors"—were "much less fashionable than formerly" (fig. 5).[19]

The specificity of Calkins's plates—page upon page of leather-covered Turkish rockers, doorstops shaped like dogs, banquet lamps with ruffled shades, and lace curtains woven to give the illusion of festoons and tassles—and Holloway's examples of unsuitable furnishings suggest that both critics still found much to react against in the typical front room of the ordinary household. Indeed, the upholstery of living rooms between 1910 and 1930 was an intriguing blend of old and new. Sometimes the changes in the forms and materials were accommodations to changes in house design. In 1909, *The Furniture Worker* published an article called "The Bungalow's Effect on Draperies," noting that the style, with its lower ceilings and short but wide window enframements, encouraged the use of simple curtains of "scrim or madras," stenciled cotton, or English chintz or cretonne. The article noted that "elaborate draperies" still were appropriate for "French" or "period" rooms in grander houses.[20] Such practical matters as the installation of domestic systems also changed home upholstery. Window treatments, for example, often consisted of the same elements —valance, side panels, sheer curtains, and shades—but they might be cut short to accommodate radiators (figs. 6 and 7).

The ideal of matching furnishings survived, but the prized parlor suite became the living room suite in the 1910s and 1920s. It was a

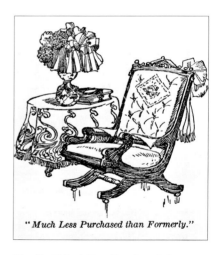

"*Much Less Purchased than Formerly.*"

Fig. 5. "Much Less Purchased than Formerly," engraving in Household Discoveries *(1909).*

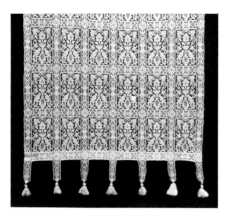

Fig. 6. Lace window shade, 1910-1930. Lace window shades were a simplified solution for housekeepers who still wished to retain drapery panels, valances, and sheer curtains on windows.

bulky, overstuffed three-piece group that still sometimes included a rocking chair. Ideas about the three-piece living room set displayed continuity with ideas about the hierarchy of forms in parlor suites. Illustrating a living room in "good taste," *The Modern Priscilla Home Furnishing Book* noted that the "big easy chair" was intended for a father, a medium-size "women's chair" for mother, and the "davenport" for the children.[21]

The economics of factory-organized upholstery, perfected by the 1890s, were put to good use in such furniture, especially when no wood that required careful finishing (or that simply was required to be of the same kind) was exposed to view. In the three pieces of a set from the 1920s, the large form is not full of stuffing but consists of a shallow deck of springs and stuffing constructed over a deep hollow well, like the box couch and "Roman divan." Such pieces could have had long finished wooden legs, but instead they are largely empty wooden boxes with fabric covers, implying the presence of layers of upholstery that do not actually exist (fig. 8; plate 46). Such sets also continued to meet popular requirements for richness and detail through their fabric covers. Better pieces sometimes employed "modern" interpretations of nineteenth-century upholstery techniques. A sofa made by the Wolverine Upholstery Company of Grand Rapids, Michigan, around 1930, demonstrates interest in detail by including ruffling and large plush buttons on its arms, as well as decorative loose cushions with contrasting patterned tops, even as it fulfilled new requirements for large, comfortable living room furniture (fig. 9).

Popular preferences for upholstery that had rich, deep colors and texture and displayed a certain amount of elaboration and detail survived into the 1920s (fig. 10). Exotica also continued to be popular, in both novel materials and upholstery colors and design. Turkish pattern in rugs and fabrics was acceptable to adherents of the

Fig. 7. "Three-Piece Colonial Curtains," illustration in Montgomery Ward and Company Catalog No. 97, Fall and Winter (1922-1923). Meant to be hung flat, without impromptu festoons made from the folded-over tops, these lace curtains were short enough to hang clear of steam radiators below windows.

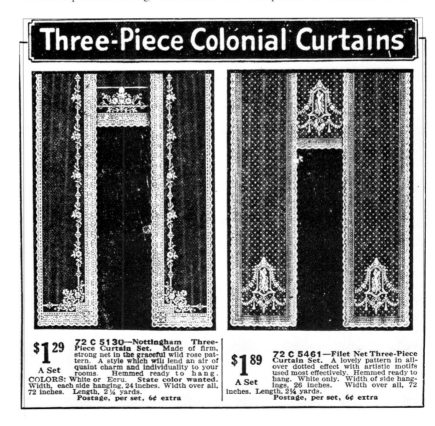

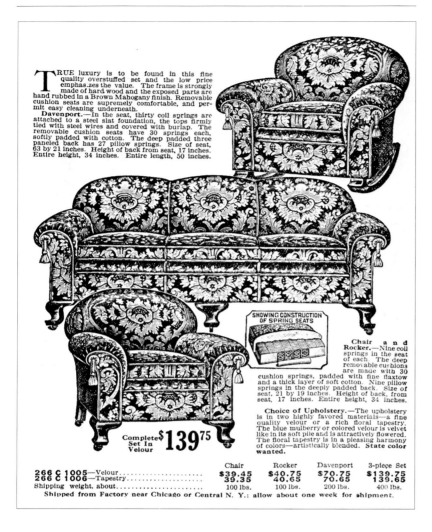

TRUE luxury is to be found in this fine quality overstuffed set and the low price emphasizes the value. The frame is strongly made of hard wood and the exposed parts are hand rubbed in a Brown Mahogany finish. Removable cushion seats are supremely comfortable, and permit easy cleaning underneath.

Davenport.—In the seat, thirty coil springs are attached to a steel slat foundation, the tops firmly tied with steel wires and covered with burlap. The removable cushion seats have 30 springs each, softly padded with cotton. The deep padded three paneled back has 27 pillow springs. Size of seat, 63 by 21 inches. Height of back from seat, 17 inches. Entire height, 34 inches. Entire length, 50 inches.

SHOWING CONSTRUCTION OF SPRING SEATS

Chair and Rocker.—Nine coil springs in the seat of each. The deep removable cushions are made with 30 cushion springs, padded with fine flaxtow and a thick layer of soft cotton. Nine pillow springs in the deeply padded back. Size of seat, 21 by 19 inches. Height of back, from seat, 17 inches. Entire height, 34 inches.

Choice of Upholstery.—The upholstery is in two highly favored materials—a fine quality velour or a rich floral tapestry. The blue mulberry or colored velour is velvet like in its soft pile and is attractively flowered. The floral tapestry is in a pleasing harmony of colors—artistically blended. **State color wanted.**

Complete Set In Velour **$139⁷⁵**

	Chair	Rocker	Davenport	3-piece Set
266 C 1005—Velour	$39.45	$40.75	$70.75	$139.75
266 C 1006—Tapestry	39.35	40.65	70.65	139.65
Shipping weight, about	100 lbs.	100 lbs.	200 lbs.	400 lbs.

Shipped from Factory near Chicago or Central N. Y.: allow about one week for shipment.

Fig. 8. "Big Values in Overstuffed Sets," illustration in Montgomery Ward and Co. Catalogue No. 97, Fall and Winter (1922-1923).

modern living room, although not for its exotic associations. However, popular taste approved of and enjoyed new forms of domesticated exotica in such diverse forms as "tropical" motifs, rayon, and other novel materials (plates 47-49).

Concerns about sanitation did not spell the end of inviting piles of elaborately stitched sofa pillows, lace curtains, and other now-traditional kinds of upholstery. Consumers probably heeded these concerns selectively, consigning the worst offenders to the attic as they continued to use other types of upholstery. Even though chenille disappeared as a portière fabric, portières were used in houses through the mid-1920s, even the purely ornamental rope portière.[22] Drapery still made living room furnishings more ceremonial in character.

Neither did popular interest in historical revivals in furniture disappear. Rather, it was channeled in new directions. By the 1920s, consumers typically could purchase "Jacobean" and "Spanish" or "Italian Renaissance" (the forerunner of contemporary "Mediterranean") furniture. They also could purchase "colonial," which often had much in common with Jacobean revival furnishings. Better furniture makers sometimes made historical revival upholstery quite accurate in appearance (figs. 11 and 12; plate 50). "French" and "Turkish" furnishings generally had disappeared from ordinary catalogs and furniture stores, although relatively expensive versions of eighteenth-century French forms were available for those consumers

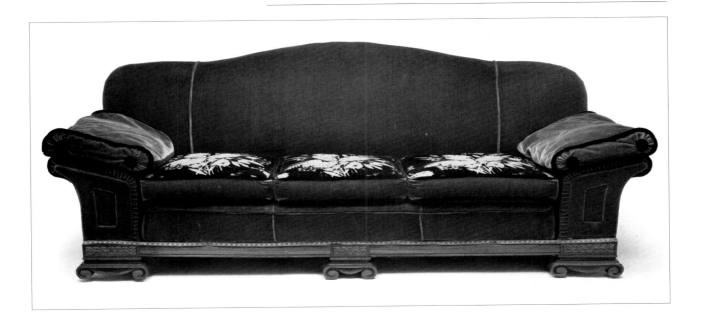

Fig. 9. Sofa, maple, mohair plush, Wolverine Upholstery Company, Grand Rapids, Michigan, about 1930. This sofa attests the continuing popularity of mohair plush and the use of Victorian techniques to create visual interest in upholstery: ruffling (on the arms), contrasting trims (here, cording covered with back mohair plush), and contrasting fabrics in the reversible seat cushions with a design of tropical plants in black, red, and shades of yellow on one side. Courtesy Grand Rapids Public Museum.

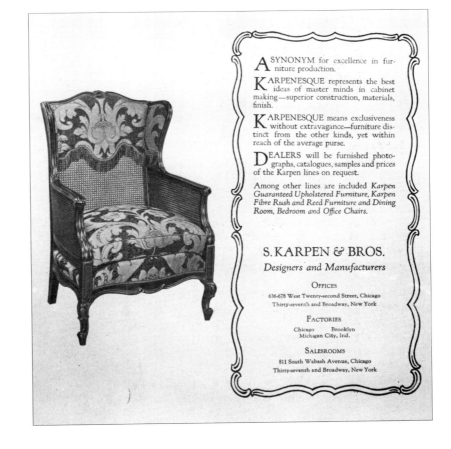

A SYNONYM for excellence in furniture production.

K ARPENESQUE represents the best ideas of master minds in cabinet making—superior construction, materials, finish.

K ARPENESQUE means exclusiveness without extravagance—furniture distinct from the other kinds, yet within reach of the average purse.

D EALERS will be furnished photographs, catalogues, samples and prices of the Karpen lines on request.

Among other lines are included *Karpen Guaranteed Upholstered Furniture, Karpen Fibre Rush and Reed Furniture and Dining Room, Bedroom and Office Chairs.*

S. KARPEN & BROS.
Designers and Manufacturers

OFFICES

636-678 West Twenty-second Street, Chicago
Thirty-seventh and Broadway, New York

FACTORIES

Chicago   Brooklyn
Michigan City, Ind.

SALESROOMS

811 South Wabash Avenue, Chicago
Thirty-seventh and Broadway, New York

Fig. 10. Advertisement for S. Karpen and Brothers, Chicago, Illinois, published in the Grand Rapids Furniture Record *(February 1919). Karpen's eclectic interpretation of a colonial wing chair featured upholstery on the chair's back intended to look like a fringed window valance. Courtesy Grand Rapids Public Library.*

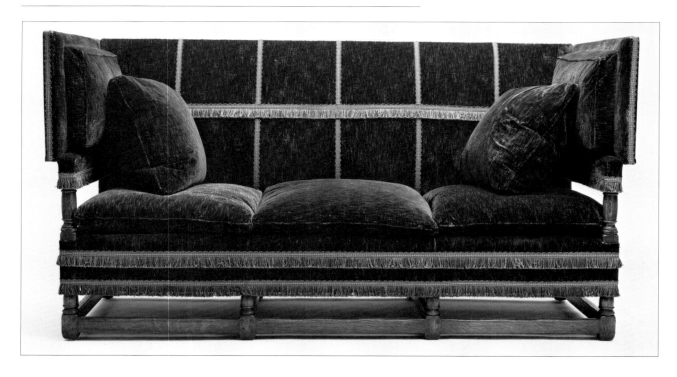

who still wished to create gala rooms for themselves from manufacturers of furniture of high quality, such as S. Karpen and Co. in Chicago.

In Jacobean and American colonial furnishings, the two most popular historical styles through the 1920s, the point of reference for furniture manufacturers and consumers seems to have shifted from French to English models. Given the nineteenth-century contrast of French formality and fashion with Anglo-American domesticity and comfort, this change may indicate some resolution of the tension in points of cultural reference. It may also have been one signal of the gradual waning of Victorianism, with its insistence that more things, and more complicated-looking things, signaled refinement and the progress of civilization. Not having experienced the direct shock of World War I's destruction of lives and land, Victorian culture in the United States faded more slowly than it did in Europe. On the continent, the lingering effects of the four-year slaughter provided a fertile field for the design revolution of Corbusier, the Futurists, and the Machine Age, as well as one final decorative reinterpretation of French eighteenth-century furniture in the *Style Moderne* (Art Deco), popularly introduced in the Paris *Exposition International des Arts Decoratifs et Industriels Modernes* of 1925.

The appearance of much upholstery in the ordinary living room of the 1920s actually contributed little to the room's sense of style, although sometimes historical fabrics and modern forms were mixed in incongruous ways (figs. 13-15). Ultimately, the upholstery of typical living rooms had little to state about the softening, polishing effects of culture. Nonetheless, living room furnishings suggested greater informality and bodily comfort even as they played a smaller role in the less home-centered world view of post-Victorian America.

Among manufacturers and consumers with no particular axe to grind, the term "living room" replaced "parlor" gradually. In furniture advertising, the former term was common by around 1910. By 1919, it had completely replaced "parlor" in articles in the *Grand Rapids Furniture Record*, a trade magazine for the furniture business.

Fig. 11. Couch, oak, cotton velveteen with silk trim, Century Furniture Company, Grand Rapids, Michigan, 1925-1930. The Century Furniture Company (1900-1940) produced a wide range of cabinetwork and upholstery in both "modern" and historical styles. Its reproduction furniture often closely copied existing pieces, as did this version of a famous ratchet-arm sofa at Knole in England dating from the reign of Charles II. The Century version contains springs in its deck below the loose cushions and in its back, however, and the adjustable arms employ stainless steel ratchets. The upholstery velvet was woven with dyed faded places and a repeated pattern of distress marks. Century sold this piece direct from the factory for $360 in 1928; it represents the highest quality of "Jacobean revival" upholstered furniture available in the 1920s. Courtesy Grand Rapids Public Museum.

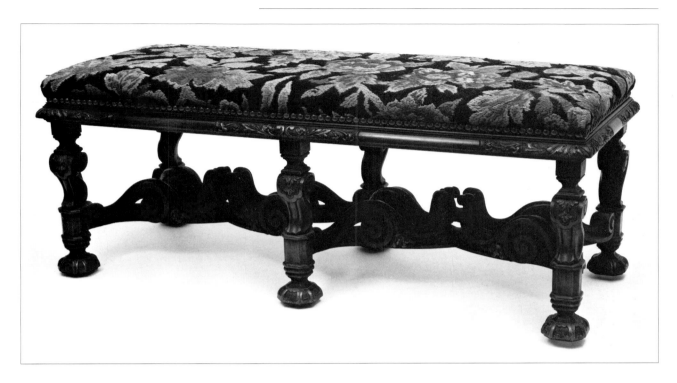

Fig. 12. Bench, walnut, hooked cotton on canvas, Century Furniture Company, Grand Rapids, Michigan, 1920-1935. Sold as a "Jacobean hearth bench," the Century Furniture Company provided an interpretation of seventeenth-century upholstery on this piece. Courtesy Grand Rapids Public Museum.

However, through the first thirty years of the twentieth century, houses continued to have parlors, even if they were called living rooms (or sometimes "front rooms," a designation that was especially apt in urban apartments where the parlor was the only room facing the street). Furnished with the best pieces in the house, they continued to be reserved for occasions of state.

The age of a family sometimes accounted for such continuity in habits of use. The Ruth family of Lebanon, Pennsylvania, occupied a Georgian revival house built in the early 1890s that featured the traditional pair of parlors connected by a wide doorway. The room facing the street served as a formal parlor (and the term "parlor" was always used) until around 1956. It contained a sofa covered in horsehair (a colonial revival upholstery), several small chairs, a pier glass with a table that held a lamp whose crystal drops reflected light, a chandelier, and a baby grand piano. The back parlor, which had been decorated with mission furniture before 1910, was the "library" or "study." As the Neupert family of Buffalo, New York, and the Yearick family of Konnarock, Virginia, also had done, the Ruths customarily sat in this back room every day. The parlor, enframed by the wide doorway, became a vignetted view, a reminder of their most formal social selves.[23] Recent ascension to economic status that permitted furnishing a parlor also accounted for the creation of formal rooms that saw little everyday use, as social workers noted in reports on working-class life in the early twentieth century.

The desire to maintain traditions of use may also have contributed to decisions to keep formal parlors. In rural communities, such rites of passage as funerals (including laying out the dead) were not delegated to new settings such as funeral parlors but continued to take place at home well into the twentieth century. John Arnold, who was born and raised in the north central Pennsylvania community of Warren, recalls the laying out of his grandfather in the parlor in 1930. So that the old man's last night at home would not be spent alone, fourteen-year-old John was required to spend the night in the parlor with the coffin, sleeping on a fully reclined Morris

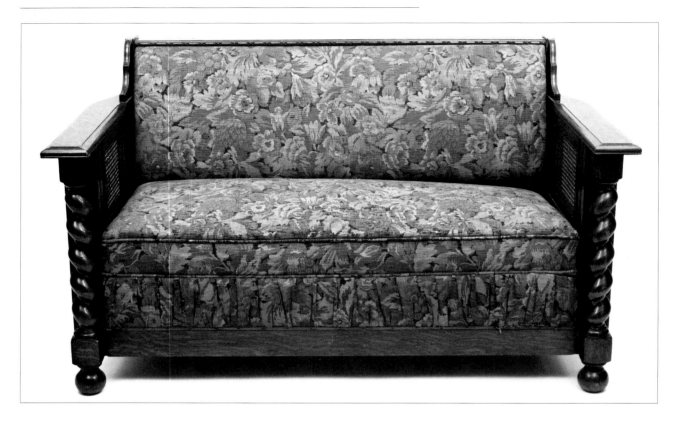

chair. Arnold recalls that the same room also was the site for courtship and holiday celebrations in the house.[24]

Even when the room was called a living room and furnished in an informal fashion, it was sometimes treated as a formal parlor. The house in which Robert Vance Stewart grew up in the teens and twenties had been constructed by his grandfather in 1887 and contained three generations of the family. The first floor contained a "living room," dining room, kitchen, pantry, and a small bedroom. The kitchen saw the most daily use and contained a couch, two sewing machines, and a rocking chair as well as the usual appliances and kitchen furniture. The living room, on the other hand, "wasn't used very much on a day to day basis. Saturdays, Sundays, and holidays, when we had company. When Eleanor [his sister] was taking piano lessons she went in there every day to practice." The room contained a sofa, chairs, the piano, a gramophone, desk, bookcase, and a library/center table, which still was used as the locus for reading and other activities.[25]

Thus, patterns of room use, the requirements of changing domestic architecture and housekeeping routines, and the forms and aesthetic qualities of upholstery associated with the living room changed gradually and unevenly between 1910 and 1930. Some families continued to have parlors in spirit, if not in name. This tradition still survives; in South Philadelphia, for example, Italian-American families continue to keep parlors with wall-to-wall carpeting, overstuffed furniture draped with antimacassars, and elaborate ruffled draperies. Modern suburban house plans that distinguish a "den" or "family room" from the "living room" follow, in essence, the distinction between everyday "sitting room" and "parlor" to which many Victorian families adhered.

Even so, these modern-day parlors differ from their Victorian predecessors in the ways their owners thought about them.

Fig. 13. Sofa bed, oak, cotton tapestry, Kindel Bed Company, Grand Rapids, Michigan, 1912-1915. Charles J. Kindel had developed the first shorter sofas that folded out into long beds at the turn of the century. This Kindel "Parlor Bed" (a term used in the firm's advertising) is typical of most Jacobean revival furniture of the 1910s and 1920s. Its style is signaled mainly by the twist turnings below the arms; the floral tapestry cover was one of the most popular upholstery fabrics of those decades, although its soft, unmercerized cotton fibers absorbed dirt and became dingy fairly quickly. Apart from the woven pattern, the upholstery is decorated only by ruffling across the front. Courtesy Grand Rapids Public Museum.

Figs. 14 and 15. *Tub chairs, mahogany, mohair frisé, Century Furniture Company, Grand Rapids, Michigan, 1930-1935. The lines of these small armchairs reflect developing interest in streamlined-looking furniture by 1930. They also carry style information in their looped pile upholstery; the patterned freize makes one chair "Jacobean" while the other is "modern." All the Century Furniture Company pieces illustrated here are in excellent condition because they were purchased by a Saginaw, Michigan, couple in the early 1930s for a planned house that was never built. A large collection of Century Furniture remained in storage until it was given to the Grand Rapids Public Museum in 1982. Courtesy Grand Rapids Public Museum.*

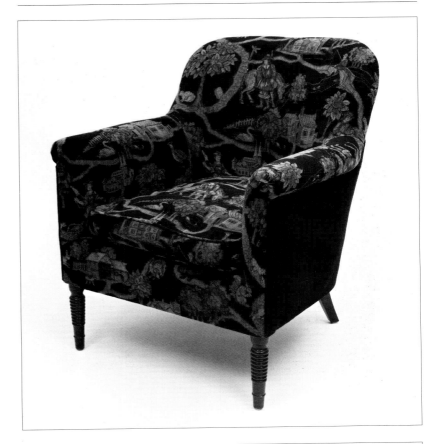

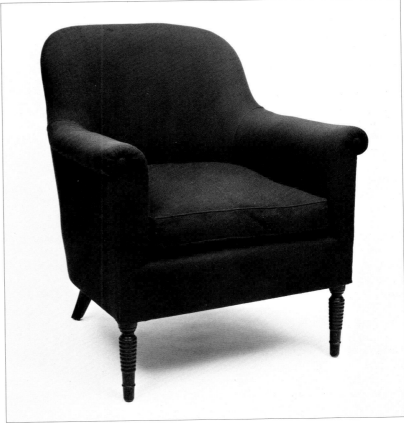

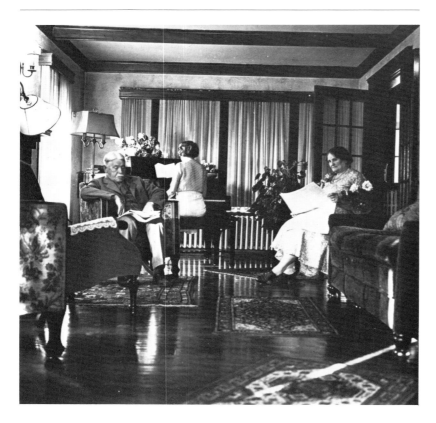

Fig. 16. *"Living room in home of Mr. A. Gilford Rounsdell, West Roxbury, Massachusetts," about 1930. The Rounsdell family used its living room much as the Appleton family had used its parlor in the 1870s (see chapter 2, fig. 1). The families presented themselves for their photographs in strikingly similar ways as well.*

Something more fundamental than the chair types and the appearance of window drapery had changed. The parlor's power as a central location for symbols lessened as families turned outward and linked themselves to urban and suburban communities that could provide new services and entertainments. The Victorian cast of mind, embellishing and commercializing the eighteenth-century concept of gentility and finding meaning in the progressive refinement of the world, did not disappear by 1930, but it probably had a generational boundary. It was a dying world view.

If anything, belief in the desirability of owning things was even more widespread, and their skillful use for the purposes of self-presentation counted just as much in 1925 as it had in 1875 (fig. 16). Being middle class—having that state of mind both compelled and repelled by consumption as a form of rhetoric, seeking a balance between culture and comfort—may be a fundamental component in a dynamic consumer society. The constant tension between purchasing and saving, restraint and desire must always be present, even if the cultural framework that shapes questions about what is valuable and worthy evolves over time. In the context of a developing consumer society, both the Victorian polarity of cultured self-display and sincere domestic comfort were articulated through forms of consumption, through furnishing as well as through the rhetoric of popular literature. In the post-Victorian era, the era of the living room, a different dynamic tension framed questions about domestic consumption and self-presentation.

A GLOSSARY OF TEXTILE TERMS

This glossary presents contemporary definitions of the textiles used for upholstering seating furniture between 1850 and 1930. Six sources have been used to compile these definitions, each of which will be followed by the source's short title and its publication date.

Brown, C. M., and C. L. Gates. *Scissors and Yardstick; or, All about Dry Goods.* Hartford, CT: C. M. Brown and F. W. Jaqua, 1872. "A Complete Manual, Giving a Detailed Description of Each Article Included in the Several Departments, Together With Upholstery and House-Furnishing Goods; Also, A List of All the Principal Dry Goods Manufacturing Cities and Towns Of the World."

Cassell's Domestic Dictionary: An Encyclopedia for the Household. London, Paris, and New York: Cassell, Petter, Galpin and Co., 1878.

Cole, George A. et al. *Cole's Dictionary of Dry Goods.* Rev. ed. Chicago: W. B. Conkey Co., 1892.

Denny, Grace Goldena. *Fabrics and How to Know Them.* 3d ed. Philadelphia: J. B. Lippincott Company, 1928.

Hunter, George Leland. *Decorative Textiles: An Illustrated Book on the Coverings for Furniture, Walls and Floors.*...Philadelphia and London: J. B. Lippincott Company, 1918.

Spitzli, Alfred. *A Manual for Managers, Designers, Weavers, and All Others Connected with the Manufacture of Textile Fabrics.*...West Troy, NY: A. and A. F. Spitzli, 1881.

Artificial Leather. *See* Leather Cloth.

Armure. Drapery fabric with designs woven on a rep foundation, or a figure weave. Plain or mixed colors usually of cotton. Uses: couch covers, portieres. Weave—Jacquard. Width, 50"....Name derived from French "Armoires" meaning coat-of-arms.
Fabrics (1928)

Brocade. A rich silk fabric, ornamented and enriched with flowers, fruits, and other designs, wrought in gold and silver. This is of very ancient manufacture, and now, by reason of its great expense, it is imitated in silk, *colors* being used to represent the gold and silver.
Scissors and Yardstick (1872)

Brocatel. A fabric composed of a fine linen warp and coarse woollen woof. It is woven in damask patterns, stripes, etc., either plain or colored. The surface of the figure or stripe is twilled. This figure is formed by the warp, which in the cheapest grades is usually black. A superior quality is composed entirely of wool, and called "wool damask."
Scissors and Yardstick (1872)

Brocatel. A coarse or inferior brocade or figured fabric, commonly made of silk or cotton, or sometimes of cotton only, but having a more or less silky surface; used chiefly for curtains, furniture-covering, tapestry linings, and linings for carriages.
Cole's (1892)

Buckram (or Burlap). A coarse, hempen cloth, woven plain. It is very heavy, and stiffened with glue.
Scissors and Yardstick (1872)

Carpet Upholstery. *See* Moquette; Tapestry, Brussels.

Chenille. French for caterpillar. 1. Name for a yarn having a pile protruding all around at right angles. Used for filling in cloth, also for fringe and tassels. May be of silk, wool, mercerized cotton or rayon. 2. Cloth made with Chenille yarn for filling, used for hangings and couch covers. 3. Kind of carpet or rug reversible (Smyrna type) or single faced. Plain color or designs. Good quality, rich looking and durable.
Fabrics (1928)

Chintz (Hindoo *chhint*, spotted). Cotton cloth printed with flowers or other patterns of bright colors, and finished with a glaze. The only difference between Chintz and Cretonne consists in the glazing of the former, which is effected by calendering. Chintz is also known under the name of *furniture print*, from its extensive use in covering furniture. About 1850 glazed chintz was greatly used for furniture, and some of the patterns which have survived are quite surprisingly bad. For this reason, and the fact that chair covers were gone out of fashion, the majority of the world got tired of Chintzes, when some enterprising manufacturer saw the beauty which might lie in a fabric called Cretonne—which is simply a Chintz without a glaze. It is a question whether Chintz is ever either suitable or salable in a town. Its extreme daintiness seems as out of place in the grime and grind of a city as the innocent chat of a country cousin seems almost like a reproach to the short-haired advocate of "women's rights." But the soft tints and darker shades of Cretonne are always harmonious, and it is asserted by artists there is no fabric with the exception of Brocade which looks so well for upholstery purposes. Chintzes are all block-printed, the principal dyes being madder, weld and indigo.
Cole's (1892)

Chintz. Chintz is the English word, cretonne the French word, for drapery prints. Consequently, when the two words are used side by side, we are apt to find the English prints, particularly those of many colours, fine texture and small floral designs, called chintzes, whilst the French prints of larger design on heavier cloth are called cretonnes. The chintzes used in England are often glazed, but the difficulty of having them freshened by re-glazing in America, has prevented glazed chintzes from becoming popular here. Murray's great dictionary defines chintz as "Originally, name of painted or stained calicoes imported from India; now, cotton cloths fast printed with designs of flowers, etc., generally not less than five colours and usually glazed."

Decorative Textiles (1918)

Cottons, Furniture. Various cotton weaves [are] used by American printers to secure various effects. The obvious peculiarities of the weaves are: (1) *Homespun*, fine warp with coarse, irregular weft, that gives a ribbed and homespun look to the surface. (2) *Swansdown*, an open, plain weave with fuzzy yarn that gives a fleecy surface. (3) *Almos silk*, a silkoline embossed to increase the lustre. (4) *Ticking*, a firm and heavy warp twill for hard wear, as the name implies. (5) *Crepoline*, a sateen embossed to increase lustre and give crepy effect. (6) *Scrim*, a plain, open weave. (7) *French rep*, fine warp and coarse weft that produces the rep effect. (8) *Antoinette rep*, a coarse, flat rep produced by inserting the coarse wefts in pairs. (9) *Voile*, like scrim, but finer and harder spun. (10) *Tuileries cloth*, a cotton taffeta figured by floating the wefts. (11) *Marquisette*, a net formed by warps twisting in pairs around the wefts. (12) *Krinkle cloth*, a plain, open weave embossed to give the crinkly effect to Austrian shades. (13) *Standish cloth*, a firm and durable plain weave with diagonal ribs formed by coarse wefts that interlace pairs of warps. (14) *Terry cloth*, a shaggy, irregular weave with twisted and uncut warp pile. (15) *Madras*, marquisette (see above) figured by weaving in pairs of soft extra wefts and then cutting away the floats. The rough side is the right side. (16) *Silkoline*, a cheap, plain, open weave of fine yarn, finished to look as silky as possible. (17) *Dimity*, warp twill stripes in relief on ground of plain weave. (18) *Crash*, plain, loose weave of irregular yarn. (19) *Sateen*, a coarse cotton satin with weft instead of warp surface. (20) *Norman cloth*, a cotton taffeta with tiny relief figures formed by floating the wefts.

Decorative Textiles (1918)

Cretonne (derived from the name of the first maker, *M. Cretonne*, of Paris). Originally a strong white fabric of hempen warp and linen weft, with various textures of surface, sometimes plain but oftener twilled or "momied." Forty years ago, when chintzes went out of fashion an enterprising Philadelphia manufacturer saw the beauty which might lie in printing the white cretonne with delicate patterns and finishing it with a glaze, and forthwith placed his inspiration upon the market. The fabric came into immediate and permanent popularity. It is used for many household purposes, chiefly however for curtains, chair and sofa coverings.

Cole's (1892)

Damask. A fabric originally made at Damascus, in imitation of brocade. It is composed of silk, or silk and linen; wool, and sometimes cotton, is also employed in its manufacture. It has two sets of woof threads, the one of linen, double, and the other single, of silk, which appear upon the surface only around the raised figures. The warp is of silk, very slightly twisted. It forms the figures in relief upon the surface by overlapping the woof. Damask is usually made of one plain color, but sometimes two or more are employed. It is used for curtains, furniture covering, etc. Single and double fold. Width, 21 inches to 7-4.

Scissors and Yardstick (1872)

Damask. A textile fabric woven in elaborate patterns, of various designs, as flowers, leaves, foliage, etc., woven in the loom. So called not because of having been originally woven at Damascus (as is so often stated) but on account of the perfection at one time attained by the Damascene weavers….At present the term signifies either of two entirely different materials: (1) *Curtain Damask*, which is made of silk and wool or silk and cotton, in large vari-colored patterns woven up in the loom, used chiefly for curtains, portieres and furniture covering; and (2) *Table Damask*, which is a fine twilled linen fabric, used solely for table linen….It is, with a few exceptions, ornamented with a pattern that is shown by the opposite reflections of light from its surface, without contrast of color.

Damasked. Fabrics ornamented on the surface with flowers or other patterns having a running figure, produced by weaving and not by printing or stamping. The word "damasked" when applied to linen textures or to mixed materials when used for upholstery purposes, has much the same meaning as "brocaded" when applied to silk and wool textures.

Cole's (1892)

Fringes. This form of trimming and decoration for dress and furniture is of very ancient date, and is mentioned in the Pentateuch in connection with the hangings of the Tabernacle and Temple, and the vestments of the priests. It is formed of ends of silk, linen, worsted, and gold or silver twist, according to circumstances, and depends from a band of the same material. The length of the fringe depends on the article it is designed to decorate. For furniture it varies from two to four inches in depth, and there are three descriptions—plain head, plain head and bullion, and gimp head. For dress their depth varies from half an inch to two or three inches. The epaulettes of naval and military officers are of bullion.

Cassell's (1878)

Frisé. From the Latin "crispare (crispus, frisé)" to curl. Pile fabric (usually mohair) of uncut loops. Designs may be produced by contrast of cut and uncut loops, by different colored yarns or by printing the surface. *Friezette** is a trade name. Use: upholstery. Weave—pile. Width, 27″, 28″.

Fabrics (1928)
Fig. 1

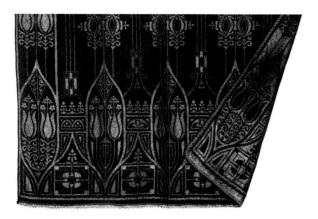

Fig. 1. *Detail of portière, mohair and silk frisé, probably Europe, 1900-1930.*

Gimp (from Fr. *guipure*, to whip round with silk). A flat trimming made by twisting silk or worsted threads round a silk foundation of wire; more or less open in design; used for borders of curtains and furniture trimmings, ladies' dresses, etc.

Cole's (1892)

Hair Cloth [also horsehair, hair-seating]. A fabric woven of the hair of horses' tails, used for sofa coverings, seatings, etc., and for stiffening of ladies' dresses. The hair used in this manufacture (which composes only the weft) is procured from South America and Russia. All the black and gray hair is dyed a deep lustrous black for the making of black hair cloth for covering furniture, while the light is reserved for dyeing the brighter hues, such as green, claret, crimson, etc. According to the length of the hair, so can this cloth be made in widths varying from 14 to 40 inches. The quality, as well as the brilliancy and permanency of the colors depend in a great degree on the nature of the warp, which may be either cotton, linen or worsted.

Cole's (1892)

Hair Cloth. Stiff, wiry fabric made of cotton, worsted or linen warp (usually cotton) and filling of horsehair. Fabric as wide as the length of a hair (horse's mane). One pick of the filling formed by a single hair. Black, white or gray. Uses: stiffening interlining, upholstering. Weave—plain or twill (herringbone). Width, 15", 18", 30".

Fabrics (1928)

Horsehair [also "hair manufacture"]. The various uses to which hair of different sorts is applied are familiar to every one. To prepare the curled hair for stuffing cushions, pillows and mattresses, short horse hair is carded between "teeth" or combs, beaten in a heap with a cane; curled and twisted round a cylinder of wood in cold water, then boiled and heated in an oven. It is then opened by partial uncurling in an opposite direction, and towzled or picked into curling pieces, by which operations they acquire a remarkable springy quality.

Cole's (1892)

Leather Cloth [also artificial leather, "American Cloth," "vegetable leather"]. A substitute for leather made by coating a cotton fabric with a nitro-cellulose preparation and embossing the surface to imitate leather. Various effects produced by kind of fabric foundation and the color and finish of surface. A good grade of manufactured leather is more durable than a poor grade of split leather. Sold under trade names as *Pantasote, Leatherwove, Fabrikoid, Zapon,* etc. Uses: upholstering, suit cases, millinery and dress trimmings.

Fabrics (1928)

Mohair. Mohair is the hair of the angora goat. The word is a corruption of the German *mohr* (a Moor). The material was first introduced into Spain by the Moors, and from thence brought into Germany. Under the head of ANGORA will be found a full account of the origin and production of this fiber. The following table indicates the amount of mohair fiber imported by this country for the last five years and the average price of same:

	Pounds.	Avg. price. Cents.
1887	842,527	26 5/8
1888	455,215	28 4-9
1889	1,841,312	28 3-10
1890	1,110,520	28 2-5
1891	1,679,599	26

Cole's (1892)

Mohair. "The silvery fleece." *Mohair* (Angora fleece) is *not a substitute for sheep's wool,* but occupies its own place among the textile fabrics. It has the aspect, feel and luster of silk without its suppleness. It differs materially from wool in the want of the felting quality, so that the stuffs made of it have the fibres distinctly separated and always brilliant. They do not retain dust or spots, and are thus particularly valuable for furniture goods. The fibre is dyed with great facility, and it is the only textile fibre that takes equally the dyes destined for all its tissues. On account of the stiffness of the fibre, it is rarely woven alone; that is, when used for filling, the warp is usually of cotton, silk or wool, and the reverse....The qualities of luster and elasticity peculiarly fit mohair for its chief use, the manufacture of Utrecht velvets commonly called furniture plush, the finest qualities of which are composed principally of mohair, the pile being formed of mohair warps, which are cut in the same manner as silk warps in velvets. Upon passing the finger lightly over the surface of the best mohair plushes, the rigidity and elasticity of the fibre will be distinctly perceived. The fibre springs back to its original uprightness when any pressure is removed. The best mohair plushes are almost indestructible. They have been in constant use on certain railroads in this country for twenty years without wearing out. They are now sought by all the best railroads in the country as the most enduring of all coverings.

A Manual (1881)

Moreen (formerly *moireen*, from moire). A fabric of mohair or wool filling and cotton warp; formerly made in imitation of moire silk, for purposes of upholstery. It was sometimes plain, but more commonly "watered" with embossed patterns by passing the cloth over a hot brass cylinder, on which was engraved various flowers and other fancy figures. At present it is manufactured to some extent and used for petticoats, bathing dresses, etc., and the heavier qualities for curtains.

Cole's (1892)

Moquette [also carpet upholstery]. (French *moquette*, tuft of wool.) A variety of carpeting, with a soft, velvety nap of wool, and a warp of hemp or linen.

Cole's (1892)

Plush. A term derived from French *peluch*, which in turn is derived from Latin *pilus*, hair, from the fact that when plush was first manufactured it was made with a worsted foundation and a pile of goat's hair or mohair. The use and manufacture of plush in Europe dates from the sixteenth century, though it is highly probable that a fabric similar in appearance has been woven in China from time immemorial. Plush may be roughly described as long napped velvet, and any kind of fiber may be used in its manufacture, the distinction from velvet being found in the *longer* and *less dense* pile upon the surface of plush....There are no plushes composed entirely of silk manufactured in this country, although cotton-back and mohair plushes are produced in fairly good qualities; in some instances being equal if not superior to the goods of Europe. This is especially true of the furniture plushes woven in Pennsylvania and Connecticut, and the exquisite seal plushes, woven in wide widths for winter cloaks and caps. The railroads of the United States consume about 40,000 yards of the best mohair plush for car seats every year, which large quantity up to the present time has been almost entirely supplied by our home mills. Crimped and embossed plush for furniture coverings are being produced in large quantities since the passage of the McKinley tariff act....Plush is embossed by means of large steel rollers, on the surface of which a pattern is cut in relief.

Cole's (1892)
Fig. 2

[By 1892, the date of this definition, wool plush had been largely replaced for upholstery use by mohair plush. —AUTHOR.]

Rayon (Fr. ray of light). Name adopted in 1924 for artificial silk. Formerly called manufactured silk, fibre silk and, for a short time, glos. Lustrous textile fibre made by converting cellulose (wood pulp or cotton linters), into a filament by means of a chemical and mechanical process. More lustrous and stiffer than silk; not so strong but less expensive; dyes readily. *Celanese**, made by the cellulose-acetate process has distinct characteristics. It appears and feels more like silk, responds only to special dyes, stronger when wet than other rayons, absorbs more slowly, is finer than viscose rayon (the process most commonly used) but costs more....Rayon yarns, used extensively in knitted goods, trimmings, laces, dress fabrics, alone or in combination with silk, cotton or wool. Many novelty fabrics are know by trade names as *Milo Sheen**, *Luminette**, and *Trico Sham**. Rayon dress fabrics have a tendency to hold wrinkles.

Fabrics (1928)

Rep. A heavy, woollen fabric, used for covering furniture; for curtains, lambraques, etc. It derives its name from its repped or corded appearance. This rep is formed by the coarse woof, which is composed of several threads twisted together, and is covered and concealed by the warp. Both surfaces are exactly alike, and about equally finished. In all except the very best qualities the woof is of cotton. Reps are made in all plain colors, but usually in colored stripes. Double fold. Width, 6-4.

Scissors and Yardstick (1872)

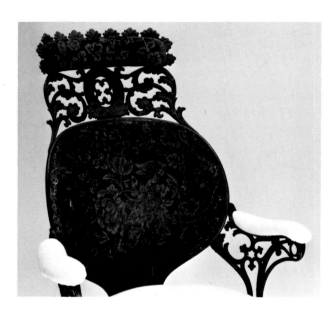

Fig. 2. *Centripetal spring chair, Thomas Warren, American Chair Co., Troy, New York, cast iron, sheet metal, wood, embossed wool plush upholstery, 1850-1860.*

Rep (corrupted from rib). A style of weaving in which the surface presents a transverse-ribbed appearance, by close, round twills or cords extending in a diagonal direction across the web. *Furniture rep* is a flowered cotton goods woven in this manner. *Worsted rep* is used for upholstering and curtains, and is 1½ yards wide, dyed in solid colors. *Silk rep* is used for ladies' dresses, ecclesiastical vestments, etc., and is narrow, usually 22 inches. The word is also applied to a thin worsted dress goods. In a general sense rep is used to describe any transversely-ribbed cloth, as distinct from "cords," which are of similar structure, but extending lengthwise of the fabric.

Cole's (1892)

Rep (repp) (probably a corruption of word "rib"). Closely resembles poplin. Rep has a heavier cord (filling yarn) and is a wider fabric used for hangings and upholstering. Cotton rep is usually mercerized. Piece- or yarn-dyed. Silk or wool may be used in combination with each other or with cotton. Variations in effect are produced by dyeing warp one color and filling another or by using an unevenly spun filling which gives variety in texture as Shiki rep. When a Jacquard figure is introduced on a rep background it is called armure. Uses: upholstery and drapery purposes. Lighter weight, skirts and suits.

Weave—plain. Width 27", 36", 50".
Fabrics (1928)
Fig. 3

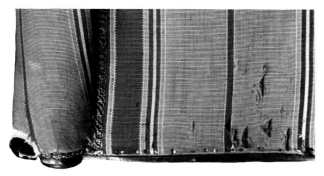

*Fig. 3. Detail of lounge, attributed to Alexander Roux,
New York, New York, walnut, striped wool rep, about 1870
(see chapter 7, fig. 18, for a full view of the lounge).*

Satin. A smooth and glossy fabric made of fine silk and
woven in a particular manner, so that one surface is
smooth and shining. The gloss and lustre of satin are
gained by the irregular manner in which the warp and weft
threads are taken in connection with one another.
Ordinarily a web is made by the alternate crossing of these
threads, but in the case of satin the greater proportion of
warp threads appear on the surface. The material is passed
over heated cylinders when it comes out of the weaver's
hands. A great many uses are made of satin, but the fabric
is not in great demand, because it is not serviceable; it
cannot be cleaned or dyed satisfactorily, and it is liable to
fray. Satin presents a very handsome, and ranks with velvet
in richness of, appearance; where economy has not to be
considered it is wisely chosen for dresses and for
trimmings....There are several kinds of satin; brocaded
satins are the richest in appearance. Satin de Bruges is
made of silk and wool, and is used for furniture purposes.
Cassell's (1878)

Tapestry, Brussels. Kind of carpet imitating body
Brussels. Yarn for pile printed, before weaving, to make
design.
Fabrics (1928)

Tapestry. Gobelin's [is] a fine, figured worsted fabric,
remarkable for strength, elegance of design, and beautiful
harmony of colors. It is ornamented with animals,
landscapes, fruits, flowers, etc. The finest paintings are
copied, and eminent artists are employed to prepare
designs. The warp is white, and the woof colored, to form
the figures. Gobelin's manufactory, where these goods are
made, is situated near Paris. This tapestry is used
principally for curtains, hangings, etc....[Beauvais tapestry]
is like the Gobelin, with this difference: the colored woof
is silk. The figures also are not as elegant, being limited to
flowers, medallions, etc. This manufactory is located near
Gobelin's.
Scissors and Yardstick (1872)

Tapestry, *Neuilly* or *Jacquard*. Made on the Jacquard
loom, in imitation of that of the Gobelins. In these goods

the design is brought out entirely by means of the weft,
the warp-threads being used only as binders to hold the
threads of the weft together. In the tapestry loom, with
the Jacquard attachment, there are sometimes used 24 or
more colors of weft—each in a different shuttle. These
shuttles are passed to and fro through the warp by the
hand of the weaver as the proper warps are raised by the
Jacquard machine, which at the same time indicates the
particular shade of weft to be used by the workman.
Cluny tapestry is a strong thick cloth, made of wool and
silk, especially for hangings and curtains, the manufacture
of which was introduced into England in 1875. *Tapestry
cloth* is a corded linen cloth prepared by tapestry painting.
Cole's (1892)

Tapestry. If you ask for a tapestry in a wall paper shop,
the salesman will show you a paper called tapestry or
verdure, because modelled after *jacquard* verdure
tapestries. The jacquards themselves you can see in the
upholstery section of any large department store....These
are the goods ordinarily called tapestries in the
merchandise upholstery trade. The all-cotton ones are
very expensive, even those with landscape and figures in
addition to verdure....Other imitation tapestries are those
block-printed by hand, like "hand-blocked" chintzes and
wall papers, but on a coarse horizontal rep in simulation of
real tapestry texture. The general effect is much more
tapestry-like than that of the jacquards, all but the simplest
of which resemble *petit point* needlework, having a square
point with lines running both ways instead of strongly
marked ribs....They also are very inexpensive.
Decorative Textiles (1918)

Tapestry. Originally a hand woven fabric made with a
bobbin worked from the wrong side on a warp stretched
vertically or horizontally. The bobbin is carried only to
the edge of the pattern and not from selvage to selvage.
The Gobelin tapestries in France are most famous; used for
wall hangings in cathedrals and palaces. The same
methods are used in making tapestries to-day. Original
designs are employed and historic patterns are reproduced.
A machine reproduction of tapestry is yarn-dyed, figured
fabric composed of two sets of warp and filling yarns
woven on a Jacquard loom. Power loom drapery fabrics
imitate real or bobbin tapestries. The wrong side is
smoother than in a hand-woven tapestry. Wool, cotton,
silk, rayon, and mixtures. Use: upholstery and wall
hangings. Weave—Jacquard. Width, 50".
Fabrics (1928)

Terry. A heavy, woollen fabric, resembling rep, and
mistaken by many in consequence of this resemblance.
The coarse woof is of cotton, each thread of which is
composed of several smaller threads twisted together, and
is covered by, but not interwoven with, the warp. It is
held in place by a small thread, which passes under, and is
interwoven with the warp, thus giving the fabric the
appearance of being all wool. In short, the face is all wool,
and the back all cotton. Terries are used for the same
purposes generally as reps. A superior article is made,
having a worsted woof and a silk warp. It is woven in the
same manner as the wool terry, and is called "silk terry."
It sometimes bears upon its surface raised figures of

flowers, etc., which are formed like those of damask. This variety is much more durable and expensive than the ordinary wool terry.

Scissors and Yardstick (1872)

Ticking. A heavy, twilled cotton fabric, woven with alternate blue and white stripes. It is used for coverings for beds, mattresses, pillows, etc.

Scissors and Yardstick (1872)

Utrecht Velvet. Mohair furniture plush. Formerly this fabric was manufactured exclusively at Utrecht, Holland, hence the name; but more recently the trade has centered at Amiens, France, and in Connecticut. The latter state supplies over one-half the amount required for domestic use by this country. It is used chiefly for upholstering railway cars and office furniture. It has a mohair pile woven into a linen foundation and is an exceedingly durable material.

Cole's (1892)

Velour. A French term signifying velvet, being derived from Latin *villosus*, shaggy. Among old English writers, and in the entries made in the lists of the royal wardrobes of England, the terms *velure* and *velures* are found, as well as *vallonettes*, mentioned by Chaucer. At this time the fabric was a species of linen plush. At present, velour denotes a cotton curtain fabric, woven with a coarse stiff pile on the terry cloth principle, alike on both sides, and dyed in solid colors.

Cole's (1892)

Velure. A cotton fabric woven with a thick and soft pile, used for curtains.

Cole's (1892)

Velour or velours (Fr. pr. ve-loor). 1. General term for pile fabrics. 2. Drapery fabric with short pile, usually of mercerized cotton; also mohair and silk may be pressed flat (panned) or in figures. Rich looking and durable. Uses: hangings, couch covers, upholstery. Weave—pile. Width, 50", 54".

Fabrics (1928)

Velvet (from Italian *velluto*, shaggy). A silken fabric having a short dense piled surface. It is the type of the numerous forms of piled fabrics now made....Of the country whence it first came, or the people who were the earliest to hit upon the happy way of weaving it, nothing is known. We are probably indebted to Central Asia, or perhaps China for velvet as well as satin....The peculiar properties of velvet, the splendid yet softened depth of dye-color it exhibited, at once marked it out as a fit material for ecclesiastical vestments, royal and state robes, and sumptuous hangings; and among the most magnificent fabrics of mediaeval times were Italian velvets. These were in many ways most effectively treated for ornamentation, such as by varying the color of the pile, by producing pile of different lengths (pile upon pile, or *double* pile), by brocading with plain silk, with uncut pile,

or with a ground of gold tissue....Until quite recently velvets in the United States have been an exclusive foreign fabric. At present, however, there are several factories in active operation, having been brought into existence by the increased duties on velvet under the late tariff act, which enables them to produce velvets in this country at a profit.

Cole's (1892)

Velvets, Upholstery. Ordinarily by velvets we mean warp velvets of the kind originated in silk, and do not even include the coarse woollen and worsted velvets woven for floor coverings, such as brussels and wilton carpets and rugs. Upholstery velvets are usually called *velours* (the French word for velvet), whether the pile be in silk or flax or wool or cotton....When only part of the pile is to be cut, in other words when the velvet is to be *cut and uncut*, the cutting is done with a hand knife....A modern way of making velvets without the use of wires is to weave two cloths together face to face, with special pile warps working back and forth between them and joining them. The cutting of this common pile by a knife that travels back and forth across the loom, produces two velvets economically and with a minimum of effort. Recently, an American manufacturer has invented a way of figuring these double-woven velvets in two-tone, by inserting the pile warps thicker in the figures than in the ground.

Decorative Textiles (1918)
Fig. 4

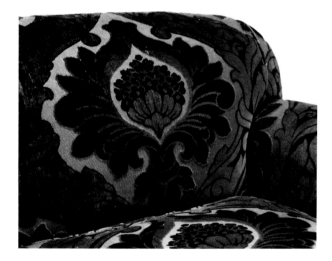

Fig. 4. *Detail of sofa, maple, upholstery velvet, United States, 1925-1930.*

Webbing. A coarse, hempen band, woven plain. It is not bleached, but the natural color of the material. It bears a black stripe near each edge, which is formed by colored threads in the warp. Width, about 4 inches. A narrower variety is made, having a herring-bone twill. The warp is black, and gives the fabric a mixed appearance. Width, about 1½ inches.

Scissors and Yardstick (1872)

NOTES

Introduction Notes

1. Janet E. Ruutz-Rees, *Home Decoration: Art Needlework, and Embroidery; Painting on Silk, Satin and Velvet; Panel Painting; and Wood-Carving* (New York: D. Appleton and Company, 1881), 57, 42.

2. Professor Walter R. Houghton et al., *American Etiquette and Rules of Politeness* (New York: Powers and LeCraw, 1886), 13, 20.

3. While the Anglo-American link is indeed important, examination of continental bourgeois culture in the same period suggests that the definition should perhaps be broadened, at least in relation to material culture. See, for example, the extraordinary collection of American, English, and Continental middle-class interiors in Peter Thornton, *Authentic Decor: The Domestic Interior 1620-1920* (New York: Viking Penguin Inc., 1982), especially those chapters covering the years between 1820 and 1920, and Daniel Walker Howe, "Victorian Culture in America," in Daniel Walker Howe, ed., *Victorian America* (Philadelphia: University of Pennsylvania Press, 1976), 3-26.

4. Richard A. Wells, *Manners, Culture and Dress* (Springfield, MA: King, Richardson and Co., 1891), 11.

5. "Home" seems to have been one of at least three "symbol sets" that had distinct identities in nineteenth- and early twentieth-century America and that mark the boundaries of Victorian culture in America. Although much remains to be done before the dimensions and character of each set are fully outlined, the scholarship of John Kasson, Leo Marx, Richard Hofstadter, Henry Nash Smith, and others suggest that one symbol set revolves around the concepts of technology and the image of the machine as the vehicle for civilization's progress. Another is the bundle of popular thinking and associations that may be designated by the image of the wilderness and what Leo Marx has termed the "middle landscape" of the cultivated garden. The classic texts that began charting the dimensions and meanings of these symbols include John Kasson, *Civilizing the Machine: Technology and Republican Values in America, 1776-1900* (New York: Grossman Publishers, 1976); Leo Marx, *The Machine in the Garden* (New York: Oxford University Press, 1964); and Henry Nash Smith, *Virgin Land: The American West as Symbol and Myth* (1950; reprint, New York: Vintage Books, 1961).

6. Julia McNair Wright, *The Complete Home: An Encyclopædia of Domestic Life and Affairs* (Philadelphia: Bradley, Garretson and Co., 1884), 3.

7. Rev. W. K. Tweedie, *Home; or, The Parents' Assistant and Children's Friend* (Norwich, CT: The Henry Bill Publishing Company, 1873), 34-41.

8. Emily Dickinson cited in Robert Craft, "Amorous in Amherst," *The New York Review of Books*, 23 April 1987, 21.

9. Catharine E. Beecher and Harriet Beecher Stowe, *The American Woman's Home* (New York: J. B. Ford and Co., 1870), 18-19, 24.

10. As anthropologist Victor Turner has noted, such a relocation of symbols should be expected to occur in societies that have become complex and in which religion is pluralistic and a matter of choice: "Symbols once central to the mobilization of ritual action, have tended to migrate directly or in disguise, through the cultural division of labor, into other domains, esthetics, politics, law, popular culture, and the like." Turner, "Variations on a Theme of Liminality," in Sally F. Moore and Barbara Myerhoff, eds., *Secular Ritual* (Amsterdam, The Netherlands: Van Gorcum, Assen, 1977), 36.

11. Richard L. Bushman, "Family Security in the Transition from Farm to City, 1750-1850," *Journal of Family History* (Fall 1981): 250-251.

12. Bushman, "Family Security," 250-251; see also Stephan Thernstrom, *Poverty and Progress: Social Mobility in a Nineteenth Century City* (Cambridge, MA: Harvard University Press, 1964).

13. Mrs. Lydia H. Sigourney, *Letters to Mothers* (Hartford, CT: by the author, 1838), 15.

14. Harriet Beecher Stowe [Christopher Crowfield, pseud.], "Woman's Sphere," in *The Chimney Corner* (Boston: Ticknor and Fields, 1868), vol. 8 of *The Writings of Harriet Beecher Stowe* (Cambridge, MA: Riverside Press, 1896), 252. Tweedie also discussed what he termed "The Republic of Home" in *Home*, 38.

15. Almira Seymour, *Home: The Basis of the State* (Boston: A. Williams and Company, 1869), 7.

16. Books of architectural advice from the middle decades of the nineteenth century made much of the connection between domestic architecture and character. In a representative statement, Lewis F. Allen, author of *Rural Architecture* (1852), argued, "As the man himself—no matter what his occupation—be lodged and fed, so influenced, in a degree, will be his practice in the daily duties of his life. A squalid, miserable tenement, with which they who inhabit it are content, can lead to no elevation of character, no improvement in condition, either social or moral, of its occupants." Allen, *Rural Architecture* (New York: C. M. Saxton, 1852), xii.

17. Beecher and Stowe, *American Woman's Home*, 84.

18. "The Domestic Use of Design," *The Furniture Gazette* 1, 1 (12 April 1873): 4.

19. Harriet Beecher Stowe, *We and Our Neighbors* (New York: J. B. Ford and Company, 1875), 152.

20. Stowe, *We and Our Neighbors*, 152.

21. Clarence Cook, *The House Beautiful* (New York: Scribner, Armstrong and Company, 1878), 49.

22. Gwendolyn Wright, *Moralism and the Modern Home* (Chicago: University of Chicago Press, 1980). American utopian communities, which mirrored the larger interests and concerns of the society for which they proposed themselves as alternatives, were often as compelled by the symbol "home" as were ordinary people. Architectural historian Dolores Hayden has argued, "When communities issued tracts or posters to recruit new members, they often illustrated them with sketches of their dwellings as tangible proof of their achievements." The motto on the masthead of Oneida's *American Socialist* was, "devoted to the enlargement and protection of home." Hayden, *Seven American Utopias: The Architecture of Communitarian Socialism, 1790-1975* (Cambridge, MA: The MIT Press, 1976), 9, 24.

23. Siegfried Giedion discusses the effects of the "mechanization of adornment," for example, as a process that devalued symbolic ornament (as in the application of the classical symbols of power to many kinds of furnishings). In his argument, the meaning of objects themselves deteriorated, since the meaning of ornament and the connection between craftsmanship, rarity, and value was broken through mechanized production. Giedion, *Mechanization Takes Command: A Contribution to Anonymous History* (New York: Oxford University Press, 1948), 338-346.

24. According to Clifford Geertz, a symbol is "any object, act, event, quality, or relation which serves as a vehicle for a conception—the conception is the symbol's meaning." Geertz, "Religion as a Cultural System," in *The Interpretation of Cultures* (New York: Basic Books, 1973), 91.

25. Lawrence J. Taylor, "Death in Godey's: Women and Death in Nineteenth-Century America" (Paper presented at the Winterthur Museum, April 1982), 16. Taylor has noted that the theory of associations was first formulated as part of an eighteenth-century epistemology, but evoking the chain of associations was at that time viewed as an act of cognition and reason alone. In later forms, including the popular verse published in *Godey's*, associations were more intuitive and emotional, and the ability to feel them was "a natural inclination, and like 'influence,' a feminine characteristic." While men could, and did, perceive chains of associations, women especially were empowered.

26. "Miss Cook," "The Old Arm-Chair," *Godey's Lady's Book*, March 1855, 273.

27. Cook, "The Old Arm-Chair," 273.

28. Victor Turner, "Symbols in Ndembu Ritual," in *The Forest of Symbols* (Ithaca, NY: Cornell University Press, 1970), 19.

29. A brief discussion of Geertz's understanding of "sensibility" may be found in his essay, "Art as a Cultural System," in *Local Knowledge* (Berkeley, CA: University of California Press, 1983), 96, 99.

30. Historians of science and technology interested in innovation recognize this boundary and how it is sometimes consciously employed when they discuss problem-solving through the "mind's eye," where problems are analyzed and solved without translation into a verbal form. See Eugene S. Ferguson, "The Mind's Eye: Nonverbal Thought in Technology," *Science*, 26 August 1977, 827-836.

31. In an essay on the phenomenon of the "miniature," Susan Stewart has also perceived and described the limits of such description: "We find that when language attempts to describe the concrete, it is caught in an infinitely self-effacing gesture of inadequacy, a gesture which speaks to the gaps between our modes of cognition—those gaps between the sensual, the visual, and the linguistic." She notes further that attempts at such description "threaten an infinity of detail that becomes translated into an infinity of verbality" without describing the experience of perceiving miniatures. Stewart, *On Longing* (Baltimore: The Johns Hopkins University Press, 1984), 52.

32. Daniel Biebuyck has defined this term in "Symbolism of the Lega Stool," in *Working Papers in the Traditional Arts 2 & 3* (Philadelphia: Institute for the Study of Human Issues, 1977), 7-37. He analyzes the way objects used in ceremonies, in this instance the stool, are described and classified in relation to Lega aesthetic and cultural values.

33. Wells, *Manners, Culture and Dress*, 441-450.

34. Mrs. H. O. Ward, *Sensible Etiquette of the Best Society, Customs, Manners, Morals, and Home Culture*, 16th ed. (Philadelphia: Porter and Coates, 1878), xv.

35. *Social Culture; A Treatise on Etiquette, Self Culture, Dress, Physical Beauty and Domestic Relations* (Springfield, MA: The King-Richardson Co., 1903), 7.

36. Communications-based approaches to the study of artifacts that also have had recourse to analogies with language may be found in the literature of cultural anthropology that discusses the visual arts; for a survey of the anthropology of art which includes communications-based approaches see Robert S. Layton, *The Anthropology of Art* (New York: Columbia University Press, 1981). The work of Mary Douglas and Baron Isherwood in *The World of Goods* is particularly apropos. They argue that the abstract concepts employed by a culture are "difficult to remember, unless they take on a physical appearance." Hence, "Goods assembled together in ownership make physical, rational statements about the hierarchy of values to which their chooser subscribes." Douglas and Isherwood, *The World of Goods: Towards an Anthropology of Consumption*

(New York: W. W. Norton and Company, 1979), 5.

37. According to the *Oxford English Dictionary*, rhetoric, the art of using language in order to persuade or influence other people, consists of "a body of rules to be observed by a speaker or writer in order that he may express himself with eloquence." When a person makes a rhetorical statement, he or she may be understood by the receiver of the message even if the receiver does not believe or accept the content of that statement. Family portraits make a clearly rhetorical statement about that family's happiness and health, even when an observer of that portrait knows the "truth" about the family's personal problems. *Oxford English Dictionary*, s.v. "rhetoric."

38. Walter J. Ong, a scholar of rhetoric and the structure of knowledge and thought in literate and oral cultures, has argued that critical differences exist between the interpretation of images and texts: "Although we look both at pictures and at texts, we don't read pictures as we read texts. A text encodes specific words for you to say. Pictures do not do this...We are so locked into literacy, and literacy is so tremendously helpful, enabling us to do all kinds of things, that we use the term 'text' to characterize everything that contains information or calls for interpretation." "Syntax is simply our English version of the Greek term for putting together in order," Ong has argued, although he considers visual syntax as relating to "conventions rather than grammars in any verbal sense." "Interview with Walter J. Ong," *Exposure* (Winter 1985): 20. See also Ong, *Orality and Literacy: The Technologizing of the Word* (New York: Methuen, 1982).

39. Neil Harris, *The Artist in American Society: The Formative Years, 1790-1860* (New York: Simon and Schuster, 1966), 42-43.

40. On the hunting symbolism associated with dining in nineteenth-century America, see Kenneth L. Ames, "Murderous Propensities: Notes on Dining Iconography of the Mid-Nineteenth Century," in Nancy H. Schless and Kenneth L. Ames, eds., *Three Centuries, Two Continents* (Watkins Glen, NY: American Life Foundation, 1983).

41. For a study of popular iconography that employs the idea of "paraphrasing," see Hedvig Branden Johnson et al., *Visual Paraphrases: Studies in Mass Media Imagery* [(Acts Universitatis Upsaliensis *Figura* New Series 27) (Stockholm, Sweden: Almquist and Wiksell International, Uppsala, 1984)].

42. *Oxford English Dictionary*, s.v. "emulation."

43. Thorstein Veblen, *The Theory of the Leisure Class* (1899; reprint, New York: Vanguard Press, 1922), 34.

44. Johnson et al., *Visual Paraphrases*.

45. "A Visit to Henkels' Warerooms in Chestnut Street Above Fifth," *Godey's Lady's Book*, August 1850, 126.

46. Francis Salet, "Introduction," in Genevieve Souchal,

Chefs-d'oeuvre de la tapisserie du XIV au XVI siecle (*Masterpieces of Tapestry From the Fourteenth to the Sixteenth Century*), trans. Richard A. H. Oxby (New York: Metropolitan Museum of Art, 1973), 17-18; see also Penelope Eames, "Furniture in England, France and the Netherlands from the Twelfth to the Fifteenth Century," *Furniture History* 13 (1977).

47. Rolla Tryon, "The Transition from Family-to-Shop and Factory-made Goods," and "The Passing of the Family Factory," in *Household Manufactures in the United States, 1640-1860* (Chicago: University of Chicago Press, 1917), 242-376.

48. Daniel Webster, "Lecture before the Society for the Diffusion of Useful Knowledge," in Michael Brewster Folsom and Steven D. Lubar, eds., *The Philosophy of Manufactures: Early Debates over Industrialization in the United States* (Cambridge, MA: MIT Press and Merrimack Valley Textile Museum, 1982), 395; *Eighty Years' Progress of the United States*, vol. 1 (Hartford, CT: L. Stebbins, 1867), 286.

49. *Niles Weekly Register* 21 (1821), 35, cited in Tryon, *Household Manufactures*, 284.

50. Tryon, *Household Manufactures*, 276.

51. *Eighty Years' Progress*, vol. 1, 291.

52. Gladys Palmer, "Labor Relations in the Lace and Lace-Curtain Industries in the United States," *Bulletin of the U.S. Bureau of Labor Statistics* 380 (November 1925); A. F. Barker, *Textiles* (New York: D. Van Nostrand Co., 1910), 257-258.

Chapter One Notes

1. *Humphrey's Journal of Photography* 5, 1 (15 April 1853): 10-11.

2. See, for example, Neil McKendrick, John Brewer, and J.H. Plumb, *The Birth of a Consumer Society: The Commercialization of Eighteenth-Century England* (Bloomington, IN: Indiana University Press, 1982), for a discussion of the spread of habits of consumption beginning with the adoption of items of fashionable clothing by working people.

3. McKendrick et al., *Birth of Consumer Society*, xx. Students of Anglo-American and French culture of the eighteenth and nineteenth centuries have begun the process of reconstructing both the economic aspects of the growth of consumer culture and have focused particularly on the department store and on international exhibitions, beginning with the Crystal Palace of 1851. Since 1980, excellent books have been published on the Bon Marché, a Parisian dry goods establishment that evolved into perhaps the first department store in the world in the 1850s; on the French expositions and the response of French intellectuals to consumer culture; and on consumer culture in the fiction of Balzac and Zola. See Michael B. Miller, *The Bon Marché* (Princeton, NJ: Princeton University Press, 1980); Rosalind B. Williams,

Dream Worlds: Mass Consumption in Late Nineteenth-Century France (Berkeley, CA: University of California Press, 1983); and Rachel Bowlby, *Just Looking: Consumer Culture in Dreiser, Gissing and Zola* (New York: Methuen,1985). Similar studies of American department stores include John Hower, *History of Macy's of New York 1858-1919* (Cambridge, MA: Harvard University Press, 1943); Neil Harris, "Museums, Merchandising, and Popular Taste: The Struggle for Influence," in Ian M. D. Quimby, ed., *Material Culture and the Study of American Life* (New York: W. W. Norton, 1977), 140-174; and Daniel J. Boorstin, *The Americans: The Democratic Experience* (New York: Random House, 1973). A number of dissertations-in-progress are reported to be examining similar topics in American consumer culture. Still, some of the oldest monographs on single businesses, such as John Hower's on Macy's, stand as seminal works. Harris's important essay linked department stores, expositions, and museums as nineteenth-century tastemakers, but no research since has expanded upon his initial observations. Boorstin's work, one of the pioneering attempts at interpreting the first monographic studies of department stores, advertising, mass media, and other elements of American consumer culture, is also correct in citing the department store and the exposition as key nineteenth-century expressions of consumer culture.

4. McKendrick et al., "The Consumer Revolution," in *Birth of Consumer Society*, 20-21.

5. Eames, "Furniture in England, France and the Netherlands," xvii.

6. Ibid., 57-58.

7. For an analysis of this changing concept of unified decor and architecture, which included more complicated furnishings, see Thornton, *Authentic Decor.*

8. Williams, *Dream Worlds*, 8-9.

9. *The American Cabinet Maker, Upholsterer and Carpet Reporter* contained in virtually every issue a statement like this one in the November 25, 1876, issue: "The demand for novelties in cabinet-work require a manufacturer to be constantly on the look-out for something fresh and new." 14, 2 (25 November 1876): 4.

10. Richard Donald Jurzhals, "Initial Advantage and Technological Change in Industrial Location: The Furniture Industry of Grand Rapids, Michigan" (Ph.D. diss., Michigan State University, 1973), 95-98; James Stanford Bradshaw, "Grand Rapids, 1870-1880: Furniture City Emerges," *Michigan History* 45, 4 (Winter 1971): 332.

11. Martha Craybill McClaugherty, "Household Art: Creating the Artistic Home, 1868-1893," *Winterthur Portfolio* 18 (1983): 1-26.

12. Fanny Kemble, *The Journal of Frances Anne Butler, better known as Fanny Kemble*, vol. 1 (1835; reprint, New York: Benjamin Blom, 1970), 74.

13. See Richard Sennett, "The Fullness of Life..." and "Little Islands of Propriety...," in *Families Against the City: Middle Class Homes of Industrial Chicago 1872-1890* (Cambridge, MA: Harvard University Press, 1970), and Sam Bass Warner, *Private City: Philadelphia in Three Periods of Its Growth* (Philadelphia: University of Pennsylvania Press, 1968).

14. "A Bargain: Is a Penny Saved, Twopence Got?," *Gleason's Pictorial Drawing-Room Companion*, 2 September 1854, 150 (hereafter cited as *Gleason's*).

15. "A Bargain: Is a Penny Saved," 151.

16. *Catalogue of Handsome Household Furniture, to be sold by Bleeker and Van Dyke on Thursday, April 22, 1841, at No. 2 Albion Place* (New York, 1841). *Catalogue of Genteel Household Furniture, for Sale at Auction, by Henry H. Leeds and Co., on Friday, April 29, 1853, at Half-past Ten O'Clock, at No. 231 East 10th Street* (New York, 1853).

17. Ann Sophia Stephens, *High Life in New York. By Jonathan Slick, Esq. of Weathersfield, Conn...* (New York: Bunce and Brother, 1854), 269.

18. Winston Weisman, "Commercial Palaces of New York, 1845-1875," *The Art Bulletin* 34 (December 1854): 285-302.

19. "Charleston Hotel," *Gleason's*, 24 April 1852, 265; "The Girard House, Philadelphia," *Gleason's*, 21 February 1852, 113.

20. Reuben Vose, *Reuben Vose's Wealth of the World Displayed* (New York: by the author, 1859), 5, 40.

21. Vose, *Reuben Vose's Wealth of the World*, 181-182.

22. "Boarding Out," *Harper's Weekly*, 7 March 1857, 146.

23. *Humphrey's Journal of Photography* (15 April 1853): 11.

24. "The Girard House," 113. Other descriptions of commercial parlors later in this chapter are additional examples.

25. Nicholas B. Wainwright, ed., *A Philadelphia Perspective: The Diary of Sidney George Fisher Covering the Years 1834-1871* (Philadelphia: The Historical Society of Pennsylvania, 1967), 116.

26. See Costard Sly [pseud.], *Sayings and Doings at the Tremont House in the Year 1832, Extracted from the Notebook of Costard Sly, Solicitor and Short-Hand Writer, of London. And Edited by Dr. Zachary Vangrifter*, 2 vols. (Boston: Allen and Ticknor, 1833) for a "factual account" of social life in the hotel's setting.

27. Francis J. Grund, *The Americans in Their Moral, Social and Political Relations*, vol. 2 (1837; reprint, New York: Augustus M. Kelley, 1971), 234.

28. Grund, *The Americans*, 234.

29. Anthony Trollope, *North America*, vol. 2 (1862; reprint, London: Dawson's of Pall Mall, 1968), 328.

30. Jefferson Williamson, *The American Hotel: An Anecdotal History* (New York: Alfred A. Knopf, Inc., 1930), 12.

31. Russell Lynes was the first social historian to call attention to the enthusiasm of the American public for these hotels and the power of their image as "palaces of the people" in *The Tastemakers* (1954; reprint, New York: Grosset and Dunlap, 1972), 81-96. See also Williamson, *American Hotel*, 301.

32. "American House, Boston," *Gleason's*, 10 July 1852, 24.

33. Trollope, *North America*, 314.

34. *A Description of Tremont House* (Boston: Gray and Bowen, 1830), 41.

35. *Description of Tremont House*, 12.

36. *Boston Legal Advertiser* (1829), unpaginated.

37. E. Page Talbot, "The Furniture Industry in Boston, 1810-1835" (M.A. thesis, University of Delaware, 1974), 73.

38. "La Pierre House," *Gleason's*, 8 October 1853, 225, 239.

39. "New Furniture," *Godey's Lady's Book*, February 1850, 152-153, and "A Visit to Henkels' Wareroom," 123-124.

40. *Catalogue of Furniture, George A. Henkels, City Cabinet Warerooms, 173 Chestnut St.* (Philadelphia, 1855?), Winterthur Museum.

41. For a discussion of Henkels' "Antique" furniture, an analysis of a group of surviving examples, and a brief business history, see Kenneth Ames, "George Henkels, Nineteenth-Century Philadelphia Cabinetmaker," *Antiques*, October 1973, 641-650.

42. "Fashion Plates for Decorating Parlor Windows, The Latest Styles," *Godey's Lady's Book*, February 1854, 97, 166.

43. Nicholas Dean, "An Exquisite Victorian Puzzle," *Historic Preservation*, October 1985, 40-45; correspondence with Arlene Palmer Schwind, Victoria Society of Maine, 6 February 1986.

44. Sly [pseud.], *Sayings and Doings at the Tremont House*, 220.

45. Ibid.

46. "C. M." [Charles Mackey], "Transatlantic Sketches—The Mississippi River," *The Illustrated London News*, 10 April 1858, 378.

47. Trollope, *North America*, 328-329.

48. "The Waverly Hotel," *Rochester* (NY) *Daily Advertiser*, 6 May 1848, 2.

49. Grund, *The Americans*, 2, 236.

50. *Eighty Years' Progress*, vol. 2, 261.

51. Eliza Leslie, *The Ladies' Guide to True Politeness and Perfect Manners; or, Miss Leslie's Behavior Book* (Philadelphia: T. B. Peterson and Brothers, 1864), 108, 116.

52. "William Brown," "American Homes in New York Hotels," *Harper's Weekly*, 26 December 1857, 824-825; "Boarding Out," 146.

53. "Boarding Out," 146.

54. Ibid.

55. Carl D. Lane, *American Paddle Steamboats* (New York: Coward-McCann, Inc., 1943), 11.

56. David Lear Buckman, *Old Steamboat Days on the Hudson River* (New York: The Grafton Press, 1907), 34-55.

57. Donald C. Ringwald, *Hudson River Day Line: The Story of a Great American Steamboat Company* (Berkeley, CA: Howell-North Books, 1965), 12.

58. The French traveler Michel Chevalier commented on the appearance of such vessels: "The Western steamboats look very much like the Vigier baths on the Seine; they are huge houses of two stories...In the interior they have that coquettish air that characterizes American vessels in general; the cabins are showily furnished, and make a very pretty appearance. The little green blinds and the snugly fitted windows, pleasingly contrasting with the white walls, would have made Jean-Jacques sigh with envy." See Chevalier, *Society, Manners, and Politics in the United States* (1839; reprint, New York: A.M. Kelley, 1966), letter XX, 17.

59. Marianne Finch, an 1853 traveler, quoted in Lane, *American Paddle Steamboats*, 82.

60. Mrs. Caroline M. Kirkland, "Mrs. Pell's Pilgrimage," in *A Book for the Home Circle* (New York: Charles Scribner, 1853), 144-161; Kemble, *Journal of Fanny Kemble*, vol. 2, 97-98.

61. J. Howland Gardner, "The Development of Steam Navigation on Long Island Sound," *Historical Transactions 1893-1943: The Society of Naval Architects and Marine Engineers* (New York: by the Society, 1945), 104, 107.

62. Wainwright, ed., *Philadelphia Perspective* [diary entry for 24 September 1847], 198. For information on the operation of palace steamers on the East Coast, see George W. Hilton, *The Night Boat* (Berkeley, CA: Howell-North Books, 1968).

63. Erik Heyl, "The 'City of Buffalo': Last of the Great Lakes' Palace Steamers,'" *Niagara Frontier* 4, 1

(Spring 1957): 10-11. Published by the Buffalo Historical Society.

64. Mark Twain, *Life on the Mississippi* (1883; reprint, New York: Library of America, 1982), 457, 461.

65. Thomas Curtis Clarke, John Bogart et al., *The American Railway: Its Construction, Development, Management, and Appliances* (New York: Charles Scribner's Sons, 1889), 240.

66. John White, author of an exhaustive history of the American railroad car, has documented the development of comfortably equipped, elegantly decorated passenger cars so thoroughly that a lengthy chronological recapitulation is unnecessary. White, *The American Railroad Passenger Car* (Baltimore: Johns Hopkins University Press, 1978).

67. *Rochester* (NY) *Evening Post*, quoted in American Railroad Journal (15 June 1842), as cited in August Mencken, *The Railroad Passenger Car: An Illustrated History of the First Hundred Years, with Accounts by Contemporary Passengers* (Baltimore: The Johns Hopkins University Press, 1957), 16-17.

68. White, *The American Railroad Passenger Car*, 208.

69. *Buffalo City Directory* (1880), unpaginated.

70. White, *The American Railroad Passenger Car*, 209.

71. Ibid., 378, 381; Alfred Spitzli, *A Manual for Managers, Designers, Weavers, and All Others Connected with the Manufacture of Textile Fabrics...* (Troy, NY: A. and A. F. Spitzli, Publishers, 1881), 126.

72. "Princely Parlor Furniture," *Sears, Roebuck and Co. Catalogue No. 104, 1897* (1897; reprint, New York: Chelsea House, 1976), unpaginated.

73. Benjamin Franklin Taylor, *The World on Wheels and Other Sketches* (Chicago: S. C. Griggs and Co., 1873), 157-158.

74. "Centennial Passenger Coaches," *The National Car-Builder* 7, 6 (June 1876): 86.

75. *The Modern Priscilla Home Furnishing Book: A Practical Book for the Woman Who Loves Her Home* (Boston: The Priscilla Publishing Company, 1925), 2.

76. *Gleason's*, 1 April 1854, 208.

77. *Rochester* (NY) *Daily Advertiser*, 3 March 1848, 1.

78. Advertisement for the Emporium Daguerreotype Gallery, *Rochester* (NY) *Daily Advertiser*, 3 March 1848, 1.

79. Advertisement for "Powelson's Photographic Rooms," *Rochester Directory* (1864).

80. Peter E. Palmquist, "Behind the Scenes: A Potpourri of Western Photographic Studios and Darkrooms 1850-1950," *The Photographist* 66 (Summer 1985): 10-25.

81. H. J. Rodgers, *Twenty-Three Years under a Sky-Light* (1872; reprint, New York: Arno, 1973), 150.

82. Robert Taft, *Photography and the American Scene* (1938; reprint, New York: Dover Publications, Inc., 1964), 76.

83. *The Daguerreian Journal* 1, 4 (1 January 1851): 58; Advertisement for the Emporium Daguerreotype Gallery, *Rochester* (NY) *Daily Advertiser*, 3 March 1848, 1.

84. Richard Rudisill, *Mirror Image* (Albuquerque, NM: University of New Mexico Press, 1971), 203.

85. M. A. Root, *The Camera and the Pencil* (Philadelphia: by the author, 1864), 45.

86. E. K. Hough, "Expressing Character in Photographic Pictures," *American Journal of Photography* 1, 14 (15 December 1858): 211.

87. Harris, "Museums, Merchandising, and Popular Taste," 145.

88. Williams, *Dream Worlds*, 58.

89. Ibid., 59.

90. See, for example, the "panoramic" wood engraving of the New York Crystal Palace of 1853 published in *Gleason's*, 4 February 1854, 73-80, where fabrics are clearly displayed as "waterfalls" of color and texture.

91. James D. McCabe, *The Illustrated History of the Centennial Exhibition...* (Philadelphia: The National Publishing Company, 1876), 376.

92. This account of the New England Kitchen and possible sources of influence is condensed from Rodris Roth, "The New England, or 'Olde Tyme,' Kitchen Exhibit at Nineteenth-Century Fairs," in Allen Axelrod, ed., *The Colonial Revival in America* (New York: W. W. Norton, 1985), 159-183.

93. Walter Smith, *Industrial Art*, vol. 2 of *The Masterpieces of the Centennial International Exhibition, Illustrated* (Philadelphia: Gebbie and Barrie, n.d.), 123.

94. McCabe, *Illustrated History of the Centennial Exhibition*, 375-377. See also *Gems of the Centennial Exhibition: Consisting of Illustrated Descriptions of Objects of an Artistic Character...* (New York: D. Appleton and Company, 1877), 139-140. An engraving of the exhibited room appears on page 138.

95. See Thornton, *Authentic Decor*, 188, 194, 195.

96. Walter Smith, *Industrial Art*, 121; Frank H. Norton, *Illustrated Historical Register of the Centennial Exhibition, Philadelphia, 1876, and of the Exposition Universelle, Paris, 1878* (New York: American News

Co., 1879), 384-385.

97. *Artistic Houses* (1883; reprint, New York: Benjamin Blom, 1971).

98. Smith, *Industrial Art*, 122.

99. "Union Hall," *Ballou's Pictorial Drawing-Room Companion*, 3 January 1852, 73.

100. "New York Atheneum," *The Daguerreian Journal* 1, 2 (15 November 1850): 59.

101. "C. M." [Charles Mackey], "Transatlantic Sketches—American Firemen," *Illustrated London News*, 23 January 1858, 92.

102. Ibid.

103. Thomas L. McKenney cited in Ringwald, *Hudson River Day Line*, 96.

104. Kemble, *Journal of Fanny Kemble*, vol. 2, 172. See also Charles Dickens, *American Notes for General Circulation* (1842; reprint, Boston: Ticknor and Fields, 1867).

105. Taylor, *World on Wheels*, 156-157.

106. This statement has been attributed to Pullman by Mrs. Duane Doty, as quoted in *The Town of Pullman Illustrated: Its Growth with Brief Accounts of its Industries* (1893; reprint, Pullman, IL: Pullman Civic Organization, 1974), 23.

107. David Lear Buckman, *Old Steamboat Days on the Hudson River* (New York: Grafton Press, 1907), 55; Lynes, *The Tastemakers*, 126.

108. Buckman, *Old Steamboat Days*, 84-87.

Chapter Two Notes

1. Cook, *House Beautiful*, 47. Basing his definition on the work of Erik Erikson, sociologist Richard Sennett provides a concise definition of the term social identity: "the meeting point between who a person wants to be and what the world allows him to be…, one's place in a landscape formed by the intersections of circumstance and desire." This definition seems particularly appropriate to the study of consumer culture and consumer aspirations involved in creating parlors. Richard Sennett, *The Fall of Public Man* (New York: Vintage Books, 1978), 107.

2. Ethel Spencer, *The Spencers of Amberson Avenue: A Turn-of-the-Century Memoir* (Pittsburgh: University of Pittsburgh Press, 1983), 16.

3. Cook, *House Beautiful*, 98-99.

4. Correspondence of Mrs. George Ware Fulton, George Ware Fulton Papers, Barker History Archive, University of Texas, Austin, TX.

5. Spencer, *Spencers of Amberson Avenue*, 17.

6. Edith Wharton and Ogden Codman, Jr., *The Decoration of Houses* (New York: Charles Scribner's Sons, 1897), 124.

7. This information relies on Thornton, "1670-1720" and "1720-1770," in *Authentic Decor*. Mark Girouard describes the elaborate plans of the largest Victorian country houses in England as the most exaggerated form of the impulse to segregate varieties of activity. In his words, they were "enormous, complicated and highly articulated machines…Victorian country houses were complicated partly because they had to contain so many people, to a lesser extent because of the new mechanical devices that were incorporated in them, but mainly because the activities and interrelationships of their occupants were so minutely organized and subdivided. In an age when government was organized into departments, the middle classes into professions, science into different disciplines and convicts into separate cells, country house life was divided up into separate parcels." See Girouard, *The Victorian Country House*, rev. ed. (New Haven and London: Yale University Press, 1979), 27-28.

8. Thornton, *Authentic Decor*, 50, 93.

9. Adam, quoted in ibid., 145.

10. As Richard Bushman has argued, "In those marvelously adorned public rooms we can picture them displaying their clothing, their wit and worldly knowledge, their fine manners and physical grace—all within a beautiful space suitable for a civil and refined society." Bushman, "American High-Style and Vernacular Cultures," in Jack P. Greene and J. R. Pole, eds., *Colonial British America* (Baltimore: The Johns Hopkins University Press, 1984), 351-352.

11. *The Century Dictionary*, vol. 4 (New York: The Century Company, 1890), 4295.

12. Beecher and Stowe, *American Woman's Home*, 86.

13. Henry T. Williams and Mrs. C. S. Jones, *Beautiful Homes; or, Hints in House Furnishing* (New York: Henry T. Williams, 1878), 110.

14. Williams and Jones, *Beautiful Homes*, 110.

15. Noah Webster, *American Dictionary of the English Language*, rev. ed. (Springfield, MA: G. and C. Merriam, 1882), 950.

16. Calvert Vaux, *Villas and Cottages* (New York: Harper Brothers, 1864).

17. Frank Luther Mott, *A History of American Magazines, 1865-1885*, vol. 3 (Cambridge: The Belknap Press, 1970), 7.

18. *Montgomery Ward and Co. Catalogue No. 57, Spring and Summer, 1895* (1895; reprint, New York: Dover Publications, Inc., 1969), 45. In the author's private library is a copy of the unnumbered 1900 edition of Reed's book, bearing a small bookplate that identifies

the source of purchase as Sears, Roebuck and Co.

19. Samuel B. Reed, *House-Plans for Everybody* (New York: Orange Judd and Co., 1878), 63-64.

20. Reed, *House-Plans for Everybody*, 51-55.

21. Ibid., 54, 65-66.

22. "New Furniture," 152-153; see also Fanny N. Copeland, "Draperies, Blinds and Curtains," *Peterson's Magazine*, April 1860, 269-272.

23. "New Furniture," 153.

24. Ibid., 152.

25. Kirkland, *Book for the Home Circle*, 110.

26. Rodd L. Wheaton, "High Style in Montana: The Kohrs Parlor," in Kenneth L. Ames, ed., *Victorian Furniture*, published as *Nineteenth Century* 8, 3-4 (Philadelphia: Victorian Society in America, 1982): 245.

27. "Daisy Fields," "How We Furnished the Parlor," *The Household*, June 1882, 180-181.

28. *The Household*, December 1881, 265; September 1881, 193; December 1881, 279.

29. Wainwright, ed., *Philadelphia Perspective*, 76.

30. See *Social Culture*; Emily Thornwell, *The Lady's Guide to Perfect Gentility* (New York: Derby and Jackson, 1856); *Etiquette for Ladies; with Hints on the Preservation, Improvement, and Display of Female Beauty* (Philadelphia: Lea and Blanchard, "successors to Carey and Co.," 1838; Appendix dated 1856.)

31. The author remembers being astonished at an enormous collection of calling cards used by the citizens of several small southeast Texas towns, surviving in the collection of a state historic site—cards used by people who obviously knew each other, given the size of the communities.

32. *Etiquette for Ladies*, 23, 25.

33. Houghton et al., *American Etiquette*, 127.

34. Karen Halttunen has made extended use of the metaphor of theater in her discussion of the "genteel performance" in manners and dress in what she has termed "sentimental culture" between 1830 and 1870. Her thesis centers on the discomfort which middle-class people felt in the new urban world of strangers, and their efforts to define an ideal of "sincere" manners between 1830 and 1850. Karen Halttunen, *Confidence Men and Painted Women: A Study of Middle-Class Culture in America, 1830-1870* (New Haven: Yale University Press, 1982), 186.

35. Catharine Harbeson Esling, *The Book of Parlour Games* (Philadelphia: Peck and Bliss, 1854), 20-23, 110-111, 248; Frank Bellew, *The Art of Amusing* (New York: Carleton; London: S. Low, Son and Co., 1866). Halttunen also has taken the craze for parlor pastimes as evidence of the decline of sentimental culture, and a corresponding acceptance and enjoyment of the theatricality of parlor social life by middle-class people who once were preoccupied with its possible "hypocrisy." See Halttunen, "Disguises, Masks, and Parlor Theatricals...," in *Confidence Men and Painted Women*.

36. Bellew, *Art of Amusing*, 10-11.

37. M. E. Dodge, *A Few Friends and How They Amused Themselves* (Philadelphia: J. B. Lippincott and Co., 1869), 11.

38. Caroline L. Smith (Aunt Carrie), *The American Book of In-Door Games, Amusements, and Occupations* (Boston: Lee and Shepard, 1873), 89.

39. Esling, *Book of Parlour Games*, and Smith, *American Book of In-Door Games*, 112.

40. See Smith, *American Book of In-Door Games* and Bellew, *Art of Amusing*.

41. See, for example, Mary D. Robertson, ed., *Lucy Breckenridge of Grove Hill: The Journal of a Virginia Girl 1862-1864* (Kent, OH: Kent State University Press, 1979), 117.

42. See Robertson, ed., *Lucy Breckenridge*.

43. Although manners books usually devoted much attention to mourning dress and customs, the display of the body in the parlor and the execution of the actual funeral ceremony were rarely discussed. A few manners books do document the role of parlors in death preparations: "If guests are invited to go from the house to the church, the corpse is usually exposed in the drawing-room, while the family are assembled in another apartment," Richard Wells noted in his 1891 volume *Manners, Culture and Dress*. "No one should call upon a bereaved family while the dead remains in the house." Wells explained at length the differences in behavior associated with funerals at home in the parlor and at churches, which suggests that recent changes in traditional practices now required such specific advice. See Wells, *Manners, Culture and Dress*, 314-315.

44. See Stowe, *We and Our Neighbors*.

45. Alice Hughes Neupert, "In Those Days: Buffalo in the 1870's," *Niagara Frontier* 24, 4 (Winter 1977): 77-78. The author of this memoir died in 1953 at the age of 73. The manuscript, which seems to have been produced for the entertainment of her family, was submitted to the journal by her daughter-in-law.

46. Neupert, "In Those Days," 77-79.

47. This kind of careful preservation also is recorded in other family histories, such as Edith Spencer's memoir of growing up in Pittsburgh. Spencer, *Spencers of Amberson Avenue*, 17.

48. A. C. Steele, *Aunt Teeks in Memory Land*, vol. 1 (Windsor, MA: The Progressive Club, 1959), 9.

49. Katherine Yearick Foster Cavano, interview with author, Pennington, NJ, March and December 1986.

50. Spencer, *Spencers of Amberson Avenue*, 17.

51. Margaret Frances Byington, *Homestead: The Households of a Mill Town* (1910; reprint, New York: Arno Press, 1969).

52. Louis Bolard More, *Wage-Earners' Budgets: A Study of Standards and Cost of Living in New York City* (New York: Henry Holt and Company, 1907), 133-134.

Chapter Three Notes

1. Invoice of Meader Furniture Co., Cincinnati, OH, 27 December 1876, George Ware Fulton Papers, Barker History Archive, University of Texas, Austin, TX.

2. [George A. Martin], *Our Homes: How to Beautify Them* (New York: O. Judd and Co., 1887), 43.

3. Mary Gay Humphreys, "The Parlor," *The Decorator and Furnisher* 11, 5 (May 1888): 52.

4. Ada Cone, "Aesthetic Mistakes in Furnishing—The Parlor Centre Table," *The Decorator and Furnisher* 17, 4 (January 1891): 132.

5. Williams and Jones, *Beautiful Homes*, 56. Who the intended audience was for such advice books is a vexing question, but an important one to try to answer. Careful reading can often divulge to whom an author chose to write, as can observation of the quality of the book itself, its cost when new (if it can be known), and the kinds of other titles the publisher advertised in a book's front and back matter. The survival of numerous copies of the book in research libraries can suggest its widespread distribution, if not its specific readership. Furnishings advice books that seem to have been directed to audiences in rural areas, audiences with small disposable incomes, or new consumers include Williams and Jones, *Beautiful Homes*; [Martin], *Our Homes: How to Beautify Them*; Louis H. Gibson, *Convenient Houses, with Fifty Plans for the Housekeeper, Architect and Housewife…* (New York: T. Y. Crowell and Co., 1889); and *Household Conveniences; Being the Experience of Many Practical Writers* (New York: Orange Judd Co., 1884). Their advice seems to express many of the most conventional ideas about furnishing houses and the meanings of those furnishings, because it is introducing ideas about interior decoration to consumers with limited budgets, living away from centers of fashion.

6. See *Sears, Roebuck and Co. Catalogue No. 104, 1897*, unpaginated.

7. Neupert, "In Those Days," 77-79.

8. See Turner, "Symbols in Ndembu Ritual," 30. "Ritual, scholars are coming to see, is precisely a mechanism that periodically converts the obligatory into the desirable. The basic unit of ritual, the dominant symbol, encapsulates the major properties of the total ritual process which brings about this transmutation. Within its framework of meanings, the dominant symbol brings the ethical and jural norms of society into close contact with strong emotional stimuli…Norms and values, on the one hand, become saturated with emotion, while the gross and basic emotions become ennobled through contact with social values. The irksomeness of moral constraint is transformed into the 'love of virtue.'"

9. Following the lead of Arthur M. Schlesinger in *Learning How to Behave: A Historical Study of American Etiquette Books* (1946), Halttunen has suggested this change in American understandings of gentility in her analysis of etiquette books dating between 1830 and 1870. See *Confidence Men and Painted Women*, 84-85.

10. Arthur Martine, *Martine's Handbook of Etiquette, and Guide to True Politeness* (New York: Dick and Fitzgerald, 1852, 1866), title page; John A. Ruth, *Decorum: A Practical Treatise on Etiquette and Dress of the Best American Society* (New York, Boston, Cincinnati, Atlanta: Union Publishing House, 1881; and Chicago: Chas. L. Snyder and Co., 1881), 1.

11. Florence Hartley, *The Ladies' Book of Etiquette, and Manual of Politeness* (Boston: G. W. Cottrell, 1856), 151-152, 149.

12. *Etiquette for Ladies*, 19.

13. This account of "sincere" etiquette in sentimental culture draws on Halttunen, "Sentimental Culture and the Problem of Etiquette," in *Confidence Men and Painted Women*.

14. Ibid., 93.

15. Hartley, *Ladies' Book of Etiquette*, 149.

16. *Chesterfield's Art of Letter-Writing Simplified, to which is appended the Complete Rules of Etiquette, and the Usages of Society* (New York: Dick and Fitzgerald, Publishers, 1857, 1860), 41.

17. Norbert Elias, *The History of Manners*, vol. 1 of *The Civilizing Process* (New York: Pantheon Books, 1978), 35-50. Originally published as *Uber den Prozess der Zivilisation* (Switzerland: Haus zum Falken, 1939).

18. Jonathan Swift, "Good Manners," *The Tatler No. 298* (London: William Harrison, 1711), reprinted in Diarmuid Russell, ed., *The Portable Irish Reader* (New York: Viking Press, 1946), 10.

19. Edwin Harrison Cady, "The Gentleman: Traditions and Meanings," in *The Gentleman in America: A Literary Study in American Culture* (Syracuse, NY: Syracuse University Press, 1949), 9-14.

20. Kasson discussed the ambivalence of American thinkers toward technology in *Civilizing the Machine.*

21. Harris has discussed the dimensions of this debate over virtue, fashion, and luxury as it affected the arts and architecture in *Artist in American Society,* although I would not agree that the argument had "solved itself by the 1830s."

22. Halttunen, *Confidence Men and Painted Women,* 89.

23. Sigourney, *Letters to Mothers,* 157.

24. "Boarding Out," 146.

25. "A Parlor View," *Gleason's,* 11 November 1854, 300.

26. For a discussion of the "French renaissance" styles with further illustrations of the type, see Ames, "George Henkels, Nineteenth-Century Cabinet-maker." Just as French etiquette and culture were considered the most refined in the world, so too, since the eighteenth century, its fashion and taste in furnishing represented to members of American elites the most cultivated vision of parlor life.

27. Mrs. Parkes, *Domestic Duties or, Instructions to Young Married Ladies…,* 3d ed. (New York: J. and J. Harper, 1829), 59.

28. Williams, *Dream Worlds,* 38.

29. John Cornforth, *English Interiors 1790-1848: The Quest for Comfort* (London: Barrie and Jenkins Ltd., 1978), 13.

30. See Cornforth, *English Interiors;* see also the illustrations of middle-class rooms in Scandinavia, Austria, Germany, and Holland in Thornton, *Authentic Decor.*

31. Kirkland, *Book for the Home Circle,* 197.

32. This concern seems to have had a regional character, for it is clear that the gentry of the South were not worried about these issues. Rather, many seem to have been aligned firmly with the "aristocratic" taste.

33. Harriet Beecher Stowe [Christopher Crowfield, pseud.], *House and Home Papers* (Boston: Fields, Osgood, and Co., 1869), 21.

34. Alice B. Neal, "Furnishing; or, Two Ways of Commencing Life," *Godey's Lady's Book,* November 1850, 299-305.

35. Stowe, *House and Home Papers,* 40, 34.

36. Catharine Beecher, *Miss Beecher's Domestic Receipt Book,* 3d ed. (New York: Harper and Bros., 1858), 274.

37. Beecher, *Domestic Receipt Book,* 275.

38. Henry William Cleaveland, William Backus, and Samuel D. Backus, *Village and Farm Cottages: The Requirements of American Village Homes Considered and Suggested…* (New York: D. Appleton and Co., 1856), 132.

39. Seymour, *Home: The Basis of the State,* 57.

40. Emma Wellmont, *Uncle Sam's Palace; or, The Reigning King,* 2d ed. (Boston: Sanborn, Carter, Bazin and Co., 1853), 180.

41. Cleaveland et al., *Village and Farm Cottages,* 131.

42. Between 1836 and 1853, about 10,000 patents were issued in the United States; by 1876, more than 200,000 had been granted. By 1873, more than 2,000 patents had been issued for improved clothes washers alone. William and Marlys Ray, *The Art of Invention: Patent Models and Their Makers* (Princeton, NJ: The Pyne Press, 1974), 35. While devices and objects associated with improved bodily comfort proliferated, patterns of domestic consumption also changed. One manifestation of changing values was creation of an up-to-date parlor.

43. Kirkland, *Book for the Home Circle,* 208. This recognition of the dual physical and psychological nature of "comfort" actually accords with its history as a concept. The lexicography of "comfort" reveals that using the term to designate a physical condition or state is almost unknown before the eighteenth century. Rather, "comfort" relates to succor, moral or spiritual strengthening, heartening, and supporting in trouble or grief. The *Oxford English Dictionary's* eighth definition of the verb "to comfort"—"to bring into a comfortable state (of body and feelings), allay physical discomfort, make comfortable"—notes that this understanding is "App. only of modern use." Its sixth definition of the noun "comfort"—"a state of physical and material well-being, with freedom from pain and trouble, and satisfaction of bodily needs…" —is supported by examples of use no earlier than 1818, although the use of the word in this sense can be found several decades earlier. While psychological state still is factored into such definitions, it is now secular ("a tranquil enjoyment") rather than a condition of moral or spiritual solace.

44. Seymour, *Home: The Basis of the State,* 57.

45. Kirkland, *Book for the Home Circle,* 198-199.

46. Cleaveland et al., *Village and Farm Cottages,* 129. See also Stowe, *House and Home Papers.*

47. Cleaveland et al., *Village and Farm Cottages,* 133.

48. Harriet Beecher Stowe, *Uncle Tom's Cabin; or, Life Among the Lowly in Three Novels* (1852; reprint, New York: The Library of America, 1982), 162.

49. "Boarding Out," 146.

50. See the introduction to [Miriam Berry Whicher], *The Widow Bedott Papers* (New York: J. C. Derby, 1856), 2, for the use of this term. The genre also includes more famous examples as in Richard Haliburton's "Sam Slick" stories and Anne S. Stephens's *High Life*

in New York.

51. [Whicher], *Widow Bedott*, 223.

Chapter Four Notes

1. Allen, *Rural Architecture*, 59.

2. John Bullock, *The American Cottage Builder* (New York: Stringer and Townsend, 1854), 122.

3. Cleaveland et al., *Village and Farm Cottages*, 132; Allen, *Rural Architecture*, 238, 239.

4. William C. Richards, *A Day in the New York Crystal Palace, and How to Make the Most of It* (New York: G. P. Putnam and Co., 1853), 44.

5. Eames, "Furniture in England, France and the Netherlands," 181-214; Thornton, *Seventeenth-Century Interior Decoration in England, France, and Holland* (1978; reprint, New Haven: Published for the Paul Mellon Centre for Studies in British Art by Yale University Press, 1983), 192-196.

6. *Oxford English Dictionary*, s.v. "ease." In this definition, *transf.*, or "transferred sense," refers to a broadening of meaning.

7. A "conversation piece" is defined as "a portrait group in a domestic or architectural setting in which the sitters are engaged in conversation or social activity of a not very vigorous character. Conversation pieces are usually, though not always, small in scale. They were produced in large numbers in Britain during the eighteenth century, but the use of the term is not confined to British painting or to this period." Harold Osborne, ed., *The Oxford Companion to Art* (Oxford: Oxford University Press, 1971), 278.

8. See, for example, the illustrations in Gervase Jackson-Stops, "Johan Zoffany and the Eighteenth-Century Interior," *Antiques*, June 1987, 1264-1279.

9. See, for example, Georges Duby, *William Marshall: The Flower of Chivalry*, trans. Richard Howard (New York: Pantheon Books, 1986). William Marshall, a knight and baron who served three English kings including Richard the Lionhearted, was described in ballad as tall and straight, part of a code of conventional description applied to people of quality. His posture and bearing were considered an important signal of his honest and courageous nature.

10. Hartley, *Ladies' Book of Etiquette*, 152.

11. Silas Lapham experienced the torments of this perilous no-man's land between the easy manner of etiquette and the crude self when he, his wife, and his daughter were invited to a dinner party at the home of the Boston Brahmin Corey family. After the agonies of escorting Mrs. Corey to the dining room, Lapham "fetched a long sigh of relief when he sank into his chair and felt himself safe from error if he kept a sharp lookout and did only what the others did." By doing so, however, Lapham took wine with each course (something he never did at home) and humiliated himself by becoming drunk at dinner. William Dean Howells, *The Rise of Silas Lapham*, in *William Dean Howells: Novels, 1875-1886* (1885; reprint, New York: The Library of America, 1982), especially chapter 14, 1034-1054.

12. Eliza Leslie, *The Housebook: or, A Manual of Domestic Economy* (Philadelphia: Carey and Hart, 1840), 198.

13. Leslie, *The Housebook*, 194. Recall British actress Fanny Kemble's comment that the "vibratory motion" of rocking chairs in ladies' parlors on American steamboats of the 1830s contributed to an overall sense of tumult in these rooms.

14. *Chesterfield's Art of Letter-Writing Simplified*, 20-21.

15. Hartley, *Ladies' Book of Etiquette*, 152.

16. Stephens, *High Life in New York*, 22.

17. "An Erect Position," *Gleason's*, 28 August 1852, 142.

18. "How to Sit on a Divan," *The Decorator and Furnisher* 18, 5 (October 1891): 8.

19. For histories of nineteenth-century underwear, see Cecil Saint-Laurent, *The Great Book of Lingerie* (New York: The Vendome Press, 1983); Nora Waugh, *Corsets and Crinolines* (New York: Theatre Arts Books, 1954); and C. Willett and Phyllis Cunnington, with revisions by A. D. Mayfield and Valerie Mayfield, *The History of Underclothes* (Boston: Faber and Faber, 1951, 1981).

20. The lessening constraints of masculine parlor clothing suggest that their social roles lay somewhere other than in parlor culture. In comparison, eighteenth-century gentlemen's tailored clothing constrained their movements at a time when they, as members of the upper classes, were also considered conservators and expressors of civility.

21. Unattributed quotation cited in Willett and Cunnington et al., *History of Underclothes*, 114.

22. *Montgomery Ward and Co. 1894-1895 Catalogue and Buyers Guide No. 56* (1894; reprint, Northfield, IL: The Gun Digest Company, 1970), 85. The U.S. Patent Office also issued a number of patents addressing this problem, such as in William A. Nettleton's 1882 patent for "corset stiffeners" made from short sections of horn or whalebone and wrapped together with thread so that they could "break joints in the manner specified" and return to shape when the sitter rose or straightened. Patent No. 265,534 in *Official Gazette, U.S. Patent Office* 22 (1882): 1220.

23. Saint-Laurent, *The Great Book of Lingerie*, 120. Long corsets not only altered sitting and "lounging" but changed the nature of a fashionable woman's gait as well. An advertisement for Warner's '98 Model Corsets explained to readers, "For grace of figure when walking the form should bend slightly forward from the line of waist, and unless Nature has given

this art it can only be produced by raising the bust, thereby tapering the waist and forcing the shoulders erect. The hips are next in importance. They should be well rounded to the centre, then sloping toward the back, which is accomplished by drawing in the abdomen with the aid of the corset." Advertisement for Warner's '98 Model Corset in *The Ladies' Home Journal*, November 1897, 32.

24. Hartley, *Ladies' Book of Etiquette*, 77.

25. For more specific information on seats structures before the advent of the spring seat, see Lizanne Landis, "The Regulator's Art: Early American Upholstery 1660-1930," *Antiques and The Arts Weekly*, 15 April 1883, 1-2, 40; Andrew Passeri and Robert F. Trent, "Two New England Queen Anne Easy Chairs with Original Upholstery," *Maine Antiques Digest*, April 1983, 26A-28A; Karin M. Walton, "The Golden Age of English Furniture Upholstery, 1660-1840" (Catalog of an exhibition at Stable Court Exhibition Galleries, Temple-Newsam House, Leeds, England, 15 August-15 September 1973).

26. Construction and use of cushion seats is discussed in chapter 9.

27. George Himmelheber, *Biedermeier Furniture*, trans. and ed. Simon Jervis (London: Faber and Faber Limited, n.d.), 89-90.

28. Dorothy Holley, "Furniture Springs," *Furniture History* 7 (1981): 64-67. There is also inconclusive evidence that French furniture makers, ever on the cutting edge of their craft, experimented with the use of "elastic springs" inside seating furniture during the reign of Louis XV. See Roger de Félice, *French Furniture Under Louis XV*, trans. Florence Simmonds (New York: Frederick A. Stokes, [1920]), 25-26.

29. Badly tempered springs apparently remained a problem worthy of particular note for decades after their common use in chairs. In its article "Easy-Chairs That Are Easy," *Cassell's Household Guide* praised the springs of chairs provided by C. and W. Trapnell, of Bristol, England: "Being made of the best charcoal wire they retain their elasticity, and will not snap, which is frequently the case with springs made of ordinary hard-drawn wire." "Easy-Chairs That Are Easy," in *Cassell's Household Guide*, vol. 3 (London and New York: Cassell, Petter, and Galpin, about 1870), 308-309. Rhoda and Agnes Garrett, *Suggestions for House Decoration in Painting, Woodwork, and Furniture* (Philadelphia: Porter and Coates, 1877), 64.

30. John Claudius Loudon, *Loudon Furniture Designs from the Encyclopedia of Cottage, Farmhouse and Villa Architecture and Furniture, 1839* (East Ardsley, Yorkshire, and London: S. R. Publishers Ltd. and The Connoisseur, 1970), 336. This edition reprints sections of the *Encyclopedia* and retains the original's pagination.

31. Fern Tuten, "American Domestic Patented Furniture 1790-1850: A Compendium" (Ph.D. diss., Florida State University, 1969; Ann Arbor: University Microfilms, 1969), 74-75.

32. Tuten, "American Domestic Patented Furniture," 83. See also Giedion, *Mechanization Takes Command*, 382-385, for a discussion of Samuel Pratt's 1827 and 1828 English patents for springs associated with shipboard furniture. These were intended to relieve seasickness.

33. Morrison H. Heckscher, *In Quest of Comfort: The Easy Chair in America* (New York: Metropolitan Museum of Art, 1971), 10-11; Thornton, *Seventeenth-Century Interior Decoration in England, France, and Holland*, 196-197; Shirley Glubok and Evelyn Hofer, "Glimpses of Holland's Golden Age: Two Seventeenth-Century Dollhouses Celebrate Daily Life in Old Amsterdam," *The Connoisseur*, December 1984, 112-118. One of the realistic doll houses discussed in the Glubok and Hofer article contains a lying-in room furnished with a tilt-back chair designed for pregnant women.

34. Loudon, *Encyclopedia of Cottage, Farmhouse and Villa Architecture and Furniture*, 322.

35. *The Marks Improved Adjustable Folding Chair* (New York: Marks Improved Adjustable Folding Chair Company, n.d.); Spencer, *Spencers of Amberson Avenue*, 70, 73.

36. See the advertisement for Boston furniture dealer Sherlock Spooner in *The Boston Directory* (Boston: Charles Stimpson, Jr., 1829), unpaginated.

37. Advertisements for J. Hancock and Co. in *Desilver's Philadelphia Directory, and Stranger's Guide* (Philadelphia: Robert Desilver, 1831 and 1833), unpaginated; advertisement for Davis and Scholes in *Matchett's Baltimore Director, 1833* (Baltimore: Richard J. Matchett, 1833), 7.

38. Jane Williams Insley, "Once Upon a Time" (Typescript of memoir delivered in 1943 at a meeting of the Indianapolis, Indiana, Fortnightly Literary Club, 12). A copy was obtained from the author's granddaughter, Elizabeth Insley Traverse.

39. See, for example, the advertisement for Joseph Crook, upholsterer and paper hanger, in *Matchett's Baltimore Director, 1831* (Baltimore: Richard J. Matchett, 1831), unpaginated advertisement. In this advertisement, "Spring Seat Sofas; Patent Spring Seat Rocking Chairs" are separated from the other upholstered furniture offered. Other upholsterers' ads in the same edition do not mention spring upholstery yet.

40. Edwin T. Freedley, *Philadelphia and Its Manufactures: A Hand-Book* (Philadelphia: Edward Young, 1858), 272.

41. Loudon, *Encyclopedia of Cottage, Farmhouse and Villa Architecture and Furniture*, 322.

42. "New Wagon Springs," *Scientific American*, 31 July

1847, 355; *Scientific American*, 27 October 1849, 3.

43. "Elasticity of Bodies," *Scientific American*, 9 April 1846, page not indicated; "Improved Blind-Fastenings," *Scientific American*, 20 March 1847, 204; "Sundry Improvements," *Scientific American*, 10 April 1847, 228.

44. Charles C. Quick, *Tufting Secrets* (Los Angeles: American Book Institute, 1954), 49. In a discussion of "Buttoning as Ornament," John W. Stephenson noted, "The buttoning of upholstering was not alone intended to assist in creating greater comfort in connection with curved and softly-filled surfaces but it was also to serve as a means of ornamentation, the placing of the buttons creating pipes and diamond or bisquit-shaped spaces which were stuffed up so that pleats were formed from button to button." John. W. Stephenson, "Furniture Upholstering," in William J. Etten, ed. *Manual of the Furniture Arts and Crafts* (Grand Rapids: A. P. Johnson Company, 1928), 508.

45. John Phin, author of *The Practical Upholsterer*, noted: "There has been a decided revolution in upholstery work during the past few years. Artistic forms, combined with French luxuriousness, are much sought after...This style of work is upholstered very soft, and can only be done with a good quantity of hair, otherwise it will lose its proper shape before it has been in use any length of time." [John Phin], *The Practical Upholsterer* (New York: The Industrial Publications Company, 1891), 41.

46. *How to Build, Furnish and Decorate* (New York: Cooperative Building Association: 1889), 6.

47. "How to Sit on a Divan," 8.

48. "Among the Stores," *The Decorator and Furnisher* 3, 3 (December 1883): 102.

Chapter Five Notes

1. *The Oxford English Dictionary* defines "formal" used in this context as "pertaining to the outward form, shape, or appearance (of a material object); also, in immaterial sense, pertaining to the form, arrangement, external qualities (e.g. of a work of art, a composition, etc.)." *Oxford English Dictionary*, s.v. "formal."

2. In the Crystal Palace of 1851, for example, papier-mâché was the object of particular admiration, particularly when the paper was transformed into large pieces of furniture such as beds, sofas, and pianos, "as was slate enamelled in imitation of costly marble." See *The Great Exhibition of the World's Industry*, vol. 2 (London and New York: John Tallis and Company, 1851), 209-219. A library table made with marble top of glass by Baccarat for the 1878 Paris Universal Exposition, was a tour de force of this kind of transformed material. The table is in the collection of the Corning Museum of Glass, Corning, New York. In his important essay "High Victorian Design," Nikolaus Pevsner discussed this "pride in

ingeniousness" with understanding, if not complete approbation. Pevsner, "High Victorian Design," in *Victorian and After*, vol. 2 of *Studies in Art, Architecture and Design* (New York: Walker and Company, 1968), 47.

3. Sofa cushion design in *Godey's Lady's Book*, June 1872, 566.

4. Mrs. Jane Weaver, "Ornamental Bracket," *Peterson's Magazine*, September 1877, 217. See also, by the same author, "Ornamental Bracket, Valence [*sic*], Chair-Back, etc.," *Peterson's Magazine*, January 1862, 77; and "Bracket," *Peterson's Magazine*, May 1852, 419.

5. The term "lambrequin" appears to be an Americanism adapted from a French nineteenth-century decorating term. The original French meaning of "lambrequin" was "a scarf or piece of stuff worn over the helmet as a covering. In heraldry represented with one end (which is cut or jagged) pendant or floating." *Oxford English Dictionary*, s.v. "lambrequin."

6. Mrs. Pullen, "Elegant Whatnot," *Peterson's Magazine*, December 1856, 412, 413.

7. "Fashion Plates for Decorating Parlor Windows," 166.

8. Williams and Jones, *Beautiful Homes*, 57.

9. *Sears, Roebuck and Co., 1908, Catalogue No. 117: The Great Price Maker* (1908; reprint, Northfield, IL: Digest Books, 1971), 901.

10. J. R. Pugh, "The Best Room. Its Arrangement and Decoration at Moderate Cost," *The Decorator and Furnisher* 13, 1 (October 1888): 19.

11. For discussion of design economics in the nineteenth-century furniture industry, see Michael J. Ettema, "Technological Innovation and Design Economics in Furniture Manufacture," *Winterthur Portfolio* 16, 2/3 (Summer/Autumn 1981): 197-223.

12. *Sears, Roebuck and Co. Catalogue No. 104, 1897*, unpaginated.

13. *Sears, Roebuck and Co. Catalogue No. 111, 1902*, 787.

14. Ibid., 784, 785.

15. In his essay "Art as a Cultural System," Clifford Geertz argues that no culture's art forms can be studied and made intelligible by only "inter-aesthetic" (internal) analysis of its forms and rules. He writes, "The means of an art and the feeling for life that animates it are inseparable." The problem, for Geertz, is how to place "aesthetic force," in whatever form it takes, "within the other modes of social activity"—to recognize that the aesthetic system of a culture "grows out of a distinctive sensibility the whole of life participates in forming." See Geertz, "Art as a Cultural System," 97-98. "Sensibility," as Geertz uses the term, may be defined as the character

of a particular culture's general awareness, or mental perception, of itself in the world. For Geertz, the most profitable analysis of any culture's art forms compares many forms of expression and leads inevitably to the broadest questions of how people make meaningful "the profusion of things that happen to them." Exploring an art form by analyzing the ways in which it is connected to other forms of cultural expression is ultimately an exploration of the "collective formulation" which is the sensibility of a culture. For Geertz, art objects express the meaning of collective life; they "materialize a way of experiencing, bringing a particular cast of mind out into the world of objects, where men can look at it" (ibid., 99).

16. Ibid., 98.

17. See Daniel P. Biebuyck, *The Lega: Art, Initiation and Moral Philosophy* (Berkeley: University of California Press, 1973); Biebuyck, "Symbolism of the Lega Stool," 1-36.

18. Biebuyck, "Symbolism of the Lega Stool," 20. The association does this through levels of codified knowledge, each requiring tutoring and initiation ceremonies involving music and dance, proverbs and stories, and the manipulation of a variety of artifacts such as ivory carvings and stools and natural objects such as large snail shells.

19. He also discusses how some aspects of painting, particularly the formal geometry of pictures, could be meaningful to men who knew the complicated mathematics of "gauging" for commercial purposes, and how the colors used in paintings, particularly blue and gold, were legible signals of the wealth of the patron. Michael Baxandall, *Painting and Experience in Quattrocento Italy* (Oxford, England: Clarendon Press, 1972), 56-64.

20. Michael Baxandall is developing this work further, and some of the information above was presented in a recent lecture, "Renaissance Art Criticism," delivered 28 August 1986 at the Institute for the Study of Critical Theory held at Hobart and William Smith Colleges, Geneva, New York.

21. Two other related kinds of associations also emphasized the ways in which the outside world of Western civilization, including commerce and technology, was brought into the service of the parlor. One consisted of a loosely understood set of historical and exotic meanings that encompassed ornament and historical style. The other emphasized the transformation of the world's material resources into parlor objects. In this way, the parlor became not only a site for domestic associations but also a memory palace of culture, history, and technology—a museum. These particular associations will be discussed in the context of the late nineteenth-century interest in French and Turkish taste.

22. [Martin], *Our Homes: How to Beautify Them*, iii.

23. See Halttunen, "Sentimental Culture and the Problem of Etiquette," in *Confidence Men and Painted Women*, 92-123, for a discussion of proper feeling in manners.

24. Wells, *Manners, Culture and Dress*, 297.

25. *Manual of Politeness, Comprising the Principles of Etiquette and Rules of Behavior in Genteel Society, for Persons of Both Sexes* (Philadelphia: W. Marshall and Co., 1837), 15.

26. Williams and Jones, *Beautiful Homes*, 179.

27. *Eighty Years' Progress*, vol. 2, 245, 260.

28. "An Antiquarian," "Our Home: Its History and Progress, with Notices of the Introduction of Domestic Inventions," *The Household Journal*, 28 September 1861, 407.

29. Benjamin Butterworth, comp., *The Growth of Industrial Art* (Washington: G.P.O./U.S. Patent Office, 1892), 80.

30. Historically, many different social and economic factors have contributed to making certain furnishing fabrics especially desirable. Rarity and difficulty in obtaining large yardages sometimes made what now seem to be ordinary textiles intensely desirable; the printed cottons imported to Europe from India in the late sixteenth and seventeenth centuries were expensive and only appeared in wealthy, fashionable households both in England and on the continent. Thornton, *Seventeenth-Century Interior Decoration in England, France, and Holland*, 116.

31. See Eames, "Furniture in England, France and the Netherlands."

32. Kirkland, "Fashionable and Unfashionable," in *Book for the Home Circle*, 102-129.

33. These do-it-yourself upholstery projects are discussed in detail in chapter 9 of this book.

34. Yi-Fu Tuan, *Segmented Worlds and Self: Group Life and Individual Consciousness* (Minneapolis: University of Minnesota Press, 1982), 115. The term "proximate senses" is used by Tuan to designate the senses that require direct bodily contact in order to function.

35. *How to Build, Furnish and Decorate*, 8.

36. [Phin], *The Practical Upholsterer*, 41.

37. Howells, *Rise of Silas Lapham*, 968.

38. "Editor's Easy Chair," *Harper's New Monthly Magazine*, July 1854, 262; *Sears, Roebuck and Co. Catalogue No. 117, 1908*, 901.

39. [Martin], *Our Homes: How to Beautify Them*, 43.

40. Copeland, "Draperies, Blinds and Curtains," 269-272.

41. *Victor Manufacturing Co. Special Up-to-Date*

Catalogue (Chicago, 1899), unpaginated.

42. "A Visit to Henkels' Warerooms," 123.

43. "Mosaic Hearth Rug," *Frank Leslie's Ladies' Gazette of Paris, London, and New York Fashions*, September 1854, 167.

44. Stephens, *High Life in New York*, 20, 92.

45. Charles L. Eastlake, *Hints on Household Taste in Furniture, Upholstery and Other Details* (London: Longmans, Green, and Co., 1872), 94-95.

46. James Carruthers, "Dry Goods Stores as Furnishing Emporiums," *The Decorator and Furnisher* 19, 2 (November 1891): 51.

47. Carroll L. V. Meeks, *The Victorian Railroad Station* (New Haven: Yale University Press, 1964), 3-5.

48. "A Chapter on Book Illustrations," *The Ladies' Repository and Home Magazine*, October 1869, 259.

49. C. T. Hinkley, "The Art of Engraving," *Godey's Lady's Book*, August 1859, 109, 110.

50. "A Chapter on Book Illustrations," 259.

51. Daguerreotyping was introduced to American inventors just weeks after Daguerre's introduction of the process in Paris, and, with no patent restrictions to prevent its widespread adoption, photography in America became an inexpensive, popular process of picture-making by the 1850s. See Taft, *Photography and the American Scene*.

52. Oliver Wendell Holmes, "The Stereoscope and the Stereograph," in Vicki Goldberg, ed., *Photography in Print: Writings from 1816 to the Present* (New York: Simon and Schuster, 1981), 107-108.

53. Baxandall, *Painting and Experience*, 24.

54. *History of the Brooklyn and Long Island Fair, February 22, 1864* (Brooklyn: The Executive Committee [of the Fair], 1864), 38. See also Richards, *Day in the New York Crystal Palace*, a small guidebook that gave readers a tour of the exhibits item by item in a text that also implies the pleasures of so much visual experience gathered together in one location.

55. *History of the Brooklyn and Long Island Fair*, 47.

56. *How to Build, Furnish and Decorate*, 10.

57. Daniel Biebuyck, for example, suggests that symbolic objects may serve as "cosmic or historical archives" or as vehicles for expressing and elaborating moral philosophy. Objects bearing symbolic meaning in Victorian culture may serve these functions but also bear other kinds of meaning; they may also be repositories of sentiment, expressions of social ideals, or expressions of the nature of sex roles. Biebuyck, "Symbolism of the Lega Stool," 28; Biebuyck, *The Lega*, 234.

58. Biebuyck offers an observation about Lega ascription of meaning to art objects that would seem to have broad application to the study of any form of material culture as a form of communication. He notes, in the case of Lega use of ceremonial stools in ritual, that the manipulation of meaningful objects is part of a highly redundant communications process of stories, proverbs, dances, and objects. See Biebuyck, "Symbolism of the Lega Stool," 28.

59. Facing a similar phenomenological problem in his observations on the "cognitive style" of Renaissance people looking at paintings, Baxandall qualifies his observations by offering a useful set of "boundaries." He argues that three "culturally relative" variables are employed in the interpretation of visual data—"a stock of patterns, categories and methods of inference, training in a range of representational conventions, and experience, drawn from the environment, in what are plausible ways of visualizing what we have incomplete information about." Because perception skills are both culturally relative and learned, not all Quattrocento viewers of pictures possessed all the skills that would enable them to enjoy a particular picture. Conversely, not all pictures contained all the elements such as body postures and paint handling that made up the repertoire of artistic aesthetic options. Instead, understanding and enjoying a picture was, in part, a question of matching two mental sets of the language of painted signs, one held by the painter and the other in the viewer's educational background. Baxandall writes, "To sum up: some of the mental equipment a man orders his visual experience with is variable, and much of this variable equipment is culturally relative, in the sense of being determined by the society which influenced his experience. Among these variables are categories with which he classifies his visual stimuli, the knowledge he will use to supplement what his immediate vision gives him, and the attitude he will adopt to the kind of artificial object seen. The beholder must use on the painting such visual skills as he has, very few of which are normally special to painting, and he is likely to use those skills his society esteems highly. The painter responds to this; his public's visual capacity must be his medium. Whatever his own specialized professional skills, he is himself a member of the society he works for and shares its visual experience and habit." Baxandall, *Painting and Experience*, 32, 34, 40.

60. See the discussion of window shades painted with landscapes in chapter 8.

61. The painting techniques graining and marbleizing, which created artificial surfaces resembling expensive woods or stone on inexpensive materials such as pine or slate, enjoyed widespread popularity during the first half of the nineteenth century, although they continued in use throughout the century.

62. Copeland, "Draperies, Blinds and Curtains," 269-272. The same article, with no author named, appeared as a three-part series in *Godey's Lady's Book*, March 1860, 78; April 1860, 325; and June 1860, 506-509.

63. "Hints and Notions," *The Decorator and Furnisher* 12, 1 (March 1888): 198.

64. Calvin Tomkins, *The Bride and the Bachelors: Five Masters of the Avant Garde* (New York: Penguin Books, 1976), 19.

Chapter Six Notes

1. Untitled notice in *The Statesman*, Yonkers, New York, 3 August 1877. The article is used as a handout at Trevor's house, which is restored and belongs to the Hudson River Museum.

2. See chapter 7 for a discussion of the apparent significance of tufting to consumers and how this preference led to the development of the tufting machine.

3. Eleanor Pearson DeLorme, "The Swan Commissions," *Winterthur Portfolio* 14, 4 (Winter 1979): 374. Gentility has been defined as "not only a theory of excellence and a set of responsibilities, but a full blown way of life with its beau monde, for the first time significantly independent of the Court, in which to express itself." See Cady, *The Gentleman in America*, 8.

4. Kenneth L. Ames, "Designed in France: Notes on the Transmission of French Style to America," in Ian M. G. Quimby, ed., *Winterthur Portfolio 12* (Charlottesville, VA: University Press of Virginia, 1978), 103-114.

5. *Cummings Telegraphic Evening Bulletin* 38, 1144, Philadelphia, Pennsylvania, 1 January 1854, 3.

6. Phillip M. Johnston, "Dialogues between Designer and Client: Furnishings Proposed by Leon Marcotte to Samuel Colt in the 1850s," *Winterthur Portfolio* 19, 4 (Winter 1984): 257-276.

7. The émigré decorators Auguste and Gabriel Elleau seem to have provided blue chintz slipcovers for a parlor suite described in an auction notice of 1841. A small upholstered tub chair, sold with only its white muslin undercover and slipcovers, survives in the collection of Peter Strickland in Philadelphia, Pennsylvania. See *Catalogue of Handsome Household Furniture, to be sold by Bleeker and Van Dyke on Thursday, April 22, 1841, at No. 2 Albion Place* (New York, 1841).

8. An advertisement of Colie and Sons, Buffalo, New York, in the *Grand Rapids Furniture Record* of August 1911 depicted an easy chair fully covered in a print fabric, with a ruffled skirt and separate seat cushion. The text introduced the chair as part of the firm's new "boudoir suites," now available with "glove-fitting removable Wash Covers." The text noted further, "There's an appeal to Milady in the continued freshness of these easily laundered chintzes." *Grand Rapids Furniture Record* 23, 3 (August 1911), 450.

9. Theodore Child, "Decorative Art in Paris," *The Decorator and Furnisher* 1, 3 (December 1882): 91.

10. "French Arrangement of a Fireplace," *The Decorator and Furnisher* 16, 1 (April 1890): 20.

11. "New Furniture," 153.

12. Kirkland, *Book for the Home Circle*, 208.

13. "The French at Home," *Godey's Lady's Book*, November 1856, 431.

14. "How They Live in Paris," *Godey's Lady's Book*, May 1859, 385, 442-443.

15. Harriet Beecher Stowe, *Pink and White Tyranny* (Boston: Roberts Brothers, 1871), 126-127.

16. Harriet Beecher Stowe, *The Little Foxes* (Boston: Ticknor and Fields, 1866), 229-230.

17. Ibid., 230, 232.

18. Ibid., 232.

19. Eastlake, *Hints on Household Taste*, 9, 71.

20. Cook, *House Beautiful*, 320-321.

21. Like design reform, the renewed interest in French style was transatlantic. In an article "Among the Upholsterers of Paris," a reprint from the London publication *The Cabinet Maker* that appeared in the May 1890 issue of the *The Decorator and Furnisher*, J. William Benn lamented, "It did seem some ten years ago that, so far as the appointments of English homes were concerned, British furnishers were prepared to shake off the thraldom which has certainly existed for the greater part of the Victorian era. Several of our leading houses set aside the twists and curves of the French modes, and went in for straight lines and palpably honest construction…But all this is over when looking at that which we sent from this country to the last Paris Exhibition. One is compelled to say with Shakespeare, 'What a falling off was there!' So far as the drawing room and the boudoir are concerned, it is perfectly clear that Paris has succeeded in regaining the position of mentor to our furnishers which she held prior to the time when Talbert and Eastlake invented their straight beaded and spindled furniture." Benn noted that "seats and fancy articles" were enjoying particular success among English furnishing firms. J. William Benn, "Among the Upholsterers of Paris," *The Decorator and Furnisher* 16, 1 (May 1890): 43.

22. "The Louis Quinze," *The American Cabinet Maker, Upholsterer and Carpet Reporter* 14, 3 (2 December 1876): 10.

23. Regarding modern use of historical architectural detail, A. J. Downing maintained that "still, even in very modest cottages, there are certain simple lines and forms, indicative of various styles of building, which may be introduced, with no more cost—provided the workmen who execute the plans

are familiar with them—than any other simple lines and forms. A degree of cultivation is necessary, perhaps, to appreciate all the enjoyment which grows out of this attention to details; but, as it is a large and enduring source of pleasure, it should receive attention in all country houses of considerable importance." Downing, *The Architecture of Country Houses* (New York: Appleton and Company, 1850; New York: Dover Publications, Inc., 1969), 365-366.

24. Michael Levey, *Early Renaissance* (New York: Penguin, 1977), 15.

25. For a useful discussion of this phenomenon, as well as an excellent and useful compendium of illustrations, see Richard Guy Wilson et al., *American Renaissance, 1876-1917* (Brooklyn, NY: The Brooklyn Museum, 1979).

26. For a survey of some of the artifactual results of this search for identity among the American business and industrial elite, see Wilson et al., *American Renaissance*. For more on this self-imaging process, see also Edward Chase Kirkland, *Dream and Thought in the Business Community* (New York: Quadrangle Books, 1956).

27. Humphreys, "The Parlor," 52.

28. "Editor's Easy Chair," *Harper's New Monthly Magazine*, 9, 50, July 1854, 261. For discussion of historical associationism in commercial architecture of the mid-nineteenth century, see Winston Weisman, "Commercial Palaces of New York, 1845-1875," *The Art Bulletin* 34 (December 1954): 285-302.

29. John Tallis, *Tallis's History and Description of the Crystal Palace*, vol. 1 (London and New York: John Tallis and Co., [1851-1852]), 62-63.

30. F. J. B. Watson, *Louis XVI Furniture* (1960; reprint, New York: Saint Martin's Press, 1973), 37. Summarizing the French seating types throughout the eighteenth century, Watson has noted that "the evolution of furniture and particularly of the seat in all its forms was dictated to a remarkable extent by these two factors: comfort and the facilities of conversation."

31. Theodore Child, "French House Furnishing. The Salon," *The Decorator and Furnisher* 3, 2 (November 1883): 49. At the same time, Child worried that the importance of attaining these particular two qualities in furniture lead to a decline in the best furniture, which had what he termed "an intense and matchless elegance."

32. For example, the unknown decorator J. W. Bliss of Providence, Rhode Island, won a prize from *The Decorator and Furnisher* for his "Louis Seize Drawing-Room," which received a full page illustration in *The Decorator and Furnisher* 17, 5 (February 1891): 161.

33. A number of surviving late nineteenth-century

schemes of interior decoration for new houses follow this formula of the French drawing room, as in the house of the John H. Ballantine family (of Ballantine brewing fame) of Newark, New Jersey, now part of the Newark Museum, Newark, New Jersey. Built between 1883 and 1885, the town house was decorated by the New York firm of D. S. Hess and Company, the drawing room,also called the "White Room," had cream-colored paneling with gold leaf details and cream-colored silk wall covering. The chairs were Louis XVI and Turkish, and the bay window drapery featured a valance of large swags with deep Turkish fringe. See Phillip H. Curtis, "The Ballantine House: Preserving a Newark Tradition," *The Newark Museum Quarterly* 27, 4 (Fall 1976): 10, 12.

34. Mrs. Barnes-Bruce, "Some Graceful Centrepieces," *Ladies' Home Journal* 12, 7, June 1895, 12-13; Helen Mar Adams, "Louis XV Embroidery Designs," *Ladies' Home Journal* 12, 9, August 1895, 11.

35. *Montgomery Ward Co. Catalogue and Buyers' Guide No. 57, Spring and Summer, 1895*, 510.

36. *Sears, Roebuck and Co. Catalog No. 110, Fall, 1900* (reprint, Northfield, IL: DBI Books, Inc., 1970), 1078.

37. Thornton, *Authentic Decor*, 52.

38. Richards, *Day in the New York Crystal Palace*, 44.

39. A chair that employs real Oriental carpet cut up and used as its upholstery is in the collections of the National Museum of American History, Smithsonian Institution, in the division of domestic life.

40. "Meister Karl" [pseud.], "Turkish Proverbs," *Godey's Lady's Book*, March 1855, 272-273, reprinted thirty-three proverbs and offered several sources for more.

41. "Turkish Bag in Wool Work," *Godey's Lady's Book*, September 1856, 260; "Turkish Purse," *Godey's Lady's Book*, October 1856, 360.

42. For an overview of the types of upholstery associated with Eugenie, including oriental "comfortables" and *Louis XVI a l'Imperatrice*, see Colette Lehman, *Mobilier Louis-Philippe Napolean III* (Paris: Editions Ch. Massin, n.d.).

43. Philipp Jullian, *The Orientalists: European Painters of Eastern Scenes*, trans. Helga and Dinah Harrison (Oxford: Phaidon Press, 1977), 77.

44. For a discussion of artists' and writers' travels in the Orient, and an analysis of the cultural products—painting, fiction, travel accounts, and theatrical production—resulting from this contact, see Edward W. Said, *Orientalism* (New York: Pantheon Books, 1978).

45. The sexual ideology of such pictures has been explored by Linda Nochlin in "The Imaginary Orient," *Art in America*, May 1983, 119-131, 186-

191.

46. Constance Cary Harrison, *Woman's Handiwork in Modern Homes* (New York: C. Scribner's Sons, 1890), 160.

47. *Gems of the Centennial Exhibition*, 43.

48. The passage continues, providing an example of the cosmopolitan experience ordinary visitors received at the fairgrounds outside the main buildings:

"We will give one day as an example of our travels.

"We enter an Egyptian structure and behold an oriental barber shaving one of his countrymen. Egypt cannot teach us anything about shaving our countrymen; we do not linger here. As we leave the building, a Russian britzska, a carriage invented especially for the use of American spelling bees, dashes by us drawn by the very cream of Tartar steeds. We catch on behind until we reach a Persian bazaar. We gaze upon the long bearded native men, and the shrouded native women, busily engaged in their national occupation of going to sleep, and became wrapped up in shawls of imagination...

"We pause for a moment before the French restaurant, enraptured, looking at the pretty girls and other dainties served up there. We decline the invitation of a Chinese drummer, hanging around to inveigle parties into the restaurant established by his country, with a long rigamarole about 'Kittens fried in castor oil,' and enter the Main Hall.

"We land in the desert of Sahara, but desert Sahara and step over to Spain...We pass through Portugal; more wine, fruit, and olive oil. We hop through Japan, change a ten cent note for a bushel of their "hard money," and sachey on. We linger for hours in fair France, principally in the Paris department. We saunter through Austria...then through Germany and Switzerland, until we reach Great Britain." See "Daisy Shortcut" and "'Arry O'Pagus" [pseuds.], *Our Show: A Humorous Account of the International Exhibition in Honor of the Centennial Anniversary of American Independence...* (New York: The American News Company; Philadelphia: Claxton, Remsen and Haffelfinger, 1875), 63-65.

49. *What Ben Beverly Saw at the Great Exposition* (Chicago: Centennial Publishing Company, 1876), 147-148.

50. Frank H. Norton, *Frank Leslie's Illustrated Historical Register of the Centennial Exposition, 1876* (New York: Frank Leslie's Publishing House, 1877; New York: Paddington Press, 1974), 107.

51. Map in Dorsey Gardner, ed., *United States Centennial Commission. Grounds and Buildings of the Centennial Exhibition, Philadelphia, 1876* (Philadelphia: J. B. Lippincott and Co., 1878), 146.

52. "Turkey: Its Past Condition and Promised Reforms," *Frank Leslie's Popular Monthly* 1, 2, February 1876, 129.

53. Catalog of S. C. Small and Co. (Boston, MA, about 1880), 10-16; *Supplement to Bub and Kipp's Illustrated Catalogue of 1885*, 32-33.

54. *Catalogue of Jordan, Marsh and Company, Fall and Winter, 1889* (Boston, MA, 1889), 30-31, 33, 35-36.

55. Hubert Howe Bancroft, *The Book of the Fair: An Historical and Descriptive Presentation of the World's Science, Art, and Industry, as Viewed through the Columbian Exposition at Chicago in 1893...* (Chicago: Bancroft Company, 1893), 855.

56. S. M. Putnam, "Draperies and Embroideries in the East," *The Decorator and Furnisher* 19, 1 (October 1891): 20-21.

57. Harvey Green has discussed the prolonged force and vitality of such arguments in his *Fit for America: Health, Fitness, Sport, and American Society* (New York: Pantheon Books, 1986).

58. James Thomson, "Cozy Corners and Ingle Nooks," *Ladies' Home Journal* 10, 12, November 1893, 27. Thomson offered five plans for do-it-yourself cozy corners, made from boxes and printed jute, denim, or cretonne for informal rooms, "figured silk, satin damask, plush or brocatelle" with silk festoons for parlors.

59. Catalog of Bishop Furniture Co. (Grand Rapids, MI, about 1910), 126.

Chapter Seven Notes

1. Philip M. Johnston, "Dialogues Between Designer and Client: Furnishings Proposed by Leon Marcotte to Samuel Colt in the 1850s," *Winterthur Portfolio* 19, 4 (Winter 1984): 268.

2. *Catalogue of Genteel Household Furniture, for Sale at Auction, by Henry H. Leeds and Co., on Friday, April 29th, 1853.*

3. Household inventory of George Clinton Latta, Charlotte, NY, 1856, Rare Books Collection, University of Rochester. Thanks to Joan Sullivan, who transcribed the inventory, and to William Siles for calling it to my attention.

4. Gail Dennis, "Factory-Made Parlor Suites, 1870-1901" (MA thesis, Winterthur Program in Early American Culture, University of Delaware, 1982), 9-11. Ms. Dennis did a statistical analysis of sixty furniture trade catalogs and price lists for the years 1871-1901. The sample was slightly biased toward the first fifteen years of her scope (thirty-seven examples). In her analysis of the 924 parlor suites offered for sale, 687 consisted of seven pieces, a sofa and a selection of chair types. She identified and discussed nine "salient characteristics" of parlor suites: 1) inclusion of a sofa; 2) two or more pieces of furniture; 3) seating furniture only; 4) associated with the parlor; 5) visually related pieces of furniture; 6) spring upholstered; 7) range of prices (fifteen to four hundred dollars, with most from forty to two hundred dollars); 8) choices of style; 9) options

available in decoration rather than in types of forms.

5. *Catalogue of Furniture, George J. Henkels City Cabinet Warerooms, 173 Chestnut St.* The range of prices for sets is based on calculating the prices presented for each piece offered in the catalog. Henkels' business, and the styles of furniture he offered, have been discussed by Kenneth L. Ames in "Designed in France: Notes on the Transmission of French Style in America," *Winterthur Portfolio* 12 (Charlottesville, VA: University Press of Virginia, 1977): 103-114. Henkels' store was described several times in fiction and articles published by *Godey's Lady's Book* during the 1850s. See "A Visit to Henkels' Warerooms" and Neal, "Furnishing."

6. P. P. Gustine, *Wholesale Price List of Furniture* (Philadelphia, 1 February 1867), Winterthur Museum. The only "suits" offered were a range of "Cottage" and "Full French" bedroom furniture. An 1870 supplement to the trade catalog put out by the Boston furniture concern F. M. Holmes and Co. depicted one such suite, consisting of a "Tete," two "Easy Chairs," and four armless "Parlor Chairs." The suite's number "45" suggests that it was an addition to a larger line; at $185 wholesale, it probably retailed for about twice the price of the Tucker family's eight-piece set. An unillustrated 1871 price list from the large New York City furniture concern of M. and H. Schrenkeisen offered fifty such suites for sale. These suites ranged in wholesale price from forty-eight dollars for the "No. 0 Suit, Plain or Carved Top" to two hundred dollars for the "Grand Duchess," which had carvings of women's faces on the chair and sofa arms, extra-fancy piping, and extra hair stuffing. See *Catalogue Supplement, F. M. Holmes and Co.* (Boston, 15 October 1870); price list of M. and H. Schrenkeisen Co. (New York, 22 March 1871).

7. Price list of Baxter C. Swan (Philadelphia, PA, 1 May 1880), National Museum of American History, Smithsonian Institution.

8. Catalog of furniture and carpets of Jordan and Moriarty (New York, NY, 1883).

9. *Montgomery Ward and Co. Catalogue and Buyers' Guide No. 57, Spring and Summer, 1895.*

10. Boris Emmet and John E. Jeuck, *Catalogues and Counters: A History of Sears, Roebuck and Company* (Chicago: University of Chicago Press, 1950), 187-195. For an influential article on working-class material culture at the turn of the century, see Lizabeth A. Cohen, "Embellishing A Life of Labor: An Interpretation of the Material Culture of American Working-Class Homes, 1885-1915," *Journal of American Culture* 3, 4 (Winter 1980): 752-775. Ms. Cohen's interpretation of some aspects of working-class material culture, particularly parlors, differs from my own.

11. See More, "The Standard of Living, General" and "The Standard of Living: Typical Families," in *Wage-Earners' Budgets.*

12. More, *Wage-Earners' Budgets,* 145-146.

13. Watson, *Louis XVI Furniture,* 37.

14. For a discussion of set-back arms, see Watson, *Louis XVI Furniture,* 34. See also Roger de Félice, *French Furniture Under Louis XIV,* trans. F. M. Atkinson (New York: Frederick A. Stokes Company, n.d.), 135-136. For images of women's informal accommodations in order to sit in armed chairs with voluminous skirts, see figures 110, 139, and 141 in Thornton, *Authentic Decor,* all of which date from the 1720s and 1730s.

15. *Price List of Parlor Furniture, Lounges, Mattresses, &c., Mackie and Hilton* (Philadelphia, 1883).

16. Frank R. and Marian Stockton, *The Home: Where It Should Be and What to Put in It* (New York: G. P. Putnam and Sons, 1872), 47.

17. The only exception known to the author is one suite offered by the Chicago firm of McDonough, Wilsey and Co. in 1878. This firm was also one of the first to offer rocking chairs and other chair novelties as part of suites.

18. de Félice, "Seats," in *French Furniture Under Louis XIV,* 88. For a lucid explanation of the concept of precedence, see Eames, "Furniture in England, France and the Netherlands."

19. *Chesterfield's Art of Letter-Writing Simplified,* 15-16.

20. Deportment suggested by parlor furniture is discussed in more detail in chapter 3.

21. The appearance of such novelties in suite chair forms was analogous to the novelties in silver flatware that appeared at about the same time. This urge to create objects with specialized uses, however spurious, is one of the underlying cultural characteristics of Victorian popular thought; it is discussed in further detail in chapter 5.

22. *Catalogue of Furniture, George J. Henkels City Cabinet Warerooms, 173 Chestnut St.,* 12.

23. For a detailed history of the rocking chair, including parlor rockers in various forms, see Denker and Denker, *Rocking Chair Book.*

24. Price list of Gerrish and O'Brien (Boston, MA, 7 August 1880).

25. Parlor rockers also became the object of elaborate needlework projects at midcentury, their seats covered with raised Berlin work and beading. These chairs, which may never have been actually used, are discussed in more detail in chapter 9.

26. See chapter 6 for more information on Turkish furniture and chapter 4 for discussion of seated comfort.

27. Peter Thornton, *Seventeenth-Century Interior Decor-*

ation in England, France, and Holland, 103-104.

28. Stockton and Stockton, *The Home*, 47.

29. Beecher and Stowe, *American Woman's Home*, 87-90; [Martin], *Our Homes: How to Beautify Them*, 146-148.

30. Wheaton, "High Style in Montana," 243-254.

31. *Sears, Roebuck and Co. Catalogue No. 111, 1902*, 780-781; *Catalogue of McDonough, Wilsey and Co.* (Chicago, IL, 1878).

32. See, for example, Sharon Darling, "Upholstered Parlor Furniture, 1873-1917," in *Chicago Furniture, 1830-1980* (Chicago and New York: The Chicago Historical Society and W. W. Norton and Co., 1984) and Thornton, *Authentic Decor*, 359, 373-375, 405.

33. Thornton, *Seventeenth-Century Interior Decoration in England, France, and Holland*, 134-135.

34. In 1910, A. F. Barker, author of the technical manual *Textiles*, noted, "So little was the success of the Jacquard power-loom known outside the Bradford district, however, that the writer well remembers in the year 1884 or 1885 a supposed authority on the trade questioning whether it ever could be a success as a power loom, i.e. twenty or thirty years after it was running by the hundred, or perhaps the thousand, in the Bradford district. Today the tapestry loom…is employed upon the simplest kinds of tapestries, consisting of little more than reversed warp and weft sateens, up to imitations of the Gobelin tapestries." See Barker, *Textiles*, 257-258. Cole's *Dictionary of Dry Goods* for 1894 describes Jacquard loom tapestry as "Neuilly tapestry" or "Jacquard tapestry," woven in imitation of Gobelins. Its description of production suggests that weaving was only partly mechanized by that date, still requiring the presence of the weaver to pass the weft shuttles through the warp. "Carpet tapestry," also called moquette, was commonly used on lounges and hassocks in the last quarter of the nineteenth century. It is discussed in chapter 4, along with lounge production. George S. Cole, *A Complete Dictionary of Dry Goods…*, rev. ed. (Chicago: J. B. Herring Pub. Co., 1894), 348.

35. Wholesale price list of Samuel Graves and Son (Boston, MA, 1878), National Museum of American History, Smithsonian Institution.

36. Katherine Yearick Cavano was able to recall the lounge's appearance and its location in the dining/sitting room vividly because she fell against it as a small child, breaking her nose against the raised end. Cavano, interview with author, Pennington, NJ, March and December 1986.

37. Ella Rodman Church, *How to Furnish a Home* (New York: D. Appleton and Company, 1881), 86. Every bedroom of the Grange, the Codman family house in Lincoln, Massachusetts, operated by the Society for the Preservation of New England Antiquities, was equipped with a lounge for daytime resting.

38. *Christmas Gifts* (Fred Macey Company: Grand Rapids, Michigan, about 1910). The Fred Macey Company advertised itself as "Makers of Office and Library Furniture." The three leather Turkish lounges advertised in this catalog retailed at prices from $59 to $80, making them too expensive for most consumers.

39. Bed lounges are even more rare than are common lounges today, either because they wore out and were discarded or because they were too eccentric a form of furniture to be retained in the twentieth century. Fern Tuten has noted that sofa-bedsteads were "the most frequently patented single item" among all forms of convertible furniture (reclining chairs, table-chairs and so on) before 1850. Tuten, "American Domestic Patented Furniture," 78.

40. Talbot, "The Philadelphia Furniture Industry," 107, 109.

41. Ibid., 82, 115.

42. "Lasting" was a sturdy cotton and wool blend fabric used most typically for coat linings and gaitors. Offered in black, or sometimes in plain colors, it had a shiny twilled surface that offered some of the same visual characteristics of horsehair and satin, but was softer than one and cheaper than the other. Price list and catalog of Rand and McSherry (Baltimore, MD, 14 May 1872). Sofa prices in *Price List and Illustrated Catalogue of J. W. Hamburger* (New York, 1874), 4.

43. Advertisement for Mueller and Slack Co. in *Michigan Artisan* 14, 12 (June 1894): 31.

44. See Michael J. Ettema, "Technological Innovation and Design Economics in Furniture Manufacture," *Winterthur Portfolio* 16, 2/3 (Summer/Autumn 1981): 199. In his recent article on the economics of design for furniture woodworking, Ettema proposed a broader understanding of the appearance of inexpensive furniture, setting aside the question of "quality" in favor of another that applied Thorsten Veblen's understanding of "emulation" and "ostentation" to "high-style" objects, those whose materials and craftsmanship are not constrained by the necessity to keep production costs and retail prices low: "A desire to emulate makes high-style artifacts models for the entire scale. The less expensive objects are not naive imitations of inferior quality, they are less labor and material intensive, and therefore are simplified objects designed in the same style…Since costs are, in part, dependent upon the labor intensity of their technologies, manufacturers must design pieces with the capabilities of their tool in mind, constantly compromising between cost and style."

45. *1890 Catalogue for the Buffalo Upholstering Co.*, 1, 14; *1890 Price List for the Buffalo Upholstering Company*.

46. Tuten, "American Domestic Patented Furniture," 116-119.

47. A centripetal spring chair by the American Chair Company of Troy, New York, dated about 1855, is one of the earliest known examples of tapestry carpet used as upholstery. It is in the collections of the National Museum of American History, Smithsonian Institution.

48. *Edward W. Vaill, Forty-First Semi-Annual Catalog of Fine Folding chairs, Autumn and Winter 1882-1883* (Worcester, MA, 1882), 3.

49. The author of *The Practical Upholsterer* provided estimates of the amount of fabric required for "an ordinary parlor suite with mouldings on the seat rails and plain seats" (probably having simple buttoning on the back) and "a similar suite with buttoned [button tufted] seats and backs":

Velvet or plush	18-20 yards	20-26 yards
Rep	8-9 "	10-12 "
Tapestry	8-9 "	10-12 "
Cretonne	14-16 "	18-20 "
Cord	22 "	22 "
Gimp	36 "	36 "
Buttons	1/2 gross	2 gross

[Phin], *The Practical Upholsterer*, 40.

50. Peter A. Stone and John Newton Thurber, *The Upholsterers' International Union: Story of the First 75 Years*. Vol. I, *Early Beginnings, Craft and Trade Unionism, "Voluntarism" and Struggle for Legality 1882-1932* (Philadelphia, PA: "Proposed for Publication in Early 1956," typescript on deposit with the Library of Congress), 16, 48. Factory upholsterers were once again able to command better salaries and more control of their working conditions, at least in Grand Rapids, when the burgeoning mass production of automobiles created new demand for their skills.

51. "Came to Blows: Striking Employees of the Paine Bedding Company. A Strict Blockade Is Being Maintained by the Insurgents Around the Factory," *The Evening Post*, Grand Rapids, Michigan, Wednesday, 25 May 1898, 1.

52. Stone and Thurber, *Upholsterers' International Union*, 56.

53. The first patent for a tufting machine, called an "Upholstering Device," appears to be one filed by Henry B. Pitner of Princeton, Illinois, on December 6, 1892. He received Patent No. 511,649 for what appears to be a board for mattress tufting, a way of placing a number of buttons at once; see *Official Gazette, U.S. Patent Office* (6 December 1892), 2024. In 1895, several devices for tufting mattresses and cushions received patents, as in G. K. Bagby's Patent No. 549,840 for a machine that tufted mattresses using needles and clamps on a grooved table; see *Official Gazette, U.S. Patent Office* (12 November 1895), 1095. Alfred Freschl, eventual owner of the Novelty Tufting Machine Company of Chicago, first appears as a patent holder in 1895 for a cushion tufting device; see Patent No. 537,385 in *Official Gazette, U.S. Patent Office* (9 April 1895), 271.

54. Stone and Thurber, *Upholsterers' International Union*, 56.

Chapter Eight Notes

1. Caroline Cowles Richards, *Village Life in America, 1852-1872, As told in the Diary of a School-Girl* (Williamstown, MA: Corner House Publishers, 1972), 84.

2. Cleaveland et al., *Village and Farm Cottages*, 130.

3. Copeland, "Draperies, Blinds and Curtains," 271.

4. "Parlor Draperies—New Designs," *Godey's Lady's Book*, August 1854, 170-171.

5. Johnston, "Dialogues Between Designer and Client," 268.

6. Receipt of Doe, Hazelton and Co., Boston, MA, 20 November 1858; receipt of Lawrence, Wilde and Co., Boston, MA, 17 March 1860, Castle Tucker, Wiscasset, ME.

7. *Godey's Lady's Book* featured illustrations and articles about curtains chiefly during two periods, 1854 to 1858 and 1869 to 1873.

8. Eastlake, *Hints on Household Taste*, 100-101.

9. "Oriental Curtains," *Peterson's Magazine*, May 1877, 382.

10. *Catalogue of Lord and Taylor, 1881*, reprinted as *Clothing and Furnishings, Lord and Taylor, 1881* (Princeton, NJ: The Pyne Press, 1971), 160. Because jute fibers deteriorate rapidly, no examples of this type of curtain are known to survive.

11. Philip B. Scranton, *The Philadelphia System of Textile Manufacture, 1884-1984* (Philadelphia: Pennsylvania Humanities Council, 1984).

12. *Part III: Selected Industries,* in *Report on Manufacturing Industries in the United States at the Eleventh Census, 1890* (Washington, D.C.: Government Printing Office, 1895), 217,203; Palmer, "Labor Relations in the Lace and Lace-Curtain Industries," 7.

13. Frank A. Moreland, *Practical Decorative Upholstery* (Boston: Lee and Shepherd, 1889), 10.

14. See the catalog of the brassworks of A. W. Gillett, Birmingham, England (about 1829), in the collections of the Winterthur Museum, for a selection of patterns for cornices, curtain pole ends, and curtain bands. These designs still are representative of hardware available at midcentury.

15. Richard Carter Barret, *Bennington Pottery and Porcelain* (New York: Bonanza Books, 1958), 136-137; Jane Shadel Spillman, *The Knopf Collectors' Guides to American Antiques: Glass Bottles, Lamps,*

and Other Objects (New York: Alfred A. Knopf, 1983), 234.

16. Janet R. McFarlane, "Shades of Our Forefathers," *Antiques Magazine*, August 1959, 124.

17. Edgar Weld King, "Painted Window Shades," *Antiques Magazine*, December 1939, 289. Catherine Lynn illustrated one such illusionistic paper shade and discussed paper curtains briefly in her 1980 volume *Wallpaper in America*. Lynn notes that the British commissioners attending the New York Crystal Palace in 1853 considered paper shades a peculiarity of the American wallpaper business and a product intended largely for use in the West. She also illustrates in passing a set of printed paper curtains with paper drapery loops, manufactured in England in the 1870s. She has, however, found no documented use of this kind of "paper curtain" in the United States. See Lynn, *Wallpaper in America: From the Seventeenth Century to World War I* (New York: W. W. Norton, 1980), 328, 365-366.

18. Cleaveland et al., *Village and Farm Cottages*, 129-130.

19. Kirkland, *Book for the Home Circle*, 110.

20. Catalog of W. A. Currier's Kitchen, House Furnishing, and Stove Warehouse, Nos. 14 and 16 Main St. (Haverhill, MA, about 1862), 7, Winterthur Museum.

21. King, "Painted Window Shades," 290-291.

22. *Catalogue of Lord and Taylor, 1881*, 163-164.

23. *Montgomery Ward and Co. Catalogue and Buyers' Guide No. 57, Spring and Summer, 1895*, 347-348.

24. Untitled article, *Godey's Lady's Book*, May 1848, 224.

25. "The History of Lace," *The Household*, November 1881, 224.

26. Mrs. Bury Palliser, *A History of Lace*, 3d ed. (London: Sampson, Low and Searle, 1875; Detroit: Tower Books, 1971). For other sources of information on developments in lace technology, see Patricia Wardle, *Victorian Lace* (New York: Frederick A. Praeger, Inc., 1968); Santina Levey, *Lace: A History* (London: Victoria and Albert Museum, 1983); William Felkin, *Felkin's History of the Machine-Wrought Hosiery and Lace* (Newton Abbot, Devon: David and Charles, 1967); and Pat Earnshaw, *Lace Machines and Machine Laces* (London: B. T. Batsford Ltd., 1986).

27. *Montgomery Ward and Co. Catalogue and Buyers' Guide No. 57, Spring and Summer, 1895*, 347.

28. *Daniell and Sons Catalogue, Spring and Summer, 1885*, 71.

29. Byington, *Homestead*. See also More, *Wage-Earners' Budgets*.

30. Williams and Jones, *Beautiful Homes*, 50; Church, *How to Furnish a Home*, 103.

31. Henry Ward Beecher, *Star Papers; or, Experiences of Art and Nature* (New York: J.C. Derby; Boston: Phillips, Sampson and Co., 1855), 291.

32. Williams and Jones, *Beautiful Homes*, 50.

33. Carroll L. V. Meeks suggested that there was a distinct "picturesque" preference in the play of light on architecture that preferred the drama of varied lights and darks. Meeks, *Victorian Railroad Station*, 4, 10.

34. "The Bay Window," *Frank Leslie's Illustrated Monthly Magazine*, November 1876, 611.

35. Harriet Beecher Stowe, "How Do We Know?," *The May Flower and Miscellaneous Writings* (1855; reprint, Boston: Houghton, Mifflin and Company, 1894), 241.

36. King, "Painted Window Shades," 290.

37. Wharton and Codman, *Decoration of Houses*, 72.

38. Thornton, *Seventeenth-Century Interior Decoration in England, France, and Holland*, 134-135.

39. A group of stereographs of the Lockwood-Mathews Mansion, in the collections of the Society for the Preservation of New England Antiquities, does include one image of drapery across a window bay.

40. See Thornton, *Authentic Decor*, for illustrations of door drapery used over a long span of time; and figure 1b in Harriet Spofford, *Art Decoration Applied to Furniture* (New York: Harper Brothers, 1877), 118.

41. Eastlake, *Hints on Household Taste*, 102.

42. Williams and Jones, *Beautiful Homes*, 53.

43. Smith, *Industrial Art*, 64-66.

44. *Frank Leslie's Illustrated Record of the Centennial*, 230.

45. Harrison, *Woman's Handiwork*, 160.

46. F. A. Moreland, *Practical Decorative Upholstery* (Boston: Lee and Shepherd, 1890), 179.

47. Spencer, *Spencers of Amberson Avenue*, 18.

48. Ibid.

49. *Catalogue of Lord and Taylor, 1881*, 160.

50. *Daniell and Sons Catalogue, Spring and Summer, 1885*, 71.

51. An article on curtains appearing in a 1859 issue of *Godey's Lady's Book*, described the most popular colors then as "solid crimson" and crimson red and maroon

used together, a combination that still found favor in the 1876 parlor furniture catalog of McDonough, Price and Co. See "Curtains for Parlor or Drawing-Room," *Godey's Lady's Book*, September 1859, 265; catalog of McDonough, Price and Co. (Chicago, IL, 1876), 33.

52. See figure 10 in *Sears, Roebuck and Co. Catalogue No. 104, 1897*, unpaginated.

53. Harrison, *Woman's Handiwork*, 163.

54. *Catalogue of Lord and Taylor, 1881*, 166.

55. John J. McFarlane, *Manufacturing in Philadelphia, 1683-1912* (Philadelphia: Commercial Museum, 1912), 20.

56. *Dockham's American Report and Directory of the Textile Manufacture and Dry Goods Trade* (Boston: C. A. Dockham and Co., 1891), 206-222.

57. Clarence D. Long, *Wages and Earnings in the United States 1860-1890* (Princeton: Princeton University Press, 1960; New York: Arno Press, 1975), 94.

58. See *Montgomery Ward and Co. Catalogue and Buyer's Guide No. 57, Spring and Summer, 1895*; and *Sears, Roebuck and Co. Catalog No. 123, 1911*, 531-534.

59. Untitled article, *The Decorator and Furnisher* 2, 2 (May 1883): 52.

60. Mabel Turk Priestman, "Portières for the Country House," *Country Life in America*, January 1906, 321.

61. See examples of rooms furnished by the Yearick and Hughes families in chapter 2, and the Ruth family in the concluding chapter.

62. *Oxford English Dictionary*, s.v. "vignette."

63. "Curtains and Draperies," *The Decorator and Furnisher* 1, 3 (December 1882), 81.

Chapter Nine Notes

1. "The Unexpected Visitor," *Godey's Lady's Book*, January 1859, 15.

2. Beecher and Stowe, *American Woman's Home*, 85.

3. Ibid.; see also Wright, *The Complete Home*, 158-165, for a discussion of value in furnishing much like Catharine Beecher's.

4. Downing, *Architecture of Country Houses*, 413-415.

5. Cleaveland et al., *Village and Farm Cottages*, 132-133, 130.

6. Loudon, *Encyclopedia of Cottage, Farmhouse and Villa Architecture and Furniture*, 298.

7. Cook, *House Beautiful*, 138, 139-140.

8. [Martin], *Our Homes: How to Beautify Them*, 53.

9. A sampling of such articles from *The Household* includes those with a straight how-to slant and advice on parlor making that takes the form of short stories. These latter were meant to be particularly encouraging to overworked farm wives. See, for example, E. M. Arnold, "Jeanette's Parlor," *The Household* 12, 4, April 1879, 73-74; Elsie Donald, "The Prettiest Room," *The Household* 13, 10, October 1880, 217-218; and, in the same issue, "Eva A.," "Our Sitting Room," 218; and Daisy Field, "How We Furnished the Parlor," *The Household*, June 1882, 181-182. In this last story, a city woman who has moved to the country helps her neighbor make a parlor with fifty dollars in cash and elbow grease.

10. Almon C. Varney, *Our Homes and Their Adornments* (Chicago: People's Publishing Company, 1885), 220, 221.

11. Varney, *Our Homes and Their Adornments*, 281. Other such volumes include Mrs. John A. Logan [Mary Simmerson Logan], *The Home Manual: Everybody's Guide in Social, Domestic, and Business Life* (Chicago: H. J. Smith and Co., 1889); and *Treasures of Use and Beauty: An Epitome of the Choicest Gems of Wisdom, History, Reference and Recreation...* (Detroit: Dickerson, 1885).

12. For examples of such needleworkers and their products, see Susan Burrows Swan, *Plain and Fancy: American Women and Their Needlework, 1700-1850* (New York: Holt, Rinehart and Winston, 1977); and Betty Ring, ed., *Needlework: An Historical Survey* (New York: Main Street Books, 1975).

13. Mrs. Henry Owen, *The Illuminated Book of Needlework...* (London: Henry G. Bohn, 1842), 397-398.

14. Wheaton, "High Style in Montana," 245-246.

15. *A Record of the First Exhibition of the Metropolitan Mechanics' Institute, Held in the East Wing of the Patent Office, February and March, 1853* (Washington, DC: H. Polkinhorn, 1853), 32-40.

16. Cited in Molly G. Proctor, *Victorian Canvas Work: Berlin Wool Work* (New York: Drake Publishers Inc., 1972), 63.

17. [Phin], *The Practical Upholsterer*, 45.

18. Jane E. Wells, "Tufted Embroidery," *The Household*, 15, 8 August 1882, 234.

19. These two chair seats are examples of a much larger, unstudied body of rocking chairs, rococo revival side chairs, and Grecian chairs embellished with the same or related needlework techniques and rendered "unsittable." The collections of the Kemmerer Museum, Allentown, Pennsylvania, contain two rococo revival chairs with tufted Berlin work upholstery. The Harris County Heritage Society in

Houston, Texas, owns an armless Turkish chair, 1890-1910, which has a completely beaded seat and back; its pristine condition suggests that it was never put to the use for which it was ostensibly designed.

20. See Ellen Gehret, Tandy Hersh, Alan G. Keyser, and Frederick S. Weiser, *This Is The Way I Pass My Time* (Birdsboro, PA: The Pennsylvania German Society, 1985).

21. Beecher and Stowe, *American Woman's Home*, 89.

22. See "Living Room in Southern Germany, c. 1817," plate 272 in Thornton, *Authentic Decor*, 205.

23. See Downing, *Architecture of Country Houses*, 413-414.

24. "L. C. C." of Ogdensburg, New York, wrote in an 1882 issue of *The Household* that she had made a "useful and ornamental" box lounge because she needed more closed space as well as the seating. "A Home-made Lounge," *The Household*, October 1882, 300.

25. Beecher and Stowe, *American Woman's Home*, 30.

26. [Martin], *Household Conveniences*, 214-215.

27. "Home-Made Furniture," *Peterson's Magazine*, June 1870, 472.

28. Williams and Jones, *Beautiful Homes*, 225.

29. "L. D. Mc.," "Lath and Lambrequins," *The Household*, October 1879, 220.

30. Downing, *Architecture of Country Houses*, 414; Cleaveland et al., *Village and Farm Cottages*, 132.

31. Wright, *The Complete Home*, 158, 464.

32. Williams and Jones, *Beautiful Homes*, 227.

33. Ibid., 97-98. According to Williams and Jones, "Mr. Conway" is apparently M. D. Conway, who wrote for *Harper's Weekly*.

34. See "How to Re-Upholster and Make Slip Covers," in *Modern Priscilla Home Furnishing Book*, 251-260.

35. *The Workwoman's Guide* (London: Simpkin, Marshall, and Co., 1840), 190. This encyclopedia of home sewing seems to have had a substantial circulation in America and survives in several research libraries, including those of the Winterthur Museum and Gardens and the Strong Museum. Only two of the twenty-six plates at the back of the book cover the subject of household upholstery.

36. Helen Anderson, "About Window Draperies," *The Decorator and Furnisher* 15,1 (October 1889): 87.

37. Copeland, "Draperies, Blinds and Curtains," 271.

38. [Martin], *Our Homes: How to Beautify Them*, 43.

39. H. M. Poole, "Artistic Draperies," *The Decorator and Furnisher* 16, 4 (June 1890): 103-104.

40. "The Queen of Prussia's bedchamber, Berlin (1810)," plate 252, p. 194; "Queen Hortense's Tented boudoir, Paris (1811)," plate 253, p. 195; "Princess Augusta's 'Muslin Closet' in Berlin (1829)," plate 323, p. 248; "A dressing-room in Austria (1820s)," plate 340, p. 262; one of "Two plates from a Parisian journal (1840)," depicting a Turkish smoking room, plate 346, p. 262, in Thornton, *Authentic Decor*.

41. See Diane Fagan Affleck, *New From the Mills* (North Andover, MA: Museum of American Textile History, 1986).

42. For 1875 domestic print prices, see *Montgomery Ward and Co. Catalogue No. 13, Spring and Summer, 1875*. For calico as a furnishing fabric, see "Home-Made Furniture," *Peterson's Magazine*, June 1870, 472. For a comparison of cotton drapery print prices see *Clothing and Furnishings, Lord and Taylor, 1881*, 161; and *Montgomery Ward and Co. Catalogue No. 57, Spring and Summer, 1895*, 15.

43. "A Bedchamber in a rich burgher's house, Holland, c. 1630," plate 16 in Peter Thornton, *Authentic Decor*, 27.

44. See chapter 2, figure 33, "Interior of a Sussex Farmhouse," signed FDH 185?, in James Ayres, *The Shell Book of the Home in Britain: Decoration Design and Construction of Vernacular Interiors, 1500-1850* (London: Faber and Faber Limited, 1981), 41.

45. Wainwright, ed., *Philadelphia Perspective*, 116.

46. *A Record of the First Exhibition of the Metropolitan Mechanics' Institute*, 55.

47. Cook, *House Beautiful*, 126-127.

48. Reed, *House-Plans for Everybody*, 51.

49. Cook, *House Beautiful*, 11.

50. Ibid., 121.

51. "Mrs. H. Emmons, Box 70, Swampscott, Mass.," *The Household*, July 1881, 146.

52. "Lenaria," "Wonderings," *The Household*, October 1880, 218; Elsie Donald, "The Prettiest Room," *The Household*, October 1880, 217; Lucy Lee, "Lambrequins," *The Household*, January 1882, 11. Lee recommended burlap, finished with a strip of black ribbon and embroidered with "red Germantown wool," for draping a mantel.

53. Harrison, *Woman's Handiwork*, 22; *Montgomery Ward and Co. Catalogue No. 57, Spring and Summer, 1895*, 350.

54. The 1875 Montgomery Ward and Co. catalog offered "Tycoon Reps. for wrappers and dressing gowns" at a cost of twenty to twenty-five cents per yard.

55. C. M. Brown and C. L. Gates, *Scissors and Yardstick; or, All About Dry Goods* (Hartford, CT: C. M. Brown and F. W. Jaqua, 1872), 114; *Montgomery Ward and Co. Catalogue No. 13, Spring and Summer, 1875*, 12.

Chapter Ten Notes

1. "The Sacrificial Parlor," in Susan Anne Brown, comp., *Home Topics: A Book of Practical Papers on House and Home Matters* (Troy, NY: H. B. Nims and Company, 1881), 488, 490. This book contains articles from *Scribner's Monthly* and *St. Nicholas* magazines. At least three articles were devoted to attacking parlor making—"The Sacrificial Parlor," "Outdoor Parlors," and "Best Parlors."

2. *Vogue's Book of Etiquette: Present-Day Customs of Social Intercourse with the Rules for Their Correct Observance* (New York: Condé-Nast Publications, 1924), 173.

3. Mary D. Chambers, *Table Etiquette, Menus and Much Besides* (Boston: The Boston Cooking-School Magazine Co., 1929), unpaginated introduction, 177.

4. Reed's *House-Plans for Everybody* was first published in 1878 but revised and reprinted with a new title in 1900. His estimated costs for plumbing, ranges, and boilers are generally lumped together and fall between $250 and $400. This sum could purchase an additional room or two; in fact, Reed's two-room starter cottage itself cost only $250 to construct. See Samuel B. Reed, *Modern House-Plans for Everybody* (New York: Orange Judd Company, 1900).

5. "Series D722-727. Average Annual Earnings of Employees: 1900 to 1970," in *Historical Statistics of the United States: Colonial Times to 1970*, vol. 1 (Washington, DC: Department of Commerce, Bureau of the Census, 1975), 168.

6. Ruth Schwartz Cowan, *More Work for Mother: The Ironies of Household Technology from the Open Hearth to the Microwave* (New York: Basic Books, 1983), 83.

7. *Modern Priscilla Home Furnishing Book*, 97.

8. Charlotte Wait Calkins, *A Course in House Planning and Furnishing* (Chicago: Scott, Foresman and Company, 1916), 46.

9. Cowan, *More Work for Mother*, 69-101.

10. *Modern Priscilla Home Furnishing Book*, 162.

11. Hazel H. Adler, *The New Interior: Modern Decorations for the Modern Home* (New York: The Century Company, 1916), 38.

12. Helen Koues, *How to Be Your Own Decorator* (New York: Good Housekeeping, 1926), 24, 25.

13. Ekin Wallick, *Inexpensive Furnishings in Good Taste* (New York: Hearsts International Library Company, 1915), 39.

14. Emily Post, *The Personalilty of a House: The Blue Book of Home Design and Decoration* (New York: Funk and Wagnalls, 1930).

15. Adler, *The New Interior*, 38.

16. Calkins, *Course in House Planning*, 55.

17. Ibid., 63.

18. Edward Stratton Holloway, *The Practical Book of Furnishing the Small House and Apartment* (Philadelphia: J. B. Lippincott and Company, 1922), 79.

19. Sidney Morse, *Household Discoveries: An Encyclopedia of Practical Recipes and Processes* (New York: The Success Company, 1908, 1909), 33-34.

20. "The Bungalow's Effect On Draperies," *The Furniture Worker* 54, 2 (25 December 1909): 65.

21. *Modern Priscilla Home Furnishing Book*, 134.

22. Even the sanitation argument against parlors—that their contents were dusty, difficult to care for, and unhealthy—is a variation of arguments made by the comfort theorists. Harriet Beecher Stowe's Christopher Crowfield and others argued that cleaning parlor upholstery required too much work—although the consideration was not the presence of germs but the desire to preserve furnishings that were actually beyond the sensible means of ordinary families.

23. Interview with Anna F. Grier, November 1987.

24. John Arnold, Rochester, New York, interview with author, 21 January 1988.

25. Robert Vance Stewart, "When Grandpa Was a Boy: Reminiscences of Robert Vance Stewart," 1982, 7. Typescript in the collections of the Genesee Charlotte Lighthouse Historical Society.

INDEX

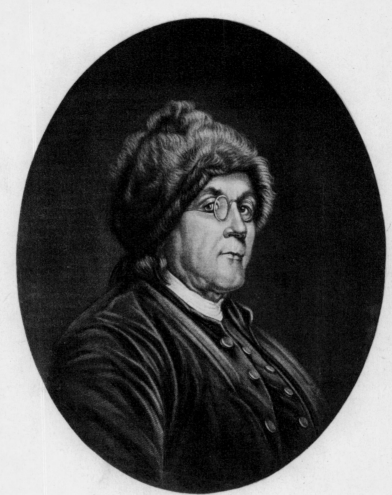

After Drawing by C.N.Cochin.1777

Benj Franklin

BENJAMIN FRANKLIN

The First Civilized American

PHILLIPS RUSSELL

Profusely Illustrated

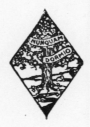

BRENTANO'S · PUBLISHERS
NEW YORK   MCMXXVI

Manufactured in the United States of America

CONTENTS

CONTENTS

ILLUSTRATIONS

ILLUSTRATIONS

BENJAMIN FRANKLIN

The First Civilized American

Prefatory Catechism

Who was the first civilized American?
Benjamin Franklin.

Why do you call him so?
Because at an American period eminent for narrowness, superstition, and bleak beliefs he was mirthful, generous, open-minded, learned, tolerant, and humor-loving. Because he was the first American man of the world in the sense that he was the first American world-man.

What was his age as compared with that of George Washington, John Adams, and Thomas Jefferson?
He was a mature man with a record of achievement when they were still swaddled infants. He was 26 years older than Washington, 30 years older than Adams, and 37 years older than Jefferson.

What was Franklin's most marked characteristic?
A gusto for living.

What was his avowed aim?
To " do good " and live a satisfying life.

Did he succeed?
Abundantly.

Were there any inconsistencies in his career?
Many.

Can you specify?
He disregarded his own maxims as uttered by " Poor Richard " and lamentably failed to observe the principles set up in his own " Art of Virtue."

--•⊰ 1 ⊱•--

Was Franklin a good man?

Most of his associates, including various clergymen, so regarded him; others deemed him sinful.

Where and when was he born?
Boston, 1706, old style.

Where and when did he die?
Philadelphia, 1790, at the age of 84.

Who were his parents?
Josiah Franklin, an immigrant dissenter from the doctrines of the Established Church in England, and Abiah Folger, daughter of one of New England's first settlers.

In what terms did Benjamin Franklin refer to his parents after their death?
On the marble he placed over their grave in Boston his father was described as " a pious and prudent man," his mother as " a discreet and virtuous woman."

To what age did they live?
His father died at 89, his mother at 85.

Where did the Franklin family originate?
Records pertaining to it have been traced back to 1555, in the village of Ecton, or Eton, Northamptonshire, England.

Are there any facts of interest relating to Benjamin Franklin's forebears?
On his father's side the eldest sons were bred as smiths for several generations back. Benjamin's paternal great-grandfather was once imprisoned a year and a day " on suspicion of his being the author of some poetry that touched

the character of some great man." [1] His maternal grandfather wrote in 1675 some " home-spun verse " favoring
liberty of conscience and exhorting the authorities to repeal
the laws against Baptists, Quakers, and other persecuted
sects. Franklin's paternal grandfather, Thomas, was a
" scrivener," public-spirited citizen, and " a chief mover for
the county or town of Northampton." [2]

What was Josiah Franklin's trade?
In England he was a dyer, but in America he became a
tallow chandler and soap boiler.

Had Josiah Franklin other children besides Benjamin?
Yes, he was the father, by two wives, of seventeen children, thirteen of whom survived.

What was peculiar about Benjamin's birth in relation to
preceding generations?
He was the youngest son of the youngest son for five
generations.

Had he any schooling?
For two years. He was placed in a grammar school at
the age of 8, and later a school for writing and arithmetic.

Was he an apt pupil?
Yes, in the grammar school he soon rose from the middle
to the head of his class.

What was his chief weakness?
He failed in arithmetic.

What occupation was chosen for him?
As the tithe of his father's sons, he was intended for the
ministry.

[1] Letter from Josiah Franklin to his " loving son," Benjamin, 1739.
[2] Autobiography.

How long after leaving school did he work for his father?
Two years.

What happened then?
At the age of 12, he was apprenticed to his brother James to learn the printing business.

Chapter I

The Moulding of a Young Chandler

I

THE evidence is that Benjamin Franklin, born in 1706, first "came alive," as the saying is, about the year 1718. Let us consider, then, his small and somewhat pudgy person at the age of twelve.

From his parents, whom he never knew "to have any sickness but that of which they dy'd,"[1] he has inherited a healthy and vigorous body and under their tutelage has had his attention turned to what is "good, just and prudent in the conduct of life." At the family table, where the food is regarded as secondary, he has listened to the discussions of ingenious and useful topics by the sensible friends and neighbors whom his father, "pious and prudent man," has invited for the edification of his multitudinous children.

The first incident which we know of concerning the canny influence of his relatives on the childish Franklin occurred when he was seven years old. Friends had given him some coppers, with which he sought a toy shop. There he was charmed with a whistle. He gave all his money for it. When the disturbance he created at home with the whistle led to a discovery of the price he had paid for it, his relatives made great fun of him, and told him he had paid four times what it was worth. They at the same time pointed out to him the good things he might have bought with the rest of the money. It is on record that little Ben "cried with vexation." He then and there resolved never again

[1] Autobiography.

to " give too much for the whistle," as he afterwards related to his charming Parisian friend, Madame Brillon, in the famous essay entitled " The Whistle."

On walks with his father, Franklin has been coached to watch joiners, bricklayers, turners, braziers and other artificers, at their work. This has stimulated in him a desire to learn the use of tools, an accomplishment which later enabled him to do little jobs about his own home without depending on dilatory workmen, and what was more important — to use his own words — " to construct little machines for my experiments, *while the intention of making the experiment was fresh and warm in my mind.*" [2] He has cut candle wicks, filled the moulds, tended the chandler's shop, run errands, and otherwise assisted that father of whom he stands in awe and whom he obeys with filial piety. But despite his exacting duties, little Benjamin has found time to play. He has gone a-fishing for minnows, learned to swim well, and has discovered his first labor-saving device by using the pulling power of a kite to draw himself across a pond. He has also exhibited that capacity for resourceful leadership which, as might have been expected, has manifested itself in an escapade.

One day Benjamin joins his fellows on a fishing expedition to a mill pond bounded by a marsh. They cannot fish in any comfort because of the quagmire which bogs their feet. The other boys make the best of the situation. Not so Benjamin. He has been taught that eyes are made to observe with. He looks around. Nearby some house builders have left a heap of stones. Eagerly he calls to his companions. He points. They do not understand.

" These will keep our feet dry," he explains.

" They'll only sink in the mud," they object.

" No, don't you see? We'll build a wharf with them."

[2] Autobiography.

" How? "

" Fetch the stones. I'll show you."

Benjamin, you see, has observed stone-masons at their work. He knows, and knows he knows. Soon the little wharf is built. The minnow-fishermen stand upon it comfortably, with dry feet. They congratulate themselves on their cleverness. Benjamin does not resent their failure to give him the credit; he has done no more than is to be expected from a loyal gang member; but in his heart there stirs a quick, warming pride. His first job of construction is a success; he feels a germ of the grown man's joy in the work of his hands.

And do their elders, discovering this boyish achievement, praise the young builders for their energy, vision and initiative? No, the history of Elder vs. Younger incessantly repeats itself. The workmen, returning the next day, call them downright nuisances, and the fathers of the ingenious fishermen, having received complaints and instituted a grave inquiry, summon the small masons into a dark corner, question them, lecture them, and finally, declaring no doubt that this hurts them more than their sons, birch them. Benjamin is one of the victims thus " corrected."

Probably this is one of the first incidents which serves to disillusion the youthful Franklin as to the justice and wisdom residing in the parental mind. Seeing his father as, after all, inconsistent and therefore merely human, he begins to tug at the ligatures which bind him to the overcrowded home and exacting shop. Gradually he asserts his individuality. Though still a young bird, he peeps over the edge of the nest. He day-dreams of the pulsing world beyond the rim of humdrum little Boston. He openly displays his dislike of his father's trade. He refuses to consider the clergyman's habit in which his father had hoped one day to see him clothed. One day he causes the elder

Franklin to stand aghast by announcing that he means to resort to that avenue of escape desired at some stage by all vigorous and restless boys — the sea.

Father and son face each other, the elder " well set, very strong; "[3] the son no less so.   But the father is a little bowed from much work and small pay; his eyes have the liquid sorrowing look of the idealist and religious devotee; he is bewildered by the sudden obstinacy of this his youngest, and up to now, his most obedient son.

Little Benjamin stands before him not truculently, but firmly.   His thin little lips, the lower projecting slightly, are pressed together.   His head is thrown back, revealing his high, rounded forehead, his oval but long and powerful chin in which there is a marked cleft.   His is not an attractive face, but it is relieved from commonplaceness by a gleam of drollery in the slightly protruding eyes rolling under heavy, drooping lids.

The struggle of wills results in victory for neither side. Benjamin fails to obtain consent to go to sea,[4] but his father, on his side, fails to obtain the son's adherence either to the chandler's shop or the Church.   Benjamin is ordered to bed, while Josiah, sorrowing, goes in to consult Abiah and conspire with her, in the manner of parents of that time, to defeat the desires of their son's heart.

Josiah emerges from the conference with a new idea. His brother, Benjamin, for whom the little Franklin is named, has a son named Samuel, who, after learning the cutler's trade in London, has set himself up in Boston.   To Samuel Josiah takes the younger Benjamin and leaves the lad in the cutler's shop " on liking."   But Samuel, though

---

[3] Autobiography.

[4] It is a curious fact that Franklin's son partly succeeded where his father failed.   When a small boy, he ran away from home and got on board a privateer, whence he was fetched home by his, let us hope, remembering father.

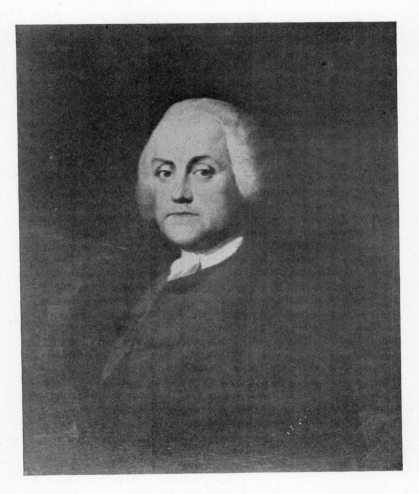

PORTRAIT OF BENJAMIN FRANKLIN AT THE AGE OF 53,
PAINTED IN LONDON IN 1759 BY BENJAMIN WILSON

RETURNED TO THE PEOPLE OF THE UNITED STATES
BY EARL GREY IN 1906.

a relative, is a business man first. He intimates that he does not, for his health's sake alone, teach boys the cutler's trade, and that he expects a fee. That word, to the father of seventeen children, is annoying. Josiah withdraws Benjamin, his son, from the house of Samuel.

Now what to do?

A moment critical in the life of the rebellious and ambitious young Franklin has arrived. His career is at a turning point. But before we discover what direction it takes, let us relate Benjamin, small though he is, to the large affairs of the world. What are the great currents which, rising mysteriously and whirling off into unknown spaces, may affect the destinies of this little chip afloat on a dark ocean?

II

In England Queen Anne is the reigning monarch. In 1706, the very year of Franklin's birth, Daniel Defoe, after a fulsome address to the queen, published in London his *Juno Divino*. It bore this strange and significant dedication:

"To the most Serene, most Invincible, and most Illustrious Lady,

"REASON,

" First Monarch of the World, Empress of the East, West, North and South; Hereditary Director of Mankind; Guide of the Passions; Lady of the Vast Continent of Human Understanding; Mistress of all the Islands of Science; Governess of the Fifteen Provinces of Speech; Image of, and Ambassador Extraordinary from, the Maker of all Things; the Almighty's Representative and Resident in the Souls of Men; and one of Queen Nature's Most Honourable Privy Council."

Thus was sounded the "keynote" of the Eighteenth Century, when it was firmly believed that henceforth Reason was to govern all human motions. Men might still flatter monarchs with their lips, but in their hearts they were already questioning the divine right of kings.

In the latter part of the preceding century, John Locke had been in the habit of meeting five or six friends informally to discuss certain philosophical questions. As a result of these discussions he set himself the task of sketching the "limits of human understanding." He naïvely thought he could do it on a single sheet of paper. But the limits in question proved to be so elastic that one sheet led to another, and finally there emerged the then monumental *Essay on Human Understanding*, issued sixteen years before Franklin's birth and read by young Ben sixteen years afterward. By this and other works Locke established himself as the philosopher of civil and religious liberty, the foe of abstract speculation, and the upholder of the rights of reason and of experimental verification in the quest after the retreating thing called truth.

Other odd people, things and events were being born into the world, including Dr. Samuel Johnson of London. Almost at the same time that young Franklin was facing his father in a struggle of wills, a lad in France, who was later to clasp hands with Franklin under dramatic circumstances, was skirmishing with his own parent in a similar combat. This was young Voltaire, who was passionately resisting his father's decision to send him into the law. While Franklin was still cutting candle wicks, Voltaire, twelve years the elder, was serving a sentence in the Bastille for writings objectionable to the authorities of his time and country. Six years later than Franklin were born two other heretical men of the period — Jean Jacques Rousseau, whose *Contrat Social* was to lay down the disturbing principle that all government must be based on the consent of the governed; and Frederick the Great, of Prussia, who accepted and taught the new theory that " a king is the first servant of the people." New forces, uncomfortable theories, and undreamed of discoveries were making themselves felt. Newton had already established a novel science of theoretical mechanics; Watt was shortly to discover the steam engine; Spinoza had written a new philosophy in Holland, and the skeptical writings of Lord Shaftesbury and Anthony Collins were finding an ever-widening circle of readers. It was a day of questionings and dim doubts. Men felt an uneasiness of the spirit without knowing its origin, for the flowers of authoritarian evil had not yet bloomed. Long afterwards the author of *The Education of Henry Adams* wrote concerning this century, of which Franklin saw nearly the whole: " Evidently a new variety of mind had appeared . . . Not one considerable man of science dared face the stream of thought; and the whole number of those who acted, like Franklin, as electric conductors of the new forces from nature to man, down to the year 1800, did not exceed a few score, confined to a few towns in Western Europe. Asia refused to be touched by the stream, and America, except for Franklin, stood outside."

Let us see what Henry Adams, keen-witted descendant of that ponderous John Adams whose relations with Franklin at a later period shall be described hereafter, meant by saying " America stood outside."

At the time when the infant Franklin was uttering his first cry, the most conspicuous writer in the American colonies was the Rev. Cotton Mather. While teachers in other lands were urging men to listen to the voice of reason, he was calling on the faithful to beware of witches. Only a few years before Franklin's birth, the mischief set afoot by eight silly and illiterate Massachusetts girls, who used to meet and giggle hysterically in the dark of the moon, had reached a maniacal climax in the Salem witch persecutions of 1692. Cotton's father, Increase Mather, and Solomon Stoddart were meantime issuing pamphlets of quarrelsome theology dealing with such questions as these:

" Is it lawful to wear long hair? "

" At what time of evening does the Sabbath begin? "

" Can baptized persons destitute of religion come to the table of the Lord? "

The ten American colonies, containing less than half a million inhabitants all told, were perched timidly on the rim of the Atlantic Ocean, the shore of which was the nearest thing to England. Loosely strung settlements hung southward from Boston, divided from each other by vast tracts of lonely land traversed at intervals by dim trails and gully-washed roads. Boston, with 10,000 inhabitants, regarded itself as a bustling city, but near the Old South Church still stood the village pillory and stocks. Probably nowhere in New England did men or women go to bed at night with minds at ease, for the shadows cast by the Indian-haunted forests on sparsely-yielding fields were deepened by that which overhung the spirits of the people. The Mathers and their kind, disagreeing with St. John, taught by precept and example that God was Fear. Fears huddled in the corners of human hearts, and toil and uneasiness imparted that grimness to the human countenance which is pathetically evident in early American portraits.

III

This is the world with which the hardy little Franklin is about to come to grips. In muscle and sinew he is, as has been explained, well equipped. But what is the furniture of his young mind? With what ideas is his immature brain garnished? From the first he has been an avid reader, gluttonous for knowledge. One by one he has pulled out the books in his father's meagre library. He seeks bread for his imagination, but receives the stone of polemic theology. He afterwards wrote feelingly of his regret that "more proper books" had not fallen in his way, much as a staid adult of today might wish that he had, in his inquisitive youth, wasted less time on dime novels.

Franklin's first purchased book was Bunyan's *Pilgrim's Progress,* that doleful volume which has probably given nightmares to more children than any other ever written. Franklin, however, says he was pleased with it, owing to its brisk plot and graphic dialogue. It moved him to make a collection of Bunyan's works. These, however, he was soon willing to part with; he sold them and replaced them with R. Burton's *Historical Collections,* forty or fifty small chap-books, of which Dr. Johnson once remarked, "They seem very proper to allure backward readers." Then came Plutarch's *Lives.* These impressed him more. He read in them abundantly. Over half a century later he wrote, "I still think that time spent to great advantage."

It was indeed time well spent, Benjamin; it taught you that beyond Boston, beyond even that England which to your father was the universe, were remote lands where in a dim antiquity men, prodded by some inner *daimōn,* strove and wrestled with each other, with Nature, and with their own reluctant spirits, finally pushing through to what their fellows called success.

Then came a book of Defoe's called *Essays Upon Several Projects.* Of this James Parton [5] says: "It is questionable if there is any other book that has so benefited mankind in the practical manner as this little essay by the author of Robinson Crusoe." Parton's estimate is exaggerated; but

[5] Life and Times of Benjamin Franklin.

no doubt Franklin derived from these papers by the brilliant and unhappy Defoe the seeds of certain ideas which later took concrete form in some of the most celebrated of Franklin's own projects. For example, one of Defoe's essays deals with banks and banking, another with insurance, a third with the organization and operation of Friendly Societies for mutual aid and joint self-help, and still another with academies for instructing the female mind as well as the male.

And then Franklin read the little book " which perhaps," he wrote afterwards, "gave me a turn of thinking that had an influence on some of the principal future events of my life." [6] This was Cotton Mather's " Essay upon the Good that is to be Devised and Designed by those who Desire to Answer the Great End of Life, and to Do Good While they Live," by Franklin called *Essays to Do Good*. Let us note the two last words of this title particularly, for we shall find them cropping up repeatedly throughout Franklin's career. Dr. Mather wrote these hortatory essays in one of his kindlier moods, when he was neither wrestling on the floor of his locked study with the re-embodiment of Jacob's angel nor inciting the superstitious to harry the wretched people upon whom, as condemned witches, the Massachusetts population vented its fears and pent passions. Dr. Mather's theme, in general, was the necessity, in order to enjoy the good life, of carrying the thought of God into the activities of one's every-day occupation. His premises granted, his reasoning was sound, his enthusiasm, as he warmed to his writing, contagious. Franklin accepted Mather's hortations. So deeply impressed was he that many years later he again referred to his debt to Dr. Mather in a letter written in 1784 to Cotton's son, Samuel, as follows:

" When I was a boy I met with a book entitled *Essays to*

[6] Autobiography.

do Good, which, I think, was written by your father. It had been so little regarded by a former possessor that several leaves of it were torn out, but the remainder gave me such a turn of thinking as to have an influence on my conduct through life; for I have always set a greater value on the character of a *doer of good* than on any kind of reputation; and, if I have been, as you seem to think, a useful citizen, the public owes the advantage of it to that book."

Candid Benjamin! Already, perhaps, he was aware of certain frailties; he felt a premonition of those weaknesses which were to assail him in his lonely adolescence; those "errata" which he was later to lament on the printed page; and so he made up his youthful mind that though he might not quite succeed in his ambition to *be* good, he could at least *do* good.

It was about two years later that he encountered another cluster of books which influenced him profoundly. One was Locke's essay *Upon the Human Understanding*, previously referred to, and *The Art of Thinking*, by Messieurs of the Port Royal, a group of French Jansenist laymen now no longer recollected except as the teachers of Racine. The Autobiography says little about these two books, which offer hard going to any youthful reader, but it is possible that Locke's practical teachings and dislike of mystical speculation appealed strongly to Franklin's earthy mind, and that both volumes encouraged that independence in thinking to which the small American philosopher was already inclined by temperament.

It was Shaftesbury and Collins who made him "a real doubter" of the theological dogmas which then dominated New England thought. Of the two writers, Shaftesbury, with his grace and ease, probably pleased the impressionable lad most. It is to be noted that Shaftesbury was the author of two essays which doubtless came into Franklin's hands — *Inquiry Concerning Virtue* and *Essay on the Freedom of Wit and Humor,* and that in the former the freethinking earl wrote: " The Wisdom of what rules and is *First* and *Chief* in nature has made it to be according to the private interest and good of every one to work toward the *general good.*"

Franklin also had a second battle with his old enemy, arithmetic, and this time he triumphed over it by easily going through Cocker's *Book of Arithmetick.* Thus fortified, he then took up books on navigation, but on encountering the part dealing with geometry, sighed and gave it up.

An English grammar was the means of acquainting him with a book which caused him to drop the " abrupt contradiction and positive argumentation " common to youth in favor of a more winning method of dealing with his fellow man. This was Xenophon's *Memorable Things of Socrates.* From that time Socrates became one of the boy's heroes, and the Autobiography gives with immense gusto a recital of Franklin's victories over the disputatious through the Socratic method of humble but artful questions.

At this early age a book by one Tryon converted Franklin to the advantages of a vegetable diet, enabling him to brag about his consequent " greater clearness of head and quicker apprehension." But at a later period there was a deplorable fall from vegetarian grace, for Franklin spent an old age groaning with the gout.

IV

The supreme book, however, of Franklin's youth and the one which, to a far greater extent than perhaps even he, with all his self knowledge, realized, was *The Spectator* of Addison and Steele. Something of the excitement he felt at his discovery of an odd volume of the series surges up as

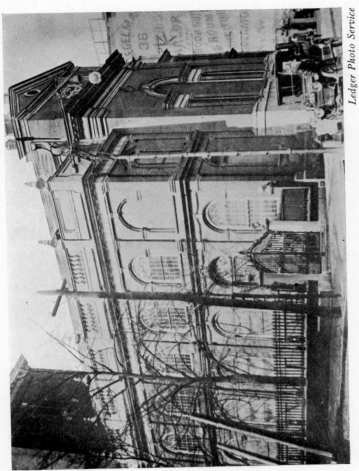

CHRIST CHURCH, PHILADELPHIA

LONG ATTENDED BY DEBORAH AND SARAH FRANKLIN, AS IT STANDS TODAY.

he writes: " It was the third. I had never before seen any-of them. I bought it, read it over and over, and was much delighted with it. I thought the writing excellent, and wished, if possible, to imitate it."

With the old thrill humming through his language, he relates how he studied the book, made notes on the various papers, laid them by, and then tried to rewrite them in a form as good as the original. Comparison showed him his defects. He carried his practice even further and finding his vocabulary needed enrichment, turned the tales into verse and back again into prose. These experiments apparently occupied him for a considerable period; the resulting benefit was perceptible. He at last fancied that in certain particulars, he had improved the method or the language, and this encouraged him to think he " might possibly in time come to be a tolerable English writer."

But in the papers of *The Spectator* the absorptive Franklin discovered much more than the merits of a graceful style, far-ranging vocabulary, and masterful construction. He discovered a new world. It was a world peopled by a society created in Queen Anne's reign and recreated by Joseph Addison, wherein was no wrestling over meticulous moral problems, no groanings of the spirit over abstruse theological dogmas, no grey didactics, nothing funereal, oppressive or depressive, but a tolerant urban world made interesting by human foibles. Whatever its failings, this world was not dull, not narrow, not mean. Human existence to *The Spectator's* contributors was not a moral problem, but a pageant to be regarded with comprehending sympathy marked by an occasional tear and more frequent smiles. To Addison, Steele and their associates life was not a thing to be hated or abstained from, but to be lived, even in its more disagreeable aspects, with a stout heart and a sustaining humor. Life in England under Queen Anne as portrayed by *The Spectator* was sometimes rather broad in its humor, its amusements were sometimes boisterous, but its manners were urbane and it did not forget to be kind.

Franklin studied this attitude as mirrored in the pages of *The Spectator* and the more he regarded it, the more he admired. It gave him a sense of release. It freed him from whatever uncertainty still remained as to whether in being good it was necessary also to be doleful.

While Franklin was trying, in the endeavor to penetrate to the secret of their charm, to rewrite the papers of Volume III of *The Spectator*, certain passages must have stamped their thought deeply upon his retentive memory. For example, perhaps this from essay No. 179:

" I may cast my readers under two general divisions, the Mercurial and the Saturnine. The first are the gay part of my disciples, who require speculations of wit and humor; the others are those of a more solemn and sober turn, who find no pleasure but in papers of morality and sound sense . . . I make it therefore my endeavour to find out entertainments of both kinds."

Since the New England cast of thought at that time was undoubtedly saturnine, and since Franklin at an early age showed himself so little in sympathy with it, it would not be strange if he chose that " gay part." He did choose it; he, as we shall see, definitely aligned himself with the Mercurial Division of the human race, who reconcile themselves to the trials of existence with saving speculations of wit and humor. After the roast beef, fruit and flowers! After the dirge the saraband!

But Franklin was too canny to permit his enthusiasms, however great, to gallop off with him. He did not overlook the necessity, for an editor, of providing " entertainments of both kinds."

In No. 197 of *The Spectator* occurs another passage

which must have given pause to our young-man-in-search-of-improvement:

" Avoid disputes as much as possible . . . if you are at any time obliged to enter an argument, give your reasons with the utmost coolness and modesty . . ."

Up to this time Franklin had been a contentious, some-what self-satisfied youth, much given to contradiction. He so confesses in his description of the argument with his boy friend, John Collins, about the propriety of educating the female sex. " I had caught it," Franklin records, " by reading my father's books of dispute about *religion*." [7] In the dispute with Collins, Franklin, as a reader of Defoe's *Projects*, took the side of the women, but failing to prevail, put his arguments on paper and sent them to Collins, who replied. Three or four letters had thus passed when Franklin's ever-critical father, discovering the correspondence, shook his head over his son's papers, pointing out that Benjamin had fallen " far short in elegance of expression, in method and perspicuity." Benjamin, by now desiring elegance above all things, began to mend his combative ways. The result is reflected in this passage of Franklin's Autobiography, closely paralleling *The Spectator:*

. . . " I wish well-meaning, sensible men would not lessen their power o*f doing good* [8] by a positive, assuming manner, that seldom fails to disgust, tends to create opposition, and to defeat every one of those purposes for which speech was given to us, to wit, giving or receiving information or pleasure."

He even abandoned the Socratic method in the course of time, " retaining," he relates, " only the habit of expressing myself in terms of modest diffidence."

[7] Autobiography.
[8] Italics ours.

V

If the style and sentiments of a book could so greatly in-fluence an impressionable boy, would not its *characters* influ-ence him no less, or even more? In *The Spectator*, which Franklin apparently studied more exhaustively than any other book of his life, the people are types rather than per-sons, but there is one character who, with a touch here by Addison and a stroke there by Steele, becomes round, alive and human. This is Sir Roger de Coverley.

Franklin could not have been content merely with Vol-ume III of *The Spectator*. He doubtless obtained the rest of the series as they appeared from 1710–11 nearly through 1714. A set of *The Spectator* and of Steele's earlier jour-nal, *The Tatler*, " handsomely bound," were among the effects disposed of by Franklin's will. He therefore must have followed the views and fortunes of Sir Roger from his first appearance until his lamented death at the hands of his creators. The sturdy knight scarcely could have failed to impress himself on Franklin's ambitious imagination.

Every boy between the ages of 12 and 16 is unconsciously seeking among the men he knows a model after which he can build himself. Often the model is the boy's father. But Franklin had already become antagonistic towards his father's beliefs and leanings. What more natural, then, at a period when he was spending almost the whole of his snatched leisure among books, that he should have found his model man in the book which he had read " over and over " ?

Woodrow Wilson says Franklin was " half peasant, half man of the world." [9] Franklin might have remained wholly a peasant, at least in attitude and outlook, had not his early reading made him wish to acquire the elegance, wit, poise

[9] Introduction to Franklin's Autobiography, Century Classics.

and *savoir faire* of superior men. It is not likely he could find these qualities among the grim Puritans he met in the Boston candle shop or in his father's house, and he had already conceived a barely suppressed dislike for men like the Mathers and other graduates of Harvard College.[10] But the character of the worthy Sir Roger de Coverley he could admire wholly.

It seems altogether probable, then, that in boyhood Franklin took Sir Roger de Coverley, as limned and sculptured by Addison and Steele, as the pattern of the man he some day hoped to be, and that all his life Franklin, subconsciously, strove to shape his own character after that sturdy, independent and kindly figure.

So far as we know, none of the previous biographers of Franklin, all observant and studious men, has noticed the striking likeness between the fictional character of Sir Roger de Coverley and that of Franklin in his riper years; at least none has pointed it out. But let us proceed to the evidence. No. II of *The Spectator* papers, entitled " The Club " — a group of Queen Anne gentlemen who met informally to discuss whatever topics, worldly or abstract, appeared to be interesting, contains, in outlining the personality of Sir Roger, this passage:

" He is a gentleman that is very singular in his behaviour, but his singularities proceed from his good sense, and are contradictions to the manners of the world only as he thinks the world is in the wrong. However, this humour creates no enemies, for he does nothing with sourness or obstinacy; and his being unconfined to modes and forms makes him but the readier and more capable to please and oblige all who know him . . . he is now in his 56th year, cheerful, gay, and hearty; keeps a good house both in town and country; a great lover of mankind; but there is such a mirthful cast

[10] Vide Silence Dogood papers.

in his behaviour that he is rather beloved than esteemed.[11] His tenants grow rich, his servants look satisfied, all the young women profess love to him, and the young men are glad of his company."

In the 6th paper an observation from Sir Roger's own mouth is quoted as follows:

" ' I lay it down therefore for a rule, that the whole man is to move together; that every action of any importance is to have a prospect of public good; and that the general tendency of our indifferent actions ought to be agreeable to the dictates of reason, of religion, of good breeding.' " The same paper continues:

" I have observed . . . that my friend Sir Roger, amidst all his good qualities, is something of an humourist, and that his virtues as well as his imperfections are, as it were, tinged by a certain extravagance, which makes them particularly *his*, and distinguishes them from those of other men. This cast of mind, as it is generally very innocent in itself, so it renders his conversation highly agreeable, and more delightful than the same degree of sense and virtue would appear in their common and ordinary colors."

In No. VII, dealing with the harmony found in the Coverley household, is the following:

" This proceeds from the humane and equal temper of the man of the house. . . . This makes his own mind untroubled, and consequently unapt to vent peevish expressions, or give passionate or inconsistent orders to those about him. Thus respect and love go together. . . ."

In No. XX is this:

" My worthy friend Sir Roger is one of those who is not only at peace within himself, but beloved and esteemed by all about him. He receives a suitable tribute for his universal benevolence to mankind in the returns of affection

---

[11] " Esteemed " is used here in the old sense of regarded coldly.

and good will which are paid him by every one that lives within his neighbourhood."

And finally in No. XXIV the gypsy girl who tells Sir Roger's fortune says to him:

" ' Ah master, that roguish leer of yours makes a pretty woman's heart ache; you ha'n't that simper about the mouth for nothing.' "

Let us see how these descriptions of the amiable Sir Roger match the impressions we derive of Dr. Franklin's character, after it had been long mature, as it appeared to the friends who had had long opportunity to study him. Madame Brillon, the fascinating Frenchwoman who perhaps learned to know him better than any other woman in the world, once said to Franklin in a letter: " You always know how to combine a great measure of wisdom with a touch of roguishness." And again: " Your letter . . . has given me keen pleasure: I found in it that gayety and gallantry which make all women love you, because you love them all." And again: " You combine with the best heart, my lovable Papa, when you wish, the soundest ethics, a lively imagination, and that roguishness, so pleasant, which shows that the wisest man in the world allows his wisdom to be perpetually broken against the rocks of femininity."

Almost at the close of Franklin's life, his sister, Jane Macom, the " baby " of his mother's children, wrote to him:

" This day my dear brother completes his 84th year. You cannot, as old Jacob, say, Few and evil have they been; except those wherein you have endured such grievous torments latterly, yours have been filled with innumerable good works, benefits to your fellow creatures, and thankfulness to God, that notwithstanding the distressing circumstances before mentioned, yours must be esteemed a glorious life. Great increase of glory and happiness I hope await you. May God mitigate your pain and continue your patience yet many years, for who that knows and loves you can bear the thought of surviving you in this gloomy world? "

The Rev. Manasseh Cutler, a scholar and botanist, who visited Franklin in his old age, thus wrote of him: " His voice was low, but his countenance open, frank, and pleasing. . . . His manners are perfectly easy, and everything about his seems to diffuse an unrestrained freedom and happiness. He has an incessant vein of humor, accompanied with an uncommon vivacity, which seemed as natural and involuntary as his breathing."

And finally there is the celebrated letter of George Washington, written to Franklin in 1789:

" If to be venerated for benevolence, if to be admired for talents, if to be esteemed for patriotism, if to be beloved for philanthropy, can gratify the human mind, you must have the pleasing consolation to know that you have not lived in vain."

If it be true, then, as we believe, that Franklin sought to make his character conform to that of Sir Roger de Coverley as an ideal, who can deny that he thunderously succeeded?

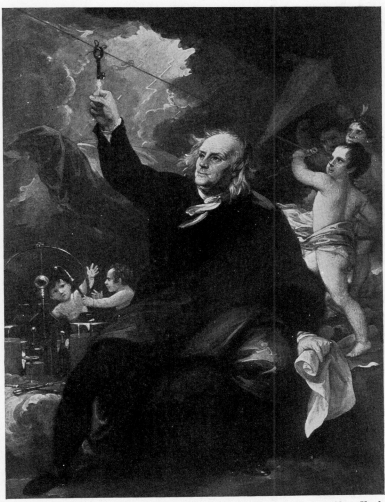

ALLEGORICAL PAINTING OF FRANKLIN DISCOVERING
THE IDENTITY OF LIGHTNING AND ELECTRICITY
BY BENJAMIN WEST

Chapter II

"The Business of Life is with Matter"

— Thomas Jefferson

I

IT is Benjamin's bookish inclinations that eventually determine Josiah Franklin to make a printer of his smallest son. Benjamin's older brother, James, is already established in the printing trade. It is respectable enough and not an ungodly business like going to sea. But Benjamin, no doubt to the disgust of his patient father, hangs back on the halter. He still, because he is a water-bred boy and also perhaps because he dreams of beholding those thousand oddities of the world described in Burton's *Historical Collections,* hankers for the ocean wide. At last, though, he dutifully gives in, and signs the indentures which bind him until he shall be 21 years old, to James, a choleric and jealous-natured young man with whom the saucy Benjamin almost at once gets into rows.

To the printing-house, however, the 12-year-old Benjamin becomes soon reconciled. It enables him to meet booksellers' apprentices, who filch for him an occasional book, though only " a small one," from their masters' stocks. Ben returns these borrowed volumes " soon and clean," thus becoming one of the few book-borrowers of that kind known to history. He also borrows books from a kindly tradesman, a customer of his brother.

Ben's time for reading is at night, before and after work during the day, and on Sundays, when he manages to avoid church by inventing excuses to go to the print-shop, where he can be luxuriously alone. According to the theological teachings of the time, this Sabbath-breaking should have been penalized by Heaven, and Benjamin's first literary Sunday is doubtless passed with some apprehension of lightning from above. But when another Sunday comes and no angry stroke falls, he breathes — and reads — more easily. Long afterwards he wrote to a friend, describing the amusements and gayeties of a Sunday in Flanders:

" I looked around for God's Judgments, but saw no signs of them. The cities were well built and full of inhabitants, the markets filled with plenty, the people well-favoured and well clothed, the fields well tilled, the cattle fat and strong, the fences, houses, and windows all in repair, and no Old Tenor (early American paper money) anywhere in the country; which would almost make one suspect that the Deity is not so angry at that offence as a New England Justice."

II

Benjamin now feels the first stirs of adolescent blood, which still retains the strain contributed to it by his versifying maternal grandfather, Peter Folger. He writes verses.

Enters the printing brother. He sees the commercial possibilities of the thing, and induces Ben not only to write ballads, but when printed to hawk them about Boston's streets. One is called " The Lighthouse Tragedy "; the other records the capture of Blackbeard, the pirate. The event makes " a great noise." [1] It is the germ of Tin Pan Alley and American popular song-making, since become a major industry. Little Benjamin beams with that vanity, the obtrusions of which he struggles to subdue for the rest of his life. Enters the lowering villain. It is Ben's father. He sets about the favorite New England pastime of killing youthful joy. Leave poetry to loafers. There's no money

[1] Autobiography.

in it. Verse-makers are "generally beggars." [2]   Stick to business. Get on. "The business of life is with matter."

"So," wrote Franklin at the age of 65, with an almost perceptible sigh, "I escaped being a poet, most probably a very bad one."

III

When Benjamin is about 15 years old, James Franklin begins to issue a newspaper, the *New England Courant*. The first number is dated August 17, 1721. The Autobiography calls it the second in America. But it was actually the fourth. The first American newspaper, regularly issued, was the *Boston News-Letter*, which appeared April 24, 1704, two years before Franklin was born. James's friends shake their heads over his project; one newspaper is all that America (population 400,000) can support. But the paper continues, partly due to the contributions of several humorous young Bostonians, mostly medical men, who like thus to amuse themselves. Ben, when not setting type, running the press and delivering the papers, looks on with envy. Remembering his success with the ballads, he itches with a desire to write a few pieces himself, in that prose which he feels is sometimes almost as good as *The Spectator's*. He does so, but knowing the contemptuous disposition of his brother, he dares not offer them directly, but slips one, written in a disguised hand, under the door of the printshop at night. It is signed, significantly, with a woman's name — "*Silence Dogood.*" Let us note well these two words. We shall hear of them again.

James Franklin and his advisers read it the next morning. They deem it good. They guess at the author, naming men known in the community for ingenuity. Little Benjamin, pretending to potter busily about the shop, listens greedily

[2] *Autobiography.*

to their comments, his whole being suffused with an "exquisite pleasure." Benjamin Franklin, journalist and writer on public affairs, is born.

The first paper by Mistress Silence Dogood is followed by several others, also slipped in via the door crack. They duly appear. They create talk. The small author's colonial hat can no longer contain his head. He divulges his secret. He expects a slap on the back from his brother. He gets something to the contrary.

"What! You wrote those pieces? On *my* time, too, I'll wager. You think you're smart, don't you? You'll be getting the swell-head now. Get back to your type. The customer's waiting for that job. Silence Dogood indeed! Your name ought to be Talkative Dobad."

Benjamin goes back to the composing case in silence. All the rest of the day he and his brother do not speak. Fifty years later he wrote:

"I fancy his harsh and tyrannical treatment of me might be a means of impressing me with that aversion to arbitrary power that has stuck to me through my whole life."

But the Dogood papers, though scorned by James, raise Benjamin in the estimation of James's friends, and they eye the small round figure moving silently among the type cases with a curious interest. "You never can tell," they say, "about these Franklins."

IV

Since the "Silence Dogood" pieces were the first of those papers, essays and disquisitions of which Franklin was so prolific during a long life, they merit more than casual study. It is, in the first place, a curious fact that Franklin should have chosen to make his first appearance in the press disguised, so to speak, as a woman.

Franklin had a pronounced feminine element in his nature and personality. This feminine element was visible even in his physical structure. His face was round. His shoulders were round. His limbs were round. Symbolists would say that Franklin typified the circle — all round. As he matured, he became conciliatory, non-combative, and preferred to please rather than antagonize. He exhibited none of the harsh angularities characteristic of such associates as Washington and Jefferson. All his life he showed his undisguised pleasure in the society of women. He frequently appeared happier and more at ease in his correspondence with feminine friends than with his masculine ones. If any great man has ever understood women, Franklin did.

As "Silence Dogood" he described himself, in terms of his ideal Sir Roger de Coverley, as handsome and good-natured, frequently witty, and always courteous and affable. Also as "a hearty lover of the Clergy and all good Men, and a mortal Enemy to arbitrary Government and unlimited Power." One of the very first Dogood letters, entitled "Dream," is a satire at the expense of Harvard College, whose graduates are described as prone to heed the beckoning finger of the goddess *Pecunia*. "Every peasant, who had wherewithal, was proposing to send one of his children, at least, to this famous place; and in this case, most of them consulted their own purses instead of their children's capacities. So that I observed a great many, yea, the most part of those who were traveling thither, were little better than blockheads and dunces."

Another Dogood paper reveals that sympathy for women, rare among the men of Franklin's time, which had previously been exhibited in Benjamin's boyish debates with his chum Collins. "Their Youth," says Mrs. Dogood, using almost the exact words of Defoe's *Essay on Projects*, "is spent to teach them to stitch and sew, or make Baubles.

They are taught to read indeed and perhaps to write their names, or so; and that is the Heigth of a Woman's Education." With that inconsistency frequently described as truly feminine, Mrs. Dogood then turns around and, in another paper, abuses her sex for indulging in the monstrous hoop-petticoats of the period. She asks " whether they, who pay no Rates or Taxes, ought to take up more Room in the King's Highway, than the Men, who yearly contribute to the Support of the Government."

Other letters deal with freedom of speech — " Who ever would overthrow the Liberty of a Nation, must begin by subduing the Freeness of Speech; a *Thing* Terrible to Publick Traytors "; with hypocrisy in religion, it being a question whether a commonwealth suffers more from hypocritical pretenders to religion or from the openly profane; with drunkenness; and with night walkers on Boston Common, a subject no doubt suggested to Franklin by a paper in the *Spectator* relating a nocturnal adventure of Sir Roger de Coverley's in London.

Still another Dogood paper owes its origin to Franklin's study of Defoe's *Essay on Projects;* it offers a plan for the insurance of widows, concluding, in the words of Silence: " For my own Part, I have nothing left to live on, but Contentment and a few Cows; and tho' I cannot expect to be reliev'd by this Project (*sic*), yet it would be no small satisfaction to me to see it put in practice for the Benefit of Others." The next letter contains a bit of the Franklinian drollery which persisted in most of his writings to his dying day. Margaret Aftercast, a spinster, begs Mrs. Dogood also to form a project for the relief of " all those penitent Mortals of the fair Sex, that are like to be punish'd with their Virginity until Old Age, for the Pride and Insolence of their Youth." Franklin was ever concerned about women; married and unmarried, elderly spinsters, fruitful mothers, bereft widows and blooming maids — he liked them all; and when he could, made love to them all.

At 16, then, we find Franklin to be a free thinker, a foe of religious intolerance, a potential rebel against powers arbitrarily exercised, and a defender of women's rights. He has revealed his abilities as a printer, a verse-maker, a humorous writer, and a journalist. He is getting on.

CHAPTER III

The Boy Publisher

I

SOON after becoming apprenticed to his brother, Benjamin concludes with him a deal betraying that canny practicality which later enables him to conquer situations that another kind of nature might have accepted supinely. Benjamin has found that he can maintain himself very comfortably on a meatless diet. He therefore goes to James and offers to find his own food if James will give him half the money that Benjamin's board is costing him. James agrees instantly. So while the other apprentices are absent at their meals, Benjamin remains in the shop holding in one hand a raisin sandwich and in the other one of the precious books which he is now able to buy. He is putting into books half the money obtained from James.

This abstemiousness, added to other independent traits exhibited by his younger brother, arouses James's dislike. Benjamin isn't docile, he isn't " regular." James becomes surly and critical. Benjamin resents his slurs. These fraternal disputes are brought before their father. Benjamin tries out his modest Socratic method of presenting the case. He wins. This naturally doubles James's rage. In secret he falls upon Benjamin and beats him, not once but often. Ben, miserable but silent, bides his time. He awaits an opportunity to tear his indenture papers to pieces and fling them in James's lowering face. Fate and the Massachusetts Council come to the rescue.

II

The quarrels between the Franklin brothers have not hampered the growth of the *New England Courant*. It is a success. It is condemned as sensational, and worthy folk, who otherwise would ignore it, buy it to see just how sensational it is. The clergy denounce it, and almost at once the circulation goes up by the dizzy figure of 40. A furious letter, attributed to Cotton Mather, appears in the rival *News Letter*. It compares the *Courant* contributors to the Hell Fire Club in England, whose members are said to have erected an altar to the Devil. It is probable that Benjamin has never heard of the Hell Fire Club before. The name interests him; he has a liking for clubs. We shall see what becomes of this interest.

Dr. Mather goes on to denounce the *Courant* as " full freighted with nonsense, unmanliness, railery, prophaneness, immorality, arrogance, calumnies, lies, contradictions, and what not, all tending to quarrels and divisions, and to debauch and corrupt the minds and manners of New England." Increase Mather announces that he has ceased to buy the paper. The *Courant* replies that this may be so; nevertheless he sends a boy around for it. But the impudence of the paper has irritated the authorities and one day they nail it.

The issue of June 11, 1792, contains a hoax story — possibly originating with Benjamin, who loved hoaxes — about a pirate ship seen off Block Island. " We are advised from Boston," says the *Courant*, " that the government of the Massachusetts are fitting out a ship, (the Flying Horse,) to go after the pirates, to be commanded by Captain Peter Papillon, and 'tis thought he will sail some time this month, wind and weather permitting."

The humor of the concluding phrase is enhanced for those who know that *papillon* is French for butterfly. They laugh, and eagerly pass the paper around. The Council has stood many things from the *Courant*, but it cannot stand being laughed at. James and Benjamin are summoned for an examination. They refuse to give the name of the story's author. James, as the publisher, is sent to jail. A week there is enough for him. He pleads to be let out. He grovels. He confesses that he has sinned, and, besides, his health is very bad. In a month he is released. Benjamin, the kid brother, meantime gets out the paper. He enjoys the opportunity. He gives the colony's rulers a few extra rubs. The rubbing continues freely for another six months. Finally the authorities explode.

The province is bossed by Governor Samuel Shute, one of those far-flung dunderheads who through the years have done so much to start seams in the British Ship of State. He has quarreled with the Massachusetts General Court, and in a dudgeon is off home to tell mama about it. The *Courant* asks this question: If, as many contend, the Governor means to hurt the province, are not the ministers who pray for the success of his homeward voyage, praying in effect for the destruction of the province? [1] This leads the *Courant* writer — whose style and thought are much like the irreverent Benjamin's — to a consideration of too-muchness in religion, which is deemed " worse than none at all. The world abounds with knaves and villains; but of all knaves, the *religious knave* is the worst; and villainies acted under the cloak of religion are the most execrable. Moral honesty, though it will not of itself, carry a man to heaven, yet I am sure there is no going thither *without it*. And however such men, of whom I have been speaking, may palliate their wickedness, they will find that *publicans and harlots will*

[1] John Bach McMaster in " Benjamin Franklin As a Man of Letters."

enter the kingdom of heaven before themselves." The italics are the *Courant's*.

The Council at once issues an order forbidding James Franklin " to print or publish the New England Courant, or any other pamphlet or paper of the like nature, except it be first supervised by the Secretary of this Province."

In Boston's respectable circles the ban placed on the *Courant* is doubtless approved. It is high time to put a damper on those young Franklins. Their writings, once merely foolish, have become inflammatory. But one voice is raised in defense of the Franklins. It comes from Philadelphia.

Philadelphia! It is a name which thereafter is sweet in the ears of that Benjamin who rarely forgets anything.

The Philadelphia *Weekly Mercury*, established in 1719, thus comments satirically on the drastic order laid against James:

" An indifferent person would judge, from this conduct, that the Assembly of Massachusetts were oppressors and bigots, ' who made religion only an engine of destruction to the people.' " It concludes with this comment: " By private letters from Boston, we are informed, that the bakers were under great apprehensions of being forbid baking any more bread, unless they will submit it to the Secretary as supervisor-general and weigher of the dough, before it is baked into bread and offered for sale."

However, the ban is maintained. James, as publisher and printer of the *Courant,* is done for. Who shall carry on the paper? A council of war is held in the print-shop. All the liveliest contributors are there. Their eyes fall on Benjamin, working tranquilly before his type cases. They already have a respect for Benjamin. He can write, he knows how to get out the paper, and he isn't afraid. Benjamin is clearly the man. Unanimously they choose him.

Thereafter the *Courant* appears with a new name at the masthead.

Benjamin Franklin, publisher, is born. Age 17.

III

The first issue of the *Courant* under Franklin sounds a " keynote " unquestionably Benjaminesque: " The present undertaking . . . is designed purely for the diversion and merriment of the reader . . . to entertain the town with the most comical and diverting incidents of human life which, in so large a place as Boston, will not fail of a universal exemplification: Nor shall we be wanting to fill up these papers with a grateful interspersion of more serious morals, which may be drawn from the most ludicrous and odd parts of life."

It is thus that Benjamin announces himself as the American *Spectator*. He even proclaims that the paper is now issued by a " club," which exists " for the Propagation of Sense and Good Manners among the docible part of Mankind in His Majesty's Plantations in America," under the guidance of the good Dr. Janus. Dr. Janus is simply Sir Roger de Coverley Americanized. He is set forth as " a chearly Christian . . . a man of good temper, courteous Deportment, sound Judgment; a mortal Hater of Nonsense, Foppery, Formality and endless Ceremony."

IV

One of Benjamin's first issues contains a letter from a supposed reader warning the editor against casting reflections on the Boston clergy. " But," continues the paper, " tho they are the *Best of Men*, yet they are but Men at the best, and by consequence subject to like *Frailties* and

Passions as other Men; and when we hear of the *Impru-dencies* of any of them, we should cover them with the mantle of Love and Charity. . . ."

Since Benjamin is already being " pointed at with horror as an infidel or atheist," [2] this passage may be taken as a mere fling at the Boston clergy in general. On the other hand, is anything specific aimed at? Did Franklin have in mind any particular incident deserving the mantle of charity?

Let us see. We know that one of the lad's hostile critics is the Rev. Cotton Mather, the witch-hunter, to whose excoriating sermons in the Old South Church, near his home in Milk Street, he has probably often listened when he would prefer to be locked luxuriously in an attic reading books.

Mather's first wife died in 1702. Some time later a young lady, " accomplished and comely," called to see him. She wished to become better acquainted with him, she said, for the purpose of religious improvement. Mather temporized; he said he feared their colloquies might be misunderstood. But the lady persisted. She came again. And again. There came upon Mather a racking trial. In his Diary he confessed his " sore distresses and temptations " concerning her. The lady continued to call.

Talk ensued. The community buzzed. Mather, seeing the danger but unable to forbid her the house, finally, with a mighty effort, wrote to her mother. The young lady came no more. Soon afterward, at the suggestion of friends, Mather took a second wife, a widow.

Did Franklin know about this incident? He, a newspaper man in a small town, with ears alert to gossip? He, the target of Mather's blazings? We must assume that he did. And, having his little vein of malice, he could scarcely

[2] Autobiography.

forbear to make subtle use of it. And there would be readers who would forgive him for it.

V

Not content with this, the democratic *Courant* soon afterward appears with another fantastic piece which must have shocked the strict religious folk and political rulers of Boston, — all piously loyal to England and England's customs — no less. It deals with the discussion by the Club of " Hat Honour " and proceeds:

" Adam was never called Master Adam; we never read of Noah Esquire, Lot, Knight and Baronet, nor the Right Honourable Abraham, Viscount Mesopotamia, Baron of Canaan; no, no, they were plain Men, honest Country grasiers, that took care of their families and their Flocks. Moses was a great Prophet, and Aaron a priest of the Lord; but we never read of the Reverend Moses, nor the Right Reverend Father in God, Aaron, by Divine Providence, Lord Arch-Bishop of Israel; Thou never sawest Madam Rebecca in the Bible, my Lady Rachel; nor Mary, tho' a Princess of the Blood after the death of Joseph, call'd the Princess Dowager of Nazareth; no, plain Rebecca, Rachel, Mary, or the Widow Mary, or the like; It was no Incivility then to mention their naked Names as they were expressed."

There is no signature to this paper, but the hand, even to the elided *e* in the past tense of verbs, is Esau's. It is also readily identifiable in this extract from another essay:

" Upon the whole, Friend Janus, we may conclude, that the *Anti-Couranteers* are a sort of *Precisians*, who mistaking Religion for the peculiar whims of their own distemper'd Brain, are for cutting or stretching all men to their own

Standard of Thinking . . . Sir Thomas Hope Blount in his Essays, has said enough to convince us of the Unreasonableness of this sour Temper among Christians: and with his words I shall conclude:

" ' Certainly (*says he*) of all sorts of men, none do more mistake the Divine Nature, and by consequence do greater mischief to Religion, than those who would persuade us, that to be truly religious, is to renounce all the Pleasures of Humane Life; As if Religion were a *Caput Mortuum*, a heavy, dull, insipid thing; that has neither Heat, Life or Motion in it. . . .' Whereas (really) Religion is of an Active Principle, it not only elevates the mind and invigorates the Fancy; but it admits of Mirth, and pleasantness of Conversation, and indulges us in our Christian Liberties; and for this reason, says the Lord *Bacon*, *It is no less impious to shut where God Almighty has open'd, than to open where God Almighty has shut.*" The italics are the author's.

We quote this *Courant* editorial at length because it states the creed to which Franklin adhered, in the main, during his life of 84 years. For him the religion of *active* principle. For him the religion of heat, life and motion. For him the religion which neither invades the shut nor ignores the unshut.

VI

The *Courant* thrives. Its price is raised from three to four pence, and a Publick Notice is printed that Advertisements will be inserted at a moderate price. The boy publisher is exhilarated. The future widens before him, glorious, free, subscription-lined. He becomes, as he admitted later, a little " saucy and provoking." And then falls the long-poised blow from Heaven.

When Benjamin became editor of the *Courant*, James,

to avoid further penalties from the authorities, cancelled his brother's old indenture papers, but got Benjamin's signature to new ones, which were kept secret. This arrangement was almost sure to cause trouble. It did.

James, keenly conscious of his own recent cowardice and bitterly envious of Benjamin's mounting success, suffers from that complex so frequently associated with the word inferiority. Unable to prevail over his younger brother by force of will or character, he again resorts to beatings. Ben, reminding him of the cancelled indentures, proclaims a declaration of independence. In short, he quits.

Almost instantly the gales of fate, so long withheld, burst upon the saucy Benjamin. He can find no work elsewhere, for James has already had him blacklisted. His father takes sides with James. Fair friends turn cool. Boston, saying "Aha!", predicts a scandalous end for a presumptuous youth. Everywhere Benjamin encounters concealed hostility, open sneers. He turns a little sick. He suddenly wants to get away from it all. He thinks he will hate the human race less in New York. But in his bewilderment, his soreness, he can devise no plan. For relief he turns to the friend he most looks up to — the facile, the ingenious Collins. Collins has his defects; he despises women, a trait which Benjamin dislikes, and is a little irresponsible, but in scheming he is a perfect Tom Sawyer. Collins is enchanted. "Leave it to me." Holding in his mirth, he goes to one of his numerous low-life friends, the skipper of a New York sloop. He arranges the passage, gravely informing the sympathetic skipper that Benjamin — studious, straitly-reared, philosophical Benjamin — has got a girl into trouble!

Ben's books have already done him several good turns. They now do him another. They are converted into the cash which every voyager to foreign shores must have. Se-

Mathematicks
Ward's Introduction. 2d Edm
Dechalls Euclid —
L'Hospital's Conic Sections
Ozanam's Course Math 5 Vol.
Hayes upon Fluxions
Keil's Astronomical Lectures

Morality
Spectators
Guardians
Tatlers
Puffendorf's Law of Nature
Addisons Works in 12
Memorable Things of Socrates
Turkish Spy

Anatomy
Drakes Anatomy

Nat. Philosophy
Abridgt of Phil. Tran. 5 Vol.
Gravesende's Nat Philosoph. 2 Vol
Boerhaave's Chymistry

Politicks
Sidney on Governmt
Cato's Letters
Messrs du Port Royal Mor. Essays

The Compleat Tradesman

Logic
Crousa's Art of Thinking
Locke's Essay on Humane Understandg
Sidney on Government
Cato's Letters

Philology
Bayley's Dictionary
English Gramar. Brightland's
Homer's Iliad & Odyssey
Greenwood's Grammar
Monsr Bayles Critical Dictionary
Drydon's Virgil

Catalogues —

PORTION OF A LIST OF BOOKS FOR THE PHILADELPHIA
LIBRARY IN FRANKLIN'S HANDWRITING

CONSPICUOUS IN THIS LIST ARE THE BOOKS WHICH MOST INFLUENCED
THE YOUTHFUL FRANKLIN. IT IS TO BE NOTED THAT VOLUMES OF "THE
SPECTATOR" ARE RECOMMENDED UNDER THE HEAD OF "MORALITY."

From the Ford collection in the New York Public Library.

cretly Collins slips him aboard the ship. Anchor is weighed. The sails fill. Boston's low houses grow dim. Adam is driven forth from the garden. Mohammed begins his hegira. But Benjamin, after all, has won his wish. He has gone to sea.

Chapter IV

Exile

I

IT takes three days to make the voyage of 300 miles from
Boston to New York, but the weather is good, the early
autumn air cool and limpid, and Benjamin's spirits,
never long in a slump, bound upward. Characteristically,
he begins to look about him for things to be observed.
During a calm off Block Island he finds the sailors amusing
themselves by fishing for tomcod. Put on the galley fire,
these fish give forth a savoury odor. It curls appetizingly
about the nostrils of the boy passenger. Up to now he has
been a devout vegetarian. The spirit continues sturdy, but
the flesh hankers after the fish pots.

It is, as we have observed, the beginning of the Age of
Reason. Benjamin, being a man of his period, therefore
surveys the subject of vegetarianism in the light of the new
dawn. Upon examination he finds that the fish which are
hauled on deck contain other fish within them. He ration-
alizes the situation. It is clear that the caught fish deserve
no mercy. The vegetarian theory slides overboard with a
rattling crash. He falls upon the guilty fish with relish.

" So convenient it is," he remarked later, " to be a *reasonable* creature, since it enables one to find or make a reason
for everything one has a mind to do."

Sly Benjamin! Already you are observing the workings
of human nature, in yourself and others, with that canny
humor which is to teach you to get along with your fellow
men in a spirit of accommodation which provides charity
for all.

II

He lands upon the jutting cobbles of New York streets in October, that month in which the climate, regretting the unreasonable heats and vapors of the summer, and with the dingy snows of winter yet lodged in the North, bestows upon Manhattan a lifting air which has been justly compared to the finest claret. The population of the town is about 7000. Benjamin walks about the narrow, meandering cow paths and pig promenades looped about the toe of the island which are known to the Dutch burghers as streets. The curious houses, of Low Country architecture, are built with their gable ends outward. Benjamin, with an inveterate interest in the recorded thoughts of men, looks about for a bookshop. But he sees none, because there is none. New Yorkers are intent on money and when the day's bartering is over, they wish to be abundantly amused. They import books from Europe to use as shelf-decorations; they plead they have no time to read them. But there is a printshop in the town and Ben soon finds it. It is kept by William Bradford, the first New York printer, who is one day to occupy a grave in Trinity Churchyard so that smartly dressed stenographers and pug-nosed flappers may have a noontime centre around which to eat their lettuce sandwiches, plentifully spread with mayonnaise. Bradford has been chased out of Pennsylvania for calling William Penn " ye Lord Penn " and other deeds offensive to the Assembly. " The old sophister " [1] has no work for the Boston lad, but suggests he can get a job under his son, Andrew, in Philadelphia. Ben likes the notion. Is not Philadelphia the fraternal town whose *Weekly Mercury* raised a sympathetic voice in defense of the Franklin freedom of speech?

[1] Autobiography.

He starts for Amboy, on the Jersey side, in an old tub of a boat with another passenger, a drunken Dutchman, who falls overboard. Ben drags him out and finds in his pocket a copy of *Pilgrim's Progress,* a title which must have seemed strikingly appropriate at that time. They are driven on Long Island and lie there all night wet, cold, and foodless. They reach Amboy after thirty wretched hours.

Benjamin, being, like a true exile, light in the pocket, sets out on foot for Burlington, fifty miles away. All day he tramps in a drizzling rain, a forlorn youth in a strange land where he knows not a human being. His usual cheerfulness sinks far below zero. He thinks of Boston, his friends there, the ample table spread by a careful mother, the security of his job if he had only kept his mouth shut, his pen still, his mind closed. He has thrown away everything. For what? To walk through the flat barrens of New Jersey in the rain!

III

His spirits touch bottom that night when at a poor inn he is questioned as if he were a runaway servant. He knows he looks the part. His rough, home-made working clothes are stuffed with his belongings. He has been without sleep. And he is very wet.

When things reach their lowest point, there is nowhere for them to go but up. The next day he finds a better inn, kept by a Dr. Brown, a defeated and disillusioned man. But the old fire re-kindles when Brown discovers in this bedraggled youth an alert mind, a bookish taste, an original turn of speech, and a quirky humor. They discuss the state of letters, philosophy, politics, religion, men, women. They take stock of the universe, laughing as they look down upon its antics from a far height. They return to earth and tell each other earthy stories.

The next day Benjamin finds the world recuperating. The conversation with the vagabond doctor has exorcised the evil spirits from his mind. The droll smile returns to his rounded countenance. In Burlington it wins him a woman friend, a gingerbread-seller. She cannot resist this waggish fellow. Few women can. She bids him lodge at her house, and gives him a good dinner. Money she refuses, but coyly accepts the mate to his pot of ale.

That evening he hails a rowboat headed for Philadelphia. It carries him to Market Street Wharf. He steps out with a dollar and some coppers in his pocket into a city whose life he is to widen, whose history he is to enrich, for more than half a century. The strange lad's hands are empty, his pockets nearly so, his sagging coat contains naught but stuffed-in shirts and home-knit stockings; nevertheless he comes laden with gifts.

His entry is signalized by a characteristic Franklinism. He gives all his change to the boatman. " A man," he remarks, " being sometimes more generous when he has but a little money than when he has plenty, perhaps thro' fear of being thought to have but little."

CHAPTER V

The New Home

I

IT is forty years after the landing of William Penn.
Strong colonies founded by English Quakers and
Welsh and Irish farmers line the banks of the Delaware from the falls of Trenton to Chester. Frugal and
hard-working Germans have given their village on the
Wissahickon the name of Germantown. Philadelphia is a
market town of 5,000 people, surrounded by thick forests
of hardwoods sheltering bear, deer, Indians, and an abundance of other wild game.

The Pennsylvanians have thrived since the beginning.
Their community life is not rent by religious factionalism
as in Boston, but they have an internal quarrel sufficiently
troublesome. It is between the land-owning class and the
common people. The former consists of the Proprietaries,
who originally acquired title to tracts in the vast area of
land granted to Penn by Charles II, lying between the possessions of the Duke of York, in New Jersey, and those of
Lord Baltimore in Maryland. The Proprietaries occasionally are disturbed in their serene enjoyment of ownership
by threats of taxation. They cannot bear the idea. They
become clamorous and abusive. They fence themselves in.
This fence has created a line of division between two opposing forces. Every newcomer, as soon as he acquires an influence, however small, is compelled to take one side or the
other. He must "line up." The freshly arrived immigrant from Boston, capital one dollar, is only a journeyman

printer. But if and when he makes a little money and begins to be respected by his neighbors, which side shall he choose, and what will be the consequence of that choice? We shall see.

II

The very first incident which occurs to Benjamin as, soiled, tired and hungry, he walks up from the wharf towards the market house is one of those dramatic ones which he loves. Our Benjamin has a bit of the showman's instinct. His pockets are stuffed with rolled-up shirts and coarse woolen stockings, also with not a little vanity — that confidence in himself which is to stiffen his backbone in the face of many over-awing situations. "It would not be altogether absurd if a man were to thank God for his vanity among the other comforts of life."[1]

A boy comes along carrying bread. Ben asks him where he got it. The boy tells him where to find the baker's, which is open, though it is Sunday. Ben goes to the shop in Second Street, and asks for "bisket." In Philadelphia they are not imaginative. The shop people do not see before them a hungry boy who wants food — any kind of food. They see merely a stranger, evidently from foreign parts, who has asked for "bisket." They do not trifle with bread that way in Philadelphia: they do not make such things. They shake their heads. Ben then asks for a thrippenny loaf. Another headshake. The exasperated stranger then flings downs his money and asks for bread — any name, any style, any shape — so it be bread. Ben receives three great puffy rolls. He is "surpriz'd at the quantity." He realizes he is no longer in stingy Boston. He walks away eating one of the huge rolls, and having no room in his stuffed pockets, sticks the others under each arm.

[1] Autobiography.

Now for the little drama. In Market Street, near Fourth, he passes, standing in the doorway of a respectable dwelling, a tidy young woman. She is fresh of cheek and of plump and pleasing figure. She has a childish face but a practical and prognathous chin. She has narrowed eyes which see everything. Being at the age when most of her girl friends have already won a husband, she inspects, without seeming to, the figure of the approaching young man. He is badly dressed, his long-tailed coat bulges at the sides, his heavy shoes make a clumping noise, and he is eating bread in the streets. He carries two rolls insanitarily under his arms. She loses interest. Such an awkward, boorish youth could not possibly mean anything to her young eyes. Her glance turns elsewhere. The young man walks slowly on and circles back to the wharf, where he gives his two remaining rolls to a woman and child who came down with him on the boat. On his first day in Philadelphia he does not forget to do good.

A far-seeing friend might have told the young woman in the doorway to save her sniff. In her present pride she happily doesn't know that she is to meet the awkward youth, that she is to like him, that he is to court her mildly but be so indifferent that he is to go away and forget her, that she is to marry a worthless fellow who will desert her, and that at last she is to be glad to accept the lad with the rolls, poor though he still is, at his own time and on his own terms. She is Deborah Read, afterwards Franklin's " Dear Child " for over forty years.

III

The one roll which Benjamin has eaten refreshes him. He cannot keep still. He is curious about the town. He again walks around, but tiring, having rowed all night, he drops into the historic Quaker meeting house at Second and

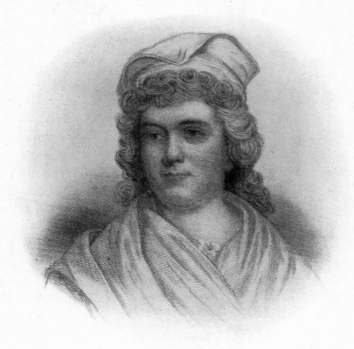

SARAH ("SALLY") FRANKLIN, DAUGHTER OF
BENJAMIN FRANKLIN

AS MRS. RICHARD BACHE SHE BECAME THE MOTHER OF A
NUMEROUS FAMILY. SHE WAS HER FATHER'S CONSTANT AND
DEVOTED ATTENDANT AS LONG AS HE LIVED.

Market Streets. Here clean-dressed, kind-faced people sit silently waiting for the Spirit to move. Benjamin cannot wait. He sleeps throughout the service — also silently, let us hope.

Still sleepy, he goes out in search of a lodging. A civil young Quaker leads him to an inn called The Crooked Billet. Here he has his first cooked meal in Philadelphia, which is marred to some extent by the sly questions of persons who, as at the tavern in New Jersey, suspect him of being a runaway. Which he is, but not the kind they have in mind.

After dinner, he lies down in his clothes and sleeps until evening, goes sleepily to supper — the evening meal was called that throughout the American colonies — and then goes to bed again and sleeps until morning.

IV

He arises betimes and goes out to look for what is so necessary to a youth who has fled from home comforts — a job. He finds Andrew Bradford's printshop, and is surprised to encounter just inside the door old man William Bradford, who has just arrived from New York on horseback. William introduces him to son Andrew. The latter has no work for the runaway, but takes him to breakfast. Here Andrew sees that this rough-looking youth from Boston is nobody's fool. He tells Benjamin to try Samuel Keimer, who has just set up a rival printery. Father Bradford sees a chance to kill two birds. He takes Ben to Keimer's place, and there they find the proprietor swearing over his single pair of type cases. He is setting up a series of verses, composed as he goes along, in memory of Aquila Rose, deceased postmaster and assembly clerk, and the poem, expanding to a great length, has used up most of the type.

Old Bradford, calling Keimer " Neighbor," introduces Ben, and then artfully draws from Keimer, whose head is almost solid ivory, the details as to his plans and prospects. Ben listens. So this is how men hornswoggle each other out in the great world! Keimer at last turns to Ben, tests his ability as a compositor, decides he will do, and says he will soon give him a job, though he has nothing just now. Ben goes back to Andrew, who gives him temporary work and takes him in as a lodger.

In a few days Keimer sends for him. Keimer has finished the Rose elegy —

" Our Rose is withered, and our Eagle's fled,
    In that our dear Aquila Rose is dead "

— and now asks Benjamin to run this off, also a pamphlet, on his wheezy and spavined press. Ben succeeds in doing so, thus making good in his first independent job. Boston can now go hang itself. He's got a job and is drawing wages. The more he examines his present prospects, the better he likes them. There are only two printers in the town, neither of them competent. Bradford doesn't know the business and is illiterate. Keimer can't run his own press. There is a future for an alert, pushful young printer in Philadelphia. He definitely decides to remain here. It is a momentous decision — far more momentous than he knows, for upon it hang the destinies not only of an obscure printer but of an embryo nation.

v

One day Keimer comes up and tells Ben he doesn't like the idea of his lodging with Bradford while working for him. He has found a room for Ben at the home of a friend, a merchant. He bids Ben be ready to go there that evening and be introduced.

Ben's chest has now arrived from Boston, and he dresses for the occasion in his best Sunday clothes. He is presented to the merchant, a Mr. Read, who receives him kindly. But before accepting him as a lodger, Mr. Read wishes him to meet his daughter. He steps to the door.

" Debby! " he calls.

" Yes, father," is the reply, and in walks a tidy young woman. She casts a startled glance at the prospective lodger, and as becomes a colonial maid, demurely lowers her eyes. She recognizes him. It is he-who-eats-rolls-in-the-street. Benjamin, enjoying the situation, says nothing; but later he says much. And Deborah Read lets it be known that she likes his present appearance better than that of a recent Sunday morning; also that his conversation is not disagreeable to her.

VI

Now ensues a period very pleasant to the exile from Boston. He meets, doubtless through Deborah Read, other young people. They are girls with whom he can flirt and boys like himself who enjoy talking of books. He works hard, spends little, and soon recovers not only his self-respect but his sense of humor. The quizzical, mirthful look, in which the girls delight, returns to his eye.

But all this time he keeps his whereabouts a secret from his people. He is still hurt and resentful. He writes not even to his mother or to his dearly loved sister, Jane. He says nothing to anyone in Boston except Collins, upon whom he imposes silence.

This is a very odd behavior on the part of Franklin, who is naturally devoted to his kindred and who rarely treasures resentment for injuries. It may be explained on the ground that he is suffering from a severe reaction against family as institution, against family censure, against family obtuseness.

It is a part of the oft-recurring revolt of the individual against the group. The only healer for such a situation is Time. The prodigal, in spirit when not in flesh, always returns. Meanwhile, blessed be he who letteth alone.

VII

Now occurs an incident which exerts a profound influence on Franklin's life and which teaches him an unforgettable lesson. Arriving at Newcastle is Robert Holmes, master of a sloop running between Boston and Delaware. He hears of Ben's presence in Philadelphia and writes to him, telling of the anxiety of his family in Boston and saying that all will be forgiven and everything done for him, if only he will return. Victory! The family runs up the white flag.

But Benjamin fails to be soothed. He replies to Holmes. He prepares the letter with great care. He writes in measured terms, combining the best Addisonian and Franklinesque styles. He points out that he left Boston not on impulse, but for carefully cogitated reasons, and that his decision is irrevocable. Holmes receives this statesmanlike document when in the company of Sir William Keith, governor of Pennsylvania. He shows the letter to Keith.

Keith is a genial, impulsive man who likes to bestow favors on his social inferiors with an air of great generosity and importance. He reads Benjamin's letter with attention.

"Well, well! And how old is this brother-in-law, pray?"

"Seventeen."

"Indeed? Evidently a remarkable young man. We shall have to look out for him, Holmes. The printers in Philadelphia are a wretched lot. Your brother-in-law has a magnificent opportunity. He should set up in business for himself. We will send him the public printing. We will advance his interests in every way possible."

A few days later Ben is working near a window with his employer. They see the governor, finely dressed, accompanied by a military officer, pick their way across the street and enter the building. The fatuous Keimer, thinking the visit is to him and having sudden visions of profit and honor, runs down to meet them, but to his astonishment, they push their way past him and approach his hobo hireling. There are stately bows on both sides.

" Have I the honor of addressing Mr. Franklin of Boston? "

Keimer stares at this " like a pig poison'd."

" Yes, your Excellency."

The governor then introduces his companion, Colonel French of Newcastle, and opens the conversation in his best manner. Darting a look of dislike at the hovering Keimer, the governor invites Benjamin to come out with him. Ben accompanies them to a tavern at Third and Market Streets. There over a bottle of Madeira, Keith renews his compliments and finally proposes that Franklin open his own printery and take advantage of the business which he and Colonel French will send him. Keith suggests that Ben's father will help him. Ben doubts it. The governor then offers to give Ben a letter to his father which will clinch the matter. Franklin is to go to Boston at once and present the letter. So it is arranged. The prodigal is about to return, but with more than swine-husks in his pockets.

Chapter VI

The Return From Exile

I

SEVEN months after leaving Boston, Benjamin, in April, 1724, makes his triumphant return to the bosom of his family. And what a difference! Where there were head-shakings and maledictions before, there are now smiles and respectful greetings. The exile returns in a genteel new suit. He wears, perhaps just a trifle ostentatiously, a watch, the mark of a gentleman. His pockets are heavy with nearly five pounds in silver, a raree show in Massachusetts, where they are still struggling with depreciated paper. Friends and former fellow journeymen gather around and say, " Prithee now, don't he look well? "

But amid the general acclaim there is one who is silent. True to form, it is the prodigal's brother. James has remained at home and worked, but has not prospered since Benjamin went away, and his printing enterprise is already on the rocks. One day Benjamin calls at the shop to see him, and possibly also to stage one of the little dramas for which he has a weakness. James receives him coolly, stares, and turns to his work. Benjamin hobnobs with the printers, shows them his watch, carelessly takes out a handful of silver, and gives them a piece-of-eight with which to have a drink all round. For James this is the final blow. He goes home and tells his mother that Benjamin has insulted him before his employees, and that he will never forget or forgive — never!

II

Benjamin's vindication is so complete that he feels good towards all the world. With great magnanimity he even goes to call on the Reverend Cotton Mather — him who only a few months before had been calling the *Courant* fierce names. The divine and the skeptic sit down and converse as if they were old comrades. On the way out an incident occurs which Franklin did not forget for sixty years. He wrote to Cotton's son, Samuel, about it from Passy, France, in 1784. On going through a low passage with a projecting beam, Doctor Mather called out " Stoop! Stoop! "

" Stoop occasionally as you go through the world, my boy, and you will miss many hard bumps."

For this saying and for the advice to do good, Franklin forgives Doctor Mather other shortcomings.

III

Benjamin has saved his chief Philadelphia trophy for a fitting moment. He now hands to his father the letter from Governor Keith. He enjoys his father's evident surprise. But Josiah Franklin is the last man to yield to impulse or pride. He puts the governor's letter in his pocket and says nothing. Privately he questions Robert Holmes, who has meantime returned home, about Keith, draws certain conclusions, and then informs Benjamin that at 18 years he is too young to launch into an independent business; that he is free to return to Philadelphia; but that if on reaching the age of 21, he is short of sufficient capital to buy his own plant, he, his father, will make up the difference. Somewhat disappointed at having his dreams thus dashed but still large with self-confidence, Benjamin again takes a sloop for New York. He carries with him many of the books he has accumulated in Boston.

Meantime Benjamin's favorite chum in Boston, the clever Collins, warmed by Franklin's account of the stir and bustle of lively Philadelphia, has quit his job in the post office and gone to New York to wait for Benjamin.

Benjamin's ship calls at Newport. Here two curious incidents occur, one of which leads to the commission of one of those " errata " which plague the perpetrator for years afterward. The other incident does not end so, but it makes Benjamin dangerously familiar with Erratum's face.

At Newport Benjamin has an affectionate meeting with his brother John. A friend of the latter's, one Vernon, asks Benjamin to collect the sum of thirty-five pounds owed to him in Pennsylvania, gives him an order, and requests him to keep the money until sent for.

Part of the cargo which the ship takes on board consists of two young women. They and Benjamin, by the merest accident, fall into conversation. They too are bound for New York. Daily he finds them on deck, where he stops for a chat and a joke or two. The trio and their merriment fall under the observation of another woman passenger — " a grave, sensible, matron-like Quaker." To the pure all things are impure. Benjamin has shown the matron a courtesy, and she feels free to draw him to one side:

" Young man, I am concern'd for thee, as thou hast no friend with thee, and seems not to know much of the world, or of the snares youth is exposed to; depend upon it, these are very bad women; I can see it in all their actions; and if thee art not upon thy guard, they will draw thee into some danger; they are strangers to thee, and I advise thee, in a friendly concern for thy welfare, to have no acquaintance with them."

Franklin thanks her and promises to take her advice.

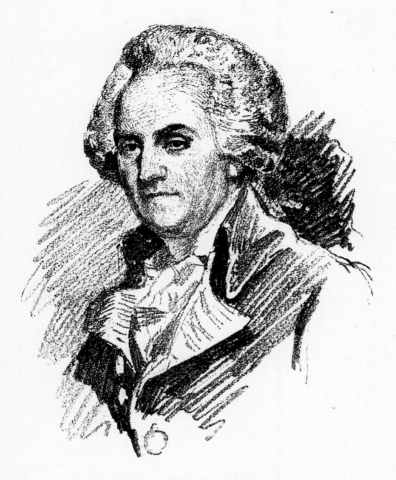

WILLIAM FRANKLIN, FIRST BORN SON OF
BENJAMIN FRANKLIN

HE BECAME THE ROYAL GOVERNOR OF NEW JERSEY. THIS REPRO-
DUCTION IS FROM A CRAYON DRAWING BY ALBERT ROSENTHAL OF A
PAINTED PORTRAIT WHICH ORIGINALLY HUNG IN THE PHILADELPHIA
LIBRARY.

He does not deny that he is ignorant of the world; he says nothing of having written an essay betraying much knowledge of the habits of the nymphs on Boston Common at night.

When the ship reaches New York, the two lady friends give him their address and invite him to come to see them. Benjamin refrains. Virtue is rewarded. The next day the two girls are arrested on a charge of stealing a silver spoon and other things from the captain's "cabbin," are convicted and punished — doubtless severely. The theft of property in these days is regarded as all but equivalent to murder.

Benjamin draws a breath of relief. He compares his escape to the close scrape, during the voyage, of the ship over a sunken rock. For comparison of similes, see the letter of Madame Brillon to Benjamin Franklin, statesman, quoted in our first chapter.

"Franklin," says the worthy James Parton, one of the earliest and most devoted of Franklin biographers, "with all his great understanding and good heart, was not able long to preserve that unconceivably precious treasure of man and woman, as precious to man as to woman, sexual integrity. But we are permitted to infer that at eighteen he was still virtuous."

IV

However, as a result of the voyage, Benjamin makes one distinguished friend. The Governor of New York, and of New Jersey as well, is William Burnet, a genial book-lover who is something of a character. His method of examining an applicant for a clergyman's license, John Bigelow informs us, is to give him a text, hand him a Bible, and then lock him in a room. If in a stated time the applicant does not produce a sermon to the governor's taste, he receives no license.

Burnet hears from the captain of the sloop about Benjamin's many books. He sends for Benjamin, shows him his library, converses with him at length about books and authors, and treats him with the utmost courtesy. "This was the second governor," writes Franklin with pride, "who had done me the honor to take notice of me; which, to a poor boy like me, was very pleasing."

Yet a little while, Benjamin, and you shall stand not only before governors but before kings. And they will be proud to know you. They will enjoy your poise and independence, your sententious wit, and the flavorous observations which already season a conversational ability well beyond your eighteen years.

v

In New York Benjamin finds Collins — the clever, brilliant Collins, who has abilities in mathematics which Benjamin, who has flunked his early arithmetic, respects. The lure of New York has been too much for Collins. Drink and gambling have got his money. He is too drunk even to accompany Ben to the house of Governor Burnet. Ben has to pay Collins's board bill and his fare to Philadelphia. On the way they collect the money due Vernon, and Franklin is compelled to dip into this, for Collins finds no work at Philadelphia and lodges there at Ben's expense. The Vernon money becomes a nightmare to Ben, for fear that the owner will suddenly demand it.

One day an incident disposes of Collins forever, much to Benjamin's relief. They and a party of friends are out rowing on the Delaware. On the way home, they take a turn about at the oars. Collins has been drinking and turns ugly. He refuses to take his turn. Ben insists. An argument follows. Collins rises and strikes at him. Ben claps him under the crotch and pitches him into the river. He then keeps the boat out of Collins's reach until the latter is thoroughly tired. When Collins is lifted back into the boat, he is sullen and refuses to speak. Soon afterward he goes to the Barbadoes as a tutor. Ben never sees him again.

VI

Benjamin, on his return, shows his father's reply to Sir William Keith. The governor is impatient.

"Then I will set you up myself," he says. "Give me an inventory of the things you need and I will send to England for them. I am resolved to have a good printer here."

Benjamin is elated. He is to be his own boss at eighteen! But he cannily says nothing about it to his friends. He is *too* canny. A friend who could tell him about Sir William's numerous unkept promises would have saved him much trouble.

Franklin, full of faith, makes out the inventory. It comes to about one hundred pounds. Sir William approves, and then has another brilliant idea. He proposes that Ben go to England and himself select the equipment. Ben's heart leaps, but he merely says that he thinks "this might be advantageous."

London! Home of Addison and Steele, and *The Spectator*. Residence of philosophers and wits and writers. Capital full of clubs and coffee houses. No, he does not want to go to London. He is perishing to do so.

"Then get yourself ready to go with the Annis," says the Governor.

But the Annis does not sail for several months yet, and Franklin, saying nothing about his impending venture, continues to work for Keimer. Keimer is a man of many erratic notions and loves to argue. He and Franklin have constant disputations, in which the younger man resorts to his trusty Socratic method. Keimer is trapped so often, and is led into so many contradictions, that he grows cautious and finally adopts the policy of asking before answering the most ordinary question:

"*What do you infer from that?*"

Keimer at length comes to have so high an opinion of Ben's debating abilities that one day he proposes they found a new sect. He perhaps purposes thus to capitalize his patriarchal whiskers, which are kept at full length because the Mosaic law has ordered: "Thou shalt not mar the corners of thy beard." Keimer is to indoctrinate the disciples and Franklin is to confound all opponents with his cunning Socratisms.

Benjamin agrees to accept Keimer's main tenets, provided his employer adopts his own doctrine of a meatless diet. Keimer is all for spiritual things, but not so much as that. He doubts if his constitution — he is a huge eater — will bear it. But Ben insists, and Keimer at last agrees.

So for three months they live on dishes in which there is neither fish, flesh nor fowl. Benjamin makes out a list of forty vegetable meals, which are prepared and brought to them by a woman of the neighborhood. The cost is only eighteen pence a week each. Both the economy and the food suit Ben, but Keimer groans in appetite. One day, being sorely tempted, he orders a roast pig. Franklin and two women friends are invited to dine with him. But before they arrive, Keimer sits down and devours the whole animal.

VII

There are other diversions for Benjamin. Since he is living in the same house, Deborah Read finds opportunities to put herself much in his path. She has quite revised her opinion of the young man with the rolls. Since he has established himself in Philadelphia and won the friendship of influential men, he has lost some of his awkwardness.

Though often fumbling and hesitating he talks with an air of authority that wins the attention of his elders, while the younger folk are delighted with his good humor and sense of fun. Deborah decides he would make a good husband. Benjamin has a "great respect and affection" for her, and finally there is talk of marriage. He tells her his great secret — his impending journey to London. Deborah agrees that it would be nice to write to him, while he is gone, as his wife.

Mrs. Read doesn't think so. Young Franklin is promising, but "a bird in the hand," etc. She counsels her daughter to wait until he is actually set up in business after his return from foreign parts. Besides, they are each only eighteen years old. The young people submit. Deborah wonders why Ben accepts the decision with so little protest.

VIII

Benjamin has meantime found a friend to replace the lost Collins. James Ralph is his name. Ben is first attracted to him because Ralph likes and writes poetry. Ben also finds Ralph to be a brilliant and eloquent talker, but above all he admires his new chum's assured and genteel manners. Franklin, the artisan, is ever fascinated with gentility.

Ralph brings along two other friends, Charles Osborne and Joseph Watson. The four of them form a group which on Sundays strolls into the woods along the Schuylkill. They read aloud from favorite books and tell each other their ambitions.

Ralph announces that one day he is going to quit clerking

for merchants and such cattle, and abandon himself entirely to poetry.

" You can't live on poetry," Osborne remarks.

" I can," says Ralph. " Moreover, I intend to make money out of it. I don't fancy this business of starving in a garret."

Jeers arise, and Osborne, who loves to tell people exactly what he thinks of them, informs Ralph that personally he considers him one of the worst poets that ever lived, and advises him to stick to his clerking job. They all turn to Ben inquiringly.

" I approve the amusing one's self with poetry now and then, so far as to improve one's language," says Franklin weightily, " but no farther."

Further arguments arise. To allay them, Ben proposes that at the next meeting each shall bring a composition which all are to criticize. It is agreed that the piece shall be a version of Psalm XVIII.

This is one of David's songs of deliverance from his enemies, especially Saul. Its best known verse is the second: " The Lord is my rock, and my fortress, and my deliverer; my God, my strength, in whom I will trust; my buckler and the horn of my salvation, and my high tower."

Ralph comes to Ben one day and announces that his piece is ready. Franklin's is not. The ingenious Ralph then proposes a trick to which Benjamin, with his love for hoaxes, delightedly agrees. Ralph explains that Osborne's habit of fault-finding will never allow him to approve his composition, and so it is arranged that Ben is to offer Ralph's piece as his own.

The meeting takes place. Watson's piece is the first disposed of. Osborne's proves to be better. But when Ben submits his performance, Watson and Osborne admit they are beaten. When Ralph confesses that, for lack of time, he has done nothing, the contest is unhesitatingly awarded to Benjamin. The only critic is Ralph, who suggests some amendments. But his voice is drowned in the applause of the other two.

Osborne and Ralph walk home together from the meeting. The former, who suspects nothing, tells Ralph in confidence of his surprise at Benjamin's extraordinary performance.

"Who would have imagined," says he, "that Franklin had been capable of such a performance; such painting, such force, such fire! He has even improved the original. In his common conversation he seems to have no choice of words; he hesitates and blunders; and yet, good God! how he writes!"

At the next meeting Ralph reveals to Osborne the trick played on him. Osborne is laughed at and doubtless cured of his hypercritical temper. But one never knows how a practical joke will end. The effect on Ralph is to raise his conceit of himself to the skies, while on Franklin there is to fall a disconcerting penalty.

Watson died a few years later in Franklin's arms, lamented as the best of their set. Osborne went to the West Indies and became rich and famous, but died young. Before his departure it was agreed between him and Franklin that the one who died first was to visit the other and inform him as to conditions in the other world. But Osborne's voice was never heard again from the West Indies, from the heavens, or any other land.

IX

The time for the sailing of the Annis to England now approaches. Governor Keith often invites Ben to his house and discusses with him the outfit that is to be bought in

London. The governor announces that he will give Franklin letters of recommendation to his numerous friends on the other side, also a letter of credit. For these Ben calls several times, but they are not ready.

At last, sailing day comes. Ben calls on the governor to take leave and to receive the letters. A secretary regretfully informs Franklin that His Excellency is busy — "in conference," no doubt, but will see him at Newcastle before the ship sails.

Ben hurriedly says good-by to friends, has a final hour with Debby Read and exchanges with her some promises. Then, with fifteen pistoles and a few curios in his pocket, he boards the ship. Here he gets a decided surprise. On the deck he finds Ralph, all dressed up for a trip. Ralph informs him that he is going to London too — to write poetry. It is not until later that Ralph discloses the fact that he is deserting his wife.

The ship stops at Newcastle. There Ben makes a final call at Governor Keith's house. Again the governor is "in conference." But the exceedingly civil secretary assures him the necessary letters will be sent on board before the ship sails. Franklin, puzzled but believing, returns to the ship. Anchor is weighed. The ship heads for the Capes. So begins the first voyage to London.

x

Ben and Ralph have to be content with the steerage. The first class cabin is occupied by more prosperous passengers. Among them is Mr. Denham, a Quaker merchant. There is also Andrew Hamilton, a famous Philadelphia lawyer, and his son. Ben also discovers on board the presence of Colonel French, who recognizes him and invites him and Ralph into the more comfortable great cabin.

Numb. XL.

THE
Pennsylvania GAZETTE.

Containing the freſheſt Advices Foreign and Domeſtick.

From Thurſday, September 25. to Thurſday, October 2. 1729.

THE Pennſylvania Gazette being now to be carry'd on by other Hands, the Reader may expect ſome Account of the Method we deſign to proceed in.

Upon a View of Chambers's great Dictionaries, from whence were taken the Materials of the Univerſal Inſtructor in all Arts and Sciences, which uſually made the Firſt Part of this Paper, we find that beſides their containing many Things abſtruſe or inſignificant to us, it will probably be fifty Years before the Whole can be gone thro' in this Manner of Publication. There are likewiſe in thoſe Books continual References from Things under one Letter of the Alphabet to thoſe under another, which relate to the ſame Subject, and are neceſſary to explain and compleat it ; theſe taken in their Turn may perhaps be Ten Years diſtant ; and ſince it is likely that they who deſire to acquaint themſelves with any particular Art or Science, would gladly have the whole before them in a much leſs Time, we believe our Readers will not think ſuch a Method of communicating Knowledge to be a proper One.

However, tho' we do not intend to continue the Publication of thoſe Dictionaries in a regular Alphabetical Method, as has hitherto been done; yet as ſeveral Things exhibited from them in the Courſe of theſe Papers, have been entertaining to ſuch of the Curious, who never had and cannot have the Advantage of good Libraries ; and as there are many Things ſtill behind, which being in this Manner made generally known, may perhaps become of conſiderable Uſe, by giving ſuch Hints to the excellent natural Genius's of our Country, as may contribute either to the Improvement of our preſent Manufactures, or towards the Invention of new Ones ; we propoſe from Time to Time to communicate ſuch particular Parts as appear to be of the moſt general Conſequence.

As to the Religious Courtſhip, Part of which has been retal'd to the Publick in theſe Papers, the Reader may be inform'd, that the whole Book will probably in a little Time be printed and bound up by it ſelf ; and thoſe who approve of it, will doubtleſs be better pleas'd to have it entire, than in this broken interrupted Manner.

There are many who have long deſired to ſee a good News-Paper in Pennſylvania ; and we hope thoſe Gentlemen who are able, will contribute towards the making This ſuch. We ask Aſſiſtance, becauſe we are fully ſenſible, that to publiſh a good News-Paper is not ſo eaſy an Undertaking as many People imagine it to be. The Author of a Gazette (in the Opinion of the Learned) ought to be qualified with an extenſive Acquaintance with Languages, a great Eaſineſs and Command of Writing and Relating Things cleanly and intelligibly, and in few Words ; he ſhould be able to ſpeak of War both by Land and Sea ; be well acquainted with Geography, with the Hiſtory of the Time, with the ſeveral Intereſts of Princes, and States, the Secrets of Courts, and the Manners and Cuſtoms of all Nations. Men thus accompliſh'd are very rare in this remote Part of the World ; and it would be well if the Writer of theſe Papers could make up among his Friends what is wanting in himſelf.

Upon the Whole, we may aſſure the Publick, that as far as the Encouragement we meet with will enable us, no Care and Pains ſhall be omitted, that may make the Pennſylvania Gazette as agreeable and uſeful an Entertainment as the Nature of the Thing will allow.

The Following is the laſt Meſſage ſent by his Excellency Governour Burnet, to the Houſe of Repreſentatives in Boſton.

Gentlemen of the Houſe of Repreſentatives,

IT is not with ſo vain a Hope as to convince you, that I take the Trouble to anſwer your Meſſages, but, if poſſible, to open the Eyes of the deluded People whom you repreſent, and whom you are at ſo much Pains to keep in Ignorance of the true State of their Affairs. I need not go further, for an undeniable Proof of this Endeavour to blind them, than your ordering the Letter of Meſſieurs Wilks and Belcher of the 7th of June laſt to your Speaker to be publiſhed. This Letter à ſaid (in Page 1 of your Votes) to incloſe a Copy of the Report of the Lords of the Committee of His Majeſty's Privy Council, with his Majeſty's Approbation and Order thereon in Council. Yet theſe Gentlemen had at the ſame time the unparallell'd Preſumption to write to the Speaker in this Manner ; You'll obſerve by the Concluſion, what is propoſed to be the Conſequence of your not complying with His Majeſty's Inſtruction (the whole Matter to by laid

Hamilton and son being suddenly recalled to Philadelphia, they quit the ship and leave their berths to the two lads.

The voyage is rough, but the discomfort from rolling seas is smoothed by the oil of conversation with a genial company. The two youths dine agreeably on the stores which Hamilton has left behind. The voyage lasts from November 2, 1724, to December 24, but the fifty-two days are never tedious. Ben, thinking of Ralph and Governor Keith, sometimes wonders at the odd conduct of human beings, but in loyalty dismisses the thought. Eight bells and all's well.

CHAPTER VII

London and "The Dangerous Time of Youth"

I

FRANKLIN, with the penniless Ralph in tow, arrives in London for the first time in his nineteenth year. The month is foggy old December, but rain and soot fail to darken his rainbow anticipations.

It is only four years since he read the third volume of *The Spectator*, and it is still The Spectator's London. It is a period prolific in poetry, essays, and plays. Pope is being eagerly read. Dryden is dead, but his works grow in esteem. James Thomson comes to London in this same year of 1724, and the next year finds Voltaire there as a visitor. The coffee-houses buzz with the arguments of literary loungers. A fresh brawl between religion and science is gathering. At night the theatres are filled with men-about-town and ladies-about-their-business. The current of the Restoration is still running strong. This to the lads from colonial America is Life. They investigate it, " going," as the *Autobiography* expresses it, " to the plays and other places of amusement." In these days plays and places of resort are very "broad" in character, relying in most cases on the appeal of sex, which was then, as now, being highly exploited. Among the spicy and popular plays of the period are those by Dryden, Wycherly and Congreve. From what we know of Benjamin at this stage, he probably enjoyed them hugely.

II

These lively occupations prevent Franklin from worrying too much about the tremendous fizzle in which his Keith-supported mission has ended.

In the Channel, before landing, the ship's captain had permitted Benjamin to search the mail bag for the letters which Franklin was sure the governor had sent aboard. None bore his name, but he picked out several which, from the handwriting, he thought might be the right ones. One was to a London stationer.

On Franklin's presenting this as coming from Governor Keith the stationer declared he knew no such person. When opened, the letter proved to be from one Riddlesden, known to Ben as a knavish Philadelphia lawyer who had half ruined Deborah Read's father. The stationer refused the letter as coming from a " compleat rascal," and turned away. Franklin, sensing something queer, looked at the other letters. None was from Keith. He had been completely befooled.

In a state of panic, Benjamin went to his friend Denham. The hard-headed merchant quickly completed Franklin's disillusionment regarding the character of the governor. Denham said no one who knew Keith believed anything he promised. Denham particularly enjoyed the joke about a letter of credit. He said Keith had no credit to give.

Here was another dismal moment for Franklin. He was in a foreign land, and not only well-nigh penniless but with his treasured hopes smashed and Ralph dependent on him for every penny.

The cheerful Denham, however, talked to him encouragingly. Denham reminded him that he ought easily to find a job in London as a printer and that when he eventually returned to America it would be as the possessor of a foreign reputation.

It was characteristic of Franklin that at this stage he at once looked about for a means of carrying out his favorite principle — to do good. One of the supposed letters from Keith disclosed what seemed to be a plot against Hamilton, the lawyer. Keith and Riddlesden were evidently concerned in it. As soon as Hamilton reached London, Benjamin went to him and told him the story. The lawyer thanked Ben heartily and later proved his gratitude to him on many occasions.

III

Franklin's next step is to get a job. It is not easy for a colonial to do this in the metropolis, but Ben soon finds work at Palmer's printing house in Bartholomew Close.

The airy Ralph declines to stoop to trade. He fancies the stage and tries to get Wilkes, the comedian, to take him into his company as an actor. Next he offers to write for a publisher a weekly paper like *The Spectator*. This sounds like Franklin's suggestion, but it doesn't work. Ralph then peddles his services as a " hackney writer," but finally relapses into idle brooding. One thing Ralph tells Ben he is decided on, and that is he is not going to return to Philadelphia.

At this time a London printer who is paid as much as a guinea [1] a week is getting a high wage. It can be imagined then, how small is the sum which Franklin and Ralph must live on. They take lodgings in a street called Little Britain at three shillings and sixpence a week. Benjamin, avid to see all of that London of which he has read so much, spends all his surplus on amusements. He must take Ralph along, of course, so there is nothing put by. Month after month

---

[1] $5.25.

passes before Benjamin saves enough even for his passage home.

His neglect of Deborah Read is astonishing. He writes her only one letter and that merely hints he is not likely to return soon. This is one of the outstanding "errata" of his life which Franklin afterwards wished he could correct.

The lodgings in Little Britain have one great advantage for Ben. They are next door to the bookshop of one Wilcox, with whom he becomes friendly. Ben makes a deal with Wilcox by which he may take out, read, and return any book. This arrangement delights Ben, and we shall see how well he remembers it.

IV

It is at Palmer's printshop that Franklin, the ever inquisitive, makes one of the first of those practical investigations into the workings of matter which are later to add to his fame. For the first time he sees a wet case of type dried before the fire. He finds the heated type agreeable to work over in cold weather, but an old workman warns him against the practice, saying it will give him the "dangles" — a kind of obscure pain in the hands. Franklin consults Mr. James, a letter founder. James ridicules the notion, contending that the malady is caused by the slovenly habits of the printers in failing to wash their hands of lead particles before eating. "This," Franklin afterwards wrote to Benjamin Vaughan, "appeared to have some reason in it."

It is at Palmer's, too, that Franklin is stimulated to write his first serious philosophical essay. The cause of this is his being employed to set up the second edition of Wollaston's *Religion of Nature Delineated*.

Wollaston was a clergyman whose writings were very popular in English religious circles at that period. He married a rich wife and being thus buttressed, obtained an abundance of leisure which he devoted to religious-literary composition. The burden of his brief argument was that nature herself laid the basis on which the rules of the Church of England were founded, saying that " the foundation of religion lies in that difference between the acts of men which distinguishes them into good, evil, indifferent."

At the time Franklin was already well soaked in the deistical writings of the period. While busy composing the Reverend Doctor Wollaston's book, he found objections to the author's contentions, and so was provoked to write a rather long pamphlet which he called " A Dissertation on Liberty and Necessity, Pleasure and Pain," and dedicated it to " Mr. J. R.," this being his still admired companion, James Ralph.

Two quotations will suffice to indicate the trend of the nineteen-year-old author's arguments. (1) God being the First Mover, "We must allow that all things exist now in a Manner agreeable to His Will, and in consequence of that are all equally Good, and therefore equally esteemed by Him." (2) Since Pleasure and Pain are inseparable and balance each other, "Every individual Creature must, in any State of Life, have an equal quantity of each, so that there is not, on that account, any Occasion for a future Adjustment."

In brief, Franklin's contention is that the Creator makes no such distinction between good, evil, and indifferent actions and things as that which Wollaston argued for.

Franklin, contrary to the popular notion, was seldom an original thinker. His ideas were mostly derivative. It is no surprise, then, to find that his essay on " Pleasure and Pain " virtually parallels that of the 183d paper in *The Spectator*, in which pleasure and pain are described as yoke-fellows.

V

Franklin afterwards condemned his pamphlet as another "erratum," but it has the present effect of raising him in the esteem of Palmer, his employer, who, however, is shocked by some of its arguments. It also brings him to the attention of Doctor Lyons, author of "The Infallibility of Human Judgment." Franklin is the source of great interest and amusement to Lyons, who takes him to a club having its headquarters at The Horns, an ale house in Cheapside, and introduces him to Bernard de Mandeville, the cynical but highly companionable author of "The Fable of the Bees." Lyons also takes Benjamin to a coffee-house, where he meets Doctor Henry Pemberton, philosopher and mathematician. Lyons, thoroughly delighted with the precocious young American, next proposes to take him to Sir Isaac Newton, but the famous scientist is very old, and the meeting never takes place.

Benjamin is now in high feather. It is small wonder that he forgets the provincial little girl back home. He is attracting the attention of influential men. He is received on equal terms by the great. He is treated with respect at the coffee houses frequented by brilliant writers. This is what he has dreamed of. He sees before him a coruscating career. Then falls an unexpected blow. It comes from the man for whom he has done so much — James Ralph. It also results in another serious Franklin "erratum."

VI

Living in the same house with Ben and Ralph at one time was a young woman, a milliner, of lively appearance and conversation. Ralph became intimate with her and was soon allowing her to support him and their child while he waited for something to turn up. After a while he tired of the ménage and took himself to Berkshire where he taught school to boys at sixpence each a week.

One day Ben got a letter from him, in which Ralph's mistress was recommended to Ben's care. It closed with a request that Ben address him as " Mr. Franklin." The lofty Ralph, not content with taking a good share of Ben's money for months, had now crowned his impudence by taking Ben's name!

Ben continued to receive letters from Ralph, each containing yard-long extracts from an endless epic poem he was composing. Perhaps this was the very one ridiculed by Pope when he wrote in the " Dunciad " :

" Silence, ye wolves! While Ralph to Cynthia howls
And makes Night hideous — answer him, ye owls."

Ben tried to scotch Ralph's muse by sending him a copy of Young's Satires, hoping that its ridicule of poetasters would stop the flow of rancid verse. But Ralph continued to draw length after length from the poetical fountain and send them to Ben by every post.

The woman whom Ralph has discarded now in her turn becomes abjectly dependent on Ben. She no longer has either friends or a business. She lives by borrowing from Franklin. He always gives her what he can spare. She looks on him as a valuable friend. Franklin one day tries to become more to her. Her emphatic repulse shows him that he has erred very decidedly; he has tried to open a door that for him is definitely shut.

The young woman at once carries the story of Franklin's behavior to Ralph. That worthy announces with a hurt dignity, that Franklin has thus cancelled all obligations between them, and that Ben has by this act showed himself unworthy of future friendship.

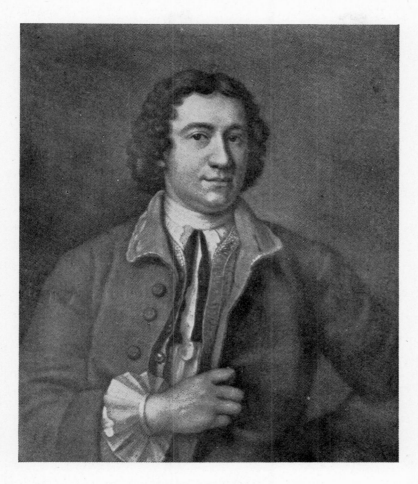

LORD DE DESPENCER

HIGH PRIEST OF THE "HELL FIRE CLUB," WITH WHOM FRANKLIN
REVISED THE ENGLISH PRAYER BOOK.

Thus does a second idol of Benjamin's fall face forward in the mud. Ralph has gone the way of Collins. In the *Autobiography* Franklin dismisses the incident as one bringing a good riddance; nevertheless it probably causes a shock, for we find him suddenly seeking a new job, changing his lodgings, and raising money by selling an asbestos purse, brought from America as a curiosity, to Sir Hans Sloane, founder of the British Museum.

VII

Benjamin next finds work as a pressman at the much larger printing house of Watts's, near Lincoln's Inn Fields, not far from the spot where now stands Bush House, the centre of American business life in London. Here Franklin pulls himself together, resumes the simple life, and is soon living serenely again, with enough incidents occurring to make existence varied and interesting.

He at once arouses the wonder and admiration of his fellow workmen by his feats of strength in carrying a large form of type up and down stairs in either hand. They carry but one in both hands. Benjamin boasts that his strength comes from his habit of drinking only water. He is instantly dubbed the "Water-American." Printers in all countries and in all ages have ever entertained a weakness for beer. Those at Watts's are a particularly thirsty lot.

"My companion at the press," writes Franklin,[2] "drank every day a pint before breakfast, a pint at breakfast with his bread and cheese, a pint between breakfast and dinner, a pint at dinner, a pint in the afternoon about six o'clock, and another when he had done his day's work. I thought it a detestable custom; but it was necessary, he suppos'd, to

[2] *Autobiography.*

—⟨ 73 ⟩—

drink *strong* beer that he might be *strong* to labor." Ben tried to convince him that the strength derived from beer lay only in its grain content, and that there was more actual strength in a pennyworth of bread with water. But Englishmen do not so readily surrender their beer; and this one went on with his " muddling liquor."

VIII

In a few weeks Ben is transferred from Watts's press room to the composing room. Here takes place another struggle of individual *vs.* group.

On Ben's entry into the new department, the men demand of him, as a newcomer, five shillings in order, no doubt, to " wet the baby's head." Ben, having paid below, refuses the tax. In this Watts backs him up. Ben is promptly excommunicated. His type is mixed up and pied, his pages are transposed, annoying accidents occur. On his complaining, the men say it is doubtless the chapel ghost at work, there being a very troublesome one in those parts. This goes on for two or three weeks, and then Ben gives in, " convinced of the folly of being on ill terms with those one is to live with continually."

Once restored to favor, Ben soon gains considerable influence among the printers, and even brings about some changes in the chapel laws.[3] He sets up a propaganda against beer for breakfast and gains patrons for his own favorite meal consisting of a porringer of hot water-gruel, nicely peppered and buttered. Its cost is the same as the price of a pint of beer — three halfpence.

He does not object to lending money to patrons of the ale house, but he charges them interest on all loans and is

[3] All the workers in the various departments of a printing house form a " chapel."

regularly present at the pay table on Saturday nights to make his collections.

His good humor and jocular abilities earn him the title of "riggite"; he is promoted to the faster and better paid work; and is soon living the cheerful life again.

IX

He now finds a more convenient lodging in Duke Street. The house is kept by a widow, who, before accepting him, "inquires his character" back in Little Britain. Satisfied, she takes him in at the same rate, 3s. 6d. a week. She is incautious enough to remark that it is worth something to have a reliable man in the house. This admission costs her something, for on Ben's talking of another and cheaper place, she lowers her rate to one shilling and sixpence per week.[4] At that price Ben remains for the rest of his stay in London. Let us hope it is with a clear conscience. Beating a lone widow down from 3/6 to 1/6 a week would seem to be poor business for a healthy young journeyman to engage in, and we might not excuse him did we not know that he is desperately saving money for his passage home.

For such a sum the widow not only lodges him but assists his education. She has been a clergyman's daughter, once knew distinguished people, and can tell anecdotes of them as far back as the gay reign of Charles II. She is glad to have Ben's company in the evening, being lame with the gout, and Ben, thirsty for such stories and being no longer given to running around o' nights, is glad to sit with her. They dine on half an anchovy each, with a strip of bread and butter, and split a half pint of ale to wash it down. But the old lady's thousand and one days among

---

[4] About 37 cents.

the great are more interesting to Ben than more substantial food. He listens eagerly, absorbing every detail and storing them away in his capacious memory.

The mistress of the house is not the only quaint character there, nor is hers the only economical supping. In the garret lives a fragile old lady, a maiden of seventy. She was once the inhabitant of a nunnery on the Continent, but being English, she was never quite at home there. And so she returned to London, choosing this garret in which to live out the rest of her nun's life. She has given all her money to charity, reserving only twelve pounds [5] a year to live on. Out of this sum she continues to give to charity, and lives on water-gruel only, never having a fire even in the bleakest weather except to boil it with. Her room contains only a mattress, a table with a crucifix and book, a stool, and a picture of Saint Veronica. Ben learns with interest that, though pale, she is never sick. This confirms him in the belief that life and health can be maintained on very little money.

A priest visits the saint every day to confess her. On being asked what she could possibly have to confess, she replied with spirit:

" Oh, it is impossible to avoid vain thoughts! "

Thus does Ben learn that no one wishes to be deemed wholly good, and that even saints take a pride in having within them at least a dash of ungodliness.

X

A temptation now comes upon Ben to abandon his steady job and seek adventures elsewhere. A fellow workman is one Wygate, an intelligent fellow who speaks French and loves books. He and Ben become friends. One day, dur-

[5] About $60.

ing a stroll, they find themselves at the Thames. Ben, the Water-American, has a swim and shows Wygate a few tricks learned in early Boston days. Wygate looks on admiringly and later tells some friends about the young American's edifying feats. They can't wait till they have taken Ben out to Chelsea, then a village well separated from the city of London, and challenged him to swim to Blackfriars. Ben, smiling a secret smile, calmly strips, plunges in, and easily covers the whole four miles, probably landing where Blackfriars Bridge now stands, a stone's throw from Ludgate Circus. Moreover, he exhibits his strength and cleverness on the way by various floating and diving tricks.

Wygate is enchanted. He immediately engages Ben to teach him how to swim and then proposes that together they tour Europe, financing themselves by giving swimming lessons. Ben, a little puffed up, almost agrees, but first mentions the matter to his friend Denham.

Denham will not hear of the notion. He tells Ben that he himself has something for him to do back in Philadelphia. Benjamin is at once all ears. He has tired of London and its loneliness. He is still a little dispirited from the Keith and Ralph incidents. He wants to be back in the simple town where he feels he belongs — Philadelphia. He rejoices when he hears that Denham purposes to make him his chief clerk in a new store there. Denham enlarges his proposals. As soon as Franklin is well versed in accounting, he is to go to the West Indies with a cargo of flour and bread and embark upon a profitable commission business.

Ben at once accepts the salary of fifty pounds a year, quits the printing house, and sets about buying and packing goods for Denham. But before he sails, once more he is sent for by one of those great men whose interest Ben is always exciting. Sir William Wyndham, bearer of a historic English name, asks him please to come and teach swimming to his two sons, who are about to travel abroad. Franklin again hesitates, but resolutely declines. He knows by now that he had rather jump upon a counter in Philadelphia than upon any throne in Europe.

He has spent a year and a half in London, made some valuable acquaintances, received several grievous shocks, widened his knowledge of the world, and recorded some more " errata." When on July 23, 1726, he turns his round face once more toward his own country, he is still only an obscure and unsuccessful young workman. If he has a moment of depression on this account, Fortune doubtless smiles at him, as we smile at the temporary disasters suffered by a hero of the stage or film. Well does Fortune know the important state in which he will return.

Philad.ª July 5. 1775

Mr Strahan,

You are a Member of Parliament, and one of that Majority which has doomed my Country to Destruction.— You have begun to burn our Towns, and murder our People.— Look upon your Hands! — They are stained with the Blood of your Relations! — You and I were long Friends: — You are now my Enemy, — and

I am,

Yours,

B Franklin

FRANKLIN'S TERSE LETTER TO HIS OLD FRIEND, WILLIAM STRAHAN, IN LONDON, BREAKING OFF RELATIONS

THE LETTER WAS NEVER ACTUALLY SENT.

CHAPTER VIII

First Studies of Men and Things

I

ON the voyage home, which lasts eighty days, Franklin sets himself a task betraying that a subtle change, long gathering, has come over him. He begins a diary. It records not only the state of his mind and feelings, but the external things of the matter-of-fact world in which he has now chosen to live.

Metaphysics has heretofore had no little fascination for him. He has at times been occupied with internal searchings and has concerned himself with the old human problem: Why am I here, and what is it all about? He no longer asks himself this question. He accepts the fact that he exists, and that he must find the means to maintain and promote that existence.

He becomes an " extrovert " — his gaze is turned from himself outward to other men and things.

II

The diary begins at Gravesend, the Thames port, which is described as " a cursed biting place." Off Portsmouth he hears of a dungeon into which the Queen's soldiers have been thrown for the most trifling offenses and partly starved. He writes down this observation:

" I own, indeed, that if a commander finds he has not those qualities in him that will make him beloved by his people, he ought, by all means, to make use of such methods as will make them fear him, since one or the other (or both) is absolutely necessary; but Alexander and Caesar, those renowned generals, received more faithful service, and performed greater actions, by means of the love their soldiers bore them, than they could possibly have done, if, instead of being beloved and respected, they had been hated and feared by those they commanded."

This is one of the earliest expressions from Franklin the humanitarian. We have seen that he is not an orthodox religionist and we shall have evidence later that he is not sure of the divinity of Jesus; but already he has chosen that better part; he means to be loved and respected rather than hated and feared.

Entry by entry that plan of life, which he says was "pretty faithfully adhered to quite thro' old age," begins to take shape. For example, here is an observation written after a game of draughts, or checkers, which he played one whole afternoon:

"Persons playing, if they would play well, ought not much to regard the *consequences* of the game, for that diverts and withdraws the attention of the mind from the game itself . . . I will venture to lay it down for an infallible rule that, if two persons *equal* in judgment, play for a considerable sum, he that loves money shall lose . . . If the player imagines himself opposed by one that is much his superior in skill, his mind is so intent on the defensive part, that an advantage passes unobserved."

Other canny reflections are provoked by the punishment of a passenger who cheated at cards. A Dutchman testified that the accused marked the cards in his presence. Ben accounted for this as follows:

"I have sometimes observed, that we are apt to fancy the person that cannot speak intelligibly to us, proportionately stupid in understanding, and, when we speak two or three words of English to a foreigner, it is louder than ordinary, as if we thought him deaf, and that he had lost the use of his ears as well as his tongue. Something like this I imagine might be the case of Mr. G——; he fancied the Dutchman could not see what he was about, because he could not understand English, and therefore boldly did it before his face."

The prisoner was sentenced to be lashed to the round top, in the view of all, and fined two bottles of brandy. On his refusing to pay, Ben and others hoisted him up, cursing and swearing, and let him hang till he was black in the face. He was then brought down, but all passengers agreed not to speak to him until he paid his fine. The victim held out for a time, but on the sixth day gave in.

Ben, the mixer, no doubt remembering his experience with Watts's printers, confided this to his journal:

"Man is a sociable being, and it is, for aught I know, one of the worst of punishments to be excluded from society. I have read abundance of fine things on the subject of solitude, and I know 'tis a common boast in the *mouths* of those that affect to be thought wise, *that they are never less alone than when alone.* I acknowledge solitude an agreeable refreshment to a busy mind; but, were these thinking people obliged to be always alone, I am apt to think they would quickly find their very being insupportable to them."

The natural philosopher as well as the moralist now begins to show himself in the twenty-year-old Benjamin. There are numerous entries in the journal dealing with marine life as observed from the ship's deck and phenomena such as eclipses. He imprisons an infant crab in a glass phial that he may study its protecting shell and draw conclusions as to its likeness to silkworms and butterflies.

III

He also records certain rules which are to govern his future conduct. He confesses that he has "never fixed a regular design in life, by which means it has been a confused variety of different scenes." He therefore begins with the following:

" 1. It is necessary for me to be extremely frugal for some time, till I have paid what I owe.

" 2. To endeavor to speak truth in every instance, to give nobody expectations that are not likely to be answered, but aim at sincerity in every word and action; the most amiable excellence in a rational being.

" 3. To apply myself industriously to whatever business I take in hand, and not to divert my mind from my business by any foolish project of growing suddenly rich; for industry and patience are the surest means of plenty."

A few days before landing he witnesses one of the first signs of the Irish invasion of America. It is the " Snow " from Dublin, with some fifty young men and women aboard who are going to enter service in New York.

He cannot see the land when the lookout first hails it. His eyes are dimmed with " two drops of joy." The date is October 11, 1726. The last entry in the diary says: " Thank God! "

Chapter IX

Franklin Begins to Find Himself

I

IN eighteen months Benjamin could not have expected to find Philadelphia much changed. Nevertheless the town had grown; immigrants were arriving steadily; the Quaker colony was expanding; new houses and shops were being built; and a burgher class of small business men was making itself felt. Among the urban population there was much talk of money, and the need for making it, saving it, and thereby becoming the head of one's own business. The respectable virtues of thrift, economy, time-saving, and industry were becoming popular, as a middle class began to arise out of elements contributed to the town by the farming population and the more enterprising artisans.

There were visible, as Franklin noted, other " sundry alterations." The facile Governor Keith had been deposed. He hung his head when Franklin passed him on the street one day, and pretended not to see the credulous youth to whom he had proposed such grandiose schemes. For this Ben did not care, but the news concerning Deborah Read was quite a blow to him. The once blooming Debby was keeping herself in seclusion. While the false and festive Ben was disporting himself in London, she had married a potter named Rogers, but had left him when she had discovered he was some one else's husband and that he was a sorry fellow, anyhow. Rogers got into debt, fled to the West Indies, and died there. Debby was therefore a widow.

Ben, however, suppressed the pang in his conscience and busied himself with mercantile pursuits. He helped Denham open his store, became his book-keeper, and perfected himself in the arts of salesmanship. Under Denham's paternal care he might in time have become the revered founder of a great American department store, had not destiny again interfered.

II

Ben was just twenty-one years old when both he and Denham were taken severely ill. Denham died, leaving a small legacy to the faithful Benjamin, but the business went into other hands.

Ben's malady was pleurisy. He sank to the point of death, and so great was his pain and weakness that he was, as he afterwards remarked, disappointed when he began to recover.

For one of Franklin's hopeful temperament this is a remarkable confession. It means that he was sick of life and had no heart to go on with it. Reading between the lines of his autobiography, it is apparent that this sickness was as much mental as physical. His misfortunes had accumulated until their weight hung heavy. Five years of hard work had brought him nowhere. He had appropriated Vernon's money to his own use. Collins and Ralph, his two dearest friends, had dealt with him treacherously. Governor Keith had played a monkeyish trick on him. He had neglected Deborah Read and caused her to plunge into a wretched marriage. His anxious months in London had been, as far as he could see, a mere waste of time. Though he had at times earned good wages, he had saved nothing. Every dream had burst into a vaporous sprinkle. Perhaps, after all, the folks back home had been right. He thought of returning to Boston and saying to Josiah, " Father, I am no more worthy to be called thy son."

He cast his mind back over his past, and resolved, as most very sick men do, to reform. He now regretted the deistical teachings which had " perverted" Collins and Ralph, and wished he could recall his London pamphlet, doubting " whether some error had not insinuated itself unperceiv'd " into his argument, " so as to infect all that follow'd, as is common in metaphysical reasonings." That he had come through " this dangerous time of youth " at all, he now thought might be due to a guardian Providence, preserving him, as he afterwards wrote, from " the hazard-ous situations I was sometimes in among strangers, remote from the eye and advice of my father, without any willful gross immorality or injustice, that might have been ex-pected from my want of religion."

Bigelow calls attention to the fact that at this point in the Franklin memoirs, the following addendum was effaced in the revision:

" Some foolish intrigues with low women excepted, which from the expense were rather more prejudicial to me than to them."

The narrative then resumes:

" I say willful, because the instances I have mentioned had something of necessity in them, from my youth, inex-perience, and the knavery of others."

It was while in this chastened frame of mind that Ben wrote one of the few of his early letters that have been pre-served. It was to his young sister Jane, then entering upon a charming young-ladyhood. It reads more like the pious admonitions of a Dutch uncle than a note from a youth who has only recently been " seeing " London. Mentioning that he has selected a gift for her, Ben writes:

" I had almost determined on a tea-table; but when I considered that the character of a good housewife was far preferable to that of being only a pretty gentlewoman, I concluded to send you a *spinning-wheel*, which I hope you will accept as a small token of my sincere love and affection. Sister, farewell, and remember that modesty, as it makes the most homely virgin amiable and charming, so the want of it infallibly renders the most perfect beauty disagreeable and odious. But when that brightest of female virtues shines among the other perfections of body and mind in the same person, it makes the woman more lovely than an angel. Excuse this freedom, and use the same with me. I am, dear Jenny, your loving brother."

Jenny was a dear, good little body. No doubt she wrote a dutiful letter of sober thanks to her big brother from abroad. And then made a face. A spinning wheel!

III

While Benjamin is thus low in his mind, an angel appears. A whiskered one. It is — of all persons — the pig-eating Keimer!

The pig-eater, carried along by the sheer current of the town's growth, has prospered despite his own foolishness. He has a new establishment with several employees and has also opened a stationery shop. He comes, full of oily smiles, and offers Ben at large wages the management of his printery, so that he can look after this shop.

Ben is not inclined to have any more to do with Keimer, but since he is penniless and fails to find a job elsewhere, he accepts. It soon becomes evident that Keimer means to have Franklin train his raw hands and then dispense with him. However, Ben puts Keimer's house in order and teaches his men what he knows. Among them is Hugh Meredith, honest son of a Welsh farmer but fond of taverns. He at once admires Ben's pluck and capacity.

Ben finds more and more work laid on his shoulders. There is no such thing as a type-founder in America, so he becomes the first. He makes a mould, contrives the matrix, and produces enough type to make up for damaged and missing letters. He also tries his hand at engraving, and even makes the ink.

IV

Meantime, Ben, the gregarious, had launched one of the most celebrated of his numerous achievements — the Junto Club.

Its purpose was to seek truth, promote good fellowship, and realize the benefits of occasional wine and song. Ben drew up the rules. It met on Friday evenings. Every member was expected to produce, in turn, " one or more queries on any point of Morals, Politics, or Natural Philosophy, to be discuss'd by the company; and once in three months produce and read an essay of his own writing on any subject he pleased." Expressions of positiveness in opinions or direct contradiction were fined. Disputation and mere desire for victory were barred.

The Junto was a success from the first and a source of immense delight to Franklin. It endured for almost forty years and was the mother of a numerous progeny of similar associations. It educated its members, made them tolerant, and vastly improved their conversation. In brief, it was a molder of civilized men.

Its first eleven members were all, like Franklin, workingmen, except Robert Grace, " a young gentleman of some fortune, generous, lively, and witty " — a type for which Franklin had a worshipful admiration; William Coleman, then a merchant's clerk, later a judge, and for two-score years Franklin's close friend; and Thomas Godfrey, of whom it was soon evident that he had got into the wrong pew. Godfrey was an able mathematician and an unendurable precisian, " forever denying or distinguishing upon trifles." His membership was brief. There was also Joseph Breintnal, a scrivener who loved poetry and was " very ingenious in little nicknackeries." We shall hear more of Godfrey and Breintnal.

There has been some disagreement among students of Frankliniana as to whence Benjamin derived the plan of the Junto. Some think he got it from Cotton Mather's scheme for a series of benefit societies in Boston. But it is more likely that he drew on other sources. It has already been revealed that Ben was a reader of John Locke, whose *Essay on the Human Understanding* grew out of discussions among friends of the philosopher who met informally; that Ben has admired the coffee-house clubs of London, and above all, that his model, Sir Roger de Coverley, was the leading spirit of that club whose doings are so often described in *The Spectator*.

Some of the queries submitted at meetings of the Junto, with " a pause between each while one might fill and drink a glass of wine," were:

" How may smoky chimneys best be cured? "

" Why are tumultuous, uneasy sensations united with our desires? "

" Can any one particular form of government suit all mankind? "

" Whether it ought to be the aim of philosophy to eradicate the passions? "

" Have you lately observed any encroachment on the just liberties of the people? "

" What new story have you lately heard agreeable for telling in conversation? "

DRAFT OF A LETTER FROM FRANKLIN TO GENERAL
GEORGE WASHINGTON

IN WHICH HE SENDS WORD THAT THE DECLARATION OF INDEPENDENCE
IS BEING PREPARED.

From the Manuscript Division of the New York Public Library.

" Have you lately heard of any citizens thriving well, and by what means? "

" Why does the flame of a candle tend upward in a spire? "

" Hath any deserving stranger arrived in town since last meeting, that you have heard of?   And what have you heard or observed of his character or merits?   And whether, think you, it lies in the power of the Junto to oblige him, or encourage him as he deserves? "

" Do you think of anything at present, in which the Junto may be serviceable to *mankind*, to their country, or to themselves? "

These queries are worth a second reading, disclosing as they do the fine American hand of Franklin himself and evidencing the very problems with which Benjamin is most concerned.

An extra query: Did Franklin form the Junto with the unconscious purpose of perhaps finding an answer to the questions which most frequently troubled *him?*

v

The end of six months found Keimer growing peevish with Benjamin.   He began to complain about Ben's high wages and hinted that he thought Ben ought to be content with less.   He found fault with his work and became daily more overbearing in his attitude.   Ben saw through this; he realized that the thoroughness with which he was teaching Keimer's men was making him more and more dispensable.

One day there was a noise near the Philadelphia courthouse.   Ben put his head out of the window and met the glowering eye of Keimer, who was in the street below. Keimer bawled out:

" Mind your own business, and you'll find less to look at outside."

He then came raging upstairs and continued his abuse. Ben, who at times had a temper of his own, replied belligerently. The row ended in Ben's being discharged. Keimer gave him three months' notice but wished aloud that he had not to give him so long a warning. Ben promptly carried out that which is the darling wish at one time or another of every man who is working for an inflated employer: he put on his hat and walked out.

As he did so he caught the sympathetic eye of Hugh Meredith. He asked Meredith to collect his things and bring them to his lodgings.

VI

Once more Ben is out of a job and "broke." Though he has had comparatively high wages for six months, he has saved barely enough to live on for a few days. He has paid none of Vernon's money back. He tries in a disheartened way to find another place, but there is no opening. His four years of absence from home have registered nothing but failure after failure. He again thinks of returning to Boston.

In the evening comes Meredith, who scouts the idea. Keimer, he says, is almost at the end of his rope, in debt, and being pressed by creditors. If Ben will stick, there will be room for another printer in Philadelphia soon. Ben pleads lack of capital.

Meredith then proposes a scheme he has had in mind. He tells Ben that his father knows about him, admires him, and is willing to put up the money for a partnership between his son and Franklin.

"I'm no good as a printer," says Meredith, "but you furnish the skill and I the stock, and we'll share equally."

Ben is so cheered by this hopeful prospect, coming at

such a moment, that he at once agrees. Meredith takes him
to his father, and the deal is arranged. The old man tells
Ben that he welcomes the opportunity to help a young fellow who has done so much to break his son of his habit of
drinking. Gaily they all make out a list of things needed,
which are to be ordered from London. By the time they
arrive, Meredith's apprenticeship to Keimer will have ex-
pired and the new printery can then open. Meantime Benjamin is to find work until the time comes to make the
announcement.

But Ben is compelled to remain idle for several days.
Again appears the knavish Keimer. He has heard that New
Jersey is about to give out a big order for printed paper
money, and since Ben is the only man in town who can
make engravings and found types, Keimer is a-tremble lest
Bradford engage him for the job. Keimer thinks it too bad
that old friends should part because of a trifling misunderstanding, lauds Ben's ability, and offers to kiss and make
up. Meredith urges Ben to accept, since it will give them
time to make their preparations.

So once more Ben returns to Keimer, who is now all respect and affection. They go to Burlington and get the job.
Ben makes a copper-plate press for it, the first in America,
and cuts the ornaments and checks. The job so pleases the
Jerseymen that they pay Keimer enough to keep him going
for some time, and the pig-eater's affection for his discharged employee returns in doubled strength.

Though Keimer gets all the money, Ben gets something
of more lasting value. He meets many public men, who
foresee a future for the bright young man. They invite
him to their houses and introduce him around, but pay little
attention to Keimer.

" My mind," says Franklin modestly, " having been
much more improv'd by reading than Keimer's, I suppose

it was for that reason my conversation seem'd to be more valu'd."

In the spring, Franklin being twenty-two years old, the press and types arrive from London. Ben and Hugh part on friendly terms with Keimer, but say nothing about the new firm of Franklin and Meredith. It is a glad spring for Benjamin. The clouds are being carried off on the shoulders of a fairer wind and he begins to see the blue.

CHAPTER X

A Young Man States His Creed of Life

I

IN 1728 Franklin is still dissatisfied with the religions with which he is acquainted, "every . . . sect supposing itself in possession of all truth," he wrote, "and that those who differ are so far in the wrong; like a man traveling in foggy weather; those at some distance before him on the road he sees wrapped up in the fog, as well as those behind him, and also the people in the fields on each side; but near him all appear clear; though in truth he is as much in the fog as any of them."

It was about this time, he says, that he "conceiv'd the bold and arduous project of arriving at moral perfection." He is, as we have seen, at work on a plan or design which will guide him through life. The impulse to complete it is probably hastened by his reflections following his recovery from the illness which brought him close to death. He feels the need of a creed which will have more positive and less negative elements than those contained in his "Dissertation" pamphlet written in London. He also wished to avoid "those articles which," as he afterward expressed it, "without any tendency to inspire, promote, or confirm morality, serv'd principally to divide us, and make us unfriendly toward one another."

He therefore begins to draw up a creed of his own and then a liturgy, because he finds innate in man the need of something to worship. Franklin carefully writes it all out in a little pocket-size book entitled "Articles of Belief and

Acts of Religion." He declares that "There is one Supreme most perfect Being, Author and Father of the gods themselves." So far as history records this is the first time that an American has stated his belief in the existence of gods subordinate to the one Deity. He proceeds: "I conceive, then, that the Infinite has created many beings or gods, vastly superior to man, who can better conceive his perfections than we, and return him a more rational and glorious praise; as, among men, the praise of the ignorant or of children is not regarded by the ingenious painter or architect, who is rather honored and pleased with the approbation of wise men and artists. It may be that these created gods are immortal; or it may be that after many ages, they are changed, and others supply their places."

This belief in a God surrounded or attended by subordinate gods is Eastern rather than Western, and to some extent parallels the teachings found in the Indian Vedantas and the Bhagavad Gita. There is no evidence, however, that at this stage young Benjamin has ever dipped into the religious lore of the Orient.

Ben goes on to state that man is happy only so far as he is virtuous, that God delights in virtue, and is pleased with human praise. "Let me not fail, then, to praise my God continually, for it is his due." It is to be noted that Franklin speaks here not simply of God but of "my God."

His liturgy opens with this Prelude: "Being mindful that before I address the Deity, my soul ought to be calm and serene, free from passion and perturbation, or otherwise elevated with rational joy and pleasure, I ought to use a countenance that expresses a filial respect, mixed with a kind of smiling, that signifies inward joy, and satisfaction, and admiration."

Worship that could be conducted with "a kind of smiling" was certainly something new in Franklin's time.

Then follows an Invocation containing these passages:

"O Creator, O Father! I believe that thou art good, and that thou art *pleased with the pleasure* of thy children. — Praised be thy name forever! . . .

"By thy wisdom hast thou formed all things; thou hast created man, bestowing life and reason, and placed him in dignity superior to thy other earthly creatures. — Praised be thy name forever! . . .

"Thou abhorrest in thy creatures treachery and deceit, malice, revenge, intemperance, and every other hurtful vice; but thou art a lover of justice and sincerity, of friendship and benevolence, and every virtue; thou art my friend, my father, and my benefactor. — Praised be thy name, O God, forever. Amen."

The liturgy next provides for readings from Ray's Wisdom of God in the Creation, or Blackmore on the Creation, or Cambray's Demonstration on the Being of a God; or for a few moments of silent contemplation. There is to follow the singing of Milton's Hymn to the Creator, and then a reading from a book "discoursing on and exciting the moral virtues."

Next comes a prelude to a litany. It expresses uncertainty that "many things, which we often hear mentioned in the petitions of men to the Deity, would prove real goods, if they were in our possession," and his hope and belief that God will not withhold from him "a suitable share of temporal blessings" if by a virtuous and holy life he conciliates God's favor and kindness. His prayers contain the following petitions:

"That I may be preserved from atheism, impiety, and profaneness; and, in my addresses to Thee, carefully avoid irreverence and ostentation, formality and odious hypocrisy, — Help me, O Father!

"That I may be loyal to my prince, and faithful to my

country, careful for its good, valiant in its defense, and obedient to its laws, abhorring treason as much as tyranny, — Help me, O Father!

" That I may to those above me be dutiful, humble, and submissive; avoiding pride, disrespect, and contumacy, — Help me, O Father.

" That I may to those below me be gracious, condescending, and forgiving, using clemency, protecting innocent distress, avoiding cruelty, harshness, and oppression, insolence, and unreasonable severity, — Help me, O Father!

" That I may refrain from calumny and detraction; that I may abhor and avoid deceit and every fraud, flattery, and hatred, malice, lying and ingratitude, — Help me, O Father!

" That I may be sincere in friendship, faithful in trust, and impartial in judgment, watchful against pride, and against anger (that momentary madness), — Help me, O Father!

" That I may be just in all my dealings, temperate in my pleasures, full of candour and ingenuousness, humanity and benevolence, — Help me, O Father. . .

The litany closes with the following: "That I may have a constant regard to honor and probity, that I may possess a perfect innocence and a good conscience, and at length may become truly virtuous and magnanimous, — Help me, good God; help me, O Father."

II

So, with a little imagination, we can picture the youthful Franklin solemnly beginning the day in his solitary Philadelphia bedroom with a recital of his creed, the singing of his Miltonic hymn, and the intonation of his litany, and then going out, perhaps with a little sigh, to resume his

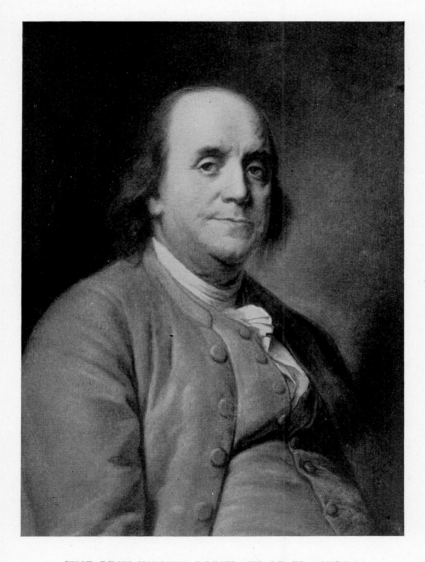

THE BEST KNOWN PORTRAIT OF FRANKLIN

PAINTED BY J. S. DUPLESSIS IN PARIS AND PRESENTED BY JOHN BIGELOW
TO THE NEW YORK PUBLIC LIBRARY.

labors before a case of cold and smudgy type. But who can contend that Franklin's religion was not, for him, a sound one? Did he not " at length become truly virtuous and magnanimous," and did he not attain a full measure of those " temporal blessings " for which he prayed?

III

To give a more complete statement of Franklin's views concerning religion, it may be well at this stage to insert an extract from his letter to President Ezra Stiles, of Yale College, written when Franklin was eighty-four years old. After stating his belief in God, who may best be served by " doing good to his children," Franklin says:

" As to Jesus of Nazareth, my opinion of whom you particularly desire, I think his system of morals and his religion, as he left them to us, the best the world ever saw or is like to see; but I apprehend it has received various corrupting changes, and I have, with most of the present Dissenters in England, some doubts as to his divinity; though it is a question I do not dogmatize upon having never studied it, and think it needless to busy myself with it now. I expect soon of an opportunity of knowing the truth with less trouble.[1] I see no harm, however, in its being believed, if that belief has the good consequence, as probably it has, of making his doctrines more respected and more observed; especially as I do not perceive that the Supreme takes it amiss, by distinguishing the unbelievers in his government of the world with any particular marks of his displeasure.

" I shall only add, respecting myself, having experienced the goodness of that Being in conducting me prosperously through a long life, I have no doubt of its continuance in

---

[1] Franklin " knew the truth " very soon; he died a few weeks later.

the next, though without the smallest conceit of meriting such goodness.

" P.S.   I confide, that you will not expose me to criticisms and censures by publishing any part of this communication to you.   I have ever let others enjoy their religious sentiments, without reflecting on them for those that appeared to me insupportable or even absurd.   All sects here, and we have a great variety, have experienced my good will in assisting them with subscriptions for the building their new places of worship; and, as I have never opposed any of their doctrines, I hope to go out of the world in peace with them all."

At another time he wrote:

" With regard to future bliss, I cannot help imagining that multitudes of the zealously orthodox of different sects who at the last day may flock together in hopes of seeing each other damned, will be disappointed and obliged to rest content with their own salvation."

IV

However, Benjamin found some time later " that the mere speculative conviction that it was our interest to be completely virtuous, was not sufficient to prevent our slipping."   What he aimed at was not a mere emotional religion for special occasions, but " a steady, uniform rectitude of conduct."

He therefore gave himself up to careful cogitation, and fixed upon thirteen virtues as being " all that at that time occurr'd to me as necessary or desirable."   To each he annexed a short precept.   These principles were to be the basis of a projected work which was never completed, " the Art of Virtue."   The famous thirteen virtues were written down as follows:

1. Temperance

Eat not to dulness; drink not to elevation.

2. Silence

Speak not but what may benefit others or yourself; avoid trifling conversation.

3. Order

Let all things have their places; let each part of your business have its time.

4. Resolution

Resolve to perform what you ought; perform without fail what you resolve.

5. Frugality

Make no expense but to do good to others or yourself; i.e., waste nothing.

6. Industry

Lose no time; be always employ'd in something useful; cut off all unnecessary actions.

7. Sincerity

Use no hurtful deceit; think candidly and justly; and, if you speak, speak accordingly.

8. Justice

Wrong none by doing injuries, or omitting the benefits that are your duty.

ing want of method . . . In truth, I found myself incorrigible with respect to *order;* and now I am grown old, and my memory bad, I feel very sensibly the want of it." [2]

Nor had he much better success with the other virtues. " I soon found I had undertaken a task of more difficulty than I had imagined. While my care was employ'd in guarding against one fault, I was often surprised by another; habit took the advantage of inattention; inclination was sometimes too strong for reason." [2]

His wrestlings continued until, at length, he decided he must organize his forces better. He therefore adopted a hint from the Golden Verses of Pythagoras, who advised his followers to give themselves a daily examination.

So Ben made himself a little book. Each page he ruled with red ink into seven columns, one for each day of the week. These columns he crossed with thirteen red lines, representing the Thirteen Virtues. His transgressions he indicated by a black spot marked in the proper place each evening before retiring. Firmly resolving to test himself by giving a week's strict attention to each virtue in succession, he began with Temperance.

In the *Autobiography* he gives us a specimen page. It shows that for one week at least, he kept his Temperance record clear. But Silence was interrupted on Sunday, Monday, Wednesday, and Friday. Order was overthrown twice on Sunday, and once each on Monday, Tuesday, Thursday, Friday and Saturday. Resolution received two black entries, on Tuesday and Friday. Frugality was fractured on Monday and Thursday. Industry was low on Tuesday. What happened to Sincerity, Justice, Moderation, Cleanliness, Tranquillity, Chastity and Humility is not recorded at all. Possibly by the time he had reached Industry, the flesh had weakened beyond repair.

[2] Autobiography.

The incessant scraping out of the black marks, so as to begin a new course, finally left the little book full of holes. He therefore transferred his tables to a set of ivory leaves, which stood erasures better. In the course of years, his self-tests became more and more infrequent, until at last they ceased entirely.

" But," adds Franklin, " I always carried my little book with me."

He consoled himself with the reflection that, at any rate, he ought not to carry his project of perfect morals to the point of foppery. " A perfect character might be attended with the inconvenience of being envied and hated," and " a benevolent man should allow a few faults in himself, to keep his friends in countenance," says the *Autobiography*.

Franklin errs, perhaps, when he asserts that it was his scheme of Order which gave him the most trouble. For it is of this time that he afterwards wrote:

" That hard to be governed passion of youth had hurried me frequently into intrigues with low women that fell in my way, which were attended with some expense and great inconvenience, besides a continual risk to my health by a distemper, which, of all things, I dreaded, though by great good luck I escaped it."

And it was about a year after the production of his liturgy that his natural son, William Franklin, afterwards the Royal Governor of New Jersey, was born.[3] Who his mother was is not certainly known. Some believe it was a strolling wench. Others have aired the charges of Franklin's enemies, that William's mother was Barbara, a servant girl, afterwards employed in Ben's home. The event is not recorded in Franklin's *Autobiography;* but this is not strange, seeing that the *Autobiography* was originally addressed to William and written for his benefit. Franklin does not

[3] Life and Times of Benjamin Franklin, by James Parton.

mention William's birth in any of his other collected writings, but he took the boy into his home and reared him with fond care. He did the same when William in his turn became the father of a natural son, William Temple Franklin. He loved both boys and tried his best to be proud of them, even when they did not deserve it.

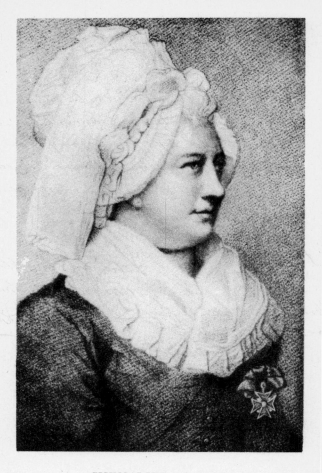

CHEVALIER D' EON

IN THE WOMAN'S CLOTHES HE CHOSE TO WEAR DURING THE LATTER
PART OF HIS LIFE.

que vous lui ferez le plaisir et l'honneur de
vous arrêter chez lui à Tonnerre, je serai
fort heureuse si je pouvois m'y trouver
dans ce tems là, et vous y donner des preuves
d'un sincère et respectueux attachement
avec lequel je suis

Monsieur

a Versailles ce 25, janvier
1778.

Votre très humble
et très obéissante servante
La Che D'Eon

PAGE OF A LETTER FROM THE FAMOUS CHEVALIER
D' EON TO FRANKLIN, WITH SIGNATURE
IN THE FEMININE.

*Reproduced by permission from the original in the possession
of the American Philosophical Society.*

Chapter XI

Philadelphia's Youngest Master-Printer

I

THE first customer for the new printing firm of Franklin and Meredith appeared almost as soon as they had opened their London-bought outfit. He was a countryman fetched by an acquaintance who had found him in the street inquiring for a printer. The job brought five shillings. Franklin says it gave him more pleasure than any crown earned afterwards, and made him the more disposed to help young beginners. The printshop occupied quarters near the old Philadelphia market on High Street, later Market Street. They paid twenty-four pounds a year for it, but eased the burden by subletting rooms to Thomas Godfrey, the meticulous member of the Junto, and his family.

One day a bearded raven stopped at the door. His name was Samuel Mickle, an elderly and prominent citizen. Seeing Benjamin's beaming countenance, he lifted up his voice and began to croak. There was no chance for the new firm to succeed, he said; the recent boom in Philadelphia couldn't last. There was nothing but ruin and desolation to look forward to. He cited at great length a list of recent failures. Then, seeing that he had reduced the hopeful Franklin to a state of misery, he resumed his walk with a satisfied feeling of having done a good day's work.

But the Junto members were already exerting themselves to recommend business to the new firm, and soon Franklin got a job, low in price but something to go on with. It consisted of forty sheets of a huge folio "History of the Rise, Increase, and Progress of the Christian People called Quakers." Meredith worked the press and Franklin set it up, a sheet a day, often working into the night. He was so determined to do a sheet a day that when by accident a form was pied, he distributed the type and set it up all over again before going to bed.

People began to notice this industry. It was remarked at the Merchants' Every-night Club that Franklin could be seen at work when the members went home at night and again the next morning before they were abroad. At length one member, wishing to reward true merit, offered to sell the firm stationery on credit, but Franklin says they did not " chuse " to open a shop.

II

Now comes George Webb, a former fellow employee at Keimer's, and wants a journeyman's job. Ben says there's nothing at present but there may be later, because he intends to start a newspaper.

At the time the only paper south of New England is Andrew Bradford's *Weekly Mercury*. It once distinguished itself by its defense of the Franklin brothers in their Boston fight, as we have seen; but most of the time, though profitable, it offers dull reading and is besides badly managed.

Webb hurries off to Keimer with the secret. The pig-eater at once sets about founding a paper of his own. The first number appears long before Franklin is ready, on December 24, 1728. It bears the grandiose title of *The Universal Instructor in all Arts and Sciences, and Pennsylvania Gazette*. A yearly subscription cost ten shillings. Advertisements were three shillings each. At one time it had as many as ninety subscribers.

Ben, thus forestalled, retaliates upon Keimer by making use of the *Weekly Mercury*. He contributes a series of satiric articles, aimed at Keimer, signed by " The Busybody."

The Busybody papers, as might be expected, are written in the vein of *The Spectator*. They are really a continuation of the " Silence Dogood " essays published in the *New England Courant*, but are better written, because Franklin has developed meantime; and are more broadly humorous in tone, because Ben no longer has in his blood the poison of his hatred for New England's dismal religiosity. In Pennsylvania he is surrounded by a people with whom he is more at home. They are like himself, half peasants, having a leaven supplied by liberal-minded Quaker influence. They love earthy pleasantries, relish allusions savoring of the barnyard, regard the existence of sex as a legitimate source of fun, and particularly enjoy jokes at each other's expense. Ben therefore instantly grips their interest when in his first paper he hints that he is going to expose " private vices " and will not ignore the fair sex, though discussing its members with " the utmost decency and respect."

Ben's second paper is directed against laughers, meaning persons who find amusement in the defects of some poor fellow's dress; he is possibly thinking of his own appearance on his arrival in Philadelphia five years before. In the third he ridicules a stuffed figure called " Cretico." Keimer takes this for his own portrait and tries to reply in a tract falsely labeled: " Printed at the New Printing-Office." Ben replies by issuing a pamphlet entitled " A Short Discourse, Proving that the Jewish or Seventh-Day Sabbath Is Abrogated and Replaced." No doubt the shot sinks home, for everybody is familiar with Keimer's Mosaic beliefs and practices.

Keimer's method of filling his own columns is simple. He merely takes Chamber's Dictionary of the Arts and Sciences, recently come from London, and begins to reprint it serially, beginning with the letter A. He fills any space left over with short news items and political addresses. It is, however, a better paper in most respects than Bradford's feeble *Mercury*, and might have supplanted it had not Benjamin's contributions filled the *Mercury* with an effervescent elixir. Ben contributes about six papers, all of which cause no end of talk in the community; the last one is a satire at the expense of the numerous inhabitants who spend all their time digging holes in the landscape in the hope of uncovering pirate gold; he then turns the column over to his Junto companion, Joseph Breintnal.

Keimer runs his paper for about nine months, when, in debt and about to flee from his creditors to the Barbadoes, he sells out for a trifle to the waiting Benjamin.

III

Ben drops most of the pompous title, and issues, in a new dress, the first newspaper under his own control on October 2, 1729, he being twenty-three years old. Its name is the *Pennsylvania Gazette*.

After explaining to his readers that he does not deem the reprinting of a dictionary a proper method of communicating knowledge, he sets down his ideals as a publisher as follows:

" We ask assistance, because we are fully sensible, that to publish a good newspaper is not so easy an undertaking as many people imagine it to be. The author of a Gazette (in the opinion of the learned) ought to be qualified with an extensive acquaintance with languages, a great easiness and command of writing, and relating things clearly and intelligibly and in a few words; he should be able to speak of men both by land and sea; be well acquainted with geography, with the history of the time, with the secret interests of princes and states; the secrets of courts, and the manners and customs of all nations. Men thus accomplished are very rare in this remote part of the world; and it would be well if the writer of these papers could make up among his friends what is wanting in himself. Upon the whole, we may assure the publick, that, as far as the encouragement we meet with will enable us, no care or pains shall be omitted that may make the *Pennsylvania Gazette* as agreeable and useful an entertainment as the nature of the thing will allow."

The first page of the *Gazette* would be considered a fine specimen of printing today. In fact, few journals of the present time surpass it in neatness, legibility, balance, spacing, and general inviting appearance. It is plainly modeled after the pattern set by *The Spectator*, that journal which has done so much to mold Franklin's taste.

One of Franklin's very first editorials causes comment and wins him many subscribers. One of those disputes is going on between Burnet, the Royal Governor of Massachusetts, and the provincial Assembly, which are heralds of the worse one about to ensue between the mother country and all her American colonies. It relates to the governor's salary, the amount of which the colonists have always maintained their right to specify " according to their sense of his merits and services." Burnet had been instructed by his government to demand a fixed salary of one thousand pounds a year. Ben gives a history of the dispute and praises the Assembly for abiding by " what they think is their right, and that of the people they represent," thus revealing " that ardent spirit of liberty, and that undaunted courage, which has in every age so gloriously distinguished Britons and Englishmen from the rest of mankind."

Bradford is still printing the laws and other public documents of Pennsylvania. He prints an address of the House to the governor in a sloppy fashion. Franklin reprints it " elegantly and correctly," and sends a copy to every member. As a result, Franklin and Meredith are chosen, with the support of Mr. Hamilton, the lawyer he met on the London ship, as printers for the House for the next year. This is one of Franklin's first important successes as an advertiser.

IV

In writing for the *Gazette* the festive Franklin richly enjoys himself. His is no squeamish public, and since his tastes are in accord with those of his subscribers, both editor and readers have rare sport with the foibles and failings of the day. He writes letters to himself as editor and answers them in the next issue. He mingles jokes and anecdotes with longer pieces of a moral, philosophical or scientific nature.

One day he describes an alleged lottery in England, in which, to further the increase and multiplication of the species, all the old maids are to be raffled for.

Again, he mentions a Bucks County farmer, who is struck by lightning, which does no damage beyond melting a pewter button on the waistband of his breeches. " 'Tis well," says the *Gazette*, " nothing else thereabouts was made of pewter."

At another time he returns to his favorite target of religious fanaticism, thus:

" I dismiss my reader with this summary Remark upon what has been said: That as the Christian Religion is the

Best of all Religions, so Christian Superstition, which is the Corruption of it, is the Worst of all Superstitions."

v

The most famous long contribution of Franklin's to the *Gazette* is " Polly Baker's Speech." It is worth quoting at length because there is evidence that Polly is mostly Benjamin. We have already seen that about this time William Franklin was born of an unrecorded mother. Polly's defense of herself as the mother of a natural child is in reality Franklin's own defense of himself made for the benefit of those critics in Philadelphia who have been saying nasty things about him. It is in keeping with what we know of Franklin's strongly feminized nature to find that for publication purposes he again assumes a woman's garb, as in the case of the Mrs. Silence Dogood papers:

" The Speech of Miss Polly Baker before a Court of Judicatory, in New England, where she was prosecuted for a fifth time, for having a Bastard Child; which influenced the Court to dispense with her punishment, and which induced one of her judges to marry her the next day — by whom she had fifteen children.

" May it please the honourable bench to indulge me in a few words: I am a poor, unhappy woman, who have no money to fee lawyers to plead for me, being hard put to it to get a living . . . Abstracted from the law, I cannot conceive (may it please your honours) what the nature of my offence is. I have brought five children into the world, at the risque of my life; I have maintained them well by my own industry, without burthening the township, and would have done it better, if it had not been for the heavy charges and fines I have paid. Can it be a crime (in the nature of things, I mean) to add to the King's subjects, in a new country that really needs people? I own it, I should think it rather a praiseworthy than a punishable action. I have debauched no other woman's husband, nor enticed any youth; these things I never was charged with; nor has any one the least cause of complaint against me, unless, perhaps, the ministers of justice, because I have had children without being married, by which they have missed a wedding fee. But can this be a fault of mine? I appeal to your honours. You are pleased to allow I don't want sense; but I must be stupefied to the last degree, not to prefer the honourable state of wedlock to the condition I have lived in. I always was, and still am willing to enter into it; and doubt not my behaving well in it; having all the industry, frugality, fertility, and skill in economy appertaining to a good wife's character. I defy any one to say I ever refused an offer of that sort; on the contrary, I readily consented to the only proposal of marriage that ever was made me, which was when I was a virgin, but too easily confiding in the person's sincerity that made it, I unhappily lost my honour by trusting to his; for he got me with child, and then forsook me.

" That very person, you all know; he is now become a magistrate of this country; and I had hopes he would have appeared this day on the bench, and have endeavoured to moderate the Court in my favour; then I should have scorned to have mentioned it, but I must now complain of it as unjust and unequal, that my betrayer, and undoer, the first cause of all my faults and miscarriages (if they must be deemed such), should be advanced to honour and power in the government that punishes my misfortunes with stripes and infamy. You believe I have offended heaven, and must suffer eternal fire; will not that be sufficient? I own I do not think as you do, for, if I thought what you

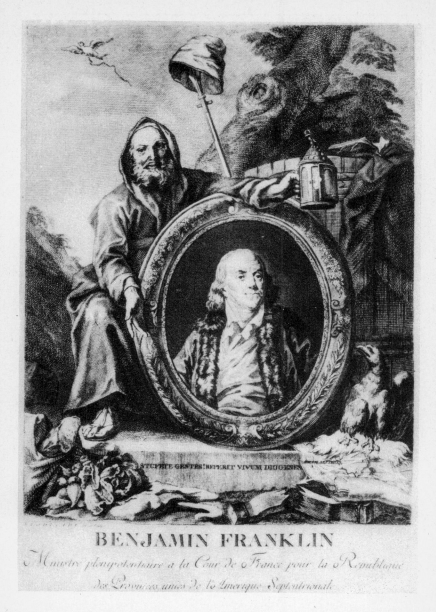

DIOGENES DISCOVERING FRANKLIN: A FRENCH PRINT
MADE IN 1780.

Reproduced from the original in the Bibliothèque Nationale, Paris.

call a sin was really such, I could not presumptuously commit it. But how can it be believed that Heaven is angry at my having children, when to the little done by me towards it, God has been pleased to add his divine skill and admirable workmanship in the formation of their bodies, and crowned the whole by furnishing them with rational and immortal souls? Forgive me, gentlemen, if I talk a little extravagantly on these matters: I am no divine, but if you, gentlemen, must be making laws, do not turn natural and useful actions into crimes by your prohibitions. But take into your wise consideration the great and growing number of bachelors in the country, many of whom, from the mean fear of the expense of a family, have never sincerely and honestly courted a woman in their lives; and by their manner of living leave unproduced (which is little better than murder) hundreds of their posterity to the thousandth generation. Is not this a greater offence against the public good than mine? Compel them, then, by law, either to marriage, or to pay double the fine of fornication every year. What must poor young women do, whom customs and nature forbid to solicit the men, and who cannot force themselves upon husbands, when the laws take no care to provide them any, and yet severely punish them if they do their duty without them; the duty of the first and great command of nature and nature's God, increase and multiply; a duty, from the steady performance of which nothing has been able to deter me, but for its sake I have hazarded the loss of the public esteem, and have frequently endured public disgrace and punishment: and therefore ought, in my humble opinion, instead of a whipping, to have a statue erected to my memory."

There are many hidden autobiographical details in this speech. For Franklin's offence in becoming the father of a natural child he might, had the law been enforced, have received twenty-one lashes at a Pennsylvania whipping post. He therefore imagines himself facing a court; but he transfers the locale to New England. He is, however, unrepentant — this is not his first offense against sexual taboos and it is not likely to be the last.

Mr. S. G. Fisher, in fact, has found evidence indicating that Franklin was the father of *two* illegitimate children, the second one being a girl, who afterwards became the wife of John Foxcroft, postmaster of Philadelphia. In a letter to Franklin dated February 2, 1772, Foxcroft specifically refers to her as " your Daughter." [1]

Franklin is not only unrepentant, but mirthful about his peccadilloes — Polly marries one of her judges and has fifteen children by him.

" I love to hear of everything," Franklin once wrote to his wife, " that tends to increase the number of good people," and his daughter Sarah said in a letter to him when in England: " As I know my dear papa likes to hear of weddings, I will give him a list of my acquaintances that has entered the matrimonial state since his departure."

Franklin, through Polly, then contends that having children, no matter by what means, is " rather a praiseworthy than a punishable action," especially "in a new country that really needs people."

Polly is poor, but possessed of " industry, frugality, fertility, and skill in economy " — the very virtues which Franklin most admires. It is no fault of hers that she is not married; she has been betrayed.

Here Franklin is probably harking back to his friend Ralph's affair with the London milliner, and his own rebuff at her hands.

Polly pleads with lawmakers not to " turn natural and

1 The True Benjamin Franklin.

useful actions into crimes." Compare this with a later direct statement from Franklin:

" Men I find to be a sort of beings very badly constructed, as they are generally more easily provoked than reconciled, more disposed to do mischief to each other than to make reparation, much more easily deceived than undeceived, and having more pride and even pleasure in killing than in begetting one another; for without a blush they assemble in great armies at noonday to destroy, and when they have killed as many as they can they exaggerate the number to augment the fancied glory; but they creep into corners and cover themselves with the darkness of night when they mean to beget, as being ashamed of a virtuous action." [2]

Franklin's summing up, in Polly's speech, is that he has done nothing of which he is ashamed; he proves this later by his care of William Franklin and the latter's natural son, William Temple Franklin; and finally asserts that instead of a whipping, he ought to have a statue erected to his memory. If statues are a proof of the acceptance of Franklin's opinions, his shade has had a thousand such proofs since, for there are at least that many statues of him now standing in his native country; and shortly after his death some French friends erected a bust in his honor bearing on its pedestal the single word:

"VIR" [3]

VI

Another witty article by Franklin in the *Gazette* is an account of an alleged witch trial at Mount Holly, New Jersey. It gives him an enjoyable opportunity for satire and burlesque at the expense of his favorite enemies, the religious

[2] Works of Franklin, by John Bigelow.
[3] Man.

fanatics who accept the Bible literally and invest the mere book itself with a superstitious power.

"It seems," says Franklin, "the accused had been charged with making the neighbour's sheep dance in an uncommon manner, and with causing hogs to speak and sing Psalms, etc., to the great terror and amazement of the king's good and peaceful subjects in the province; and the accusers being very positive that if the accused were weighed against a Bible, the Bible would prove too heavy for them; or that, if they were bound and put into the river they would swim; the said accused, desirous to make innocence appear, voluntarily offered to undergo the said trials if two of the most violent of their accusers would be tried with them."

Scales and a Bible were ceremoniously introduced. "The wizard was first placed in the scale, and over him was read a chapter out of the Book of Moses, and then the Bible was put in the other scale, which, being kept down before, was immediately let go; but, to the surprise of the spectators, flesh and blood came down plump and outweighed that great Book by abundance."

The mob then proposed trial by water. "Accused and accusers, being stripped (saving only the women their shifts), were bound hand and foot and severally placed in the water . . ." All floated except the chief male accuser. "The more thinking part of the spectators were of opinion that any person so bound and placed in the water (unless they were mere skin and bones) would swim till their breath was gone, and their lungs filled with water. But it being the general belief of the populace that the women's shifts and garters with which they were bound helped to support them, it is said they are to be tried again the next warm weather, naked."

VII

Franklin's essays in the *Gazette* are not always consistent in their teachings or tone. One of the most admired is " The Meditations on a Quart Mug," which contains a moral for chronic drinkers; but there is also a curious catalogue of slang terms and synonyms for drunkenness whose great length — if Franklin was really the compiler of it — indicates that Benjamin had more than a prohibitionist's interest in the subject of alcohol. Some of the terms are:

Addled, Boozy, Buzzey, Crocus, Cock'd, Dagg'd, Cock-Ey'd, Fettered, Glaiz'd, Hammerish, Tagg'd, Juicy, Knapt, Lappy, Momentous, Nimptopsical, Oil'd, Pungey, Raddled, Stew'd, Trammel'd, Valiant.

There is also a song originally written by him for use at Junto Meetings:

Fair Venus calls; her voice obey,
In beauty's arms spend night and day.
The joys of love all joys excell,
And loving's certainly doing well.

Chorus

Oh! no!
Not so!
For honest souls know,
Friends and a bottle still bear the bell.

Then toss off your glasses, and scorn the dull asses,
Who, missing the kernel, still gnaw the shell;
What's love, rule or riches? Wise Solomon teaches
They're vanity, vanity, vanity still.

Chorus

That's true;
He knew;
He'd tried them all through;
Friends and a bottle still bore the bell.

VIII

For a time the pair of young printers manage to keep going and their prospects are steadily improving when they are suddenly made defendants in a creditor's suit. It threatens to take away their whole enterprise.

Hugh Meredith's father has been able to advance them only one hundred pounds for their outfit, on which another one hundred pounds is still due. The youthful partners are unable to raise the money, the creditor threatens foreclosure, and once more Franklin sees another castle about to crash. He has a heart-to-heart talk with Hugh. The latter confesses that he has lost interest in printing and would prefer to follow other Welsh farmers who are settling in North Carolina. Hugh offers to sell out if Ben will take over the debts, return to his father the one hundred pounds borrowed, pay Hugh's personal debts, and give him as a bonus thirty pounds and a new saddle.

Despite these rather exacting terms, Ben is willing to meet them, for Hugh, with his fondness for tavern company, has not been a helpful partner. But he has no money.

At this juncture Ben has reason to thank his guiding Providence that he has founded the Junto, for two members now come forward separately and offer to advance to Ben all the money necessary. They are Robert Grace, the generous and witty, and William Coleman, the cool and clear-headed. Franklin accepts from each half the money offered, pays off Meredith, and becomes in 1730 sole proprietor of Philadelphia's new printing-house. He also pays off the debt long due to Vernon.

So, at the age of 24, Benjamin becomes the head of his own business, without having saved any money, without having worked unusually hard, without having omitted any of the pleasures beloved by imaginative youth, and without having lived up to any of the maxims for which he is later to become renowned.

CHAPTER XII

Money Making and Saving

I

NOW begins a period of Franklin's career which is to color his thoughts for many years. He has been a little frightened by his repeated failures; he resolves upon success. He has been forcibly reminded of the disadvantages incurred by lack of money; he therefore resolves to get some. He is the proprietor of his own business, but in name only; he wishes to pay off the loans advanced by Grace and Coleman as quickly as possible and stand forth as his own untrammeled boss. He therefore gives himself entirely to the mastery of external things; he becomes the complete extrovert and model *bourgeois*.

In doing this, he calls to his aid his showman's talents. The Autobiography tells how:

" In order to secure my credit and character as a tradesman, I took care not only to be in *reality* industrious and frugal, but to avoid all appearances to the contrary. I drest plainly; I was seen at no places of idle diversion. I never went out a-fishing or shooting; a book, indeed, sometimes debauched me from my work, but that was seldom, snug and gave no scandal; and to show that I was not above my business, I sometimes brought home the paper I purchased at the stores thro' the streets on a wheelbarrow."

II

It is noteworthy that in referring to books Benjamin uses the word " debauched." In this word is epitomized the state

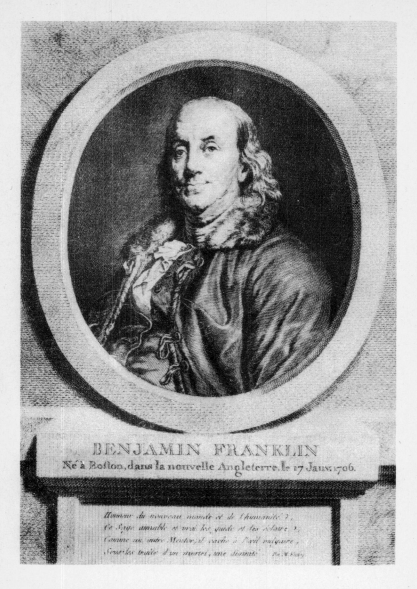

PORTRAIT OF FRANKLIN ENGRAVED IN PARIS IN 1778.

Reproduced from a print in the Bibliothèque Nationale, Paris, based on a portrait formerly belonging to Franklin's friend, M. le Ray de Chaumont.

of civilization then prevailing not only in Pennsylvania but virtually throughout America, except in Virginia, where life and leisure, if not laziness, were virtually synonymous. Philadelphia had not even a bookshop. There was little sale for anything beyond eighteen-penny pamphlets. Literature and the other delightful arts were regarded with deep suspicion. They detracted from the chief end of man, which is to get on. They were " debauching."

III

The Millet-like picture which Franklin presents to his fellow citizens has its effect.

" Thus being esteemed an industrious, thriving young man and paying only for what I bought, the merchants who imported stationery solicited my custom; others proposed supplying me with books, and I went on swimmingly."

Keimer's former apprentice, David Harry, tries for a time to maintain a rival printshop, but being " dressed like a gentleman " and therefore handicapped in wheeling a barrow, follows his former master to the Barbadoes, where Keimer becomes his hired man.

There is no competitor left except Bradford, who now having the post office, pays little attention to printing. He tries to prevent the post riders from carrying Ben's paper, but Franklin circumvents him by bribing the riders. He means to prosper; and by dint of laborious toil and careful saving, does so.

IV

Benjamin's next step is what might be expected. He thinks of marriage. He goes about it as if it were a transaction in salt pork or baled hay; still, this is in accord with the customs of the people and period. Mrs. Godfrey, whose family lives in Ben's house and with whom he boards, comes forward as matchmaker. She introduces Ben to the daughter of a relative and leaves them often together. Franklin's courtship is rapid, and the time soon arrives for talking business. Ben informs Mrs. Godfrey that he expects the girl's dowry to be enough to pay off the balance due on his printshop, about £100. Mrs. Godfrey spreads her hands, saying the amount is more than they can manage. Ben suggests that they mortgage their house at the loan-office; in a word, " hock " it. She says she will see.

When next she meets Ben, her manner is cold. They have decided the printing business is not a profitable one and that the match had better be called off. The girl is shut up and Ben is forbidden to call. Ben suspects that this is a plot to trap him into a runaway, and hence a dowerless, marriage. He makes no attempt to see his lady-love. After a time Mrs. Godfrey thaws and renews her overtures. But Ben is now in his turn frozen. He announces that he will have nothing more to do with the Godfreys or the girl either. This leads to a row, and the Godfreys move out of the house, leaving Ben there alone.

But Ben is now ready for a marriage: he also needs the money; so he tries to meet other ladies. He learns that parents think poorly of the printing business and that money is not to be expected with a daughter, unless he will take an ill-favored one. So for the time being he is compelled to remain in single state.

v

Meantime Ben has obtained one or two profitable " jobbs " of printing paper money. These come to him because of the success of his anonymous pamphlet, " A Modest

Inquiry into the nature and necessity of a Paper Currency."
For a young man of twenty-four this is a remarkable production. Its ideas, probably derived from his studies of
Locke and Defoe, are far in advance of those of the period.
For instance, Ben lays down the dictum that money is only a
medium of exchange and that the measure of its value is
labor. " Money as bullion," he says, " is valuable by so
much labor as it costs to produce that bullion." Franklin's
argument is that to promote the commerce of the country
more money is needed. He therefore becomes one of the
country's first proponents of currency inflation. His writings on money are said to have received the respectful attention both of Adam Smith and Karl Marx.

His proposals are violently opposed by the Proprietaries,
the land speculators, the money-lenders, and their satellites
among the professions. They are supported with equal
vigor by the shopkeepers, merchants, tradesmen, and small
manufacturers. The latter class being more numerous and
having more representatives in the Assembly, win the fight.
The Lords of Trade in England are defied and £30,000 in
new money is ordered printed. Much of the credit for this
victory goes to Franklin, and his prestige in the eyes of the
town burgher class is correspondingly heightened.

He procures the printing of the laws and votes of the
provincial government; opens a stationer's shop, and is soon
able to hire a compositor and an apprentice. The latter is
the son of Aquila Rose, the subject of Keimer's hand-set
threnody.

The strain of earning a mere living is considerably eased.
He commands more leisure than formerly. He now stands
solidly on the first rung of the ladder of success.

Chapter XIII

Marriage

I

AS a former lodger and a rising man of affairs, Benjamin is often consulted by the family of Mr. Read, who is now dead. He is a frequent visitor at the Read home. There he sometimes sees Deborah Read. She remains woeful of face and avoids company. Ben is conscience smitten. He resolves to repair his "erratum" in neglecting her. He again proposes marriage and is accepted.

Deborah's mother has already lamented her interference in preventing the marriage before Franklin sailed for London, and though she now welcomes the prospect of Benjamin as a son-in-law, she fears Rogers, though reported dead, may turn up some day. There is also the matter of Rogers' debts, which Ben might have to assume. But the young people have already had enough of old folks' caution and they go ahead. The date of the ceremony is September 1, 1730.

In his Autobiography Franklin does not say they were married. He says, "I took her to wife." No record of a legal marriage exists. Perhaps this was omitted because of the uncertainty of Deborah's status. Anyhow, no complications ever ensued. Debby's no-account husband never appeared, and Ben was never bothered by Rogers' creditors. Soon she is calling him "Pappy," and he addresses her as "dear child."

No better wife could have been found for a young man on the make. Debby soon recovered her spirits and eagerly helped Benjamin in all his pursuits. No doubt in her gratitude for escaping a lonely grass widowhood, she was happy to work for Franklin incessantly. She made all his linen and woolen clothing by hand. She tended the shop, helped to make ink with lamp-black, and traded in goose-feathers. She was a tireless housekeeper.

For these labors a thoughtful nature had equipped her with a sound physique. She was broadly built, and full bosomed, with a kind of vigorous beauty. The best picture of her is by Franklin himself. When in London later he wrote her of finding " a large fine jug for beer."

" I fell in love with it at sight: for I thought it looked like a fat jolly dame, clean and tidy, with a neat blue and white calico gown on, good natured and lively."

She was lively enough, as her resolute defense of her home when attacked by a mob during the negotiations with England about the Stamp Act later proved; but there is more doubt about the uniformity of her good nature. Witnesses have left testimony as to her sharp tongue, and there is evidence that at one time she became heartily tired of William Franklin's presence in the house. She deserves some excuse for this, perhaps, as William turned out to be a rather self-centred and pompous young man, who extracted high satisfaction from the fact of his own existence.

She became the mother of two children. The first was Francis Folger Franklin, whose death at the age of four still gave his father a pang when he wrote about it 50 years afterward. The boy is buried near his parents in the yard of Christ Church, Philadelphia. The other child was the amiable Sarah Franklin, afterwards Mrs. Richard Bache.

II

In that day it was not deemed good Americanism to educate the female mind, and Debby Franklin's letters show that she had merely an impressionist's view of grammar and spelling. The following specimen, from a letter dated October 29, 1773, is preserved by the American Philosophical Society:

"I shall tell you what consernes myself our yonegest Grandson is the finest child as alive he has had the small Pox and had it very fine and got abrod agen Capt All will tell you a boute him Benj Franklin Beache but as it is so deficall to writ I have desered him to tell you I have sente a squerel for your friend and wish her better luck it is a very fine one I have had very bad luck with two they one killed and another run a way allthou they was bred up tame I have not a caige as I donte know where the man lives that makes them my love to Sally Franklin — my love to all our cousins as thou menthond remember me to Mr. and Mrs. Weste due you ever hear aney thing of Ninely Evers as was . . . I am your afeckthone wife

"D. Franklin."

Debby's letters are full of household references and local gossip. For example, she writes on June 30, 1772, that "George is a widower and a dreadful crier but he is a looking out but shant mary very soon."

Franklin's letters to her contain the same kind of homely material. During his many long absences from her — there was one period of ten years in London and another of nine in Paris — he wrote her constantly and affectionately in the indulgent manner of an elder addressing a child. He never tired of praising her thrifty virtues to his friends and he even wrote a song in her honor, entitled "My Plain Country Joan." One stanza was:

" Some faults we have, and so has my Joan,
    But then they're exceedingly small;
And now I'm grown used to them, so like my own,
    I scarcely can see them at all,
        My dear friends,
    I scarcely can see them at all."

Debby regularly attended Christ Church, which practice Franklin, though not a church-goer himself, encouraged. This was the cause of a typical advertisement, evidently written by Franklin himself, which appeared one day in the *Gazette:*

" Taken out of a pew in the Church, some months since, a Common Prayer Book, bound in red, gilt, and lettered D. F. (Deborah Franklin) on each cover. The person who took it is desired to open it, and read the Eighth Commandment, and afterwards return it into the same pew again; upon which no further notice will be taken."

Though Franklin was content with her as a helpmate, he does not seem to have missed her much as a companion, when absent on his political missions; Debby was not the type of woman who could give him much intellectual stimulus or sympathy. To a versatile but slightly lethargic man like Franklin the companionship of bright and vivacious women met one of his fundamental needs, and what he could not find at home, he sought for elsewhere. He was in particularly high feather when in the society of young girls. He made friends of them wherever he went, at home, in England, and in France. His attitude towards them was that of an appreciative father and counsellor. All his life he had feminine correspondents by the score, and he liked to remember them with little notes, gifts, and delicately amorous compliments. Debby does not seem to have minded these little flirtations, and his daughter Sally was not only aware of his relishes in this respect but even encouraged them, if we may judge by these extracts from her letters to him:

" I see the girls this morning, and they begged me to send their love to you . . . There is not a young lady of my acquaintance but what has desired to be remembered to you."

An occasional husband misunderstood Franklin's fondness for stimulating feminine society, but most of the male relatives of the gay and witty women whom he liked, regarded his friendship with them indulgently. But it cannot be said to which class the French husband belonged who, witnessing his young wife's infatuation for Franklin's society in Paris, finally made her a present of a *vase de nuit* in the bottom of which was stamped the face of the American savant.

LETTER TO FRANKLIN FROM ROBESPIERRE, ONE OF
THE LEADERS AND VICTIMS OF THE
FRENCH REVOLUTION.

WRITTEN WHEN HE WAS AN OBSCURE LAWYER. HE ASKS FRANKLIN
TO ACCEPT A COPY OF HIS PLEADING IN A CASE INVOLVING LIGHTNING
RODS, CALLING HIM "THE MOST ILLUSTRIOUS SAVANT IN THE WORLD."

*Reproduced by permission from the original manuscript in the
library of the University of Pennsylvania.*

Chapter XIV

The Era of Poor Richard

I

BENJAMIN has now reached a stage in which he is ready to launch his first public project for doing good to his fellow men.

The Junto has solidly established itself and has, by a process of fission, given birth to several other similar clubs called the Vine, the Union, the Band, etc. Young Benjamin's sagacious mind soon discerns the advantages that lie in this method of organization. The Junto remains the mother club, and to it the younger clubs are required to report what goes on at their meetings. Thus Benjamin has a rare opportunity for keeping in touch with public sentiment and also for influencing opinion when necessary.

The Junto has been able to move from its tavern quarters to a little room lent by Robert Grace. There books are often brought by members who wish to prove a point in a debate. Their gradual accumulation gives Ben an idea. He proposes that members club their books together so as to form a common pool or library which may be freely consulted by all. Accordingly one end of the room is soon filled. But after a time some of the books became damaged by careless use, and their owners withdrew them.

Ben then emerges with a scheme for a public subscription library. It is probably the offspring of his experience with Wilcox, the London bookseller, who permitted him, for a fee, to take out and return books. His keen observation of human nature teaches him to set about the project cannily.

Since he must ask for subscriptions, he carefully refrains from announcing the scheme as his own, but offers it as that of "a number of friends" who have asked him to present it to "lovers of reading." The method works. Though there are few genuine book-lovers in Philadelphia and though support is asked almost exclusively from comparatively poor young workingmen, about fifty persons are found who are willing to pay forty shillings down and ten shillings annually thereafter. Ben has a plan and rules drawn up in articles of agreement prepared by a conveyancer. The library is duly founded. The date is 1731. Since almost no books of value have yet appeared in America, the stock is imported from England. After many delays the books arrive from London, where they were purchased by Franklin's friend, Peter Collinson. In 1732 the library is opened for the giving out of books once a week. Franklin himself printed the first catalogue of them, for which he was exempted from dues for two years. In its second year he was also the librarian.

The Philadelphia Library was soon imitated in other towns and provinces. This gave Benjamin much pride. He wrote in his Autobiography:

"Reading became fashionable; and our people, having no public amusement to divert their attention from study, became better acquainted with books, and in a few years were observed by strangers to be better instructed and more intelligent than people of the same rank generally are in other countries."

Franklin himself used the library an hour or two every day. The founding of the library was his attempt to remove the peasant mind from himself and the American people.

II

Reading was the only diversion which Franklin was then permitting himself. He worked indefatigably, not only because he wanted to get ahead, but as he himself says, because it was necessary. He had a debt to pay off and a young family to care for and educate. He resorted neither to "taverns, games nor frolicks." He and Debby kept no servants and ran their house with the closest economy. His breakfast consisted of bread and milk, eaten out of a twopenny porringer with a pewter spoon. His printing business gradually forged ahead. His shop, under the ministrations of the tireless Debby, increased its stock until it included besides the usual stationer's supplies, soap, cheese, tea, coffee, " very good sack," and old rags. The laying in of a stock of pocketbooks was the herald of a new day. It meant that the inhabitants were beginning to carry paper money instead of loading themselves with bulky coin or depending on barter. The inflation of the currency which Franklin had advocated was having its effect. Prices had risen, but wages had risen to correspond, so no one worried. Philadelphia had added several thousands to its population. The numerous " To Let " signs on the houses, which had been conspicuous when Benjamin first arrived, were gone, and a general stir and bustle were visible. Franklin was able to thrive largely because the town was thriving too.

One day a significant event occurred in the Franklin household. Debby called her Benjamin to breakfast, and there on the table he found his bread and milk contained in a China bowl with a silver spoon. It was Debby's little surprise. She acknowledged that the new bowl and spoon had cost " the enormous sum of three-and-twenty shillings," but was proud of it. "She thought *her* husband deserved a silver spoon and China bowl as well as any of his neighbors." In short, Debby was resolved to keep up with the Joneses.

III

It is 1732. On February, 22 of this year a male infant is born at Bridges Creek, Westmoreland County, Virginia. His name is George Washington. George II is king of England. The first colony in Georgia is being founded. The Spaniards hold Florida, and the French are consolidating their grip on Canada and the valley of the Mississippi down to New Orleans. They are extending a line of forts southward and are incessantly being charged with inciting the Indians, who, seeing themselves being constantly pushed westward by land-hungry Englishmen, probably do not need much incitement to commit an occasional massacre, for which they invariably suffer frightful reprisals. But, generally speaking, it is a time of peace and hopefulness.

It is at this favorable moment that Franklin, at the age of 26, launches " Poor Richard's Almanac." His aim is the public good. " I considered it a proper vehicle," he says, " for conveying instruction among the common people, who bought scarcely any other books; I therefore filled all the little spaces that occurred between the remarkable days in the calendar with proverbial sentences, chiefly such as inculcated industry and frugality, as the means of procuring wealth, and thereby securing virtue; it being more difficult for a man in want, to act always honestly, as, to use here one of those proverbs, *it is hard for an empty sack to stand upright.*"

Virtue is the product, result, and concomitant of wealth. It was through the medium of " Poor Richard," then, that Franklin promulgated this dictum, which was accepted at the time by the American people and religiously believed in by their descendants for nearly a century and three-quarters, until the investigations into the operations of the great insurance companies of New York by Charles Evan Hughes created the first dim doubts as to whether virtue is necessarily and under all circumstances the daughter, by immaculate conception, of grandiose financial success.

Benjamin published the first advertisement for the almanac in his Pennsylvania *Gazette* on December 19, 1732, as follows:

"Just published, for 1733, An Almanack, containing the Lunations, Eclipses, Planets' Motions and Aspects, Weather, Sun, and Moon's Rising and Setting, High Water, etc.; besides many pleasant and witty Verses, Jests, and Sayings; Author's Motive of Writing, Prediction of the Death of his Friend, Mr. Titan Leeds; Moon no Cukold; Bachelor's Folly; Parson's Wine and Baker's Pudding; Short Visits; Kings and Bears; New Fashions; Games for Kisses; Katherine's Love; Different Sentiments; Signs of a Tempest; Death of a Fisherman; Conjugal Debate; Men and Melons; The Prodigal; Breakfast in Bed; Oyster Lawsuit, etc. By Richard Saunders, Philomat. Printed and Sold by B. Franklin."

Almanacs had been highly popular in the American colonies from the first, particularly in Pennsylvania, where agriculture predominated. In Philadelphia there were no less than seven. The best known of these was one issued by a solemn individual named Titan Leeds.

Benjamin had already learned that a new publication, to succeed, must be instantly talked about. In his very first issue he therefore perpetrates one of the hoaxes that he loves and announces the forthcoming death of this same Leeds.

"Inexorable death, who was never known to respect merit," says Poor Richard, "has already prepared the mortal dart, the fatal sister has already extended her destroying shears, and that ingenious man must soon be taken from us. He dies, by my calculation, made at his request, on October 17, 1733, 3ho., 29m., P.M. . . . By his own calculation, he will survive till the 26th of the same month. This small difference between us, we have disputed whenever we have met these nine years past; but at length he is inclined to agree with my judgment. Which of us is most exact, a little time will now determine. As, therefore, these Provinces may not longer expect to see any of his performances after this year, I think myself free to take up the task."

"Poor Richard" tickled the fancy of a public grown tired of the stodgy contents of the other almanacs. Three editions were sold out in a month. At fivepence a copy this brought a good profit to the fertile Franklin. He continued to publish the almanac successfully for twenty-five years.

Titan Leeds, as Ben expected, took Poor Richard's prediction seriously. He replied by calling him names and stoutly asserted that he would be alive and writing long after Poor Richard was dead.

Poor Richard on his next appearance declares that though there is no positive proof, it is hardly to be doubted that Titan is dead. "The stars only show to the skilful what will happen in the natural and universal chain of causes and effects; but 'tis well known that the events which would otherwise certainly happen, at certain times, in the course of nature, are sometimes set aside or postponed, for wise and good reasons, by the immediate particular dispositions of Providence; which particular dispositions the stars can by no means discover or foreshow. There is, however (and I cannot speak it without sorrow), there is the strongest probability that my dear friend is no more; for there appears in his name, as I am assured, an Almanack for the year

1734, in which I am treated in a very gross and unhandsome manner; in which I am called a false predictor, an ignorant, conceited scribler, a fool and a lyar. Mr. Leeds was too well bred to use any man so indecently and so scurrilously, and moreover, his esteem and affection for me was extraordinary; so that it is to be feared that pamphlet may be only a contrivance of somebody or other, who hopes, perhaps, to sell two or three years' Almanacks still; by the sole force and virtue of Mr. Leeds' name."

Incidentally Poor Richard seizes the occasion to rejoice in the success of his venture. His wife no longer has to borrow a cooking pot but can afford one of her own. " She has also got a pair of shoes, two new shifts, and a new warm petticoat; and for my part I have bought a second-hand coat, so good that I am not ashamed to go to town and be seen there. These things have rendered her temper so much more pacific than it used to be that I may say, I have slept more, and more quietly, within this last year, than in the three foregoing years put together."

This speech was well calculated to please the farmers, for it identified Poor Richard as one of themselves and also dealt with a domestic situation familiar at a period when overwork, hardship, and absence of comfort, drove many women into ill-temper, lunacy, or the grave.

IV

Poor Richard well reflects the manners, customs, and improprieties of the period. In England, whose social observances are quickly reflected in America, there has been a reaction against Cromwellian Puritanism. It is an era when the broad allusions of Fielding and Smollet in written literature, and Gay and Congreve in the drama, offend not even the most " refained " taste. This rhyme from Poor Richard well illustrates the humor of the 18th century:

" When Robin now three days had married been,
    And all his friends and neighbours gave him joy,
This question to his wife he asked then,
    Why till her marriage day she proved so coy?
Indeed, said he, 'twas well thou didst not yield,
    For doubtless then my purpose was to leave thee:
O, Sir, I once before was so beguil'd,
    And was resolved the next should not deceive me."

It is significant that in Pennsylvania, the western part of which, at least, was never successfully included in the Puritanic belt, the ancient and respected custom of " bundling " survived until comparatively recent times. Under such free if not easy conditions Franklin was able to give full play to his love for a very racy type of humor. This did not please all the Philadelphians any more then than it would now; indeed, Mr. S. G. Fisher, the historian, is authority for the intimation that for years after his death Franklin was regarded in upper-class Philadelphia circles as a repugnant old wretch, and in his day there were certainly many parlors into which he would not have been admitted unless previously disinfected.

The following jingle from Poor Richard's Almanac for 1744 is probably flavored by the bundling custom:

Biblis does solitude admire,
A wondrous Lover of the Dark:
Each night puts out her Chamber Fire,
And just keeps in *a single Spark;*
'Till four she keeps herself alive,
Warmed by her piety, no doubt;
Then tired with kneeling, just at five
She sighs — and lets that Spark *go out.*

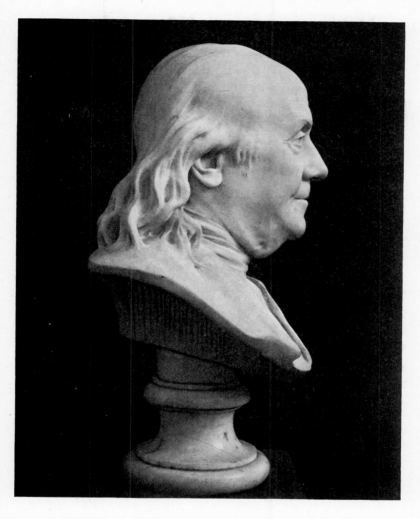

PROFILE OF BUST OF FRANKLIN BY HOUDON
IN THE METROPOLITAN MUSEUM OF ART, NEW YORK.

The italics are Benjamin's own. Ben was no poet — whatever poetry his nature originally possessed had long ago been stamped out by the stern practicality of his father's admonitions — but he was a versifier of no mean skill. The following pieces which appeared in Poor Richard from time to time will illustrate his wit, also the tastes of his subscribers:

Two or three frolicks abroad in Sweet May,
Two or three civil things said by the way,
Two or three languishes, two or three sighs,
Two or three *bless me's* and *let me dies,*
Two or three squeezes, and two or three tow-zes,
With two or three hundred pound spent at their houses,
Can never fail cuckolding two or three spouses.

Says Roger to his wife, my dear,
  The strangest piece of news I hear;
A law, 'tis said, will quickly pass
  To purge the matrimonial class;
Cuckolds, if any such we have here,
  Must to a man be thrown i' the river;
She smilingly cry'd — My dear, you seem
  Surprized; *Pray, han't you learn'd to swim?*

Old Batchelor would have wife that's wise,
  Fair, rich, and young, a maiden for his bed:
Not proud, nor churlish, but of faultless age,
  A country housewife in the city bred.
He's a nice fool, and long in rain hath staid;
  He should bespeak her, there's none ready made.

Poor Richard's prose humor, as exemplified in his prefaces to the almanac and in his numerous maxims, runs in a similar Rabelaisian vein. Explaining the duties of a star-gazer, " he spies perhaps *Virgo* (or the virgin), she turns her head as it were to see if any body observed her, then crouching down gently, with her hands on her knees, she looks wistfully for a while right forward. He judges rightly what she's about; and having calculated the distance and allowed time for its falling, finds that next spring we shall have a fine *April* shower."

Concerning eclipses, Poor Richard writes: " During the first visible eclipse Saturn is retrograde; for which reason the crabs will go sidelong and the ropemakers backward. The belly will wag before, and the —— shall sit down first."

These are some of his aphorisms:

" A ship under sail and a big-bellied woman, are the handsomest two things that can be seen common."

———

" After three days men grow weary of a wench, a guest, and weather rainy."

———

" You cannot pluck roses without danger of thorns, nor enjoy a fair wife without danger of horns."

———

" Neither a fortress nor a m——d will hold out long after they begin to parley."

v

Such pleasantries, however, were merely sprinkles of salt to make the full dish more savory. Franklin could never long resist being didactic, and the almanac gave him full opportunity to insert between the customary observations the wise saws and adages, most of them revamped from Bacon, la Rochefoucauld, and Rabelais, which made Poor Richard's name famous and for which Franklin is best known to the world at large even today. Some of them were:

Industry need not wish.
Forewarned, forearmed.
Diligence is the mother of good luck.
Keep thy shop and thy shop will keep thee.
Necessity never made a good bargain.
God heals, the doctor takes the fee.
There are three faithful friends, an old wife, an old dog, and ready money.
Fly pleasures and they'll follow you.
Let thy child's first lesson be obedience, and the second will be what thou wilt.
He that would have a short Lent, let him borrow money to be repaid at Easter.
Keep your eyes wide open before marriage; half shut afterwards.
As we must account for every idle word, so we must for every idle silence.
Let thy discontents be thy secret.
Let thy maid servant be faithful, strong, and homely.
Deny self for self's sake.
Love well, whip well.

This stock of canny maxims was greatly increased by the publication of " Father Abraham's Speech " in the Almanac for 1758. At this time the colonists of America were disgruntled because of the heavy taxes occasioned by the campaigns against the French and Indians. All sorts of schemes were proposed to remedy the hard times. Franklin's remedy was more thrift, and to emphasize his contention he put these remarks in the mouth of " Father Abraham," whose sermon he pretended had been overheard by Poor Richard at an auction:

The used key is always bright.

Early to bed, and early to rise, makes a man healthy, wealthy, and wise.

Industry pays debts, while despair increaseth them.

One today is worth two tomorrows.

The cat in gloves catches no mice.

Constant dropping wears away stones.

What maintains one vice would bring up two children.

He that goes a-borrowing goes a-sorrowing.

Experience keeps a dear school, but fools will learn in no other.

Fools make feasts and wise men eat them.

God gives all things to industry.

Lost time is never found again.

He that riseth late must trot all day.

Leisure is the time for doing something useful.

Three removes are as bad as a fire.

A small leak will sink a great ship.

Buy what thou hast no need of, and ere long thou shalt sell thy necessaries.

If you would have your business done, go; if not, send.

In Poor Richard's Almanac, then, was founded the great American Philosophy of Get-on. It was eagerly read and accepted throughout the colonies, and as " The Way to Wealth " was reprinted in many editions in foreign countries. Its maxims appeared in countless copybooks, over which young penmen toiled laboriously with small hands and moist tongues. To thousands it still recalls dismal memories of staying in after school. Poor Richardism gave to parents a bludgeon which they brought down upon the heads of all their children, regardless of their diverse natures, gifts, and predilections. It established a rock of philosophic materialism against which generations of sensitive craft beat in vain. It well nigh drove out from the spirit of the American people, all tendency to a love for leisure and a cultivation of the graceful arts, made its literature didactic and its art timid, and remained almost unchallenged until Walt Whitman hurled his shout across the roofs of the world: " I loaf and invite my soul."

VI

How to account for it?

Those who have followed Franklin's career in these pages thus far will readily see that his maxims, as aired by Poor Richard, are colored by his own experiences and difficulties up to the year 1732, when he first began to sight financial independence. Before that time he had never saved any money, never succeeded in any enterprise despite continuous hard work; never brought order into his affairs; and never lived either a moral or a regular life. When he married, became a father, and started a business, he changed his habits. He did so, because he had to. Out of this necessity he accordingly manufactured virtue, and began to preach the new gospel of work-and-save.

It was a gospel peculiarly suited to small tradesmen who were becoming employers and to farmers who wanted to grow out of tenantry into proprietorship. They took to Poor Richard's pawky teachings with avidity. And Franklin, who naturally wanted to sell his almanac, naturally gave them more and more of the same. Even in France, where Poor Richard was translated as *Bon Homme Richard,* his philosophy was eagerly accepted by the mercantile class, which had grown tired of monarchy and aristocracy, with their heavy taxes and weight on individual enterprise.

Did Franklin practice what he preached?

Yes, until he had acquired a comfortable fortune. He then as we shall see, gaily tossed overboard all his Poor Richardisms and mingled almost exclusively with the leisured class whose opportunities he had always envied, but from which he had previously been barred by the disease which Poor Richard lamented as " Lackomony." We shall see how he changed his habits shortly after he became forty years old, thus bearing out his own maxim: " At 20 years the will reigns; at 30 the wit; at 40 the judgment."

As Poor Richard he uttered this maxim:

" Women and wine, game and deceit,
Make the wealth small and the want great."

Compare this with a letter he wrote in 1761, when again in London, to his friend Hugh Roberts:

" For my own part, I find I love company, chat, a laugh, a glass, and even a song, *as well as ever.*" Our italics. We still have great respect for you, Benjamin, because of your geniality and mirth, your many abilities and achievements, but henceforth you must not expect us to regard you as the fount of all wisdom. Or of consistency.

VII

The profits from the *Gazette* and Poor Richard enable Benjamin to begin several new projects. He founds the first German newspaper in America, the *Philadelphische Zeitung;* publishes several pamphlets, chiefly sermons, and an occasional political tract; and imports fine books from England which he sells in his shop.

Hearing that a printer is wanted in Charleston, S. C., he sends one of his journeymen there and sets him up under a partnership agreement by which Franklin pays one third of the expense and receives one third of the profits. His protégé dies, but his widow, a Dutch girl, successfully continues the business, brings up a family on the profits, and eventually purchases the business from Franklin. This makes a deep impression on Benjamin. He at once decides that a knowledge of accounts is more important to young females than either music or dancing.

This experiment having worked out well, he backs other young journeymen in the same way and sends them to various provinces. " Most of them," he writes, " did well, being enabled at the end of our term (six years) to purchase the types of me, and go on working for themselves, by which means several families were raised. Partnerships often finish in quarrels; but I was happy in this, that mine were all carried on and ended amicably; owing, I think, a good deal to the precaution of having very explicitly settled in our articles every thing to be done by, or expected from, each partner, so that there was nothing to dispute, which precaution I would therefore recommend to all who enter into partnership."

It was this method of sending out young revenue producers that helped to lay the foundation of Franklin's fortune, which later invested in land, grew to considerable dimensions and enabled him to make an early retirement from money-making. For business he had an acquired rather than an innate taste, and he was glad to be rid of it.

He is in his 28th year when he pays his second visit to Boston, after an absence of about nine years. His parents are hale, with a good many more years to live. On his return, he stops at Newport to see his brother James. Poor James is weakened by ill health and is glad to be friends again with the younger brother, whom he was once accustomed to beat. He asks Ben to take home with him his small son and teach him the trade. After James's death Franklin does so, while the boy's mother, Anne, carries on the Newport printshop, with the help of her two daughters. They become skilled compositors and are probably the first women printers in America. When the boy is grown, Franklin supplies him with an outfit of new type. Thus does he repair one of the first of what he calls his " errata," in deserting James and running away to Philadelphia.

His increased leisure now enables Benjamin to take up the study of foreign languages. He learns French, Spanish, and Italian. He acquires facility in Italian by characteristic device. A friend who is also studying the language, knowing Ben's weakness for chess, entices him into many games. Ben finally refuses to play any more except on condition that the loser pay a forfeit by learning a new part of speech or doing a translation. Since their ability is about equal, they " beat one another into that language."

Soon afterwards Ben picks up a Latin Testament. He finds that he can read it fairly well. He is surprised; he thought he had forgotten all of the tongue he had learned as a boy in Boston. He concludes that the prevailing method of teaching ancient and modern languages is all wrong; that the modern, being easier, should come first and so prepare the way for the harder ancient tongues. But this is a reform against which the American school system braces itself resolutely, and decades elapse before the suggestion is adopted.

Chapter XV

First Ventures in Politics

I

BENJAMIN is 30 years old when his fellow citizens
recognize his merits by electing him to his first political post. He becomes clerk of the Pennsylvania
General Assembly without opposition. In the following
year a new member makes a speech against him in favour of
another candidate. Ben wins, but thereafter he keeps his eye
on the new member. He finds this gentleman is likely to
be a person of influence. He takes thought and hits upon a
typical scheme. He hears that this man owns a certain rare
and curious book. Ben therefore writes to him, politely requesting the loan of it. The owner sends it promptly. Ben
returns it in a week, carefully accompanying it with a letter of profuse thanks. The new member is touched. When
next he meets Ben, he speaks to him for the first time and
with great civility. He afterwards goes out of his way, to
do Ben other favours. From this Ben draws a sage con-
clusion:

" *He that has once done you a kindness will be more
ready to do you another, than he whom you yourself have
obliged.*"

It is at this moment that B. Franklin, politician, is born.

But whatever illusions he has about the thrills of par-
liamentary life are dispelled when he finds that, as Assembly clerk, he must be present and listen to hour upon hour
of tedious speeches emanating from unicellular egotists.

He is disappointed that so few members act with " a view to the good of mankind." He dreams of a " United Party for Virtue," to include the good and wise men of all nations. At other times he despairs of public life and beguiles the windy hours by figuring out " magical squares," causing the celebrated James Logan, William Penn's Secretary, to write to Peter Collinson in London:

" Our Benjamin Franklin is certainly an extraordinary man, one of a singular good judgment, but of equal modesty. He is clerk of our Assembly, and there, for want of other employment, while he sat idle, he took it into his head to think of magical squares, in which he outdid Frenicle himself, who published above eighty pages in folio on that subject alone."

In the same year Colonel Spotswood, the postmaster general, becomes dissatisfied with the accounts of Andrew Bradford, his deputy and Ben's competitor, and offers the place to Franklin, who instantly accepts. The pay is small, but the job greatly increases his facilities for gathering both news and advertisements. The circulation of the *Gazette* increases and so does its revenue. It is another sign that Ben has turned the corner of success.

B. Franklin, office-holder, now occupies an eminence from which he can observe the conduct of public affairs. He first proposes to reform the Night Watch, composed of a comic crew of ragamuffins under a guzzling constable given more to grafting than to guarding. Ben suggests that efficient men be hired and paid by taxing property-owners in proportion to the value of their possessions. This is the origin of the modern municipal system of police roundsmen.

He next organizes a volunteer fire company of thirty members, with leather bags for carrying water and bags and baskets for removing goods. As compensation for obliging the members to keep this equipment in good order, he provides a social evening once a month. Other companies spring up, finally giving rise to the Union Fire Company of Philadelphia.

Franklin's method of putting over these projects are the same in every case. He first prepares notes for a speech or paper before the Junto. Noting the effect on the members, he next publishes an article in the *Gazette*. If a scheme does not at once take hold, he lays it aside for a time, but firmly produces it later.

It was in this manner that he successfully launched an academy for the " compleat education of youth," which grew into the University of Pennsylvania, and brought about the formation of the American Philosophical Society, which has continued its honorable history down to the present day.

II

Now comes along a period of religious excitement into which Benjamin is drawn. He dislikes preachers as a class, but is always ready to exempt ingratiating individuals. For example, he has already taken part in the defense of Samuel Hemphill, a young Presbyterian, or rather Unitarian, preacher who came to Philadelphia from Ireland in 1734 and immediately brought on himself, because of his lack of dogma, the dislike of the orthodox. Hemphill vanished when it was discovered that he was repeating other men's published sermons, which he had committed to memory. As a result of the ensuing quarrel, Franklin left the congregation and never went back, though he continued his contributions for the support of the ministry.

In 1739 arrives, also from Ireland, the renowned George Whitefield. Ben at first holds aloof, but when the Philadelphia pastors begin to refuse Whitefield their pulpits, forcing him to preach in fields, Franklin is irresistibly attracted, and is soon helping Whitefield's supporters build a huge tabernacle as a free church.

Whitefield leaves Philadelphia for his historic visit to Georgia, where he finds helpless children perishing because their broken fathers are unable to make a living in the woods. Whitefield returns with a grand scheme for an orphan asylum down there. Franklin advises him to build it in Philadelphia and bring the children to it. Whitefield declines, so Ben refuses to contribute.

He goes to a Whitefield meeting one day, but with his mind made up to give nothing. The preacher begins his discourse, and Ben decides to give some coppers. The speaker adds some of the flowers of oratory and Ben thinks of giving some silver. Whitefield concludes in a glorious burst, and Ben empties his pockets, copper, silver and gold, and all.

Ben and the preacher became admiring friends. Whitefield used to pray for his conversion but in vain. Once Whitefield, after an absence, wrote that he was coming to Philadelphia but was not sure where he could lodge. Ben invited him to his home. The preacher wrote that if he had made his offer for Christ's sake, he should not fail of reward. Ben's historic reply was:

"Don't let me be mistaken; it was not for Christ's sake, but your own sake."

Franklin proves his admiration for the great preacher by bringing out his Sermons and Journals in four volumes. They are sold out in advance of publication.

In the same year, 1740, Benjamin announces another publishing venture — a magazine to be called "The General Magazine and Historical Chronicle for all the British Plantations in America." It is to be a novelty, in that no subscriptions are to be accepted. It is to be sold exclusively by " chapmen." This is probably the origin of the present-day news-stand magazine.

A quarrel breaks out between the editor-elect, John Webbe, and Franklin over a division of the prospective profits. Webbe goes over to Ben's old rival, Bradford, whose " Mercury " thereupon announces the forthcoming publication of a periodical to be called " The American Magazine, or A Monthly View of the Political State of The British Colonies." About this time the post-riders are forbidden to carry the " Mercury " any longer, and Webbe declares that Ben, as the deputy postmaster-general, is responsible for the order. " The American Magazine " beats Franklin's publication out by three days. But the former is dead in three months and the latter in six. The American colonists are not yet ready for a literary magazine.

The year 1740 beholds other broils of more consequence. War begins in Europe, and General Oglethorpe of Georgia, by laying siege to St. Augustine, begins a series of attacks which are eventually to drive the Spaniards out of Florida. Not many years longer are Americans to farm their clearings in peace.

Chapter XVI

The First Thrills from Science

I

ALL this time Benjamin continues his diligent studies at the Philadelphia Library. No matter what his duties, he spends an hour or two there every day, roaming through volume after volume. The library is growing steadily both in the number and quality of its books. Every year Peter Collinson sends over from London a well-selected assortment, and sometimes adds a few volumes of his own as a gift.

It can be imagined that one day Ben takes down from a shelf a large, well-printed book known as *Boyle's Lectures*. Robert Boyle was an English naturalistic philosopher and writer on religious topics, born in 1627 and dying in 1691. His book is a hodge-podge of observations dealing with natural phenomena and accounts of homely experiments, mingled with long theological discussions. The latter are tedious and meaningless, but his scientific observations are sharp, practical, and entertainingly described. It is evident that the good brother writes his religious essays as a kind of self-imposed duty, but that his real zest is reserved for his experimentations.

It is on record that Ben dipped into this book when he was a half-grown boy in Boston, and though it made a certain impression upon him, it is unlikely that he was able to grasp its contents fully owing to his extreme youth. Now, however, the book reawakens all his dormant curiosity.

Moreover, Boyle teaches him that the most exciting discoveries as to the workings of nature can be made simply by keeping one's eyes incessantly, open and by using apparatus no more elaborate than that which can be found in any well-equipped kitchen. From notes faithfully kept and compared, certain laws can be deduced and proved in the most thrilling manner.[1]

We can imagine that Ben goes home and sits down reflectively in front of the fireplace. It is of the good old, bad old type. It bakes the face and permits the back to freeze. It must be constantly fed with wood, which it burns wastefully. It sometimes has nervous fits, drawing badly and filling the room with smoke. Ben therefore resolves to begin with this the nearest thing at hand. The result is the invention of the Franklin stove, one of the first contrivances to banish barbarism from the American home and give it a civilizing comfort marvelled at by the world.

Franklin's reform was simple. He simply took the fireplace out of its deep recess where 99 per cent of its heat was bound to escape up the chimney and reconstructed it so as to cause it to warm the fresh air as it entered.

Franklin had no thought of making money from the invention. Experimentation in physical science was simply one of his methods of enjoying himself. He therefore presented the model to his friend Robert Grace, who owned a furnace. Grace immediately began to do a good business by casting plates for the stove. To promote the demand, Ben also wrote an advertising booklet entitled: " An Ac-

---

[1] Tending to confirm this supposition is the following verse from Poor Richard's Almanac for 1750:

" Still be your darling Sturdy Nature's laws;
And to its Fountain trace every Cause.
Explore, for such it is, this high Abode,
And tread the Paths which *Boyle* & *Newton* trod."

count of the new-invented Pennsylvania Fireplaces; wherein their Construction and Manner of Operation is particularly explained; their Advantages above every other Method of warming Rooms demonstrated; and all Objections that have been raised against the Use of them answered and obviated," etc.

Governor Thomas was so pleased with the stove that he offered to give Ben a patent on it, but Franklin declined on this ground: "that, as we enjoy great advantages from the invention of others, we should be glad of an opportunity to serve others by any invention of ours; and this we should do freely and generously."

A London ironmonger, however, did not scruple to steal the idea of the stove, and made changes in it — for the worse, and got a patent for it, from which he made a small fortune. "And this," wrote Franklin, " is not the only instance of patents taken out for my inventions by others, tho' not always with the same success, which I never contested, as having no desire of profiting by patents myself, and hating disputes."

A little later Ben, simply by noting the time of an eclipse with reference to a storm that swept over the Atlantic Coast, was able to determine that northeast storms, contrary to the popular notion, moved backwards against the wind from the southwest to the northeast. He also cuts a hole in his kitchen wall and places a little windmill there to turn the meat roaster. Unconsciously he is shaping his mind and sharpening his faculties for the discovery with which his name is to be associated for all time.

In 1744 is born Franklin's daughter Sarah. In the same year occurs the death of his father, the good but limited Josiah. About the same time son William ruptures the family inhibitions and runs away to sea. He gets as far as the deck of a privateer when father Benjamin descends upon

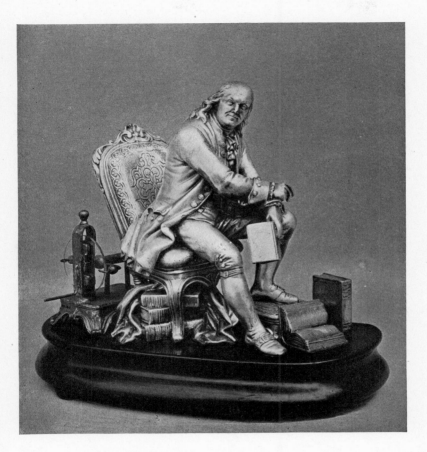

FRENCH STATUETTE OF CHINA BISQUE

SHOWING FRANKLIN SURROUNDED BY HIS BOOKS AND SCIENTIFIC
APPARATUS, AND WEARING HIS CHARACTERISTIC SHREWD SMILE.

From the Metropolitan Museum of Art, New York.

him and drags him back home again. Franklin's nephew and namesake, Benjamin Mecom, son of his sister Jane, is the next repressed Franklin to hear the call of the ocean wave. He is also brought back and placed as an apprentice in the New York shop of James Parker, one of Franklin's many partners. Franklin tries to soothe the fears of young Mecom's mother in the following letter:

"When boys see prizes brought in and quantities of money shared among the men, and their gay living, it fills their heads with notions, that half distract them, and put them quite out of conceit with trades, and the dull ways of getting money by working. This, I suppose, was Ben's case, the Catherine being just before arrived with three rich prizes; and that the glory of having taken a privateer of the enemy, for which both officers and men were highly extolled, treated, and presented, worked strongly upon his imagination. My only son, before I permitted him to go to Albany, left my house unknown to us all, and got on board a privateer from whence I fetched him. No one imagined it was hard usage at home, that made him do this. Every one that knows me, thinks I am too indulgent a parent, as well as master."

So quickly does the younger generation become the older. It has been only a very few years since Franklin was wanting to run away to sea himself.

II

We are come to the year 1745. November finds three men experimenting with a glass jar connected with a rude apparatus at the University of Leyden, Holland. They are professors Muschenbroek and Allemand and an amateur friend named Cuneus. They are trying to verify and extend the experiments of Gilbert, von Guericke, Hawksbee, and Dufay in exciting electric currents, thereby producing sparks and flashes. Several men have suspected that these flashes are the same nature as lightning, but nothing definite is known. The Dutch experimenters have progressed far in producing electricity by friction, but they have failed to find a method of collecting and retaining it. The power leaks away even as it gathers. Muschenbroek suspects that what is needed is a non-conducting container. He therefore fills a bottle half full of water. The water is a conductor, the glass a non-conductor. Into the water he dips one end of a wire leading to his friction machine. Nothing happens. Cuneus chances to touch the machine with one hand while the other is in the water. The result is a shock that not only runs around Mr. Cuneus but around the world. The first electric shock has been created by a man-made device. The two professors repeat the experiment and are promptly knocked out. There is no doubt that the workings of a mighty and hitherto mysterious force have been uncovered.

The Leyden jar instantly becomes the sensation of the scientific and near-scientific worlds. It is carried all over Europe and of course capitalized by fakers and itinerant medicine-men. Electricity is to cure all ailments, eradicate double chins, and restore lost hair. Mountebanks find the Leyden jar better than alchemy. It converts an invisible force into gold coin.

The next year Franklin pays a visit to his mother in Boston. While there he witnesses some astounding experiments performed with an electric tube which, when rubbed with buckskin, charges objects with electricity. Dr. Spence had brought the new apparatus over with him from Scotland. From that time on Benjamin is lost to all other worlds. He takes a tube sent him from London by Peter Collinson and has duplicates made at Philadelphia. With these Franklin enjoys some of the most exhilarating hours of his life.

"I never was before engaged," he wrote, "in any study that so totally engrossed my attention and my time as this has lately done; for, what with making experiments when I can be alone, and repeating them to my friends and acquaintance, who, from the novelty of the thing, come continually in crowds to see them, I have, during some months past, had little leisure for anything else."

Any task, however, which requires concentrated attention over a long period soon tires Franklin, and he suddenly turns from these engrossments to become the first Pennsylvania advocate of preparedness for war.

England's war with France has drawn in the American colonies, and a New England force has just taken the fort of Louisburg, on the island of Cape Breton. Part of the powder was furnished by the colony of Pennsylvania, under a grant of £3000 voted by the Quaker-dominated Assembly for the purchase, Franklin says, of "bread, flour, wheat and *other grain*."

A proposal is made to put Pennsylvania and Philadelphia in a state of defense. But the populace fails to become excited. Franklin then issues a pamphlet of 22 pages entitled "Plain Truth."

"What must be your condition," he said to the Philadelphia burghers, "if suddenly surprised, without previous alarm, perhaps in the night! . . . Your best fortune will be, to fall under the power of commanders of kings' ships, able to control the mariners, and so into the hands of *licentious privateers*. Who, can, without the utmost horror, conceive the miseries of the latter, when your persons, fortunes, wives, and daughters shall be subject to the unbridled rage, rapine, and the lust of negroes, mulattoes, and others, the vilest and most abandoned of mankind."

Franklin does not scruple to call in the help of his old
enemy, the clergy. He induces the Governor to appoint a
fast day, and himself writes the proclamation in New England style.

The agitation succeeds. A public meeting is called. Benjamin makes a speech, and several hundred young men sign
applications for membership in an association for defense.
In order to build a battery on the river front, Ben also proposes a lottery, which is successfully held. Not enough
cannon being available, Franklin is sent on his first diplomatic mission as a member of committee which goes to New
York to borrow some guns from Governor Clinton.

The Governor is at first obdurate; he says New York has
no cannon to spare. A dinner is held by the council. The
Governor attends. Some excellent Madeira wine is introduced. History does not say by whom; but possibly it was
no other than our sagacious Benjamin. The Governor
samples a little of the wine and sees the situation in a new
light. He thinks that after all New York can spare six
cannon to so good a neighbor as Pennsylvania. He quaffs a
few more bumpers and voluntarily raises the number to ten.
Before the evening is over, he has without solicitation offered eighteen, and is quietly removed by friends before he
strips New York's defenses bare and gives the entire contents
to Pennsylvania. The New York guns are soon transported
to Philadelphia and mounted. A nightly guard is posted, in
which Benjamin takes his turn as a common soldier, until
peace is signed at Aix-la-Chapelle.

B. Franklin, military man, is born, aged 41.

Before the war is over, however, Franklin has enough of
strutting up and down a barren and lonely earthwork and is
soon back at the fascinating sport of electrical experimentation. In this he is joined by Ebenezer Kennersley, Thomas
Hopkinson, and Philip Syng, who occasionally make experi-

ments on their own account. For this joint and simultaneous labor some authorities think that Franklin has received an undue amount of credit. However, Franklin arrived independently at what he called the " plus and minus," later known as the positive and negative, theory of electricity; and he never claimed that the group's momentous discovery that electricity is not created but only *collected* by friction, was his exclusively.. At any rate there was glory enough for all.

The year 1748 finds Benjamin no longer interested in printing, editing or publishing for commercial purposes. He therefore sells his printing office, almanac, and newspaper to his associate, David Hall, for £18000, payable in annual instalments of £1000. He already owns an estate bringing him an annual income equivalent to about $3500. His two political offices bring about $750 more. He retires with the assurance of an ample income for a good many years. He moves to the outskirts of the town at Second and Race Streets, near the Delaware.

So at the age of 42 Franklin rids himself of all business cares. Henceforth he means to devote himself to electricity, to enjoying himself, and to the public good.

CHAPTER XVII

The Challenge to the Clouds

I

FRANKLIN soon finds that his avowed plans for a life consisting entirely of philosophical studies and amusements are not approved by his fellow citizens. They have other uses for him. Wherever they find a vacant office they try to push Benjamin into it. The governor appoints him a justice of the peace. The Philadelphia corporation makes him a member of the common council and later an alderman. The citizens send him to the Assembly as a burgess.

As a judge Franklin is a failure. Court procedure bores him, and he finds excuses for withdrawing from it, pleading insufficient knowledge of the law. Being a legislator is more to his taste. He is re-elected again and again, for ten successive terms. He accepts each time, though never offering himself as a candidate. He has already made up his mind to adhere to this rule: "Never to ask for an office, never to refuse, and never to resign."

Son William, now about 20 years old, gets a job in the Assembly, too, as its clerk. Franklin does not say it was through his influence, but very likely it was. All his life Franklin looked out politically for his relatives. He was one of the earliest American exponents of nepotism.

II

At the first opportunity, however, Ben is back at the magnificent sport afforded by the fascinating jar from Leyden.

The faithful Peter Collinson has sent one over from London, and this is followed by a present to the Philadelphia Library Company of a whole set of electrical apparatus from Thomas Penn, one of the two sons of William Penn, who are the Pennsylvania Proprietaries. Meantime Franklin has bought the apparatus of Dr. Spence. With this equipment he and his friends contrive an electric battery with which they propose to send a spark through the Schuylkill River from bank to bank, using the water as a conductor. Ben's house is filled with curious idlers and headshaking skeptics. The older inhabitants predict the judgment of God on him, and when on two occasions he is knocked stonecold by rambling currents, they join in the age-old chant of " I told you so."

The phenomena which most absorb Benjamin's attention are the action of lightning and the cause of thunder. These have been mysteries since ancient days, and as far back as 1737 Franklin has mentioned them in the *Gazette*. The whole winter of 1747–1748 he gives to tests and speculations. Finally in 1749 emerges his first paper on the subject entitled " Observations and Suppositions towards forming a new Hypothesis for explaining the several Phenomena of Thunder-gusts." Later came his paper on " Opinions and Conjectures concerning the Properties and Effects of the Electrical Matter, and the means of preserving Buildings, Ships, etc., from lightning, arising from Experiments and Observations made at Philadelphia, 1749."

It is in the latter that he makes his first suggestion concerning experiments with lightning rods which are to " draw the electrical fire silently out of a cloud." Science for its own sake is all very well for some people, but not so for Benjamin the Yankee. He is not satisfied until he can put Science under the currycomb and lock her in the stable at night alongside the family cow and billygoat.

His conclusions he sent in a letter to Peter Collinson, dated July 29, 1750. The generous and loyal Collinson at once laid them before the Royal Society in London, whose members did little more than look down their noses and sniff. It was still the Age of Condescension in the mother country and gentlemanly English scientists were not going to be stampeded by any half-wild colonial. Growing impatient at their inaction, Collinson the next year published Franklin's papers in a pamphlet prefaced by Dr. John Fothergill, long one of Franklin's firmest friends.

A copy got to France and was promptly seized upon by Buffon, the natural philosopher, who procured its translation and publication. The French were delighted. From that moment Franklin's name in France became synonymous with interesting novelty. King Louis XV had every suggestion made by Franklin carried out in his presence on the grounds of the Duke d'Ayen. The French scientist Dalibard was actually the first man in the world to perform the Franklin experiment with an iron rod, thereby proving that electricity and lightning were identical. It was a month later before Franklin proved the same fact by drawing an electric current out of the clouds not with a rod but by means of the kite and key with which his name is associated for all time.

The experiment was performed on a June afternoon of 1752, in a pasture near what is now the corner of Fourth and Vine streets, Philadelphia. His only companion was his son William, who was not the fat urchin that illustrators of the alleged scene have loved to depict, but a grown young man. They sheltered themselves meantime under a cowshed. From instructions written by Franklin, we gather that his kite was made of a thin silk handkerchief fastened to a cross of cedar. From the top of the kite projected a pointed wire to act as the lightning-catcher. The conductor was the kite string of sleazy twine. Tied to the end of the twine and held in the hand was a silk ribbon, to act as a non-conductor and keep the current from shooting through the daring experimenter's body. Where the ribbon and twine joined, a key was fastened to act as a circuit breaker.

Let us try to reconstruct the scene. Father Benjamin, with Son William palpitating in the rear, goes out to the pasture on a sultry afternoon. Looms a beautiful thunder-head behind a breath of wind. It mutters in its throat and spits viciously between its red teeth. Straight up into its black face soars the tiny white kite. Nothing happens. There is a crack of thunder and a sprinkle of rain. The rain wets the kite and twine nicely, but Father Ben backs further under the shed so that the silk ribbon may be kept dry. He is put to it to keep the twine from touching the roof, knowing that otherwise there may be some fireworks not on the program. Still nothing happens. He wonders what is wrong. The cloud draws almost overhead. There is a moment of dense and racking silence. Then Benjamin, trying to show a fatherly calm before the nervous William, notices that the loose fibres of the twine are standing out straight. He runs a finger close to and parallel with them, but not touching them. The filaments wave to and fro. He holds his fist cautiously near the key. A dart of fire leaps out to his knuckles.

It is enough. They wait till the clouds pass and then pull down their kite and go home, probably to be scolded by Deborah for not having sense enough to come in out of the rain. There has been nothing astounding, nothing noisy. It has been a simple affair of a key and a kite and a cow pasture. In his *Autobiography* Franklin passes over his electrical experiments with the barest mention. But Franklin's kite did more than draw lightning quietly out of the clouds. It drew a dread from the cluster in the soul of man. It pulled one more superstitious fear from his imagination. It jerked one of the Genii from the threatening heavens and made him stand ready to spring into his collar at a lever's touch.

III

The world, its dramatic sense thrilled to the spine, rejoiced and ran for garlands. But on all occasions of public rejoicing, there must be at least one who stands apart from the feast. In France the Abbé Nollet not only pronounces Franklin's discovery all bosh, but proves to his own satisfaction that no such person ever existed. However, in that country there are other Abbés who wait to do him honor. And later two men humbly come forward to beg information about lightning and such things from the great Dr. Franklin. They do not know that one day they themselves will be known as the very sons of lightning. Their names are Marat and Robespierre.

Let us, however, keep the record clear. Franklin was not, as so many of his countrymen vaguely imagine, the discoverer of electricity. He simply dramatized it more successfully than any of his predecessors, and he later popularized it and helped to tame it. He showed more clearly than anyone that lightning was a mere manifestation of electricity, and that electric-laden clouds do not, as supposed, strike into the objects on the earth, but that the objects of the earth strike into electric-laden clouds. He achieved this by keeping his eyes open and then putting two and two together. Therein lay his superiority. Even today few are taught to keep their eyes open and fewer are capable of putting two and two together. He crowned his achievements by writing about them clearly and charmingly, using terms that even tyros could understand. We thus begin to comprehend the source of Franklin's fame: he could not only do things but get publicity for them.

Chapter XVIII
Projects Ripen and Increase

I

FRANKLIN'S nature could not endure long concentration on any one subject. His method of refreshing his mind was to skip gaily from one project to another, just as they bobbed up. In a single letter he was capable of mingling observations on politics, science, women's fashions, ventilation in bedrooms, and the price of beans, with entire unconcern. Even his *Autobiography* does not concern itself with continuity. It backs, fills, retreats, recollects itself, darts forward at increased speed, and then wanders off on by-paths only remotely connected with the subject in hand.

Hence it is no surprise to find him suddenly switching off his electric currents to go back to his scheme for an academy. He begins, as usual, by prodding up the Junto, interesting a few friends, and then printing a pamphlet entitled " Proposals relating to the Education of Youth in Pennsylvania." According to his Socratic method, he avoids mentioning it as a project of his own, but introduces it as that of " some public-spirited gentlemen." The scheme takes hold and the school is soon housed in the wooden tabernacle previously built for the Rev. Mr. Whitefield. By this time Franklin was experienced in the ways of religious sects, so to see that no one of them got the upper hand, it was provided that the trustees should consist of one representative of each Philadelphia sect. The Moravian one soon fell afoul of his colleagues. They waited patiently till he died and then refused to have another like him. A dispute arose as to the filling of the vacancy. To settle it, Franklin himself was chosen as " merely an honest man and of no sect at all."

The trustees having worn themselves out in these quarrels, they had no energy left to make the necessary changes in the building, so Franklin had to do the work himself, even purchasing the materials. Out of this academy, which was to be partly a " free school for the instruction of poor children," grew the present University of Pennsylvania, of which Franklin was a trustee for forty years.

From this occupation he suddenly plunges back into politics and becomes, with William Hunter of Virginia, postmaster-general of the colonies. Two commissioners being needed to negotiate a treaty with the Indians at Carlisle, the assembly chooses the speaker as one. The other is, of course, Franklin. The Indians open the solemn proceedings with a demand for rum. They are informed they will get none until the treaty is signed. The business is concluded with astonishing celerity. The Indians then receive their rum. They at once get howling drunk, humorously try to set fire to each other with brands plucked from a bonfire, and finish the day by coming to the commissioners' door at midnight with a thunderous demand for more rum. The next day they send three of their elder statesmen to make an apology. It was not they who did the cutting up, they said, but the rum. Franklin gives the substance of their speech as follows:

" *The Great Spirit, who made all things, made everything for some use, and whatever use he designed anything for, that use it should always be put to. Now, when he made rum, he said, ' Let this be for the Indians to get drunk with,' and it must be so.*"

It is not improbable that the waggish Franklin invented this speech himself. He has already been guilty of adding to the Book of Genesis a chapter with which he confounds the devout when he reads it to them aloud. It is not improbable, too, that out of this historic treaty made at Carlisle, on ground afterwards sacred to football, he drew the material for his caustic essay called "Remarks concerning the Savages of North America," one of the best pieces of writing he ever did and one in which the white man is proved to be no better than the savage whom he despises.

II

The next project to come before Franklin concerns a hospital for Philadelphia. One of his numerous medical friends, Dr. Thomas Bond, brings it up. He confesses that his personal efforts have had no success so far; everybody asks, " Have you seen Franklin about it, and what does he say? " Ben's interest is immediately won. He goes about the scheme with all the chuckling zeal of a conspirator. Finding that the rural members of the Assembly will not make a grant because of their jealousy of the city, he asks the legislators to appropriate 2000 pounds on condition that the city raises an equal amount. The device succeeds. The country members " now conceived that they might have the credit of being charitable without the expense," and the subscribers were told that each man's contribution would be doubled. " Thus," says Franklin triumphantly, " the clause worked both ways." So was created the Pennsylvania Hospital, which still stands.

" *I do not remember,*" adds Franklin, " *any of my political maneuvers the success of which gave me at the time more pleasure, or wherein, after thinking of it, I more easily excused myself for having made some use of cunning.*"

Such feats in money-raising are bound to draw the attention of the unsuccessful, and the next to come for help is the Rev. Gilbert Tennent, who wants to build a new meeting house for a group of Presbyterian dissenters. Benjamin flatly declines to give money or services, but offers advice instead. " Apply to all those," he said, " whom you know will give something; next to those whom you are uncertain whether they will give anything or not, and show them the list of those who have given; and lastly do not neglect those who you are sure will give nothing, for in some of them you may be mistaken." The preacher laughed but obeyed the advice; he got the church and more than enough money.

It is by similar methods, sometimes slow but always sure, that Benjamin finally induces the lethargic town to pave its filthy streets; to introduce street-cleaning; and to pattern after the example of one of its progressive citizens in placing a lamp at street doors, thus gradually " enlighting " all the city. The idea was John Clifton's, but the fertile Benjamin improved on it by inducing the town not to adopt the foul globe lamps of London, but to use his own invention of a four-sided lamp with a funnel above and air-channels at the bottom.

Franklin's efforts to find a better way of doing everything were not confined to cities alone. Having become prosperous enough to buy land near Burlington, N. J., he engaged in agricultural experiments concerning which he wrote long letters to friends. To show his fellow farmers how their soil would benefit from the application of lime, he sowed a field and then inscribed upon it in large white plaster letters: " THIS FIELD HAS BEEN PLAS-TERED." When the white letters disappeared, they emerged in a vigorous green visible at a distance. He procured samples of broom corn from Virginia and distributed the seeds among friends. He is said to have introduced the yellow willow from Europe. He encouraged the planting in Pennsylvania and Massachusetts of Rhenish grape vines. He made numberless experiments in soil-cultivation and manures. He defended this " attention to affairs of this seemingly low nature " by saying that " *human felicity is produced not so much by great pieces of good fortune that seldom happen, as by little advantages that occur every day.*"

He wrote to Whitefield: " For my own part, when I am employed in serving others, I do not look upon myself as conferring favors, but as paying debts. In my travels, and since my settlement, I have received much kindness from men, to whom I shall never have any opportunity of making the least direct return; and numberless mercies from God, who is infinitely above being benefitted by our services. Those kindnesses from men I can therefore only return to their fellow men, and I can only show my gratitude for these mercies from God, by a readiness to help his other children and my brethren."

It is greatly to Franklin's credit that he nowhere claims that his prosperity was due exclusively to his own efforts or to the " vision," " foresight," and " energy " which the obsequious ascribe to successful men. His willingness to return to his fellow men the equivalent of what he had derived from them indicates that by the time he had reached the middle forties he had become a genuinely civilized human being.

III

By now, Franklin's mother, Abiah, has attained a great age and is gradually failing, though the next year she writes that she still has " a pretty good stomach to my victuals." Addressing her as " Honoured Mother," he gives her some news of her grandchildren: " Will is now 19 years of age, a tall, proper youth and Much of a Beau. He acquired a

Habit of Idleness on the Expedition (to Canada). He imagined his Father had got enough for him, but I have assured him that I intend to spend what little I have myself. . . . Sally grows a fine girl, and is extremely industrious with her needle, and delights in her work. She is of a most affectionate temper, and perfectly dutiful and obliging to her parents, and to all."

It is this letter which closes with the celebrated remark of Franklin: " I would rather have it said, *He lived usefully,* than *He died rich.*"

When Abiah died in 1752, Franklin wrote to his sister Jenny: " I received yours with the affecting news of our dear good mother's death. I thank you for your long continued care of her in her old age and sickness. Our distance made it impracticable for us to attend her, but you have supplied all. She has lived a good life, as well as a long one, and is happy."

Franklin's memory does not seem to have received so strong a stamp from his mother as from his father. In his *Autobiography* she is barely mentioned, though his father's name is repeated many times. She seems to have been a serious-minded old lady and gazed upon the business of life rather grimly, not being cushioned with the sense of humor in which her agile son delighted. Possibly it was because one's sense of humor wears rather thin when spread over thirteen children.

IV

The next public service which Franklin examines with an eye to improvement is that of the post office. As joint postmaster-general for the colonies, he finds that current practices are slow and cumbrous. There is a mail between Philadelphia and New York only once a week. To exchange letters between Philadelphia and Boston sometimes

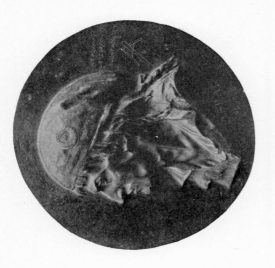

JEAN PAUL MARAT

LEADER OF THE FRENCH REVOLUTION AND VICTIM OF
CHARLOTTE CORDAY'S KNIFE, WHO ONCE ASKED FRANKLIN TO
PASS ON CERTAIN OF HIS SCIENTIFIC STUDIES.

*From a bronze plaque in the Metropolitan Museum of Art,
New York.*

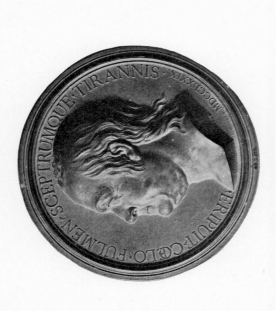

MEDALLION OF FRANKLIN BY NINI

CONTAINING THE FAMOUS SAYING IN LATIN REGARDING FRANK-
LIN ATTRIBUTED TO TURGOT: " HE HAS TORN THE LIGHTNING
FROM THE SKY; SCEPTRES FROM KINGS."

From the Metropolitan Museum of Art, New York.

requires six weeks. Post-riders go no farther north than Boston and no farther south than Charleston. In 1735 Franklin makes a tour of inspection and introduces several reforms. He creates the first penny-post known in the colonies. He straightens routes, puts on more riders, and in general speeds up the service. He opens the mail-bags to all newspapers and establishes the practice of advertising unclaimed letters. He materially increases the revenue, even up to the point where it is able to pay his own salary with a profit over. He is still engaged in this work when he is suddenly summoned to a great task.

He answers the summons laden with fresh honors. They are bestowed by Yale College, which makes him a Master of Arts, and Harvard, which recognizes him likewise.

Chapter XIX

Franklin's Humourous Year

I

BEFORE we take up the next phase of Franklin's career, a serious one in which he begins his first exercises in statecraft, we must retreat a little to the year 1745. This was one of Franklin's most mirthful years. There is a reason for it. All his various enterprises were prospering. His printery, his newspaper, his almanac and his shop were doing well and he was holding two political jobs which fattened his income. For the first time in his life, at the age of 39, he was under no money anxieties. He therefore could relax and utilize some of his increasing leisure time as he pleased. It was in this year that he wrote a few of his slyest productions. Belonging in this period is " Polly Baker's Speech," given in a previous chapter. In 1745 he wrote one of the letters which editors and biographers suppressed until the Philadelphia *Portfolio* printed it years later, in the course of an attack on Franklin for " hypocrisy." As addressed to James Read it follows:

" Dear J.

" I have been reading your letter over again, and since you desire an answer I sit me down to write you; yet as I write in the market, will I believe be but a short one, tho' I may be long about it. I approve of your method of writing one's mind when one is too warm to speak of it with temper: but being myself quite cool in this affair I might as well speak as write, if I had the opportunity. Your copy of Kempis must be a corrupt one if it has that passage as you quote, *in omnibus requiem quaesivi, sed non inveni, nisi in angulo cum libello.* The good father understood pleasure (*requiem*) better, and wrote *in angulo cum puella.* Correct it thus without hesitation."

Also in 1745 he wrote the letter to an unknown correspondent which has been called " Advice to a Young Man on the Choice of a Mistress." Like so many of Franklin's papers after his death, it was left to remain in an accumulating pile of junk until Henry Stevens, of Vermont, a bibliophile long resident in London, bought it along with a mass of other Franklin documents and kept it until in 1881 he sold his collection of Franklin manuscripts to the United States government for $35,000. It is now in the possession of the State Department at Washington. Certain writers and biographers have listed it or hinted at its existence in such a way as to excite a curiosity which they might as well have allayed. Since the letter is in a sense a public document which helps to reveal Franklin just as he was, there is no longer any reason for not publishing it in full. It follows here just as Franklin wrote it, with f's used to indicate the old-fashioned " s ":

To   PHILADELPHIA, 25 June, 1745
MY DEAR FRIEND:

I know of no medicine fit to diminifh the violent natural inclinations you mention; and if I did, I think I fhould not communicate it to you. Marriage is the proper remedy. It is the moft natural ftate of man, and therefore the State in which you are moft likely to find folid Happinefs. Your reafons againft entering into it at prefent appear to me not well founded. The circumftantial Advantages you have in view by poftponing it, are not only uncertain, but they are fmall in comparifon with that of the Thing itfelf, the being married and fettled. It is the Man and Woman united that make the compleat human Being. Separate, She wants his Force of Body and Strength of Reafon; he, her Softnefs, Senfibility and acute Difcernment. Together they are more likely to fucceed in the World. A fingle man has not nearly the value he would have in the State of Union. He is an incomplete Animal. He refembles the odd half of a pair of Sciffars. If you get a prudent, healthy Wife, your Induftry in your Proffeffion, with her good Economy, will be a fortune fufficient.

But if you will not take this Counfel and perfift in thinking a Commerce with the Sex inevitable, then I repeat my former Advice, that in all your Amours you fhould prefer old Women to young ones.

You call this a Paradox and demand my Reafons. They are thefe:

1. Becaufe they have more Knowledge of the World, and their Minds are better ftored with Obfervations, their Converfation is more improving, and more laftingly agreeable.

2. Becaufe when Women ceafe to be handfome they ftudy to be good. To maintain their Influence over men, they fupply the Diminution of Beauty by an Augmentation of Utility. They learn to do a thoufand Services fmall and great, and are the moft tender and ufeful of Friends when you are fick. Thus they continue amiable. And hence there is hardly fuch a thing to be found as an old Woman who is not a good Woman.

3. Becaufe there is no Hazard of Children, which irregularly produced may be attended with much Inconvenience.

4. Becaufe through more Experience they are more prudent and difcreet in conducting an Intrigue to prevent Sufpicion. The Commerce with them is therefore fafer with regard to your Reputation. And with regard to theirs, if the Affair fhould happen to be known, confiderate People might be rather inclined to excufe an old Woman, who would kindly take care of a young man, form his Manners by her good counfels, and prevent his ruining his Health and Fortune among mercenary Proftitutes.

5. Becaufe in every Animal that walks upright, the Deficiency of the Fluids that fill the Mufcles appears firft in the higheft Part. The Face firft grows lank and wrinkled; then the Neck; then the Breaft and Arms; the lower Parts continuing to the laft as plump as ever: fo that covering all above with a Bafket, and regarding only what is below the Girdle, it is impoffible of two Women to know an old one from a young one. And as in the dark all Cats are grey, the Pleafure of Corporal Enjoyment

with an old Woman is at leaſt equal, and frequently ſuperior; every Knack being, by Practice, capable of Improvement.

6. Becauſe the Sin is leſs. The debauching a Virgin may be her Ruin, and make her for life unhappy.

7. Becauſe the Compunction is leſs. The having made a young Girl miſerable may give you frequent bitter Reflection; none of which can attend the making an old Woman happy.

8th & laſtly. They are ſo grateful ! !

Thus much for my Paradox. But ſtill I adviſe you to marry directly; being ſincerely

Your affectionate Friend,

BENJAMIN FRANKLIN

Not even this writer, however, has the hardihood to include another of Franklin's suppressed documents. It is known as the letter " On Perfumes." It is supposed to have been addressed to the Royal Academy of Brussels and was intended as a satire on the fatuous activities of most of the scientific societies of the time. It does not deal, as not a few of Franklin's letters did, with the fact of sex in a manner sportive and jocund, but with Rabelaisian gravity lays certain proposals before the Belgian academicians regarding the creation of gases within the human system during the processes of digestion. The title of the paper suggests the nature of Franklin's remedy.

" Let it be considered," writes Franklin, " of how small importance to Mankind, have been useful those Discoveries in Science that have heretofore made Philosophers famous. Are there twenty men in Europe at this day the happier, or even the easier, for any knowledge they have pick'd out of Aristotle? What Comfort can the Vortices of Descartes give to a Man who has Whirlwinds in his Bowels? " . . .

II

Few of the biographers and commentators on Franklin's life have been able to stomach all his writings. In some cases their prudish omissions have amounted to a deliberate falsification of the genuine records. William Temple Franklin, who edited the original edition of the Autobiography, tried to alter his grandfather's short and Saxon words into a stilted phraseology of his own. The Rev. Mason Weems' life of Franklin is a collection of fairy tales. Jared Sparks, one of the earliest and most devout of biographers, could not bring himself to print the word " belly " when it occurs in Franklin's papers, but omitted it in a way that frequently changed the sense of a passage. Albert H. Smyth, the most faithful compiler of Franklin's documents, omits reference to the letter " On Perfumes," and even the blunt Sydney George Fisher fails to give the whole of " The Choice of a Mistress." Senator William Cabell Bruce [1] gives quotations accurately, but cannot refrain from accusing his subject of " moral squalor." None, however, reaches the height of prunes-and-prisms indignation attained by Charles Francis Adams, who says: " The errors of Franklin's life may be detected almost anywhere in his familiar compositions. They sprang from a defective early education which made his morality superficial to laxness, and under-mined his religious faith." [2] Even Thomas Jefferson wrote: " There are defects in the life of that great man which it is not wise to palliate or excuse." [3]

The present age, however, is one less hostile to facts. It is willing to regard a man as great despite human shortcomings. It believes with Oliver Cromwell that a portrait should include all the warts.

[1] Benjamin Franklin Self-revealed.
[2] Life of John Adams.
[3] Writings of Jefferson, edited by H. A. Washington.

CHAPTER XX

Army General and Ambassador

I

IN 1753 the American colonies hear the preliminary rumblings of the Seven Years' War which is enormously to extend the boundaries of England's empire, humiliate and weaken France, and bring Prussia into the European picture with a doughty boldness which is eventually to frighten the world into the convulsion of 1914–1918.

The Americans, being patriots all, prepare to fight for England's claim to the valley of the Mississippi. They hasten to make peace with all the Indian tribes which are not already on the side of the French, in order to prevent the latter from cutting them off from the vast tract of fertile land just granted by George II to the Ohio Company. Under this pressure the colonies make their first attempt at union. A conference is called by the English Lords of Trade to make defensive arrangements with the Six Nations. Seven colonies send delegates to Albany, New York, in June, 1754. The Pennsylvanians are John Penn, Richard Peters, Isaac Norris, and Franklin. There for the first time Franklin meets Thomas Hutchinson, of Massachusetts, with whom later he is to have something to do.

Franklin is all for union. He publishes in his *Gazette* a rough picture of a snake cut into seven pieces, having the caption " Join or Die." He submits a scheme which is to comprise all the provinces under one government, afterwards known as the Albany Plan of Union. After noisy debate, the delegates approve it unanimously. They go home feeling that they have taken the first great step towards American unity. But to their astonishment, officialdom is cold. The various colonial assemblies think the plan concedes too much to the prerogative of the King, while in England it is deemed dangerously democratic. The English Lords of Trade refuse even to consider it, but counter with a plan of their own.

In Boston Governor Shirley shows him a copy of it. Franklin at once detects a poisonous clause in it. It provides that the defense of the colonies shall be in the hands of a council of the various governors and that the expenses of war shall be repaid to the English treasury through a tax laid by Parliament. At that instant Franklin becomes one hundred per cent patriot. In letter after letter he assails the proposal for a tax laid in a mother country ignorant of American conditions.

" Compelling the colonies to pay money without their consent," he writes, " would be rather like raising contributions in an enemy's country, than taxing of Englishmen for their own public benefit; it would be treating them as a conquered people, and not as true British subjects."

This visit to Boston, however, withdraws the sting from old wounds. The Hub's citizens show him marked respect, causing him to write to Catherine Ray, one of those feminine correspondents whom he had begun to acquire, of his " unwillingness to quit a country in which I drew my first breath, spent my earliest and most pleasant days, and had now received so many fresh marks of the people's goodness and benevolence, in the kind and affectionate treatment I had everywhere met with."

This letter he closes with one of his gallant tributes:

" Persons subject to the *hyp* complain of the northeast wind, as increasing their malady. But since you promised to send me kisses in the wind, and I find you as good as your word, it is to me the gayest wind that blows, and gives me the best spirits. I write this during a northeast storm of snow, the greatest we have had this winter. Your favors come mixed with the snowy fleeces, which are as pure as your virgin innocence, white as your lovely bosom, and — as cold. But let it warm towards some worthy young man, and may Heaven bless you both with every kind of happiness."

II

There ensues a period of wrangles between governors and assemblies as to the raising of funds for defense. Governor Hamilton quits Pennsylvania and is succeeded by Morris, a character whom Franklin afterwards wrote about lovingly. He counsels Morris not to dispute with the Assembly.

"My dear friend," says Morris, "how can you advise my avoiding disputes? You know I love disputing; it is one of my greatest pleasures."

Later Franklin as a legislator is drawn into these broils and assists in writing tart and even abusive letters to the governor. Morris remains genial. He meets Franklin in the street one day and takes him home to have a laugh over a glass of wine with a merry company. Morris remarks that he admires Sancho Panza, "who, when it was proposed to give him a government, requested it might be a government of *blacks*, as then, if he could not agree with his people, he might sell them."

"Franklin," asks a member of the company, "why do you continue to side with these damned Quakers? Had you not better sell them?"

"The governor," says Franklin, "has not yet *blacked* them enough."

Morris lasts only for a time. He is succeeded by Denny. Meantime Massachusetts proposes to attack the French fort at Crown Point. Edmund Quincy comes down to ask help from Pennsylvania. The governor refuses his assent to a grant of ten thousand pounds unless the estates of the Proprietaries and their hangers-on are exempted from tax. Franklin is compelled to get the money from the provincial loan office.

" These public quarrels," he wrote, " were all at bottom owing to the Proprietaries, our hereditary governors, who, when any expense was to be incurred for the defense of their province, with incredible meanness instructed their deputies to pass no act for levying the necessary taxes, unless their vast estates were in the same act expressly excused."

III

From these activities Franklin is diverted by the arrival in Virginia of a worthy but fatuous individual who has been sent from England to show the colonials how to fight. It is General Edmund Braddock. A man less fitted for his mission was never selected by any ponderous governmental machine. He is to lead one wing of a tripartite expedition against the French and their Indian allies. With his two regiments of regular British troops, assisted by forces from Maryland and Virginia, the latter under the young Colonel George Washington, he is to attack and take Fort Du Quesne, on the site of what is now Pittsburgh.

On landing at Alexandria, Braddock marches to Fredericktown, Maryland, where he halts and vents two loud complaints, one against his government for sending him into such a horrible country without proper supplies, and the other against the American provinces for not having ready the 150 wagons necessary for moving his baggage. The

General does not know that few American farmers are able to own such a luxurious article as a wagon.

Franklin, under the guise of perfecting postal communications, is sent down to mollify him. He takes along his son William. On the journey Franklin leaves the road to make some scientific observations regarding the curious conduct of a whirlwind. He rides along with it for nearly a mile, vainly attempting to break it by striking through it with his whip. He afterwards wrote Peter Collinson a long letter about it. Franklin asked his host if such whirlwinds were common in Maryland. The reply was, "Not at all common; but we got this on purpose to treat Mr. Franklin."

On reaching Braddock's tent, Franklin finds the General, red with spleen and prejudice, cursing Virginia and Maryland because they have sent him but 25 wagons. Franklin ventures to remark that Pennsylvania might do better. Braddock turns to him eagerly.

"Then you, sir, who are a man of interest there, can probably procure them for us; and I beg you will undertake it."

It is this meeting which is described in Thackeray's novel, "The Virginians." Franklin is referred to there as "the little postmaster of Philadelphia."

Franklin undertakes the commission, and by appealing to the cupidity and fears of the farmers of Lancaster, York and Cumberland counties in a series of advertisements, raises a complete outfit of horses, wagons, and drivers within twenty days. He is compelled to advance heavy sums out of his own pocket to do so, and in addition to sign bonds.

Braddock now expands and begins to treat Franklin almost as an equal. He even invites him to dinner.

"After taking Fort Du Quesne," he says complacently, "I am to proceed to Niagara; and having taken that, to Frontenac, if the season will allow, and I suppose it will;

for Du Quesne can hardly detain me above three or four days; and then I see nothing that can obstruct my march to Niagara."

Franklin and Col. Washington warn him against possible Indian ambushes. They urge him to throw out an advance screen of friendly Indian scouts, about a hundred of which have been procured for him. Braddock smiles indulgently; are not his advisers aware that the brunt of the battle is to be borne by regular British troops, dressed in gaiters and scarlet tunics?

" These savages may, indeed, be a formidable enemy to your raw American militia, but upon the king's regular and disciplined troops, sir, it is impossible that they should make any impression."

The sequel is sufficiently known. Within a few miles of the fort Braddock's army is attacked by invisible foes on front and flanks. His officers, with their train of pack horses laden with beautiful spare uniforms, are wiped out. His huddled soldiers are riddled. His secretary is killed. As yells of panic arise and horses are cut loose from their traces, the general himself falls mortally wounded. The whole campaign ends in a fiasco. The owners of the teams sue Franklin for their losses. His claims are not settled till months afterward, and he never collects the full amount due him.

Braddock dies saying, " Who would have thought it? " But he has meanwhile spoken a good word to London about Franklin's able efforts, and when Thomas Penn complains to the Secretary of State that Franklin " is not to be depended upon to assist in promoting the public service," he receives small attention.

The Braddock defeat leaves Franklin in a thorny situation and for a time he is called ugly names. The farmers are enraged at the conduct of their defenders from overseas, who have plundered and stripped the countryside, leaving some poor families ruined and humiliated. They pour in their claims until Franklin finds himself obligated in the sum of 20,000 pounds, to pay which would have ruined him. No wonder he afterwards wrote:

"*There never was a good war, or a bad peace.*" [1]

But when public opinion veers and the Assembly gives him a vote of thanks, he is again in good humor.

When Catherine Ray writes him in this same year, 1755: "How do you do? What are you doing, Does everybody still love you? And how do you make them do it? " he replies:

. . . "As to the second question, I must confess (but don't you be jealous) that many more people love me now than ever did before: for, since I saw you I have been enabled to do some general services to the country, and to the army, for which both have thanked and praised me, and say they love me. They say so, as you used to do; and if I were to ask any favors of them, they would, perhaps, as readily refuse me; so that I find little real advantage in being beloved, but it pleases my humor."

IV

Braddock's downfall brings about a renewal of the quarrel between the Proprietaries and the Pennsylvania Assembly. The Indians, heartened by success and athirst for revenge, massacre settlers within 80 miles of Philadelphia. Bethlehem, Lancaster, and Easton are threatened. The agitation for defense arises to fever heights, but the Proprietaries remain firm on one point. Whatever lands are taxed, theirs are to be exempted. But finally Franklin, by sending word to England of their meanness, attacks the

[1] Letter to Josiah Quincy, Sept. 11, 1783.

Penns in the rear. They give way — partly, and offer to add 5000 pounds to any sum appropriated by the Assembly. As the Indian depredations have increased, the Assembly temporarily waives a tax on the proprietary estates, and votes 60,000 pounds. Franklin is appointed on the commission to spend it.

He prepares a bill for raising volunteers. It exempts the Quakers. Non-Quakers resent this and declare they will not enlist. Franklin takes a hand in the controversy by publishing in the *Gazette* " a Dialogue between X, Y, and Z concerning the present State of Affairs in Pennsylvania."

Says Z: " I am no coward, but hang me if I fight to save the Quakers."

X replies: " That is to say, you will not pump ship because it will save the rats as well as yourself."

The dialogue closes with an appeal to all parties to " unite in our country's cause, in which to die is the sweetest of all deaths, and may the God of armies bless our honest endeavors."

As the volunteers come forward, word comes of a massacre at the Moravian village of Gnadenhutten, in Northampton County. The governor asks Franklin to accept a military commission and proceed there to protect what remains of the inhabitants. Franklin accepts and becomes General Franklin. As his aide he selects his son William. Fortified by stout wraps knit by the faithful Deborah, the General leads his little army northward through the frozen forest. They are a month covering ninety miles. He puts heart and a yearning for cash into his volunteers by offering $40 for each Indian scalp, " produced with proper Attestations," and a gill of rum each per day, served half in the morning and half in the evening.

They prove to be earnest soldiers, and are prompt in attending to everything except divine service. The chaplain complains about it.   Franklin make one of his canniest suggestions:

" Deal out the rum just after prayers."

The worthy brother, seeing a great light, accepts the job as bar-tender, assisted by a few willing hands.

" Never," says Franklin sententiously, " were prayers more generally and more punctually attended."

He finds the situation at Gnadenhutten serious enough. It has been burnt down.   Around the silent ruins lie bodies gnawed by animals.   He sets to work to fortify the place, which he names Fort Allen.   He is strengthened in this task by supplies arriving from Deborah, who well knows the way to a general's heart.   They consist of roast beef, roast veal, apples, and that foundation stone of American liberty, mince pie.   The men get along on salt pork and bread.

Their commander notices something curious about his soldiers.   When they are at work they are good-natured, and spend their evenings in cheerful conversation and song, but when the weather compels them to remain idle, they become quarrelsome and fault-finding.   This reminds Franklin of a sea captain whose one aim was to keep his men at work.   One day when the mate reported that all tasks had been completed and there was nothing more for the men to do, the captain's reply was prompt:

" *Oh, make them scour the anchor.*"

Within two months Franklin has enough of military service.   When a Col. Clapham arrives to visit the fort, General Franklin hastily bestows on him his commission and returns to Philadelphia, to which he has been summoned on account of new quarrels with the Proprietaries.   At home he is acclaimed as a great leader, and the governor urges him to lead an army against Fort Du Quesne.   This Franklin modestly declines.   However, he accepts an honorary post as colonel to a new Philadelphia regiment, which boasts of six brass field-pieces. It parades in his honor and even follows him home. As a parting salute it fires several rounds in front of Franklin's door with such enthusiasm that they shake down his electrical apparatus and break the glasses.

v

In 1756 the continuous disputes between the Assembly and the governor, who acts in all cases as the deputy of Thomas and Richard Penn, reach a crisis.

The Penns have become more and more arrogant. Though under the terms of the grant of 26,000,000 acres made to their father, they have become the possessors of an estate worth $50,000,000 they still refuse to submit to taxation for defense against the Indians, saying " that is no affair of ours." At last they signify that they will receive no more direct addresses from the legislature. Franklin then attacks them in his most outspoken and satiric fashion. This draws on him the ill-will of the Philadelphia upper-class, then almost entirely Tory in sentiment. They virtually impose a social boycott on Franklin and his family. Washington, Jefferson, and Hamilton in their day are entertained in Philadelphia drawing-rooms, but never Franklin.

Finally the Assembly, tired of the rows with Governor Denny, passes a bill designed to raise funds by an excise on wine, rum, and brandy. They suppose this will be unobjectionable. But the governor refuses his assent, saying that he is bound to do so by his instructions, meaning those of the Penns in England.

The assemblymen attempt no further measures, but vote to present their grievance against the Penns to the king himself. They name two commissioners to go to England for this purpose. They are the Speaker, A. Isaac Norris,

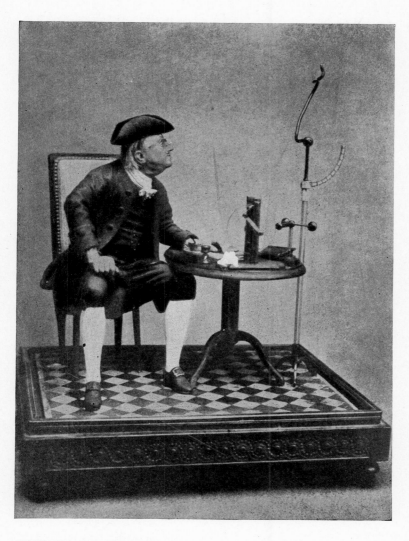

FRENCH STATUETTE BY NINI OF FRANKLIN EXPERI-
MENTING WITH HIS ELECTRICAL APPARATUS

and Franklin. Norris declines owing to his age, and Franklin offers to go alone. To pay his expenses, the sum of 1500 pounds is voted. Franklin at once prepares to sail, taking along the inevitable William.

He sends his stores to be put on board a ship at New York, but before he departs, Lord Loudoun, commander in chief of the British forces in America, arrives to have a word with him.

This noble lord was one of the most ludicrous figures ever inflicted by a British government on a meek and prayerful colony. In character he was a combination of Sir William Keith and General Braddock, but having the likable qualities of neither. Franklin wondered " how such a man came to be intrusted with so important a business." The only proper place for him would have been in the middle of a Gilbert and Sullivan comic opera.

Loudoun asks the governor and Franklin to meet him in conference. There he requests Franklin to help him patch up an understanding. Franklin yields and prepares a new bill for the Assembly, which is passed with the assertion that the province thereby yields none of its rights. Triumphantly his lordship sails away, blandly accepting all the credit for Franklin's work. Meantime the ship at New York has sailed with Franklin's stores on board.

He finds another ship early in April. But since it cannot sail without Lord Loudoun's permission, it remains in the Hudson until nearly the end of June, awaiting his lordship's dispatches. For eleven weeks of warm weather this noble cunctator keeps Franklin kicking the sides of his ship. At last permission is grandly given and Franklin's ship, with two other packets, is requested to join the English fleet waiting outside and attend Loudoun's ship until he writes a certain letter. Five days pass before his lordship's letter is ready and Benjamin's ship can steer for England. Meantime his lordship sails on to Louisburg, which he is to beseige; but he changes his mind, turns around and sails right back again, bringing with him the whole fleet with its troops on board and the two packets, with its passengers, which were to have sailed with Franklin's ship to England.

Franklin is five months reaching Falmouth from Philadelphia, but the actual crossing occupies only about 30 days. His ship is slow at first but picks up speed noticeably after her human and other freight have been shifted aft. This incident sets Franklin wondering whether more attention should not be paid to the scientific loading and sailing of ships. He afterwards prepares a paper on the subject.

Off Falmouth harbor the ship barely escapes crashing into rocks on which rests a lighthouse. Its glare saves them in time. When they land the next day, Franklin breaks his usual habit and goes to church. He gives thanks for being alive. He also vows to promote the building of lighthouses in America when he returns. He thinks that will be soon. He does not know he will not see home again for five years.

CHAPTER XXI

Conquests in England

I

IT was doubtless a contented Franklin who looked out on the streets of London on the morning of July 27, 1757. Thirty years previously he had left the murky old town as an unknown and unsuccessful youth. He now returns with his head held high. Men distinguished in science, literature and politics hasten forward to do him honor. He is a guest at the splendid home of Peter Collinson. Come Dr. Fothergill, author of the preface to the London pamphlet on Franklin's electrical experiments; Governor Shirley of Massachusetts; William Strahan, printer and publisher to Dr. Samuel Johnson, who is glad to welcome his best American customer; and finally, grinning slyly, James Ralph, Benjamin's erstwhile chum. Ralph lets it be known that he has done rather well for himself. He is a political writer selling his services for fat fees, has had the patronage of the Duke of Bedford, and has been honored by a denunciation in Pope's Dunciad.

To make himself comfortable while he waits to hear from the Penns, Franklin, with " Billy " and a white and a negro servant, finds quarters at No. 7 Craven Street, between the Strand on one side and the Thames on the other. The house is kept by Mrs. Margaret Stevenson, who at once makes the philosopher so comfortable that in later years he was never able to speak of her housekeeping without a sigh. Mrs. Stevenson's home has another great attraction — her lively daughter, Mary, better known as " Polly."

With mother and daughter Franklin maintained a life-long friendship and correspondence. For them he did some of his sprightliest bits of writing, and for years they were delighted to make the whole household revolve around the great and jocund American.

It becomes quickly evident to Franklin that he may as well make himself comfortable, for the very first statement made to him by an English statesman indicates that he has a long fight ahead. Lord Granville, to whom he is taken, informs him that the king's instructions to his governors in America are " the law of the land, for the king is legislator of the colonies."

Franklin is taken aback. " I told his lordship," he writes, " this was new doctrine to me."

His first meeting with the Penns is at Thomas Penn's house in Spring Garden. They propose that he put in writing the substance of the Pennsylvania Assembly's grievances. He does so. They hand the paper to their solicitor, one Paris, who treats Franklin with such haughtiness that Franklin announces he will deal in future with no one but the two principals. Their reply is sent not to Franklin but to the Assembly. It complains of Franklin's rudeness and demands that the Assembly send as their envoy " a person of candour."

Tedious delays convince Franklin that he will get nowhere with the stiff-necked Penns, and he turns his attention to the English politicians. He has little better success. Politicians are preoccupied with bigger games; they have no time for remote and insignificant little America. William Pitt, the Great Commoner, refuses even to see him. Pitt is too busy enjoying the adulation heaped upon him for the British victories over the French in Canada and India.

" I admired him at a distance," writes Franklin, " and made no more attempts for a nearer acquaintance. I had only once or twice the satisfaction of hearing, through Lord Shelburne, and, I think, Lord Stanhope, that he did me the honor of mentioning me sometimes as a person of respectable character."

Meantime Franklin is stricken with a severe illness, which keeps him in bed for eight weeks. His friend Dr. Fothergill tenderly ministers to him with horrible infusions of bark.

" I took so much bark in various ways," writes Franklin, " that I began to abhor it."

Nature finally revolts and rids his system of the learned doctor's nostrums. He gradually mends and resumes his war on the Proprietaries. But he makes small headway. It is a year before he is able to extract a statement out of the Penns and another year before he succeeds in getting the Pennsylvania viewpoint before English public opinion. To do this he exercises all his arts as a master propagandist. He writes pieces for the English papers and guides William into doing likewise. He pays for insertion when necessary. He and " Billy " prepare an extensive *Historical Review* of the long quarrel between the Pennsylvania Assembly and the governors, beginning with William Penn's day. William does the writing while his father supervises the work and supplies the documents. Franklin then sends a copy to every public man in England and America, to the English periodicals, and to the bookshops at home.

II

While he awaits the next move from his adversaries, he diverts himself with those agreeable occupations in which he takes most delight. He spends gay evenings with the two ladies of the house and grave ones with the philosophers and scientists who visit him or invite him to their homes.

He is ready alike for a song and a glass of wine, or a solemn discourse on the reason for and the origin of things. He has vast sport with the new and powerful electrical apparatus which he has set up in the Craven Street house.

One day he sees a new musical instrument called the Armonica, constructed from the "musical glasses" which give forth a sound when rubbed. He is enchanted, and at once has built for himself a new and improved instrument on which he gives concerts for the benefit of friends. This induces sundry reflections on the meaning and theory of music. He is not long in discovering that music and poetry, instead of being twin sisters, are bitter rivals, and that each lives with difficulty in the presence of the other. He wishes to make the melody of a song serve the words and when he finds the music of such masters as Handel overwhelming the words, he condemns the composers of the time. He clung to his beloved Armonica all the rest of his life, and it is preserved in Philadelphia to this day.

From this he turns his attention to the foulness of London's streets and submits to Dr. Fothergill a proposal " for the more effectual cleaning and keeping clean the streets of London and Westminster." He would have the dust swept up early in the morning before the shops are open — a revolutionary proposal — but he is convinced that it is a practical one; " for," he writes, " in walking thro' the Strand and Fleet Street one morning at seven o'clock, I observ'd there was not one shop open, tho' it had been daylight and the sun up above three hours; the inhabitants of London choosing voluntarily to live much by candle-light, and sleep by sunshine, and yet often complain, a little absurdly, of the duty on candles, and the high price of tallow."

This is probably the germ of the daylight-saving theory which Franklin aired at more length in Paris later, and is the cause of his receiving the credit for the daylight-saving laws of the present day.

In the summer of 1758 Franklin takes " Billy " on a tour of the provinces. This is done probably with a view to the improvement of Billy's mind. William is now a law student in the Middle Temple of the Inns of Court, intending to return to Philadelphia as a barrister. He takes readily to social life in London, and Strahan, the printer who has become Franklin's worshiping friend, thinks of him as a son-in-law, pronouncing him, in a letter to Mrs. Franklin, " one of the prettiest young gentlemen I ever knew from America."

This opinion is shared by others, notably by a London young woman, to this day unknown, who suddenly presents William, the natural son, with a natural son of his own. Thus does Franklin, at the age of 54, become a grandfather. Grandfather Benjamin is in no way disconcerted. He tranquilly welcomes the little stranger, has him tenderly brought up, names him William Temple Franklin, and when the lad is old enough, makes him his companion and secretary. It is through this same young man that the world receives, years after his grandfather's death, the famous *Autobiography*.

III

In the course of their tour Benjamin and Billy visit the University of Cambridge, where the grandfather hobnobs happily with the professors, and shows one of them, Dr. Hadley, of the chair of chemistry, a few tricks in the reduction of temperatures by the evaporation of ether. From there they go to visit their ancestral home in Northamptonshire, where only 30 miles away is Sulgrave, once the home of John Washington, grandfather of the renowned George.

The next year Benjamin and Billy have six glorious weeks in Scotland, receive the freedom of the city of Edinburgh, and are entertained by notabilities everywhere, including Hume, Robertson, and Lord Kames. The tour is crowned by the conferring upon Franklin of a doctor's degree by the University of St. Andrews. Franklin received these honors with a beaming pride.

" On the whole," he wrote to Lord Kames in Scotland, " I must say I think the time we spent there was six weeks of the *densest* happiness I have met with in any part of my life."

Amid these pleasures, however, he assures Deborah, who firmly resists all of William Strahan's efforts to tempt her to London, that he wishes he were home. He writes her:

" The regard and friendship I meet with from persons of worth, and the conversation of ingenious men, give me no small pleasure; but, at this time of life, domestic comforts afford the most solid satisfaction, and my uneasiness at being absent from my family, and longing desire to be with them, make me often sigh in the midst of cheerful company."

Deborah writes him constantly and voluminously, and he replies with spoil from the London shops. In one letter he mentions the following consignment:

China cups and bowls.

Four silver salt ladles, " newest, but ugliest fashion."

" A little instrument to core apples."

" Another to make little turnips out of great ones."

" Six course diaper breakfast cloths."

" A little basket, a present from Mrs. Stevenson to Sally, and a pair of garters for you, which were knit by the young lady, her daughter, who favored me with a pair of the same kind, the only ones I have been able to wear, as they need not be bound tight, the ridges in them preventing their slipping. . . . Goody Smith may, if she pleases, make such for me hereafter. My love to her."

Carpeting " for the best room floor."

" Two large fine Flanders bedticks."

Two pair of large superfine blankets.

Two fine damask tablecloths and napkins.

Forty-three ells of Ghentish sheeting Holland.

56 yards of cotton, " printed curiously from copper plates."

7 yards of chair bottoms, " printed in the same way, very neat. These were my fancy; but Mrs. Stevenson tells me I did wrong not to buy both of the same color."

7 yards of printed cotton, blue ground, " to make you a gown. I bought it by candlelight, and liked it then, but not so well afterwards. If you do not fancy it, send it as a present from me to sister Jenny."

" A better gown for you, of flowered tissue, 16 yards, of Mrs. Stevenson's fancy, cost nine guineas."

Snuffers, snuffstand, and extinguisher. " The extinguisher is for spermaceti candles only, and is of a new contrivance, to preserve the snuff upon the candle."

" Some music Billy bought for his sister."

" Some pamphlets for the Speaker and for Susy Wright."

" A mahogany and a little shagreen box, with microscopes and other optical instruments loose, are for Mr. Alison, if he likes them; if not, put them in my room till I return."

Two sets of books, " a present from me to Sally, *The World* and *The Connoisseur*."

7 pair of silk blankets, very fine. " You will excuse the soil on some of the folds; your neighbor Foster can get it off."

1 beer jug.

A notation regarding the latter explains that " it has the

coffee cups in its belly, packed in best crystal salt, of a peculiar nice flavor, for the table, not to be powdered."

But by the time this letter saw print in the works of Jared Sparks and James Parton, the fleshly word " belly " had been edited out. The eighteenth century could use the word; but the nineteenth resolutely refused to admit that people had such things.

IV

Three years pass and Franklin still waits in London. Then the Pennsylvania Assembly returns to the attack and passes " An Act for granting to his Majesty the sume of £100,000." It provides a sinking fund by " a tax on all estates." The Penns instantly hurl their legal battalions against it and demand its repeal. A committee of the Privy Council for Plantation Affairs in London report on it as " manifestly offensive to natural justice, to the laws of England, and to the royal prerogative." Franklin employs counsel and furnishes them with able arguments against the repeal. His contentions are so convincing that the lords of the committee waver. They offer to make a second and different report if Franklin will agree to certain amendments. The result is a compromise. The unsurveyed lands of the Penns are not taxed, but the surveyed lands are. It is a partial victory for Franklin; the stiffnecked and parsimonious Penns lose some of their prerogative and are compelled to accept the principle of a tax.

Franklin's friends back home rejoice and the Assembly votes him thanks, but the proprietary party attacks his name and reputation with ferocity. Deborah writes him disturbed letters. He replies:

" I am concerned that so much trouble should be given you by idle reports concerning me. Be satisfied, my dear, that while I have my senses, and God vouchsafes me his protection, I shall do nothing unworthy the character of an honest man, and one that loves his family."

The year is 1760. Quebec and Montreal have been taken, and France loses Canada and Guadeloupe to the victorious English. Franklin writes a pamphlet urging the retention of Canada, for there is actually a party which prefers Guadeloupe. Before the year is out, a frightful calamity befalls the conquering English: George III ascends the throne.

V

Franklin lingers on in London, enjoying his social and political triumphs. His leisure he employs in scientific experiments, arriving at conclusions which he puts in long letters to friends. Polly Stevenson, for instance, on a visit to the country receives one relating an experiment with squares of colored cloth laid on the snow on a sunny morning. The black squares, having absorbed the sun's rays, have sunk into the snow, but the white one remains unaffected. From this Franklin deduces that all summer clothes should be white, while garden walls should be painted black to retain the heat for the benefit of fruit trees and vines.

In 1761 he and William visit Germany and the Netherlands. The next year Oxford University makes Franklin a D.C.L. and Billy an M.A. In the same year William, now 32 years old, is appointed Governor of New Jersey and soon afterwards marries Miss Elizabeth Downes, of the West Indies. He returns home to take up his official residence at Burlington, only a few miles across the river from his father's home.

When at last Franklin obtains a ship home, his English friends sent him affectionate farewells. David Hume remarks that America has sent England many good things, but only one philosopher. To Polly Stevenson Franklin writes: " I fancy I feel a little like dying saints, who in parting with those they love in this world, are only comforted with the hope of more perfect happiness in the next. . . . Adieu, my dear good girl."

On the voyage he passes the time with more observations, notably the tranquilizing effect of oil on water. His attention to this is attracted by the behavior of a lamp. On arriving at Philadelphia, he finds the pleased city has made him its representative in the Assembly. Friends crowd the house to congratulate him on his achievements abroad.

He is 57 years old. He has become so round as to be portly. He no longer moves around with the old energy, but loves to linger at the table and to sit at his desk instead of exercising. Once more he dreams of a tranquil leisure, during which he can observe the curiosities of the natural world, chat with old friends, watch Sally moving to and fro, and begin his long-contemplated work on " The Art of Virtue." He writes to his friend Dr. Fothergill in London:

" By the way, when do you intend to live? i.e., to enjoy life? When will you retire to your villa, give yourself repose, delight in viewing the operations of nature in the vegetable creation, assist her in her works, get your ingenious friends at times about you, make them happy with your conversation and enjoy their society; or if alone, amuse yourself with your books and elegant collections?

" To be hurried about perpetually from one sick chamber to another is not living. Do you please yourself with the fancy that you are doing good? You are mistaken. Half the lives you save are not worth saving, as being useless, and almost all the other half ought not to be saved, as being mischievous. . . ."

It is a long time before Franklin himself can enjoy that repose which he recommends. Impending are labors beside which his former exertions will appear trifling.

Chapter XXII

Political Slings and Arrows

I

IN December, 1763, occurs one of the first of those outbursts of mob fury which have since become so common in American history and which, nearly always directed against the weak and unprotected, have so often grown into wholesale exhibitions of cowardice and bestiality.

The Indians of Pennsylvania, fired by rum and made cunning by contact with the white man, are for the most part a desperate lot, but among them are harmless tribes living in entire amity with the peaceful Quakers and Moravians. Among them is the remnant of a tribe of Conestogas living near Lancaster. There are only twenty of them, men, women and children. Early one morning a mounted band known as " the Paxton boys " surrounds their village and sets fire to it. Only six Indians are found at home. These are butchered.

Here and there a horrified protest is made, but most of the inhabitants approve the deed. Religious circles are silent when not openly commendatory. The authorities do nothing. However, the Lancaster magistrates collect the fourteen unbutchered Indians into the workhouse. The Paxton boys return to the blood-feast. A hundred of them break into the workhouse and slaughter the women and children as well as the men, carefully detaching their scalps in order to collect the provincial bounty.

The perpetrators are never found, never molested. The deed is regarded as an incident in a necessary and holy crusade, a virtuous clean-up campaign. Thus is set up one of those precedents which have virtually guaranteed immunity to mobs ever since, not only in Pennsylvania but in practically all other American States.

Thus encouraged, the Paxton boys, believing themselves latter-day Joshuas, draw to themselves new and thirsty recruits. Meantime Indians are taken to Philadelphia for protection. They are sent under escort to New York. The governor there refuses them admission and they have to march back to Philadelphia. The Paxton mob announces that it is coming to get them. The frightened governor, John Penn, runs to Franklin, takes refuge in his house, and gladly leaves the situation for him to deal with.

Franklin issues a blazing pamphlet entitled " A Narrative of the late Massacres, in Lancaster County, of a Number of Indians, Friends of the Province, by Persons Unknown." In this he lays aside his accustomed easy, droll manner, and speaks his mind in unminced words. He assails the mob not only as murderers but as violators of the historic right of sanctuary. He riddles the clergymen who have tried to justify the act as that of God-blessed crusaders. He pleads for more magnanimity towards the helpless. He might as well have used an atomizer on a gorilla. The Paxton mob arrives at Germantown, only seven miles away. Once more Franklin becomes a military commander, organizes a defense force, meets the invaders, and reads them a firm warning. The Paxtons veer off, turn the countryside into a hell, and on their return home are received by their own people as heroes.

" Governor Penn," writes Franklin, " did everything by my advice; so that, for about forty-eight hours, I was a very great man; as I had been once some years before, in a time of public danger."

A little later he notes this change in the situation: " The

fighting face we put on, and the reasonings we used with the insurgents, having turned them back and restored quiet to the city, I became a less man than ever; for I had, by this transaction, made myself many enemies among the populace."

These enemies consist of the respectable classes of the town, including the friends of the Proprietaries and the clergy dependent on them. They are enraged at Franklin's superseding the governor and his treatment of the Paxton " army of the Lord."

Factions arise, and Franklin is alternately praised and cursed. Governor John Penn, grandson of the great William, in a panic signs a proclamation enormously raising the price of Indian scalps, including those of women. His opponents declare that the proprietary government is no longer able to preserve order and put down mobs. A new demand arises for an appeal to George III, to make Pennsylvania a royal province like New York and New Jersey. Governor Penn chooses this moment to reject a bill taxing all estates alike. Bedlam ensues. The Assembly adjourns to consult the people as to a petition to the king. Franklin, when not on committees, finds time to write and print a pamphlet entitled " Cool Thoughts on the Present Situation of our Public Affairs, addressed to a Friend in the Country." It states the case for the Assembly. The legislature, on reassembling, votes to address a petition to the king praying him to make Pennsylvania a royal province. When Speaker Norris, pleading ill health, refuses to sign it, Franklin is chosen in his stead.

II

The fall elections of 1764 come on. Franklin is named on what is called " The Old Ticket " for re-election to the Assembly. A storm of pamphlets for and against the rule of the Penns floods the city. Franklin issues a satiric " Preface to a Speech " in which he ridicules the attempt of the respectable classes to shelter the Penns under the cloak of " the father, the honored and honorable father."

" The sons," he says, " have been heard to say to each other with disgust, when told that A, B, and C were come to wait upon them with addresses on some public occasion, " *Then I suppose we shall hear more about our father.*"

He proposes an inscription for an imaginary memorial to Thomas and Richard Penn beginning as follows:

> " Be this a Memorial
> Of T—— and R—— P——,
> P—— of P——,
> Who, with estates immense,
> Almost beyond computation,
> When their own province,
> And the whole British empire,
> Were engaged in a bloody and most expensive war,
> Begun for the defense of these estates,
> Could yet meanly desire
> To have those very estates
> Totally or partially
> Exempted from taxation . . ."

Franklin's enemies produce a counter-epitaph, shot through with the malicious gossip of the streets and taverns concerning the birth of William:

> " An Epitaph &c.
> To the much esteem'd Memory of
> Benjamin Franklin Esq., LL. D.

· · · · · · · · ·

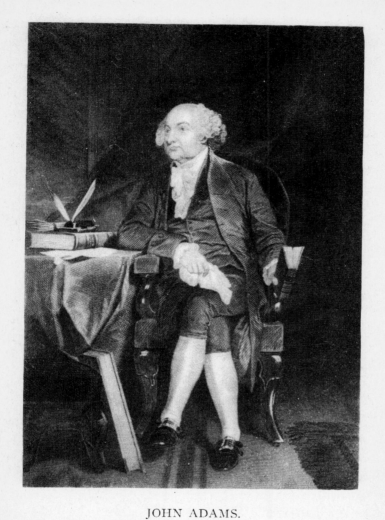

JOHN ADAMS.

THE SECOND PRESIDENT OF THE UNITED STATES, WHO, WHEN AN ENVOY
IN PARIS, QUARRELED WITH FRANKLIN.

Possessed of many lucrative offices

Procured to him by the Interest of Men whom he in-
famously treated

And receiving enormous sums from the Province for
services

He never performed,

After betraying it to Party Contention,

He lived, as to the Appearance of Wealth in moderate
circumstances;

His principal Estate, seeming to consist in his Hand
Maid Barbara,

A most valuable Slave,

The Foster Mother of his last offspring who did his
dirty work.

And in two angelic Females whom Barbara also served

As Kitchen Wench and Gold Finder, But alas the Loss!

Providence for wise tho' secret ends

Lately deprived him of the Mother of Excellency.

His fortune was not however impaired, for he piously
withheld from her Manes

The pitiful stipend of Ten pounds per Annum

On which he had cruelly suffered her To starve,

Then stole her to the Grave in Silence,

Without a Pall, the covering due to her dignity, without a tomb or even a Monumental Inscription."

On election day the Philadelphia conservatives muster
every force against Franklin. They are assisted by the
Dutch Calvinists and Presbyterians. The Church of England and Dutch Lutheran congregations are divided in sentiment. Most of Franklin's support comes from the
Quakers and Moravians.

Franklin is defeated. His fourteen years of loyal service in the Assembly come to an inglorious end in mire and

mud. The majority against him, however, is small. It is only about a score in a total vote of nearly 4000. Franklin accepts his defeat with his usual philosophic calm, but his friends rally around him strongly. They propose him as the Assembly's agent, to present the petition to the king in person. The Proprietary party breaks out into new exclamations of horror. John Dickinson, a Philadelphian of wealth and influence, declares that " no man in Pennsylvania is at this time so much the object of the public dislike as he " and that Franklin is in " the whole world the man most obnoxious to his country." Other opponents paint Franklin as an agitator and disturber of the peace. They charge him with being the author of the other Assembly measures " which have occasioned such uneasiness and distraction among the good people of this province."

Nevertheless he is elected as agent and at once prepares to sail for England for the third time. On November 7, 1764, he is escorted to his ship by three hundred mounted men, and within a month is once more in London, where Margaret and Polly Stevenson stand ready to welcome him back to his old lodgings in Craven Street.

He sends a letter of love and advice back to Sally. " Go constantly to church," he writes. . . . " I do not mean you should despise sermons, even of the preachers you dislike; for the discourse is often much better than the man, as sweet and clear waters come through very dirty earth."

This advice is the more surprising, since the rector of Christ Church, which Deborah and Sally attend, is a bootlicker to the Proprietaries and an enemy of Franklin. Our Benjamin is much like other males of the species: he may not care for sermons himself, but he is not above looking to the church to do police duty over his womenfolk.

Chapter XXIII

In London for the Third Time

I

FRANKLIN quickly finds that he must put on one side the business of getting the Pennsylvania petition into the hands of George III, and assist the other American colonial agents in London in their fight against the Stamp Act, which George Grenville, minister of the treasury, has prepared for action by Parliament. It imposes taxes on fifty-four classes of objects, from almanacs and advertisements to legal papers and college degrees. To scattered farmers living at a distance from towns it threatens to be an unmitigated nuisance, to small tradesmen it is a hardship; but the chief objection of the American colonists is that the taxes are to be imposed by a Parliament in which none of their representatives are permitted to sit. They have already had stamp taxes of their own.

"The first was imposed for one year by Massachusetts in 1755," says John Bach McMaster, "and re-enacted in 1756. The other was passed by New York in December, 1756 . . . It was against stamp duties laid without consent of the colonies that the four London agents protested vigorously on the 2nd of February, 1765." [1]

Protests are indulgently disregarded. Parliament passes the measure by a large majority. Franklin, still the loyal subject, does not seem to be greatly cast down by his defeat.

"I took every step in my power," he wrote, "to prevent

[1] Benjamin Franklin as a Man of Letters.

the passing of the Stamp Act. But the tide was too strong for us. The nation was provoked by American claims of legislative independence, and all parties joined in resolving by this act to settle the point. We might as well have hindered the sun's setting. That we could not do. But since it is down, my friend, and it may be long before it rises again, let us make as good a night of it as we can. We may still light candles. . . ."

So ready is he to submit that he buys a supply of legal blanks and sends it over to his partner, David Hall, to be stamped and sold in their stationery shop. When he hears that a young burgess named Patrick Henry has introduced in the Virginia Assembly a resolution declaring the exclusive right of that body to tax the inhabitants of the province, he writes to John Hughes, the Philadelphia merchant:

" A firm loyalty to the crown and a faithful adherence to the government of this nation, which it is the safety as well as the honour of the colonies to be connected with, will always be the wisest course for you and I to take."

This being his frame of mind, he falls readily into a trap laid for him by Grenville. The latter asks him to suggest a discreet and reputable man to act as stamp officer in Pennsylvania. Not realizing that this will virtually commit him to approbation of the act, Franklin names John Hughes. He soon hears of the effect at home. Hughes' home is threatened by a mob and he resigns the post. Franklin's enemies in Philadelphia try to provoke an attack on his own home. William hurries over from New Jersey to take the inmates away. Sally consents to go, but not the redoubtable Deborah. She barricades the house, sends for her brother to bring his gun, and prepares to repel invaders. She is still in a belligerent mood when she finds time to write Franklin about it:

" I said, when I was advised to remove, that I was very

sure you had done nothing to hurt anybody, nor had I given any offense to any person at all, nor would I be made uneasy by anybody, nor would I stir and show the least uneasiness, but if anyone came to disturb me I would show a proper resentment."

Nothing could better reveal Debby's confidence in her " Pappy," or her own sturdy and pugnacious nature. Any Philadelphia roughneck with the hardihood to set foot in Pappy's sacred study would doubtless have got not only an earful but a gunful.

II

When the news reaches Franklin that there have been riots in Boston and New York, that the homefolks are resisting the duties, and have even declared a boycott on English manufactures and are busy weaving homemade cloth on handlooms, he realizes that they are taking the situation more seriously than he. Before he can do anything, however, the Grenville ministry falls, an event celebrated with bell-ringing and cannon-firing in Philadelphia. Grenville is succeeded by the Marquis of Rockingham, whose secretary is Edmund Burke, friend of Franklin and of America.

However, the Stamp Act remains in force, and the American colonists, in a fury, adopt more drastic means of showing their resentment. Their measures are remarkably like those adopted in India during the recent *swaraj* agitation culminating in 1925. They pledge themselves to wear homespun, to import no English manufactured goods, and to eat no lamb in order to encourage the growing of American wool. Spinning and knitting become the fashion. Citizens boast of being dressed from head to foot in homemade goods. Legal proceedings are abandoned and disputes are settled by private arbitration. Stamped papers are destroyed wherever found. Franklin's newspaper, the

Gazette, announces that no stamped paper is to be had and even changes its title for a short period to " Remarkable Occurrences."

Franklin himself, despite his non-approval of the Stamp Act, still remains the loyal British subject. Aware of this, his political enemies at home make capital of it and accuse him, as a royal jobholder, of secretly working against his country's interest. A political versifier issues this quatrain:

" All his designs concenter in himself.
    For building castles and amassing pelf.
    The public 'tis his wit to sell for gain,
    Whom private property did ne'er maintain."

In England the boycott on imported goods and the attempts of the Americans to set up small factories of their own cause sundry quakings. Tall stories appear in that portion of the London press dominated by the industrialists concerning the attempts of the colonies to become independent of English factories. The Tory press, catering to the feudal land-owners, tries to allay such fears by scouting the possibility of the rise of industry in America.

Franklin is well aware that there are certain kinds of human foolishness which cannot be dealt with seriously. He therefore draws his feathered pen, dips it in a bottle filled with ridicule mixed with a little acid, and writes:

". . . Give me leave to instance the various accounts the newspapers have given us, with so much honest zeal for the welfare of *Poor Old England,* of the establishing manufactures in the colonies to the prejudice of those of the kingdom. It is objected by superficial readers, who yet pretend to some knowledge of those countries, that such establishments are not only improbable, but impossible, for that their sheep have but little wool, not in the whole sufficient for a pair of stockings a year to each inhabitant; that, from the universal dearness of labor among them, the working of iron and other materials, except in a few course instances, is impracticable to any advantage.

" Dear sir, do not let us suffer ourselves to be amused with such groundless objections. The very tails of the American sheep are so laden with wool, that each has a little car or wagon on four little wheels, to support and keep it from trailing on the ground. Would they calk their ships, would they even litter their horses with wool, if it were not both plenty and cheap? . . .

" And yet all this is as certainly true as the account said to be from Quebec, in all the papers of last week, that the inhabitants of Canada are making preparations for a cod and whale fishery ' this summer in the upper lakes.' Ignorant people may object, that the upper lakes are fresh, and that cod and whales are salt water fish; but let them know, sir, that cod, like other fish, when attacked by their enemies fly into any water where they can be safest; that whales, when they have a mind to eat cod, pursue them wherever they fly; and that the grand leap of the whale in the chase up the Falls of Niagara is esteemed, by all who have seen it, as one of the finest spectacles in nature."

III

Warned no doubt by letters from home, and encouraged by Burke, Franklin throws himself vigorously into the struggle for repeal of the Stamp Act. For several months, he is " in a continual hurry from morning till night."

At last Parliament in February, 1766, agrees to give a hearing on the subject before a Committee of the Whole House. Men of every rank and calibre who have any kind of connection with America are invited to testify. Chiefest witness of all is Dr. Franklin. During his long examination Franklin is at his best. He is cool, dignified, poised, and never at a loss for an answer. Burke said the scene reminded him of a master surrounded by a parcel of schoolboys. His friend George Whitefield, the preacher, afterwards wrote:

"Our worthy friend, Dr. Franklin, has gained immortal honor by his behavior at the bar of the House. His answer was always found equal if not superior to the questioner. He stood unappalled, gave pleasure to his friends, and did honor to his country."

There was a reason for the worthy Doctor's good showing. He had thoughtfully provided himself with a few friends in the Commons and had arranged that at the right time they should ask him questions for which he had pat answers ready. In this way he was able to get before British reactionaries the fact that America could supply 300,-000 men for a war of defense, and before the North of England trading faction the fact that America annually bought a half million pounds worth of goods from England.

Franklin was asked whether a military force could enforce the Stamp Act. "Suppose a military force sent into America," he replied; "they will find nobody in arms; what are they then to do? They cannot force a man to take stamps who chooses to do without them. They will not find a rebellion: they may indeed make one."

When asked what those colonists would do who found they could not sue for debts due them without using stamped paper, Franklin said:

"I can only judge what other people will think and how they will act by what I feel within myself. I have a great many debts due me in America, and I had rather they should remain unrecoverable by any law than submit to the Stamp Act."

There ensue several days of debate, excitement and intrigue. George III and the court faction set their faces against repeal, but the manufacturing interests, thoroughly scared by the American boycott, bring to bear powerful influences, in which cash plays its part. The Stamp Act is repealed at 4 o'clock on the morning of February 21, 1766.

The news is received in America with public rejoicing. Cheering crowds parade through the streets of Philadelphia. And Franklin's name is extolled to the stars. The Pennsylvania Assembly elects him agent for another year. In October of this year Philadelphia holds another election and the wave of enthusiasm carries Franklin back to his old seat. Sally Franklin scribbles off this note to her brother William in New Jersey:

" Dear Brother — *The Old Ticket forever! We have it by 34 votes! God bless our worthy and noble agent, and all his family,* were the joyful words we were waked with at 2 or 3 o'clock this morning, by the White Oaks. They then gave us three huzzas and a blessing, then marched off. How strong is the cause of truth! We have beat three parties; The Proprietary, the Presbyterians, and the Half-and-Half. . . ."

" As the Stamp Act is at length repealed," writes Franklin to Deborah, " I am willing you should have a new gown."

In England, however, the repeal of the Stamp Act is only a temporary reverse to the Tory party and the next year they return to their old tricks. Under Charles Townsend, Chancellor of the Exchequer, a new tax measure is introduced for the purpose of somehow extracting a revenue out of America. It lays duties on paper, paints, glass and tea, and since it is meant to raise only £40,000 annually, Parliament believes America will not object. But the result is a new storm of opposition. Franklin's position as a colonial agent becomes more and more difficult. He is able to do little except try to educate English opinion by means of letters to the newspapers signed " Pacificus," " Secundus," " Homespun," etc.

Daily it becomes plainer that the root of the difficulty is the fear in England that America will establish her own factories and set up her own industries. English hatters obtain from Parliament an act restraining the colonists from manufacturing their own hats. English steel-makers induce Parliament to forbid the construction in America of slitting-mills or steel furnaces. Americans are forbidden to import wine, oil or fruit from Portugal except through England.

It was this situation which was the real cause of the Revolutionary War; and the real enemies of American independence were not so much the king and the politicians as the nascent industrial class and the intrenched commission houses of England.

IV

Between his wrestlings with Parliament and with English public opinion, Franklin does not forget to have a good time. As soon as Parliament adjourns for the summer he is among the first to bounce over to the Continent. " Traveling," he once remarked, " is one way of lengthening life, at least in appearance." In 1766 he enjoys himself in Germany and Holland, and the next summer finds him and Sir John Pringle, the queen's physician, gaily dashing off to Paris. In one of his blithest moods Franklin writes to " Polly " Stevenson, who is a little lonely down at an aunt's home in Bromley, Kent:

" I had not been here six days before my Tailor and Perruquier had transformed me into a Frenchman. Only think what a figure I make in a little bag-wig and with naked ears!

They told me I was become twenty years younger and looked very gallant; so being in Paris where the Mode is to be sacredly followed, I was once very near making Love to my Friend's Wife."

Thus revivified, he is moved to notice some particulars regarding the fair inhabitants of France:

" The women we saw at Calais, on the road, at Boulogne, and in the inns and villages were generally of dark complexions; but arriving at Abbeville we found a sudden change, a multitude of both women and men in that place appearing remarkably fair. Whether this is owing to a small colony of spinners, wool combers, and weavers, brought hither from Holland with the woolen manufactory about sixty years ago, or to their being less exposed to the sun than in other places, their business keeping them much within doors, I know not. . . .

" As soon as we left Abbeville, the swarthiness returned. I speak generally; for here are some fair women at Paris, who, I think are not whitened by art. As to rouge, they didn't pretend to imitate nature in laying it on. There is no gradual diminution of the color, from the full bloom in the middle of the cheek to the faint tint near the sides, nor does it show itself differently in different faces. I have not had the honor of being at any lady's toilet to see how it is laid on, but I fancy I can tell you how it is or may be done. Cut a hole of three inches diameter in a piece of paper; place it on the side of your face in such a manner, as that the top of the hole may be just under the eye; then, with a brush dipped in the color, paint face and paper together; so when the paper is taken off, there will remain a round patch of red exactly the form of the hole. This is the mode, from the actresses on the stage upwards through the ranks of ladies to the princesses of the blood; but it stops there, the queen not using it, having in the serenity, complacence, and benignity that shine so eminently in, or rather through, her countenance, sufficient beauty, though now an old woman, to do extremely well without it."

Follows an account of his meeting with Louis XV, one of the five kings before whom he once boasted that he had stood:

" You see I speak of the queen as if I had seen her; and so I have, for you must know I have been at court. We went to Versailles last Sunday, and had the honor of being presented to the king, Louis XV; he spoke to both of us very graciously and very cheerfully, is a handsome man, has a very lively look, and appears younger than he is. In the evening we were at the *Grand Couvert,* where the family sup in public. The table was half a hollow square, the service gold. When either made a sign for drink, the word was given by one of the waiters: *A boire pour le Roi,* or, *A boire pour la Reine.* Then two persons came from within, the one with wine and the other with water in carafes; each drank a little glass of what he brought, and then put both the carafes with a glass on a salver, and then presented it. Their distance from each other was such, as that other chairs might have been placed between any two of them. An officer of the court brought us up through the crowd of spectators, and placed Sir John so as to stand between the queen and Madam Victoire. The king talked a good deal to Sir John, asking many questions about our royal family; and did me too the honor of taking some notice of me; that is saying enough, for I would not have you think me so much pleased with this king and queen, as to have a whit less regard than I used to have for ours. No Frenchman shall go beyond me in thinking my own king and queen the very best in the world, and the most amiable."

This last sentence is not the least interesting in this interesting letter. It reveals Franklin as still the worshipful provincial, still the devout subject. Franklin the republican is not yet born.

IV

In 1768 comes a change in the ministry which threatens a terrifying disaster to Franklin. Lord Sandwich at one time is almost on the point of depriving him of his postmastership because Franklin is "too much of an Englishman." Since David Hall has ceased his payments of £1000 annually, the purchase of the Franklin & Hall printing business having been completed, a large hole looms in Franklin's income, but the lonely and struggling colony of Georgia comes to the rescue by appointing him its agent at London at £200 a year. New Jersey follows, adding £100. Massachusetts comes next despite the opposition of Samuel Adams, with £400 a year. These sums, added to the £500 which Pennsylvania pays him, are cheerfully received. And he doesn't lose the postmastership after all.

"My enemies were forced," he writes to Jane Mecom, "to content themselves with abusing me plentifully in the newspapers and endeavoring to provoke me to resign. In this they are not likely to succeed, I being deficient in that Christian virtue of resignation. If they would have my office, they must take it."

Thus does he remain faithful to his ancient motto: never to seek an office, and never to resign one.

Chapter XXIV

Franklin Meets the High Priest of the Hell Fire Club

I

THOUGH Franklin was blandly unaware of it, in 1768 he might as well have been an earnest fly trying to butt through a window pane as to get his propaganda successfully before mass opinion in the London of that day. The reason was that, in the world of politics, the London man-in-the-street could see nothing, hear nothing, but the magic, the incandescent, figure of John Wilkes, one of the most astonishing individuals produced by the eighteenth century.

"London was illuminated," wrote Franklin to his friend, Joseph Galloway, "two nights running, at the command of the mob, for the success of Wilkes in the Middlesex election. The second night exceeded anything of the kind ever seen here on the greatest occasions of rejoicing, as even the small cross-streets, lanes, courts, and other out-of-the-way places were all in a blaze with lights, and the principal streets all night long, as the mobs went round again after two o'clock, and obliged people who had extinguished their candles to light them again. Those who refused had all their windows destroyed. The damage done and the expense of candles have been computed at fifty thousand pounds."

That wasn't all the mob did. It made "gentlemen and ladies of all ranks, as they passed in their carriages, to shout for Wilkes and Liberty, marking the same words on all their coaches with chalk, and No. 45 on every door. . . . I went last week to Winchester, and observed, that for fifteen miles out of town there was scarce a door or window shutter next the road unmarked; and this continued, here and there, quite to Winchester, which is sixty-four miles."

John Wilkes?

Wilkes and Liberty?

No. 45?

These references appear very mysterious, until we begin to investigate. Then we find that the trail leads from Wilkes to Lord Sandwich, whom we have just seen in the act of trying to shunt our worthy Doctor out of his good job in the Philadelphia postoffice. Lord Sandwich's assistant is Sir Francis Dashwood, afterwards Lord le Despencer and Chancellor of the Exchequer. Lord le Despencer is the so-called great libertine with whom Franklin solemnly produced a revision of the English Book of Common Prayer.

At this point we must quote from another letter of Franklin's addressed to son William:

" I was down at Lord le Despencer's when the post brought that day's papers. Paul Whitehead was there, too, who runs early through all the papers and tells the company what he finds remarkable. He had them in another room, and we were chatting in the breakfast parlor, when he came running into us, out of breath, with the paper in his hand. ' Here! ' says he, ' here's news for ye. Here's the King of Prussia claiming a right to this kingdom! ' All stared, and I as much as anybody; and he went on to read it. When he had read two or three paragraphs a gentleman present said, ' Damn his impudence; I dare say we shall hear by next post that he is upon his march with one hundred thousand men to back this.' Whitehead, who is very shrewd, soon after began to smoke it, and looking in my face, said, ' I'll be hanged if this is not some of your American jokes upon us.' The reading went on, and ended with abundance of laughing, and a general verdict that it was a fair hit; and the piece was cut out of the paper and preserved in my lord's collection."

We may be sure that amid the laughter no one's was more ventral than Franklin's own; for the " fair hit " was one of the most famous of his own numerous newspaper hoaxes entitled " An Edict of the King of Prussia."

We have now rounded up a group composed of Lord le Despencer, Lord Sandwich, John Wilkes, and Whitehead, with all of whom Franklin has some kind of relation, as yet not defined.

II

Let us go back a few years earlier and imagine that we have come upon this group some dark night in London. They are dressed as if for a fête, but as they come out of a house on a side street they are cloaked and hooded. As they enter a carriage, we overhear a low laugh and a quiet chuckle. We follow them out into the country where heavy trees do silent sentry duty along the banks of the Thames. We arrive at the village of Marlow, in Buckinghamshire. We pass through and take the road to Henley, of boat-race renown. The carriage slows and stops before a ruined and deserted building of an ecclesiastical architecture.

It is Medmenham Abbey, founded by a Cistercian order of monks in 1145 and now the seat of the Hell Fire Club, whose orgies and rites are presided over by the High Priest and Monk Superior, Sir Francis Dashwood.

The club's members number twelve. Besides the quartet mentioned, they include Charles Churchill, Robert Lloyd, Bubb-Dodington, George Selwyn, and at various times Ben

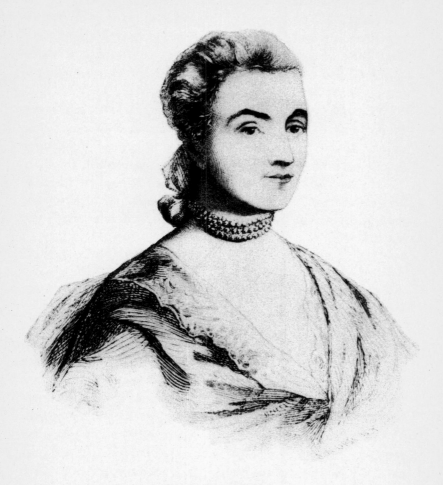

ABIGAIL ADAMS.

WIFE OF JOHN ADAMS, WHO DID NOT APPROVE OF FRANKLIN'S TASTE IN
WOMEN FRIENDS.

From an old woodcut.

Bates, Henry Lovibond Collins, Sir William Stanhope, Sir John Dashwood-King, Sir John d'Aubrey, and Thomas Potter.

Of all the numerous rakish clubs founded in England in the eighteenth century, the Hell Fire Club was regarded as the most scandalous. Ascribed to it were the most harrowing blasphemies. Stories concerning it were told by whispers in secluded corners. The prominence and unquestioned talent of its membership made it the target of loose-lipped, and sometimes envious, gossip. The following is from a contemporary chronicle:

" The Hell-Fires, you may guess, aim at a more transcendent malignity, deriding the forms of religion as a trifle with them, by a natural progression from the form they turn to the substance; with Lucifer they fly at Divinity. The third person of the Trinity is what they peculiarly attack; by the following specimen you may judge of their good will: i.e., their calling for a Holy-Ghost-pye at the tavern. . . ."

The shade of this ancient chronicler will forgive us if his horror causes us no more than a smile. Calling for a Holy Ghost pie at a tavern sounds more like the irreverent prank of a modern gang of college students than the deliberate blasphemy of seasoned criminals. The Hell Fire Club undoubtedly contained dissipated and sometimes dissolute men, but it is doubtful if their performances, in the beginning, surpassed those of any high-spirited and reckless young bucks who in any land or age, are prone to react impiously against the respectabilities and confining rigidities of their elders.

Of Dashwood, who was afterwards Franklin's frequent host at his magnificent country place at West Wycombe, Dr. Franklin wrote:

" But a pleasanter thing is the kind countenance, the facetious and very intelligent conversation of mine host, who having been for many years engaged in public affairs, seen all parts of Europe, and kept the best company in the world, is himself the best existing."

In Lord le Despencer Franklin found the kind of man which he most looked up to. His lordship was elegantly wicked, and so was possessed of a quality which Franklin admired with his whole heart. There can be little doubt that membership in the Hell Fire Club, though perhaps not accepted, would have enticed him irresistibly. We already know how he loved clubs and good company.

The very inscription over the entrance at Medmenham, taken from the Abbey of Thelème described in Rabelais, would have delighted him — *Fay ce que voudras* (Do what you like); for Franklin had been trying to observe that precept ever since he had sold his printing business and ceased, in spirit at least, to be Poor Richard.

Of the whole group the ablest and most brilliant figure was John Wilkes. There was a time when his name was scarcely less revered in Boston and Philadelphia than in London. His memory has a certain additional interest for Americans because a nephew, Charles Wilkes, became an admiral in the United States Navy.

Married in his youth to a woman half again as old as himself and totally dissimilar from her in sentiments, John Wilkes threw himself into the somewhat boisterous dissipations favored in the drawing rooms and clubs of the period. Having gifts as a political writer, he became editor of the *North Briton* in 1762. There he established his name as the "Friend to Liberty" and to the cause of the American colonists. Consequently he made himself hated by George III and the court party. In issue No. 45 of his paper he had the impudence to comment satirically on a Speech from the Throne. He was arrested for libel and imprisoned in the Tower. To put an edge on the case, the prosecution dragged in a forgotten and privately printed pamphlet, written in his youth, called, as a burlesque on Pope, *Essay on Woman*. A noble lord arose in Parliament and denounced Wilkes as having " violated the most sacred ties of religion as well as decency " by publishing this book. This was no other than the Earl of Sandwich, Wilkes's former fellow member in the Hell Fire Club! Wilkes at length went in exile, to Paris, whence he wrote the tenderest of letters to his daughter " Polly," and became the friend of Beaumarchais, playwright, business man, and friend of Franklin and of America. On returning to England, he was repeatedly rejected from Parliament, but one of fate's little ironies made this haunter of drawing rooms and boudoirs the idol of London's proletariat, and finally he was triumphantly elected Sheriff and then Lord Mayor of London. It was as Lord Mayor in 1775 that he presented to the king a remonstrance against the policy of coercing America. In person he was squint-eyed and unattractive, but made a name for himself as a boundless amorist. He once boasted that with half an hour's start he could win a woman from the best-looking man in the world. Tradition says that it was he who finally broke up the Hell Fire Club by introducing a baboon, dressed like the devil, in the midst of an after-midnight revel.

In genuine evil-doing, the Earl of Sandwich probably outranked any other member of the club. His seductions of women became so notorious that he was named " Jemmie Twitcher," after the seducer of that name in Gay's *The Beggar's Opera*.[1] He insinuated himself into the graces of George III and was promoted rapidly as a diplomat and occupant of high posts. There was high comedy in his turning on Wilkes for writing the *Essay on Woman*, for the pamphlet had been actually dedicated to him and he him-

[1] Dictionary of National Biography.

self had been previously expelled from the Beefsteak Club for blasphemy.[2] As a handy man for George III, it was not surprising that he arose in Parliament one day and denounced Franklin as " one of the bitterest and most mischievous enemies this country has ever known."

Paul Whitehead was an amiable loafer, minor poet, and hanger-on of men more highly placed in the world. Franklin's account of him as a reader and clipper of newspapers for Lord le Despencer indicates his character. Until he married money and got a small post from Dashwood, he lived by his wits and by doing political hack writing similar to that by which James Ralph, Franklin's friend, earned a tainted livelihood. The people who liked Whitehead held Dashwood responsible for getting him into bad habits. He was a pet aversion of Dr. Samuel Johnson, and was also despised by his fellow " Hell Fire " member, Churchill, who wrote this couplet about him:

" May I (can worse disgrace on Manhood fall?)
Be born a Whitehead and baptized a Paul! "

But he died peacefully among suburban neighbors who respected him. His will requested that his heart be removed and given to Lord le Despencer. He bequeathed £50 for a marble urn to contain it. Lord le Despencer, with his strong dramatic sense, interred the heart to the accompaniment of music and appropriate ceremonies in the mausoleum which he had caused to be built on his beautiful West Wycombe grounds.

Churchill was a former curate, a satiric poet of some consequence during his time, and an ardent friend and political supporter of Wilkes. His invective gifts earned him many enemies, including Hogarth, the painter, and Dr. Johnson, whom Churchill crowned with the name " Pomposo." He

[2] Lives of the Rakes, by E. Beresford Chancellor.

lived briefly and fiercely. He wrote his own inscription for his grave: " Life to the last enjoyed, here Churchill lies."

Robert Lloyd was a young scholar and writer of a fluency too facile to become distinguished. Wilkes wrote of him: " He was content to scamper round the foot of Parnassus on his little Welsh pony, which seems never to have tired." His was an impressionable nature, prone to absorb the color of his associates.

Bubb-Dodington, Lord Melcombe, left behind him a memory flavored with a kind of obscene comedy. He was fat, gross, conceited, in private life a toady, and in public a turn-coat, but always regarded himself as at heart an artist. An uncle left this son of an apothecary named Bubb an immense fortune, a great part of which the recipient spent on the erection of a gigantic villa, the very dream of a nabob in stone and marble, in which the purple-jowled owner slept in a glided bed canopied with peacocks' feathers. He lived to bask in the sun of King George's court. When, on the occasion of the royal marriage, he bent low to kiss the hand of Queen Charlotte, he burst the fastenings of his lilac-tinted silk trousers, but survived to a hale old age.[3]

George Selwyn was a wit, gambler, and man-about-town. When he attended a session of Parliament it was always to sleep tranquilly. He had two great passions: one was for his adopted daughter, Maria Fagniani; the other was for executions and the sight of dead bodies. His sayings were famous. When in his presence someone wondered at the marriage of Lord North to the enormously fat widow of the Earl of Rockingham, he remarked: " Oh, she had been kept on ice three days before the wedding! "[4]

Sir William Stanhope was another member of the Hell Fires who had a wit, but of a somewhat dryer kind. At the

[3] The Lives of the Rakes, by E. Beresford Chancellor.
[4] Idem.

coronation of George III, he objected to the removal of a table of the Knights of the Bath, to whom he belonged, on the ground that " some of us are gentlemen here."

The remaining members of the Hell Fire Club seem to have been minor and undistinguished personages, but we have already said enough concerning their companions to indicate what they were like. Franklin arrived in London for his third visit too late to have been admitted to membership, the club having been dissolved when Dashwood became Lord le Despencer in 1762; but there can be little doubt that he would have rejoiced in the company of the other members almost as much as in that of his lordship. Wit, clubbability, free-thinking, and bold gallantry — these were attributes that ever fascinated the provincial Franklin.

There was another associate member or visitor to the club, who perhaps fascinated Franklin even more. This was Eon de Beaumont, known as the Chevalier d'Eon, soldier of France, writer, poet, and diplomat, the secret of whose real sex agitated for years the gossips of the chancelleries of Europe. Indeed, the Hell Fire Club once held a mock trial to determine this very point. D'Eon was living in exile in London while Franklin was there, and there is evidence that they became friends.

The mystery concerning d'Eon involved, as an old French biography puts it, " the imperious circumstances which one day compelled him to conceal his sex." What those strange circumstances were has never been authentically disclosed, but the concealment is said to have been by the order of his king, Louis XV, whose secret correspondence with the Empress Elizabeth of Russia was in charge of d'Eon for five years. Early in his career d'Eon was the secret agent and close confidant of the king, but on somehow falling out of favor, he spent an exile of 14 years in England. He was permitted to return to France in 1775.

Two years afterwards, Count Vergennes, of whose later relations with Franklin we shall presently hear, ordered d'Eon at his home in Tonnerre, to " reassume the garments of his sex." The autopsy at his death is said to have revealed d'Eon as unquestionably male.

Bearing on this point, there is a curious letter from d'Eon to Franklin in the files of the American Philosophical Society at Philadelphia. It was written in Paris in 1778, a year after Count Vergennes had issued his queer order. The following is a translation:

" Monsieur,

" I have been to Passy to have the honor of seeing you and to felicitate you on recent events occurring in America, but you were in Paris. In your absence we drank to your health and to Liberty, at the home of your friend M. le Ray de Chaumont, who was joined by madame his wife and mademoiselle his daughter in extending to me the most agreeable reception. I hope that the health of the Liberty carried by Madlle d'Eon to three places in Versailles results in all the good possible to America. My brother-in-law, the Chevalier O'Gorman, has arrived from Burgundy. He will return next week. He hopes that when next spring you go to Dijon that you will give him the pleasure and honor of stopping with him at Tonnerre. I shall be very happy if I can be present at the same time and there give proofs of the sincere and respectful attachment with which I am

" Your very humble and very obedient servant,
" LA CHEVALIÈRE D'EON."

It is to be noted that d'Eon's signature is in the feminine. Moreover, in calling himself " servant," he uses not the usual masculine *serviteur* but the feminine *servante*. Also, on the back of the letter there is this memorandum, apparently in Franklin's handwriting and possibly for filing purposes: "Chevalière D'Eon, 24 jany, 1778" — again the feminine form. This letter heightens the mystery which even to this day is attached to the name of d'Eon.

To the last he dressed in women's clothes, and, clinging to his skirts, even took part in fencing duels. In his later years he was always careful to call himself, as in the above letter, "Mademoiselle d'Eon."

In connection with d'Eon there is a curious story told of Franklin during his residence as American envoy at Passy, now part of Paris but then a suburb. Franklin let it be known that he wished to contribute to the "blessed bread" being distributed in the parish of Passy. He offered thirteen *brioches*, or cakes, representing the thirteen American colonies, on the first of which — destined for the curé — should be inscribed, in large letters, the word "Liberty." The curé and the bishop sought to dissuade him, but it was d'Eon who caused him to renounce the project by saying: "Passy is too close to Versailles. They do not greatly care for that word there." [1]

It may have been that d'Eon, who at times manifested sportive inclinations, took it upon himself to carry the inscribed cakes to Versailles. If so, this would explain his reference to "the Liberty" in his letter to Franklin.

III

Franklin's association with the former High Priest of the Hell Fire Club led to his joining in one of the most curious enterprises in which he ever engaged. This was the revision of the English Prayer Book. Lord le Despencer did most of the work, but Franklin cut down the catechism and the reading and singing Psalms, and wrote the preface. As

[1] Archives of the Historical Society of Auteuil and Passy.

we have already seen, Franklin had an incurable fondness for criticizing and altering religious works. Of the catechism only two questions were retained: "What is your duty to God?" and "What is your duty to your neighbor?" Omitted were all reference to the sacraments, to the divinity of Jesus, the commandments in the catechism, the Nicene and Athanasian Creeds, and even the canticle, "All ye Works of the Lord." The Apostle's Creed was pared down "to the parts that are most intelligible and most essential." The *Te Deum* and *Venite* were abridged, and the services for communion, infant baptism, confirmation, visitation of the sick, marriage and burial of the dead were much shortened.

Franklin expressly approved Lord le Despencer's omissions of the Commination "and all cursing of mankind," and explained his own cuts in certain of the Psalms by saying that "they imprecate, in the most bitter terms, the vengeance of God in our adversaries, contrary to the spirit of Christianity, which commands us to love our enemies and to pray for those that hate us and despitefully use us."

The purpose of the book, as explained in the preface, was a humanitarian one — to prevent the old and faithful from freezing to death through long ceremonies in cold churches; to make the services so short as to attract the young and lively; and to relieve the well-disposed from the affliction of interminable prayers.

Theology fascinated Franklin, but it also troubled him. He could not forbear tinkering with it whenever he had the time. He sought to make it not only good, but humane. He strove to remodel it in his own kindly image. To see him, ancient enemy of New England ecclesiasticism, associated in this task with the former Abbot of the Hell Fire Club, might well have caused a smile on Olympus itself.

The book was issued by Wilkie, the bookseller in St.

Paul's Churchyard, in 1773, but, says Franklin, was " never much noticed." It was ahead of its time. In the eighteenth century, bigotry, though productive of convulsive reactions among the young, was still strong among the old, who had erected upon it institutions as precious as temples.

It is a curious fact that " Franklin's Prayer Book " was followed by his friend Thomas Jefferson's revision of the New Testament, better known as " Jefferson's Bible." This too, was a product of the reaction against reaction.

IV

The " Edict of the King of Prussia," which aroused the laughter of the gentlemen at Lord le Despencer's house, purported to be an announcement emanating from Frederick the Great. In solemn, burlesque style it cited the fact that Britain has been first settled by Saxon colonies, that it had been decided to raise a revenue from these colonies to defray the expenses of defense, and that certain measures had been ordered to be put into execution. These measures were the same which Britain had ordained for America. One command was this: " That all the thieves, highway and street robbers, housebreakers, forgerers, s-d-tes, and villains of every denomination, who have forfeited their lives to the law in Prussia, but whom we in our great clemency do not think fit here to hang, shall be emptied out of our gaols into the said Island of Great Britain, for the better peopling of that country."

Another of Franklin's newspaper contributions, which appeared about the same time, was called " Rules for Reducing a Great Empire to a Small One." It began with this statement: " A great empire, like a great cake, is most easily diminished at the edges," and then proceeded to recite, in satirical form, those acts of the British ministers and Parliament against which the American colonists had made most complaint.

Franklin was 63 years old before any of his collected writings were published in book form. In 1769 a volume called his " Works " appeared in London. It consisted chiefly of letters and papers on electrical and other scientific subjects. It was translated into French by his friend Dubourg in Paris.

CHAPTER XXV

The Attack in the Cockpit

I

MEANTIME ugly incidents have been occurring in America, particularly in Massachusetts, greatly to the annoyance of Governor Hutchinson. The seizure of John Hancock's sloop, the "Liberty," for a violation of the revenue laws, has caused a riot in Boston. British troops have occupied Faneuil Hall and the State House. A collision in King Street has caused three deaths and the trial of the officer commanding the British detachment, Captain Preston. At Providence the British revenue schooner, the "Gaspee," has been boarded and burned.

Franklin regards as particularly offensive the quartering of troops in Boston. He tells a Whig member of Parliament so. The member informs Franklin that all these forcible measures are due to the suggestions — the actual request, indeed — of prominent Americans themselves. He offers to back up his assertions with indisputable documents. He brings Franklin a packet of letters written by respectable New Englanders to William Whately, a former member of Parliament and a confidential agent for the Grenville ministry. The contents of these letters amaze Franklin. They call for a strong hand in dealing with the American populace. Six of them are by Thomas Hutchinson, written when he was chief justice and lieutenant-governor of Massachusetts. Hutchinson is not an Englishman but a native, a graduate of Harvard, and one of the earliest advocates of narrow and rigid Sabbath laws. In one letter he asserts that "there must be an abridgment of what are called English liberties."

Four of the letters are by Andrew Oliver, Hutchinson's successor as lieutenant-governor. Oliver writes in the spirit of a wretched little sycophant. He recommends that the "officers of the crown be made, in some measure, independent of the people," and even suggests that the ruling power be vested in an Order of Patricians, composed exclusively of land owners.

Franklin obtained permission to send the letters to Boston, on condition that they be neither copied nor printed, and be afterwards returned to the lender. In 1772 he sent them to the Massachusetts Assembly, where they naturally created astonishment and fury. John Adams showed them everywhere, even to his aunt, of whom he wrote: "Aunt is let into the secret, and is full of her interjections." The Assembly indignantly demanded the removal of Hutchinson and Oliver, but nothing came of their petition.

In time, of course, the letters got into print and were published in England. A demand was set up to account for their falling into American hands. William Whately was dead and his brother, Thomas, was at once placed on the defensive. He explained that William's letters, by permission, had once been examined by John Temple, former lieutenant-governor of New Hampshire, but he failed to clear Temple of suspicion. This led to a duel between Temple and Whately in Hyde Park, the combatants being separated by Ralph Izard, of South Carolina, and Arthur Lee, of Virginia, of whom we are to hear more later.

About this time occurred the "Boston Tea Party," when fifty men, disguised as Mohawk Indians, boarded English vessels at night and emptied the tea cargoes belonging to the East India Company into Boston Harbor.

In December, 1773, Franklin issued through the London *Public Advertiser* a statement saying that neither Whately nor Temple had anything to do with the arrival of the letters in America, but that he alone was responsible for sending them. He justified his action on the ground that they were not private letters, but related to public matters closely concerning the dispute between England and America.

Franklin, as the Massachusetts agent, is promptly summoned to appear before the Committee of Lords which is to consider the petition for the removal of Hutchinson and Oliver. Almost at the same time he is sued by Thomas Whately for the alleged profits made from the sale of his brother's letters. Franklin realizes that the English Tories, who have been long lying in wait for him, are about to hurl their attack. Knowing that he is to be questioned by Alexander Wedderburn, the king's solicitor, an ambitious Scotchman with an acid tongue, he engaged as his counsel the Liberal, John Dunning, afterwards Lord Ashburton, and musters his forces for the defense.

The hearing is held before the Privy Council in a room called the Cockpit. Both English and American notables are there. It is a case of standing room only. Even Franklin has to stand. He does so calmly, dressed in Manchester velvet, spotted, with a flowing wig on his head. During the whole blazing examination his tranquil countenance does not alter.

Wedderburn opens in his fiercest manner. He virtually accuses Franklin of stealing and misusing private letters. He contends that Franklin's purpose is to become governor of Massachusetts himself.

" I hope, my lord," he cries, " you will mark and brand the man for the honor of this country, of Europe, and of mankind."

Wedderburn finishes in a crescendo of invective and violent abuse, "laying on," wrote Edmund Burke, "beyond all bound and decency." Franklin, realizing that he has been summoned not for a hearing but a humiliation, declines to be questioned. The Committee of the Council throws out the Massachusetts petition, and a few days later Franklin is dismissed as deputy postmaster-general in America. Wedderburn becomes, in time, Lord Loughborough.

Wedderburn's abuse of Franklin releases a torrent of Tory ire against the impudent colonials of America. Dr. Samuel Johnson writes his pamphlet, "Taxation no Tyranny," calls Franklin "the master of mischief," and announces that he is "willing to love all mankind except an American." Press and politicians become bitter and scornful. Franklin realizes that his mission in behalf of peace and union has been a failure. He can hear the growls and curses of approaching war. He makes ready to return to that peaceful home on the Delaware from which he has been absent for ten years.

II

Meantime things have been happening there. Sally, now 23 years old, has become engaged to Richard Bache, a young merchant. Franklin receives the news without objection, but without enthusiasm. "At present," he writes Deborah, "I suppose you would agree with me that we cannot do more than fit her out handsomely in clothes and furniture, not exceeding in the whole five hundred pounds of value. For the rest, they must depend, as you and I did, on their own industry and care, as what remains in our hands will be barely sufficient for our support, and not enough for them when it comes to be divided at our decease."

Bache was not successful as a provider, and his father-in-law occasionally had to help him, but he and Sally became

231

the parents of very handsome children. One of these, Benjamin Franklin Bache, was the spoiled idol of his grandmother. She could write Franklin little else than a "history of his pretty actions." When this boy grew up, he became the bitter editor of the *Aurora*, the ardent partisan of Jefferson, and the insatiable critic of Washington.

The occasional letters which Franklin receives from son William back home are disturbing. William takes some pride in himself as the Royal Governor of New Jersey and in all cases of dispute between the crown and the colony, he inclines more and more toward the royal viewpoint. Franklin is pained, but refrains from criticism. "I only wish you," he writes William, "to act uprightly and steadily, avoiding that duplicity which, in Hutchinson, adds contempt to indignation. If you can promote the prosperity of your people, and leave them happier than you found them, whatever your political principles are, your memory will be honored."

III

It is probable that Franklin, now no longer a young man, would not have ridden out the pre-Revolutionary storm so well had he not been so well sheltered in the quiet home of Margaret and Polly Stevenson in Craven Street. "In all that time," he wrote Polly, "we never had among us the smallest misunderstanding; our friendship has been all clear sunshine, without the least cloud in its hemisphere."

It was for those who produced this unclouded atmosphere that Franklin wrote his light-hearted "Craven Street Gazette," a chronicle burlesquing the solemn events at court as devoutly reported in the newspapers. In this Mrs. Stevenson is called the Queen, Polly is the lady chamberlain, and another Sally Franklin, daughter of an English relative whom Franklin has brought down to live with him, ce jeudi matin

101

[handwritten letter in French]

is the first maid of honor. He himself is referred to as " the great person " or " Dr. Fatsides." The following are specimen passages:

Saturday, September 22, 1770.

This morning Queen Margaret, accompanied by her first maid of honor, Miss Franklin, set out for Rochester. Immediately on their departure, the whole street was in tears — from a heavy shower of rain. It is whispered, that the new family administration, which took place on her Majesty's departure, promises, like all other new administrations, to govern much better than the old one.

We hear that the great person (so called from his enormous size), of a certain family in a certain street is grievously affected at the late changes, and could hardly be comforted this morning, though the new ministry promised him a roasted shoulder of mutton and potatoes for his dinner.

.   .   .   .

We hear that the lady chamberlain of the household went to market this morning by her own self, gave the butcher whatever he asked for the mutton, and had no dispute with the potato-woman, to their great amazement at the change of times.

Sunday, September 23.

It is now found by sad experience, that good resolutions are easier made than executed. Notwithstanding yesterday's solemn order of Council, nobody went to Church today. It seems the great person's broad-built bulk lay so long abed that the breakfast was not over till it was too late to dress.

.   .   .   .

Dr. Fatsides made four hundred and sixty-nine turns to his dining-room, as the exact distance of a visit to the lovely

Lady Barwell, whom he did not find at home; so there was no struggle for and against a kiss, and he sat down to dream in the easy-chair, that he had it without any trouble.

. . . .

Monday, September 24.

This evening there was high play at Craven Street House. The great person lost money. It is supposed the ministers, as is usually supposed of all ministers, shared the emoluments among them.

. . . .

Tuesday, September 25.

At six o'clock this afternoon, news came by post, that her Majesty arrived safely at Rochester on Saturday night. The bells immediately rang — for candles to illuminate the parlor; the court went into cribbage; and the evening concluded with every demonstration of joy.

IV

During the long lulls of waiting on the movements of ministries and Parliaments, Franklin frequently found solace in his ancient love — scientific investigation and experiment. He invented a reformed alphabet with phonetic spelling; he improved a stove in the Craven Street house so that it would burn its own smoke; he recommended a scheme for the better ventilation of the Houses of Parliament; he studied colds and traced them to impure air and overfeeding; he subscribed to a project for conveying " civilized " animals and seeds to the islands of the Pacific; he wrote on rainfalls, swimming, and the Gulf Stream; he was interested in the Northwest Passage and the Aurora Borealis; he discovered that it was easier to draw a boat through deep water than through shallow; he advised upon the equip-

ment of St. Paul's Cathedral, the government powder magazines, and Buckingham Palace with lightning rods; he
went on walks carrying a cane containing oil to study the
effects of oil on water; he advised with Adam Smith while
Smith was writing " The Wealth of Nations "; he watched
three flies come to life in the sun after being drowned for
many months in a bottle of Madeira sent from Virginia,
and wrote:

" I wish it were possible, from this instance, to invent a
method of embalming drowned persons in such a manner
that they may be recalled to life at any period however distant; for having a very ardent desire to see and observe the
state of America a hundred years hence, I should prefer to
any ordinary death the being immersed in a cask of Madeira
wine, with a few friends, till that time, to be recalled to
life by the solar warmth of my dear country! "

All the time he was making friends among the great and
meeting eminent personages. He often attended the heavy
dinners of the period and followed its customs in sometimes
coming home with a thickened head. The days of Poor
Richard and his pawky maxims were far, far behind. He
was once invited to dine with Christian VII, king of Den-
mark, who was in London on a visit to his brother-in-law,
George III. He attended the salon of Mrs. Montagu,
and the meetings of numerous clubs and societies. He con-
sorted often with clergymen and physicians. The latter
had a club of which his friend, Sir John Pringle, was president. Thomas Jefferson thus quotes a story about this club
which Franklin told him one day when they were seated together listening to some wearisome discussion in early congressional days:

" I happened to be there when the question to be considered was whether physicians had, on the whole, done most
good or harm. The young members, particularly, having

discussed it very learnedly and eloquently till the subject was exhausted, one of them observed to Sir John Pringle, that although it was not usual for the President to take part in a debate, yet they were desirous to know his opinion on the question. He said they must first tell him whether, under the application of physicians they meant to include *old women;* if they did, he thought they had done more good than harm; otherwise, more harm than good."

English clergymen were charmed by Franklin's geniality, learning, and occasional jokes at their expense no less than physicians. Among men of the cloth with whom he founded solid friendships were such conspicuous figures as Dr. Richard Price, Dr. Joseph Priestley, and Jonathan Shipley, the good bishop of St. Asaph. At the bishop's country home at Twyford, Hampshire, Franklin spent many tranquil weeks. It was here that he began his oft-interrupted " Autobiography " and gained for himself the worshipful admiration of the bishop's daughters. To one of them, Georgiana, he had presented " Mungo," an American gray squirrel. On its meeting with sudden death, he wrote for its tomb one of the epitaphs which he was fond of composing in the style he liked to call " monumental."

V

One day the easy routine of life at the Craven Street house was broken by a momentous announcement. Polly Stevenson wrote him from Margate, at the seaside, that she had met a handsome and insinuating young physician. She confessed that he had made an impression on her. To the Doctor this news must have been a little saddening, for Polly was the best beloved of all of " Franklin's girls "; but he bravely mustered all the gayety with which he was accustomed to write to Polly and replied:

" There are certain circumstances in Life wherein 'tis perhaps best not to hearken to Reason. For instance, possibly if the Truth were known, I have Reason to be jealous of this same insinuating, handsome young Physician; but as it flatters more my Vanity, and therefore gives me the more pleasure, to suppose you were in Spirits on account of my safe return, I shall turn a deaf Ear to Reason in this case, as I have done with Success in twenty others."

Polly duly married her young doctor and became Mrs. William Hewson. Her devotion to the old doctor, however, remained steady, striking proofs of which we shall see at a later date. Franklin made friends easily; but he also had a rarer quality which held them constant through long silences and wide spaces of years.

Polly had become a mother and Franklin had returned to Philadelphia when one day she wrote him:

" My mother was urging me to-day to wean my little girl. I cannot tell why, for I never was in better health; I pleaded for her by saying that as she is to be your granddaughter you would be very angry if I did not let her suck a year. My mother then was silent, for absent as well as present, your opinion is her Law."

A mighty presence, this, that could make its influence felt across 3000 miles of water and determine the question of weaning a child as well as the shape of the lightning rods on Buckingham Palace.

Chapter XXVI

The Defeat of Pitt and Peace

I

IN the course of years Franklin has learned that the thing which is impossible to the go-getter, frequently comes round of its own motion to him who waits. On his previous visit to London, he had tried unsuccessfully to see the Great Commoner, William Pitt. He must therefore have smiled one of his shrewdest smiles when one morning in August, 1774, fourteen years later, he hears a knock at the door and learns that the great man is outside and craves an interview with him.

Pitt is now the august Lord Chatham; his powers are waning as his gout increases; but his is still a weighty influence throughout the land. He invites Franklin to come home with him in his carriage. He civilly questions Franklin upon the state of affairs in America. Is it true that the colonies there aim to set themselves up as an independent state, and that they particularly intend to get rid of the Navigation Acts? Franklin reassures him. He declares he has never heard the least wish for a separation; and as to the Navigation Acts, he is sure that the colonies are perfectly willing to accept the provision requiring that trade be carried on in British or plantation bottoms, that foreign ships be excluded from American ports, and that the crews be at least three-fourths British. His lordship expresses his gratification and adds that he hopes he will see Franklin again.

On September 4, the Continental Congress meets at Philadelphia. It passes measures of alternating defiance of and devotion to the British crown. It encourages Massachusetts in its resistance to arbitrary power, and calls for the complete cessation of imports from or exports to Great Britain. It passes the carefully prepared Declaration of Rights. On the other hand, it votes rather pathetic addresses to the people of Great Britain, of Canada, and America, and sends a petition to George III, calling him " the loving father of your whole people," and closing as follows:

" We therefore most earnestly beseech your Majesty, that your royal authority and interposition may be used for our relief, and that a gracious answer may be given to this petition. That your Majesty may enjoy every felicity through a long and glorious reign over loyal and happy subjects, and that your descendants may inherit your prosperity and dominions till time shall be no more, is, and always will be our sincere and fervent prayer."

Franklin sends a copy to Lord Dartmouth, the colonial secretary, and then drives out to Kent to lay a copy before Lord Chatham, who receives him " with an affectionate kind of respect." He tells Franklin that he deems the Continental Congress to be " the most honorable assembly of statesmen since those of the ancient Greeks and Romans in the most virtuous times," and that he means to address the House of Lords on the immediate and unconditional withdrawal of General Gage's troops from Boston. He invites Franklin to attend.

On the appointed day at the Lords, Franklin meets Lord Chatham, who takes him by the arm and is about to show him through a door, when they bump full into the stony face of an established British Precedent. This door, the rigid keeper informs them, can be entered by none but the eldest sons or brothers of peers. Even the mighty Chatham retreats in awe, and Franklin has to be taken back by his limping lordship to an obscure door near the bar.

Chatham makes one of his mightiest efforts. He declares that the very basis of British liberty is that no subject shall be taxed but by his own consent. He demands justice for the Americans. " Let the sacredness of their property remain inviolate, let it be taxable only by their own consent, or it ceases to be property." But " all availed," wrote Franklin, " no more than the whistling of the winds." The lords and bishops signify that they not only do not mean to withdraw the troops from Boston, but that they are thinking of sending more.

II

Chatham's defeat darkens the cloud of unpopularity hanging over Franklin in London. He is no longer invited to great houses. The press abuses him. In Parliament he is called a mischievous enemy. There are rumors that he is to be arrested for treason and in one of his letters he refers to the possibility of his reposing in Tyburn. Even in his own country he is suspected of deceit and double-dealing. Josiah Quincy is sent over from Massachusetts to take soundings, and Arthur Lee, who is to succeed Franklin as the Massachusetts agent, sends home letters full of the criticisms and innuendos that could emanate only from an imagination made turgid by a sense of superiority having no proper outlet.

The ministry's next move in the attempt either to win Franklin over or to circumvent him is to employ feminine wiles. He receives an invitation to play chess with Mrs. Howe, sister of Admiral Lord Howe. He complies, enjoys himself, and is asked to come again. Negotiations ensue, participated in by David Barclay, the Quaker leader, and Franklin's old friend, Dr. Fothergill. For discussion Franklin prepares certain "Hints," which call for the repeal of the tea duty, the granting of a large measure of autonomy to the colonies, and among other things, the right of unrestricted manufacturing. Several meetings and discussions with notabilities take place, but all come to naught. Franklin even offers to stand as security for the payment of damages inflicted by the Boston Tea Party, to the extent of £15,000, but Lord North's ministry will concede no jot. Finally a scarcely concealed bribe is offered to Franklin. He is told that if he can bring about a reconciliation with the colonies on terms suitable to the dignity of the government, he may reap a reward "beyond his expectation."

Barclay and Fothergill give up. They admit that no peace is possible except on corrupt terms. Waiting an extra year has availed nothing, and once more Franklin prepares to sail.

Before the year is out, he hears that Deborah is dead, full of years, and Sally reigns in her stead in the new house on Market Street. He sails for home March 21, 1775. On the way his ship passes another bearing a letter from a young Englishman, much battered by fortune, whom he has recommended to friends in America as an "ingenious, worthy young man." The letter is written from opposite the London Coffee House, Front Street, Philadelphia. It says:

"Your countenancing me has obtained me many friends and much reputation, for which please to accept my sincere thanks."

It is signed "Thos. Pain," without the final "e."

CHAPTER XXVII

Assistant at the Birth of a Republic

I

IT was a heavy-hearted Franklin who turned his face away from England, where he had spent ten and a half years of continuous labor, towards a Deborahless home in disturbed America. Dr. Priestley, the discoverer of oxygen and the historian of electricity, with whom he spent his final hours in London, says that the Doctor's last act was to read over some American papers from which he desired extracts to be sent to the English press, " and in reading them, he was frequently not able to proceed for the tears literally running down his cheeks."

But on the six weeks' voyage home, accompanied by William Temple Franklin, Franklin is soon happily engaged in probing the ocean. His chief comforter is the Gulf Stream. He keeps it under constant observation, sounds it and repeatedly takes its temperature, finds that it is warmer than the surrounding ocean, and concludes that it has its source in the tropics and receives its impulse from the trade winds. He also discovers that its waters are not phosphorescent. He likewise watches the navigation of the ship and concludes that it would do better if its hull were shaped so as to offer the least resistance to the water and if its rigging were so changed as to make the least resistance to the wind. He writes a piece about it, illustrated with drawings.

When he lands in Philadelphia, he learns with concern but no surprise that the embattled patriots of Concord and

Lexington have fired shots which are calling the entire thirteen colonies to arms. The next day an ode appears in the local paper dedicated " To the Friend of his Country and Mankind, Doctor Benjamin Franklin, on his Return from England, May 6th, 1775." It begins:

> " Welcome!   Once more
> To these fair western plains — thy native shore.
> Here live beloved, and leave the tools at home
> To run their length, and finish out their doom.
> Here lend thine aid to quench their brutal fires,
> Or fan the flame which Liberty inspires,
> Or fix the grand conductor, that shall guide
> The tempest back, and 'lectrify their pride.
> Rewarding Heaven will bless thy cares at last,
> And future glories glorify the past."

He finds there is a new hotel in town; it is called the " Franklin Inn." It is the first of a long line of things bearing the name of Franklin, including hotels, clubs, societies, inventions, institutes, colleges, cities, counties, and cigars. Even Tennessee tries very hard to have herself called the State of Franklin.

He instantly becomes the complete patriot, writing to Edmund Burke: " Gen. Gage's troops made a most vigorous retreat — twenty miles in three hours — scarce to be paralleled in history; the feeble Americans, who pelted them all the way, could scarce keep up with them "; but he still has a notion that he may be asked to return to England. Upon hearing this, Jane Mecom writes:

" You positively must not go; you have served the public in that way beyond what any other man can boast till you are now come to a good old age, and some younger men must now take that painful service upon them. Don't go, pray don't go. . . ."

II

On the day after his arrival Franklin is chosen to be one of Pennsylvania's three delegates to the Continental Congress, which organizes for war, with George Washington as commander-in-chief of the army. One of its first acts is to elect Franklin postmaster-general. He signalizes the event by thriftily appointing his none too prosperous son-in-law, Richard Bache, his deputy; and by changing the frank on letters from " Free — B. Franklin " to " B free Franklin," thereby setting up a precedent for making propaganda out of postmarks which other governments have been happy to follow. Being appointed on the committee charged with the production of a new Continental currency, he also thriftily procures the work of printing and engraving for Sally's husband.

Congress places him on numerous other committees: To find supplies of saltpeter; to negotiate with the Indians; to consider a conciliatory offer from Lord North; and to regulate and protect colonial commerce.

His belief that he might soon return to London was set aside when news came of the burning by the British of coast towns, and of the losses at Bunker Hill. He sat down and wrote a blunt and indignant letter breaking off relations with William Strahan, one of the oldest and most faithful of his London friends. But on cooling off, he never actually sent it, and after doing much propaganda duty, it now reposes in the files of the State Department at Washington.

In the same month — July, 1775 — he brings before Congress his Plan of Union, proposing that each colony retain its independence in internal affairs, that a Congress annually elected shall regulate external relations, and that supreme authority shall be vested in a council of twelve.

All the British colonies bordering on the Atlantic are to be invited to join, including Ireland. The Plan was referred to a committee, where it died of inattention and under-nourishment. Even at that date, a filial Congress did not wish to affront the mother country by flourishing the sundering knife, and the Episcopal clergy went right on praying for the king. These prayers gave offense to some of the hot-heads, who proposed that they be stopped. But Franklin raised a warning hand.

" The measure," he said, " is quite unnecessary; for the Episcopal clergy, to my certain knowledge, have been constantly praying, these twenty years, that ' God would give to the king and his council wisdom '; and we all know that not the least notice has been taken of that prayer. So it is plain, the gentlemen have no interest in the court of Heaven."

During the first few weeks of Congress, Franklin was absent from many sessions, due to attacks of gout. Strange ailment for the author of Poor Richard's frugal maxims! But he did much work for the Pennsylvania Committee of Safety, of which he was elected chairman, in organizing measures of defense, particularly in inventing ingenious chevaux-de-frise to block the river Delaware against the British fleet. In the autumn of 1775 he was elected to the Pennsylvania Assembly, but resigned when he was appointed a member of a committee of three to go to Cambridge, Mass., and help the despairing Gen. Washington work out a plan for raising and maintaining an army to replace the disorderly mob which had first been inflicted upon him.

III

When the year 1776 opens, there is still much confusion. The wealthier classes in America cannot bring themselves to hurl away their allegiance to the throne of England, whose ritual, traditions, and viewpoint they regard as well-nigh divine, and in Pennsylvania the reactionary following of the Proprietaries produce sordid dissensions. It is realized that a propaganda pamphlet is needed for general circulation, something ringing, something bold and dramatic. Franklin is too busy to do it. He writes to Mrs. Stevenson in London: " I am well, and as happy as I can be under the Fatigue of more Business than is suitable to my Age and Inclination. But it follows me everywhere, and I submit."

Where there is a demand, however, there is always a supply, and the supplier proves to be the young Englishman who but recently has come over with an introduction from Franklin — Thomas Paine. His pamphlet appears on January 10, 1776, published by Robert Bell in Philadelphia, price two shillings. It is entitled " Common Sense," and reaches a climax in these sentences:

" Everything that is right or natural pleads for separation. The blood of the slain, the weeping voice of Nature cries, IT IS TIME TO PART."

When soon afterwards Paine goes on a visit to New York, he carries with him this letter of introduction from Franklin to Gen. Charles Lee:

" The bearer, Mr. Paine, has requested a line of introduction to you. . . . He is the reputed, and I think the real, author of Common Sense, a pamphlet that has made a great impression here."

IV

About this time a mysterious stranger, having a military bearing, arrives in Philadelphia and after several efforts gets a message through to Congress. A committee composed of John Jay, Thomas Jefferson, and Franklin hears him in Carpenters' Hall. The stranger reveals that he speaks in the name of the King of France, who is ready to aid the Americans with arms and money. A long delay occurs before Congress is able to make up its mind to follow up the hint. It finally appoints a committee to act as a kind of secret department of foreign relations and " to correspond secretly with friends in Great Britain, Ireland, and other parts of the world." On it are John Jay, John Dickinson, Thomas Johnson, Benjamin Harrison and Franklin. On Franklin, with his trained abilities and long experience abroad, the bulk of the secret committee's work naturally falls. One of his first acts is to send a " feelout " letter to his old friend in Paris, M. Dubourg. Arthur Lee is asked to sound the foreign embassies in London, and preparations are made to send Silas Deane, of Connecticut, direct to France to act as a commission merchant and confidential agent.

Then comes the news of the dismal collapse of the expedition to Canada, with Gen. Montgomery dead on the heights of Quebec and Gen. Benedict Arnold severely wounded. Congress, having by now learned the committee habit, appoints one to go to Canada and win it for the Union. The members are Samuel Chase, Charles Carroll of Carrollton, and — of course — Franklin. Carroll's brother John, a Catholic priest, is taken along as French interpreter and propagandist.

The committee boards a sloop at New York and sets sail up the Hudson for Albany. The perils of the deep assail the little sloop, and its tired crew sight West Point only after three days. Two more days are required to reach Albany. There follows a jolting ride in a country wagon over the 32 miles to Saratoga. Franklin, now 70 years old and more suited to carpet slippers in a warm study than a wild-goose expedition to Canada in the frozen winter, dismounts at the home of Gen. Schuyler in an enfeebled and dispirited condition. He believes he will not survive. He even sits down to write to a few friends " by way of farewell." But the Schuyler home has its warming attractions, including, so Carroll notes, " two daughters (Betsey and Peggy), lively, agreeable, black-eyed gals "; and a week's rest in such company restores the frozen commissioners. They push onward by boat through the ice of Lake George and at last reach Montreal, all of them worn out. There they encounter the bitterest experience of all: they learn that lack of money, American bad manners, and resolute Tory opposition make the very notion of winning Canada hopeless. Franklin, feeling the pangs of age, cold, and gout, has had enough. He turns back to report to Congress.

The year is 1776. Comes June, nowhere more flaming than in the demurely walled gardens of Philadelphia. Franklin, looking out on the soaring roses of the month's 21st day, writes this letter to Gen. Washington:

" I am just recovering from a severe fit of the Gout, which has kept me from Congress and Company ever since you left us, so that I know little of what has pass'd there, except that a Declaration of Independence is preparing."

v

A committee of five had been elected to draft that document: Thomas Jefferson, John Adams, Robert R. Livingston, Roger Sherman, and — inevitably — Franklin. He cheerfully agreed with his colleagues in leaving the actual work of writing to Jefferson. His gout made an excellent excuse.

" I have made it a rule," he told Jefferson later, " whenever in my power to avoid becoming the draftsman of papers to be reviewed by a public body."

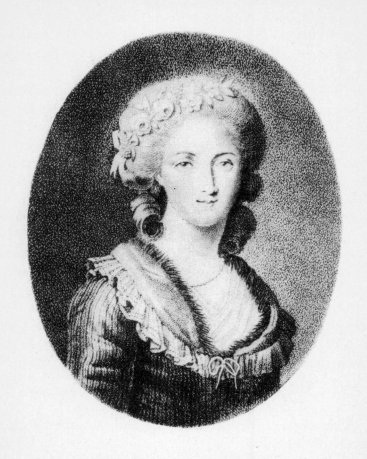

THE COUNTESS D' HOUDETOT.

ONE OF THE FRENCHWOMEN WHO HAD AN ALMOST EXTRAVAGANT
ADMIRATION FOR FRANKLIN.

From the Ford Collection in the New York Public Library.

He then related his famous anecdote of John Thompson, the hatter:

"When I was a journeyman printer, one of my companions, an apprenticed hatter, having served out his time, was about to open shop for himself. His first concern was to have a handsome signboard, with a proper inscription. He composed it in these words, *John Thompson, Hatter, makes and sells Hats for ready Money*, with a figure of a hat subjoined. But he thought he would submit it to his friends for their amendments. The first he showed it to thought the word *hatter* tautologous, because followed by the words *makes hats*, which showed he was a hatter. It was struck out. The next observed that the word *makes* might as well be omitted, because his customers would not care who made the hats; if good and to their mind they would buy, by whomsoever made. He struck it out. A third said he thought the words *for ready money* were useless, as it was not the custom of the place to sell on credit. Everyone who purchased expected to pay. They were parted with; and the inscription now stood, *John Thompson sells hats*. '*Sells* hats? says his next friend; why, nobody will expect you to give them away. What, then, is the use of that word?' It was stricken out, and *hats* followed, the rather as there was one painted on the board. So his inscription was reduced ultimately to *John Thompson*, with the figure of a hat subjoined."

When signing time came, there was some objection on the part of Southerners to the wording of Jefferson's document, particularly from fiery ones, owing to Jefferson's attack on George III for repeatedly preventing the repeal of the slave-importation law, whereupon John Hancock cried: "We must all hang together," thus giving Franklin his chance to make the celebrated observation:

" We must, indeed, all hang together, or, most assuredly, we shall all hang separately."

Robert Morris and John Dickinson failed to appear to make Pennsylvania's vote unanimous, so Franklin cast it alone for the proudest document in American history — still proud, though so unfamiliar to the country's patriotic citizenry that during the World War persons were arrested in Pennsylvania for distributing legible copies of it.

And then Franklin signed his name, adding that scroll-like flourish beneath which is well-nigh an autobiographical hieroglyph, betokening abundant vitality and a secret love for the fantastic.

VI

In the same month Franklin is elected to Congress, which at once embroils itself in a fierce debate over the question of voting by states. He fights in vain against the expedient of giving one vote to each state, regardless of size. He next goes to the Pennsylvania Constitutional Convention and is promptly elected president. It closes by voting him unanimous thanks for his able advice; but Franklin has no opportunity to take pride therein, for on its heels comes the news that his son and pride, William Franklin, has been removed from his post as Royal Governor of New Jersey and taken to Connecticut under arrest as " a mischievous and dangerous enemy." William remains an obdurate royalist for the duration of the war, and afterwards goes to England to enjoy a life pension of £800 a year voted him by an appreciative government.[1]

" Nothing," wrote Franklin, " had ever affected him with such keen sensations as to find himself deserted in his

---

[1] Elizabeth Franklin, wife of William, died of "accumulated distresses" before he was released and was buried within the chancel of St. Paul's Church, New York.

old age by his only son; and not only deserted, but to find him taking up arms against him in a cause wherein his good fame, fortune, and life were all at stake."

VII

While Washington is wondering how he is going to defend New York with his rag-tag army of 9000 men, Admiral Howe, Franklin's recent friend at the London chess table, lands on Staten Island an army of trained troops which his brother, Gen. Howe, is to command. The admiral at once sends a conciliatory letter to Franklin, together with books, parcels, and letters forwarded in his care by Franklin's still faithful English friends. A correspondence ensues during which the colonial forces lose the battle of Long Island. Finally Congress names a committee to meet the admiral. Its members are Edward Rutledge, John Adams, and — once more — Franklin. Lord Howe receives this committee in a specially built bower on Staten Island while his Grenadier Guards present arms, and spreads before them a collation including claret, ham, tongue and mutton. But nothing comes of the conference. The American commissioners insist that their country will discuss terms only as an independent power, while he admits that he is not empowered to make a definite proposal. The war goes on, the year ending gloomily for American arms. Washington is driven off Manhattan Island, evacuating Forts Washington and Lee, losing the battle of White Plains, and retreating through New Jersey. Congress in alarm quits Philadelphia for Baltimore, and Thomas Paine in " The American Crisis " writes: " These are the times that try men's souls." Only one success comes to relieve the dismal prospect: on Christmas day, 1776, Washington surprises and routs the Hessians at Trenton.

But Franklin is meantime mightily cheered by a long letter from his friend Barbue Dubourg at Paris. It begins by calling him " My Dear Master," assures him of Dubourg's interest and coöperation, and closes thus: " Adieu, fare you well, be prosperous, you and yours, and know that not one in the world is more devoted to you." Also word comes from Arthur Lee that at the court of the young Louis XVI and Marie Antoinette in France, a powerful figure has arisen marchais, playwright, musician, courtier, watchmaker and man of business. Only the year before a Paris theatre has produced his " Barber of Seville," with music by Rossini.

Congress, vastly elated, decides to dispatch a commission of three to France. Franklin is unanimously elected on the first ballot. The other members are Thomas Jefferson, now 33 years old, and Silas Deane. Jefferson excuses himself owing to the illness of his wife, and the meticulous Arthur Lee is elected in his stead. Franklin breathes a little sigh. Will he never get back to his beloved electrical devices, his library, his writing desk, his armonica, and the soothing ministrations of Sally? He rises and shakes himself, but does not think of declining.

" I am old and good for nothing," he remarks to Dr. Rush, " but, as the storekeepers say of their remnants of cloth, ' I am but a fag end, and you may have me for what you please.' "

In profound secrecy he leaves Philadelphia, with his two grandsons, William Temple Franklin and Benjamin Franklin Bache, on October 26th, 1777, and the next day boards the sloop Reprisal at Marcus Hook. But the British spy service watches every move. They know why he is going to France, but take it as a sign of the early collapse of the American rebellion.

The voyage is rough, but Franklin mitigates its horrors by a new study of ocean temperatures. He arrives at

Nantes, however, so weak that he can scarcely stand. The ladies of Nantes take one look at his peaked fur cap and rush back home to dress their hair *à la Franklin*. It augurs the success of this his last and greatest effort, begun at the age of 71. He has been midwife at the birth of the world's first great republic. He now goes to ensure its supply of certified milk.

CHAPTER XXVIII

A Fur Cap among Powdered Heads

I

SOON after establishing his residence in France, Franklin wrote two characteristic letters to feminine friends. One, to Mary Hewson in London, said:
" My Dear, Dear Polly, figure to yourself an old man, with grey hair appearing under a Martin fur cap, among the powder'd heads of Europe."

It is this fur cap which is pictured in the Franklin portrait by Cochin, reproduced as the frontispiece to this volume.

The other was to Elizabeth Partridge in Boston:
" Somebody, it seems, gave it out that I loved Ladies, and then everybody presented me their Ladies (or the ladies presented themselves) to be embrac'd, that is, to have their Necks kiss'd. For as to kissing of Lips and Cheeks, it is not the Mode here, the first is reconed rude, and the other may rub off the Paint. The French Ladies have, however, 1000 other ways of rendering themselves agreeable; by their various Attentions & Civilities, & their sensible Conversation."

Franklin was too much of a showman and had, besides, too much shrewdness and knowledge of the world, not to realize at a very early date that in France the ground had already been laid, the atmosphere already created, the settings already moved into their place, for the success of the appeals which he was about to make. He saw that all he had to do was to go slowly, to feel his way gradually, and not to make offensive mistakes.

And with it all he perceived that he was going to have the time of his life. This was the kind of *milieu* for which all his life he had craved and one for which he had unconsciously been preparing all his toilsome years in business, politics, science, and diplomacy. Here was Paris at the zenith of its exhilaration at getting rid of Louis XV and acquiring as its new monarchs the amiable Louis XVI and the charming if irresponsible Marie Antoinette. It was a Paris ready to hope and adore. It was especially in the mood to adore Franklin, and Franklin sagaciously decided to put nothing in its way. He swept his memory clean of all the shrivelling maxims of Poor Richard and gathering up the thirteen Virtues of his quondam creed — including Temperance, Silence, Order, Frugality and Moderation — he dropped them through a hole in his mind and closed the lid upon them with a barely muffled thud.

" In the midst of the effeminate and servile refinement of the 18th century," says the Count Sigur in his Memoirs, " the almost rustic apparel, the plain but firm demeanor, the free and direct language of the (American) envoys, seemed to have introduced within our walls . . . some sages contemporary with Plato, or republicans of the age of Cato and Fabius."

But the Count perhaps permitted his emotions to get out of hand. The American envoys were not quite so rustic and simple as all that. The lapse of a few months found Franklin, at any rate, installed in a comfortable villa at Passy, two miles from the centre of Paris, where he kept a carriage and a cellar full of the best wines, and whence he was soon dining out six nights a week, chiefly in the company of those ladies who had learned a thousand and one methods of rendering themselves agreeable.

As for the other envoys, they did not stint themselves, as their accounts soon showed.

II

The secret and unexpected landing of Franklin is still keeping France abuzz when a few days later he, Lee and Deane have their first interview with the Count de Vergennes, the French foreign minister. The Count is sympathetic but cautious. There are many difficulties in the way. The British ambassador, Lord Stormont, is making a fuss about the shipments of ammunition to America through the mercantile house of Roderique Hortalez & Co., which is simply another name for Beaumarchais. Treaties must be considered. France has been drained by recent wars with England. One must go slow. Meantime if Congress desires a loan of two million livres, payable after the war without interest, that can be arranged; only there must not be a word . . . not a word.

About the time of the payment of the second installment of this loan the twenty-year old Marquis de Lafayette, excited by the rapturous reception given to Franklin and athirst for adventure, sails for America, where Gen. Washington awaits him with an indulgent smile.

"He is exceedingly beloved," writes Franklin to the Secret Committee, " and everybody's good wishes attend him. . . . He has left a beautiful young wife, and for her sake particularly, we hope that his bravery and ardent desire to distinguish himself will be a little restrained by the General's prudence, so as not to permit his being hazarded much, but on some important occasion."

Lafayette's romantic deed sets up an instant fashion. All the young bloods of France and no end of out-of-work officers demand passage to America and a commission in the Continental army, it being usually specified that their rank must be one degree higher than that enjoyed at home.

" You can have no conception," writes Franklin to Dubourg, " how I am harassed. All my friends are sought out and teazed to teaze me. Great officers of all ranks, in all departments, ladies, great and small, besides professed solicitors, worry me from morning till night. The noise of every coach now that enters my court terrifies me. I am afraid to accept an invitation to dine abroad, being almost sure of meeting with some officer or officer's friend, who, as soon as I am put in good humor by a glass or two of champagne, begins his attack upon me."

Worse than men the infant republic needed money. The first French loan was a mere drop in a yawning bucket; what the American commissioners set their hearts on was ten millions of dollars, but as regards an increased loan the French remained coy if not silent. Evil news was coming through about Washington's retreat through New Jersey and the woeful winter at Valley Forge. When questioned about these events, Franklin is said to have remarked: " Ça ira, Ça ira," which freely translated means: " It will work out all right." Whether it was Franklin who thus created the slogan which a few years later was so often sounded in the French Revolution is not certainly known, but since every sententious phrase that he uttered was quickly repeated throughout France, it may have been he.

To create a favorable atmosphere for a new loan and to spread some useful propaganda, Franklin now takes his well-trained pen in hand and prepares a pamphlet containing the American state constitutions, which is translated by Dubourg. He also writes " A Comparison of Great Britain and America as to Credit in 1777 "; " A Catechism relative to the English National Debt "; and " A Dialogue between Britain, France, Holland, Saxony, and America." By day he works incessantly and laboriously, keeping William Temple Franklin busy copying his many dispatches to Congress and his evermounting correspondence with individuals; at night he recuperates by dining out.

From the records and documents he left behind, we can reconstruct a picture of him opening one day's letters as follows:

From Dr. Ingen Housz, physician to the Empress of Austria, asking Franklin to put him right regarding certain scientific experiments.

From a French chevalier who begs a few louis to avert impending starvation.

From a fellow countryman stranded at Marseilles.

From a poet asking for financial assistance in publishing an epic poem directed against the English.

From an anonymous correspondent who points out how wrong Franklin is in certain theories pertaining to lightning.

From a group of sailors on the U.S.S. Ranger complaining about the treatment received from Capt. John Paul Jones.

From Capt. Jones complaining about the behavior of the sailors.

From Arthur Lee declaring that he, Lee, is being ignored and insulted by French officials, and that he does not propose to stand for it.

From a lady asking him to locate her son believed to be somewhere in America.

From Jean Baptiste Le Roy asking for Ingen Housz's observations on Dr. Priestley's discovery relative to carbon.

From Madame Le Roy, who reminds him that she is " la petite femme de poche " — the little pocket Venus — and that he has been neglecting her shamefully, though she has loved him more than any of his other adopted daughters.

From the prior of a Benedictine abbey who has lost money gambling and begs Franklin to help him save his reputation. This letter bears a note appended by Franklin: " Wants me to pay his gaming debts and he will pray for success to our cause."

It is little wonder that after a day of such matters, Franklin fled from the house and sought refuge in genial company. Also it seems that he sometimes breakfasted as well as dined with fair guests, for it is on record that the Marquise de Crequi told horrified friends that Franklin ate his eggs cracked into a goblet and cut his melon with a knife.

III

In reality Franklin at first enjoys no greater powers than those bestowed by Congress on the other two commissioners, but his greater age and far greater prestige lead the French to regard him as the chief envoy and he was soon being treated as if he were the head of the commission. Silas Deane does not mind, but the honors and attentions lavished upon Franklin fill the egotistic Arthur Lee with a poisonous jealousy. Describing the respect shown to Franklin by the Parisians on public occasions, Deane writes home: " I confess I felt a joy and pride which was pure and honest, though not disinterested, for I considered it an honor to be known to be an American and his acquaintance "; but Lee writes to his brother: " Things are going on worse and worse every day among ourselves, and my situation is more painful. I see in every department neglect, dissipation, and private schemes." Lee even goes to the length of proposing that Franklin be sent to Vienna, and Deane to Holland, while he should be left in sole charge at Paris. He makes repeated half-veiled charges against Franklin, and soon brings on open quarrels with Deane and Beaumarchais.

The situation as regards the ten or dozen American agents in France has been made worse by the failure of Congress to define their precise duties and jurisdiction. On Sunday they all meet and dine at Franklin's home in Passy amicably enough, but during the rest of the time concealed intrigue makes the atmosphere sultry and dangerous. At this stage not even Franklin himself seems to have been made fully aware of the transactions that have taken place between Deane and Beaumarchais, with the connivance of the French government.

When the romantic Beaumarchais first proposed to the king that the Americans be supported as a means of weakening Britain, it was thought that France's assistance should be given directly, but this notion was abandoned in favor of a more crafty scheme which would hoodwink the English ambassador. Accordingly Beaumarchais got from the French treasury a million francs to set up a commercial firm which would sell war supplies to America on long terms. He was also to have the privilege of taking arms and powder from the royal arsenal and paying for them or replacing them at his convenience. Beaumarchais, then much in love with things Spanish, called this firm Roderique Hortalez & Co., and immediately began making secret shipments to America much in the spirit of a story-fed schoolboy. His great privileges are supposed to have come to him through the favor of Queen Marie Antoinette.

Beaumarchais intended to recoup himself through American shipments of tobacco, indigo, and rice, which his government was to help him dispose of. His capital was strengthened by the grant of a second million francs from Spain, and all would have gone well except that the expected cargoes from America failed to come through. This was due partly to congressional carelessness, partly to the vigilance of British cruisers, and partly to the malefactions of Arthur Lee, who led Congress to believe that the French shipments were sent as a gift.

It was arranged that the French government was to help

get Beaumarchais's ships safely out of port. Then if Lord
Stormont, the English ambassador, discovered their purpose,
it was to appear to be surprised and mortified, and stop the
ships. When the ships were brought back to port and ostentatiously unloaded, Beaumarchais was to reload them elsewhere, or pretend to sell the ships and change their names
before a new voyage was attempted. All this was to prevent an open breach with the British government, which
still held the French port of Dunkirk; and though Lord
Stormont often made a disturbance, this curious hugger-
muggery was actually carried on for two years, through an
understanding between Deane and Beaumarchais reached
before Franklin's arrival.

Beaumarchais seems to have hypnotizèd Deane. The
American found it impossible to resist the Frenchman's
powerful and reckless personality. He even permitted
Beaumarchais to foist upon him the comic but ill-fated General du Coudray, who, with a whole train of officers, went
to America with a commission signed by Deane as " General-
in-Chief of Artillery " and a letter of recommendation from
Dr. Franklin which Deane induced the doctor to write. As
Gen. Knox was already in command of the American artillery, du Coudray's arrival produced a situation which ended
only when the French artillerist was accidentally drowned in
the Schuylkill River. We shall see what a penalty Deane
paid for his excessive good nature.

IV

While Lee goes on with his jealous undermining of his
colleagues, Franklin says nothing and attends to business.
In his letters home, he never refers to Lee's constant sus-
picions of his associates and never makes any counter-
charges. But, due to the division of authority, neither he

nor his colleagues keep any accurate records or books, and there is no one who can refute Lee's charges of graft and corruption, some of which are aimed at Jonathan Williams, American naval agent at Nantes, who is Franklin's nephew. The confusion grows in the absence of orders or any other communications from home, and there must have been times when the French government wished that the entire American contingent, with the exception of Franklin, whom it trusted entirely, could be shipped back in charge of trained madhouse keepers.

Meantime the news from both home and abroad is edged with dark blue. Gen. Burgoyne has landed in America with a fresh army which is to cut off New York from New England. Gen. Howe has taken Philadelphia, and British officers are playing with the sacred electrical apparatus and stealing pictures in Franklin's own home.[1] The French loan has been exhausted, and Beaumarchais, pleading in vain for return shipments from America, is threatened with bankruptcy.

It is December 4, 1777. The American envoys are sitting in Franklin's home wondering what new appeal they shall make to the French government when a chaise is driven rapidly into the courtyard. There are shouts that it is a messenger from America, and Franklin and his colleagues hasten out to greet him. Jonathan Loring Austin, of Massachusetts, steps out with a smiling face. He brings the electrifying news that Gen. Burgoyne and his entire army have surrendered.

Within two days M. Gerard, secretary of the king's council, calls at Passy to offer congratulations. He adds that the Count de Vergennes is in a receptive mood regarding

[1] The portrait by Benjamin Wilson reproduced in this volume was taken from Franklin's home by Major André. It was returned to the American people in 1906 by Earl Grey, Governor-General of Canada, descendant of the Gen. Grey in charge of the evacuation of Philadelphia.

any proposals the commissioners may care to make. On December 8 Franklin sends an address to the king, thanking him for the loan of three million francs so far received and asking that an alliance between France, Spain, and the United States be considered.

A few days later the Count receives the envoys at a secret place outside Versailles, and on December 17 he sends word that the king has decided to conclude a treaty with the American colonies as soon as Spain is heard from. There ensue two or three weeks of negotiations, proposals, counter-proposals, visits, and the drawing up of documents, during which the fussy Lee makes more trouble than any other five men concerned. He finds fault with everything, and particularly complains about Franklin's dining out so often. It seems to have been about this time that Franklin began his twice-a-week visits to his neighbor, Madame Brillon, and took part in the other little flirtations which made him so happy and kept him in such a good humor.

v

"Do you know, my dear papa," wrote Mme. Brillon, whom the daughter of John Adams described as "one of the handsomest women in France," to the 72-year old doctor, "that people have the audacity to criticize my pleasant habit of sitting upon your knees, and yours of always asking me for what I always refuse? . . . I despise slanderers and am at peace with myself, but that is not enough. One must submit to what is called *Propriety* (the word varies in each century in each country) and sit less often on your knees. I shall surely love you no less, nor will our hearts be more or less pure; but we shall close the mouths of the malicious, and it is no small thing, even for the secure, to silence them."

VI

On Feb. 6, 1778, M. Gerard and the American commissioners meet and sign a Treaty of Amity and Commerce and a Treaty of Alliance between France and the United States. In this hour of triumph Franklin wears the suit of Manchester velvet in which he was clothed when he was the victim of the attack before the British Privy Council in the Cockpit at London. It is agreed that profound secrecy shall be maintained until word comes that the treaties have been ratified by Congress. But of course the usual leak occurs, and within a few days the whole of Europe knows about the treaties, including England, where Lord North's Conciliation Bill is brought out too late to be anything but a feeble anti-climax.

"Never have I seen a man," wrote Franklin's friend Le Roy to the Abbé Fauchet, "so happy, so joyous, as M. Franklin on the day that Lord Stormont, the British Ambassador, left Paris owing to our rupture with his court. We dined together, and he, who was ordinarily very calm, very tranquil, appeared on this day, from his exclamations of joy, to be another man."

Events follow fast. On March 20 the American commissioners are summoned to meet Louis XVI at Versailles. Deane and Lee appear in the rigidly prescribed court dress, with wig and sword; but Franklin, with a superb dignity concealing his showman's heart, emerges in clothes of plain but rich brown velvet, set off by a cascade of ruffles at breast and wrist, white silk stockings, and silver buckles.

There is a story that when ushered into the presence of the king he broke down slightly and seemed on the verge of weeping, but recovered himself when he saw that to Louis XVI, who would far rather have been in the hunting field than attending elaborate ceremonials, this was quite an

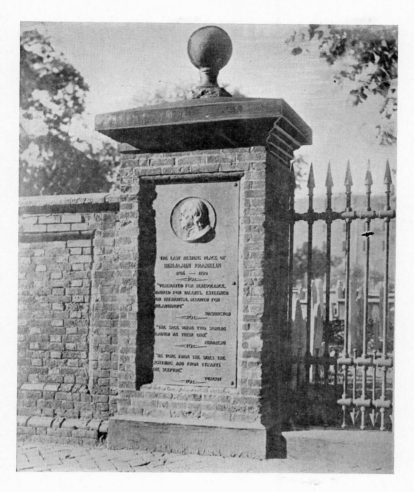

BRICK PILLAR MARKING FRANKLIN'S GRAVE,
PHILADELPHIA

IT CONTAINS QUOTATIONS FROM ENCOMIUMS BY WASHINGTON,
MIRABEAU, AND TURGOT.

ordinary occasion. In fact, Arthur Lee, who could be depended upon to have a jealous eye for details, afterwards wrote that the king's hair was hanging down upon his shoulders undressed, and that he had " no appearance of preparation." This may have been due, however, to the Count de Vergennes, who is said to have advised the king to take Franklin by the hand in English fashion and to converse with him informally.

Madame du Deffand, who kept a kind of political salon in Paris and though blind learned everything, gives a different account of Franklin's reception. In a letter to Horace Walpole, dated March 22, 1778, she wrote:

" Mr. Franklin has been presented to the king. He was accompanied by some twenty insurgents, three or four of whom wore a uniform. Franklin wore a dress of reddish brown (mordoré) velvet, white hose, his hair hanging loose, his spectacles on his nose, and a white hat under his arm. I do not know what he said, but the reply of the king was very gracious, as well towards the United States as toward Franklin their deputy. He praised his conduct and that of all his compatriots. I do not know what title he will have, but he will go to court every Tuesday, like all the rest of the diplomatic corps."

The recognition thus bestowed upon the American envoys, signalizing the fact that France is ready to begin war in support of American independence, causes an uneasy twinge in England, where there is already an undercurrent of desire to patch up a peace. Even George III writes to Lord North on March 26:

" The many instances of the inimical conduct of Franklin towards this country makes me aware that hatred of this country is the constant object of his mind. . . . Yet I think it so desirable to end the war with that country, to be enabled with redoubled ardor to avenge the faithless and insolent conduct of France, that I think it may be proper to keep open the channels of intercourse with that insidious man."

These channels are, in fact, never closed. All the time Franklin is in more or less constant communication with his faithful friends in England, who keep up a ceaseless propaganda for peace, and the British government, fully aware of the interchange of letters, does nothing to stop them. In addition, repeated efforts are made in disguised form to draw Franklin into conversation regarding terms of peace, but his invariable reply is that such hidden negotiations are useless, since nothing but complete independence will now satisfy the united colonies.

VII

Other events of interest occur in this year. Voltaire, who has greeted the beginning of Louis XVI's reign with the remark, "We are in the age of gold — up to our necks," returns to Paris from his long exile, surrounded by delirious crowds. The American commissioners pay the old eagle a visit. He converses with Franklin in English, proud of his ability to "speak in the language of a Franklin." He greets William Temple Franklin with the saying, "My child, God and liberty! Recollect those two words." A few weeks later Franklin and Voltaire are again brought together at a meeting of the Academy of Sciences. The crowd clamors for them to greet each other. They rise and shake hands. The crowd renews its clamor. "Embrace!" The two worn old veterans oblige. They take each other in their arms and kiss each other on the cheek, French fashion. The crowd shouts its ecstasy. John Adams says the cry spread over all Europe, "How charming it was to see

Solon and Sophocles embrace! " In a few weeks Voltaire is dead.

In the same year, tired and almost forgotten, dies Jean Jacques Rousseau. The mighty are falling. The end of a century approaches, and with it an epoch. After it the deluge and the hoarse cry of " Ça ira! "

Chapter XXIX

A Chapter of Altercations

I

IN the spring of 1778 Franklin writes two significant letters. One is to the president of the Continental Congress at Philadelphia. It is meant to anticipate the arrival there of Silas Deane, who has been called home to give an account of his operations as American agent in France before the coming of Franklin and Lee. John Adams has been appointed to succeed him. Franklin's letter praises Deane as " a faithful, active and able minister."

The other letter is to Lee. The old gentleman must have been choked with suppressed ire for some months, to have been able to use, even towards a trouble-making colleague, such scorching language:

" It is true that I have omitted answering some of your letters, particularly your angry ones, in which you, with very magisterial airs, schooled and documented me, as if I had been one of your domestics. I saw in the strongest light the importance of our living in decent civility towards each other while our great affairs were depending here; I saw your jealous, suspicious, malignant, and quarrelsome temper which was daily manifesting itself against Mr. Deane and almost every other person you had any concern with. I therefore passed your affronts in silence, did not answer, but burnt your angry letters, and received you, when I next saw you with the same civility as if you had never wrote them. Perhaps I may still pursue the same conduct, and not send you these. I believe I shall not, unless exceedingly pressed by you; for, of all things, I hate altercation."

If Franklin, above all things, hates strife, Lee with equal intensity hates peace. He has filled the homeward mails with insinuations against Deane; and when Congress, after a long silence, receives a packet of dispatches from Franklin and Lee which has been rifled and blank paper substituted, Lee even hints that he believes Franklin knows something about it. Congress, previously only vaguely aware of the dissensions between its envoys in Paris, becomes suddenly suspicious. Consequently, when Deane, accompanied by M. Gerard as the French envoy, reaches Philadelphia, he is treated, not like a returned hero and deserving patriot, as he expects, but more like a poor and undesirable relative. It is seven weeks before he even receives an audience. Meantime Arthur Lee has put new barbs on his accusations. He declares that Deane has kept all his transactions to himself, has refused to keep his colleagues informed, and has left his accounts in " studied confusion." He charges that Deane's private expenses have been nearly twice those of any other colleague. As a matter of fact, the records show that from December, 1776, to March, 1778, Deane, who bore all the early burdens, received on his private account $20,926; Lee $12,749; and Franklin $12,214.

However, Deane is only able to answer that all his papers and accounts are in Paris, that they will be found in order, and that he has done nothing of which his country can be ashamed. But his mysterious arrangement with Beaumarchais and the fuss made over the du Coudray affair has raised up loud and vocal critics. In December, 1778, Deane makes the mistake of publishing an angry and verbose defense of himself. It makes a bad impression on public opinion, which is scandalized by the revelation of the broils going on between the American commissioners in Paris.

Public opinion decides to "take it out" on someone; and at once does so on Deane himself. Even Thomas Paine comes out with a public letter taking the part of Lee against Deane. Not even Franklin's praise can save him.

After begging and waiting for months for the audit which will vindicate him, Deane turns bitter and ugly, develops a persecution complex, goes over to the English with his friend Benedict Arnold, and finally dies in a broody obscurity.

Almost half a century elapsed before Congress recognized the claims of his heirs. Though it was prodded into making some payments to Beaumarchais, it never met in full the claims of that romantic supporter of America's cause.

II

Second only to Lee as a trouble-hatcher is Ralph Izard, of South Carolina, who has been hanging around Paris until the Grand Duke of Tuscany, to whose court he has been appointed, shall be ready to receive him. Tuscany never does receive him, so Izard, having nothing else in particular to do, employs himself in attempts to polish up his own prestige as an envoy and in trying to make Franklin consult him on all matters pertaining to international diplomacy. He, Lee, and Lee's elder brother, William Lee, appointee to Vienna, form a cabal which suffers anguish whenever it sees Dr. Franklin enjoying the deferential attentions of the French court and people. Izard follows Lee's attempts to discredit Franklin in his letters home. He writes of Franklin's "effrontery" and "chicanery," and declares that he believes the doctor to be under no restraint of "virtue and honor."

And now comes John Adams, later the second President of the United States, to unravel the tangle and iron out the differences between Franklin and the other agents. Congress, even if it had tried very hard, could not have selected an individual less fitted for a place on the American commission to France than this honest, serious, well-meaning, detail-loving lawyer and pedant straight from the mold of the Brahmin caste in New England. He goes about his assumed business with great seriousness, first annoying the French and then causing their concealed snickers. He lends an attentive ear to Izard's tale of woe and graft, and then discharges Jonathan Williams, Franklin's nephew, from the naval agency at Nantes. He next addresses himself with pronounced ostentation to the task of sorting out and properly filing Franklin's papers in the house at Passy. In so doing, he comes very near scoring over the doctor, who, even at the age of 72, has never been able to observe that principle of Order which was No. 3 in his youthful creed. Even his admirers have protested at the manner in which he permits important documents to lie about. However, Franklin betrays no annoyance; he agrees to the discharge of Williams, even though there is no evidence of his malfeasance, and makes no objection to Adams's taking apartments in the Passy house and stowing away the papers.

Adams's third attack is on this very house, the elegant Hôtel de Valentinois. He learns that M. Ray de Chaumont, the French merchant, has lent a court of it to Franklin and has refused to accept any compensation, merely requesting that at the end of the war a souvenir in the shape of a tract of land in America. Adams is horrified: this is not regular. He writes to M. de Chaumont asking him to place a rental valuation on that part of the house occupied by the Americans. The owner declines to be businesslike. He replies politely that it is " so much the better for me to have immortalized my house by receiving into it Dr. Franklin and his associates! "

M. de Chaumont was right in foreseeing immortality for his house. One hundred and eighteen years later, on March 8, 1896, the Historical Society of Auteuil and Passy placed on the site a plaque inscribed as follows:

" Here stood a building, part of the Hôtel de Valentinois, in which Franklin dwelt from 1777 to 1789 and on which he placed the first lightning rod erected in France."

As time goes on, it becomes more and more apparent that there is only one solution to an anomalous condition: the American commission to France must have a head and in cases of dispute he must be the sole plenipotentiary. Each of the five agents is aware of this, and each so writes to Congress. Congress finally acts. In February, 1779, Gen. Lafayette arrives in Paris on leave of absence from America. He brings a commission to Franklin as the sole plenipotentiary to the court of France.

III

The French receive this news with pleasure unalloyed and undisguised. They have recognized in Franklin a man with whom they can do business and whom they understand. As their contempt for the boorish behavior of the other envoys deepens, their admiration for Franklin increases. They have learned that his more sturdy traits are unshakeable; at the same time his little foibles are those which they share and sympathize with — his love for bright women, a bottle of wine, and mellow conversation in the midst of good company. He becomes the fad, the rage, the cult of the hour. They make innumerable portraits, engravings, medals, cameos, medallions, statuettes, and busts of him, mounting his image on their jewelry and on their walls. Painters and sculptors such as Nini, Caffieri, Cochin and Houdon beg him to pose. Sophisticated women are thrilled by his notice. Statesmen, scientists, philosophers, and genial old abbés compete for his society and repeat his pawky sayings with infinite relish. If a day intervenes when there is no new Franklin anecdote, they invent one.

Envoys like John Adams attended strictly to business and failed in their mission; Franklin neglected business — at judicious intervals — and success emptied its largest cornucopias over his head.

All this incense, however, failed to affect either the size or levelness of Franklin's cranium. He was too experienced, too seasoned, in the ways of the world for that, even had his native shrewdness permitted it. There is proof in this letter to his daughter Sally:

" The clay medallion you say you gave to Mr. Hopkinson was the first of the kind made in France. A variety of others have been made since of different sizes; some to be set in the lids of snuff boxes, and some so small as to be worn in rings, and the numbers sold are incredible. These, with the pictures, busts, and prints (of which copies upon copies are spread everywhere) have made your father's face as well known as that of the moon, so that he durst not do anything that would oblige him to run away, as his phiz would discover him wherever he should venture to show it. It is said by learned etymologists that the name *doll*, for the images children play with, is derived from the word *idol*. From the number of dolls now being made of him, he may be truly said, *in that sense*, to be i-doll-ized in this country."

IV

One letter received by Franklin about this time must have given the old gentleman particular pleasure; for it was from a man in whose behalf he had assumed much responsibility and for whom he was predicting great things. It said:

" In the fullness of my heart I congratulate you on your well merited appointment, and I trust you will believe that I do now and ever shall rejoice in every circumstance that tends to the honor or happiness of a great and good man, who has taught me as well as his country to regard him with a veneration and affection which proceeds directly from the heart, and that is due only to the best of friends."

This was from John Paul Jones, Scotchman, sentimentalist, sea raider, and madcap, with some element in him of the swashbuckler which Franklin, who once longed to run away to sea himself, must have loved. Jones was then at the port of L'Orient, where he was busy preparing the *Bon Homme Richard* — " Poor Richard " — for the doughty deeds which were to thrill many generations of American schoolboys. It was a long letter that Jones wrote, containing some labored reference to a mysterious story about himself which he felt he must explain. This compelled Franklin to give an explanation in his turn, which he did in a reply which must have given at first glance some consternation to the earnest captain:

" The story I alluded to is this: L'Abbé Rochon had just been telling me and Madame Chaumont that the old Gardiner and his wife had complained to the Curate of your having attacked her in the Garden about 7 o'clock the evening before your Departure and attempted to ravish her, relating all the circumstances, some of which are not fit for me to write. The serious part of it was that three of her sons were determined to kill you, if you had not gone off; the rest occasioned some laughing, for the old woman being one of the . . . ugliest that we may find in a thousand, Madame Chaumont said it gave a high idea of the Strength, Appetite & Courage of the Americans. A day or two after I learned it was the femme de chambre of Mlle. Chaumont who had disguised herself in a suit, I think, of your Cloaths, to divert herself under that Masquerade, as is customary the last evening of Carnival; and that meeting the old woman in the garden, she took it into her head to try her Chastity, which it seems was found Proof."

v

It was well that Franklin could find recreation in composing 18th century pleasantries, for he soon found that in becoming plenipotentiary he had not rid himself of the malevolent Arthur Lee. Lee was supposed to go to Spain as envoy, but instead, he, his brother William, and Ralph Izard remained in Paris to plague Franklin. This precious trio seem to have occupied themselves in fomenting one new trouble for Franklin every day. If their ingenuity sometimes failed them, their appetites fell off and insomnia ensued. When they succeeded, they went to bed tranquil and happy.

Congress at length appointed a committee of thirteen to settle the matter once for all. It is a matter of record that only by the width of an eyelash did they escape recalling Franklin and appointing Lee in his stead! In which case the American revolt against the mother country would have ended far otherwise than it did, for Franklin alone was able to raise the money in France for which Congress was incessantly importuning him. With their withering contempt for Lee and his allies, the French were more than once inclined to close their purses, but Franklin, with his adroit persistency and humorous candor, they were seldom able to refuse, though their own finances were becoming weaker every day. The loans granted to Franklin for the United States totaled 26,000,000 francs, beginning with two millions in 1777 and ending with six millions in 1782.

The Lees and Izard were at last recalled. They went

back home to air their grievances in the presence of those who were only too ready to believe that Franklin was a grafter, a spendthrift, and an unprincipled old wretch. Franklin's hands were at last free to attend to the even greater tasks which he knew were coming. If he celebrated the passing of his late confrères at all, it was doubtless to go over to the home of his attractive neighbor, Madame Brillon, and there sing his favorite French song. The name of it was *Les Petits Oiseaux* — " The Little Birds."

Chapter XXX
Franklin and Madame Brillon

I

IN the course of the twenty-five years and more which Franklin spent abroad in the service of his country, he met many able and eminent personages. Most of them were glad to become his friends. Those who ran counter to him, or who in any way engaged in a contest with him, lived to regret it; for though he disliked strife, his mental agility, adroitness, and subtlety, added to his wide reading and observation of human nature, made him, when aroused, a sinuous and doughty opponent.

It remained for a woman of France to reveal herself as fully his equal, and at times his superior, in those very qualities in which he most excelled. She was a match for him in wit, in fantasy, in verbal fencing, and gay and sophisticated dialectics, while in subtle feeling, intuition, culture, and mastery of language, she surpassed him. During his ardent flirtations with her, though he brought to bear every atom of his skill and persistence, he never quite prevailed.

This was Madame d'Hardancourt Brillon, wife of Franklin's neighbor, a French official named Jouy de Brillon; and hostess to Franklin twice and sometimes three times weekly at her leafy home, Moulin Joli (Pretty Mill). She was the chiefest of the women who called him " dear papa "; she once wrote him, " My heart loved you from the first moment of our acquaintance "; and she sometimes almost knelt before him in a kind of humble adoration.

The 119 letters from her to Franklin which have been preserved indicate, between the lines, why she encouraged Franklin's friendship and even permitted a little of his unsubtle love-making. As the wife of a man many years her senior, who neglected her, she was lonely. As a religious and introspective woman, her mind tended towards introversion; and as a daughter who had had what pyschologists term a father-fixation, she craved affection and fatherly advice. Franklin, with the high spirits which the company of women imparted to him, with his fondness for broad jokes, and his love for material good things, offset and checked her loneliness and constant brooding, while his indulgence for human weaknesses and his gift of paternal sympathy made her beg for his presence at times as if it were the world's greatest boon.

There was one other respect in which she surpassed him in his own field. She was the superior letter writer. Beside hers, Franklin's letters are all in one key, and are a little complacent besides. Madame Brillon's letters are orchestrations. They sound the 'cello as well as the flute. They contain a higher as well as a lower gamut of notes than Franklin's. The following is one of the many specimens preserved in the library of the American Philosophical Society at Philadelphia. It was written from La Thuillerie, her mother's home, just after a week-end visit from Franklin:

" I was too happy Saturday, Sunday, and Monday, my dear papa. I was too happy. My present depression proves it. I have not yet been willing to visit your room, because everything would tell me in a manner too heartfelt that you are no longer there. But I have been in our fields. I have there seen the trace of your footsteps everywhere; the trees have seemed to me to be a sad green; the water of our

streams seems to flow more softly. These are not compliments which I pay you; it is the simple expression of my
heart to which I yield. It is to my father that his tender,
loving child speaks. I had a father, the best of men. He
was my first and my best friend. I lost him before his
time. You have often said to me, can I not take the place
of those whom you mourn? and you have told me of the
humane custom of certain savages who adopt the prisoners
they make in war, and let them take the place of their relatives who are gone. You have taken the place in my heart
of this father, whom I loved, whom I revered so much.
The harrowing grief I felt at his loss has been changed to
a sweet melancholy which is dear to me and which I owe to
you. You have gained in me a child, a friend the more. I
have come to have for you the idolatry which all have for a
great man. I had a curiosity to see you; my self-love has
been flattered by receiving you in my home; since then I
have seen in you only your soul sensitive to friendship, your
goodness, your simplicity; and I have said, this man is so
good that he will love me, and I began to love you well in
order to bind you to the same for me."

At another time she wrote:

" My papa loves me. He loves to know that I think of
him; he loves to hear me say it. My heart, which is always
ready to say it to him, guides my pen, and the word *aimer*
(to love) is always formed in the nib."

" Always formed in the nib " — Franklin could never
have said anything so delicately poetic as that. We have
seen how, during Franklin's tender years, his father permanently chilled the germ of whatever poetry then dwelt in
his nature; and at a time when Benjamin might have been
developing any poetic gifts, how circumstances found him

turning out, instead, Poor Richard's maxims for fishmongers and pawnbrokers.

A letter by Franklin to Madame Brillon, during her absence, is as follows:

" I often pass before your house. It wears a desolate look to me. Heretofore I have broken the commandments in coveting it along with my neighbor's wife. Now I do not covet it. Thus I am less the sinner. But with regard to the wife, I always find these commandments very inconvenient, and I am sorry that we are cautioned to practise them. Should you in your travels find yourself at the home of St. Peter, ask him to recall them, as intended only for the Jews, and as too irksome for good Christians."

During the eight-year friendship between Franklin and this, his neighbor's wife, he must have written her nearly as many letters as he received, for he was a faithful, if sometimes dilatory, correspondent. But only a few of them are known to exist, and these are mostly rough drafts from which he made clean and corrected copies. It is to one of these lost letters that Mme. Brillon seems to refer in the following:

" I found in it evidences of your friendship, and a tinge of that gayety and gallantry which make all women love you, because you love them all. Your proposal to carry me on your wings, as if you were the angel Gabriel, made me laugh, but I would not accept it, although I am no longer very young nor a virgin. That angel was a sly fellow, and your nature united to his would become too dangerous. I should be afraid of miracles happening, and miracles between women and angels will not always bring a redeemer. . . . If you had been at Avignon with us, it is there you would have wished to embrace people! The women there

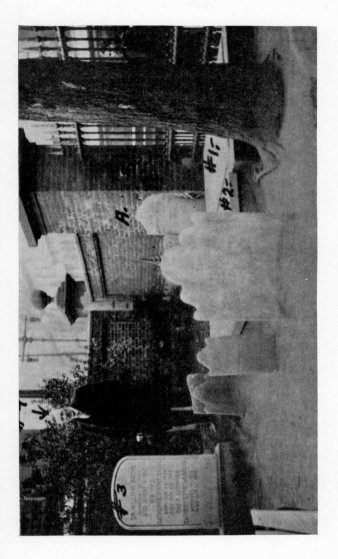

THE FRANKLIN CORNER IN THE CHRIST CHURCH BURIAL GROUND, PHILADELPHIA

A. — GRAVE OF JOHN READ, FATHER OF DEBORAH READ FRANKLIN; 1. — GRAVE OF BENJAMIN FRANKLIN AND HIS WIFE, DEBORAH; 2. — GRAVE OF SARAH FRANKLIN AND HER HUSBAND, RICHARD BACHE; 3. — GRAVE OF WILLIAM BACHE, AND HIS WIFE, CATHERINE WISTAR BACHE. ARROW INDICATES FRANKLIN BACHE HUNTINGTON, GREAT-GREAT-GREAT-GRANDSON OF BENJAMIN FRANKLIN.

are charming; I thought of you every time I saw one of them."

Madame Brillon's own wit and her appreciation of it in others stimulated Franklin to do some of the gayest and most graceful writing of his life. It was for her that he wrote many of the " Bagatelles," or short pieces, which he had set up and printed on his private press in the basement of the house at Passy. Among them were *The Story of the Whistle*, *The Ephemera*, *The Petition of the Left Hand*, *The Handsome and Deformed Leg*, *Dialogue between Franklin and the Gout*, and *The Morals of Chess*.

Franklin's addiction to chess once led him to start a game in her bathroom, it seems, and he went right on playing long after his modest hostess had finished her Saturday night splash and wished to emerge into the world again. His apology has been preserved, as follows:

Saturday, 11 at night

" On arriving at home I was surprised to find that it was nearly 11 o'clock. I fear that in forgetting everything else by our too great attention to chess, we have inconvenienced you very much by keeping you so long in the bath. Tell me, my dear friend, how you are this morning? Never again will I consent to begin a match in your bathroom. Can you forgive me this indiscretion? "

Madame Brillon could, and doubtless did; but it is terrifying to contemplate what might have happened if this indiscretion of the worthy doctor's had come to the knowledge of the stern and rockbound patriots back home. It would have lent color to the darkest insinuations of Lee and Izard.

II

The dialogue with the gout, which was reprinted in America in a bowdlerized form and not as Franklin wrote it, drew this reply from Madame Brillon:

" There would be many little things, in truth, to criticize in your logic, which you fortify so well, my dear papa. ' When I was a young man,' you say, ' and enjoyed the favors of the sex more freely than at present, I had no gout.' Therefore, one might reply to this, when I threw myself out of the window, I didn't break my leg. Therefore, you could have the gout without having deserved it, and you could have well deserved it, as I believe, and not have had it. . . ."

There was a stage in the correspondence between Franklin and Madame Brillon when he intimated that he was not satisfied with being merely her friend. He wrote:

" I am incredibly hungry . . . and you have given me nothing to eat. I was a stranger and I was almost as lovesick as Colin when you were singing. You have neither taken me in nor cured me, nor eased me. You who are rich as an archbishop in all the Christian and moral virtues, and could sacrifice a small share of some of them without visible loss, you tell me that it is asking too much, and you are not willing to do it. That is your charity to a poor wretch who once enjoyed affluence, and is unfortunately reduced to soliciting alms. . . ."

Her reply was firmly in the negative, as follows:

" You adopted me as your daughter. I chose you for my father. What do you expect of me? Friendship? Well, I love you as a daughter should love her father. The purest, the most respectful, the tenderest, affection for you fills my soul. You asked me for a ' louis.' I gave it to you, and yet you murmur at not getting another one, which does not belong to me. It is a treasure which has been entrusted to me, my good papa. I guard it and will always guard it carefully. Even if you were, like Colin, sick, I could not cure you, but nevertheless whatever you may think or say, no one in this world loves you more than I."

This should have sufficed to put a 72-year-old admirer in his place, and keep him there; but Franklin more than once returned to the charge in terms that have caused certain of the collectors and editors of his writings to denounce him as not quite a gentleman. These commentators perhaps err in taking Franklin's amorous letters too seriously. In addressing ladies in such terms, he but followed the manners of his century, which were, as already shown, rather bold and broad. His many feminine correspondents do not seem to have found fault with his gallant expressions. On the contrary, they, as the saying is, came back for more; which is sufficient proof of Madame Brillon's observation that propriety is a thing that varies from century to century and country to country.

III

Madame Brillon occasionally confessed to Franklin her difficulties with her husband. We know little of this gentleman, except that he was large and stout, was apparently of a jovial and roaming disposition, was fond of telling stories, and was himself an admirer of Franklin, to whom he apparently gave the run of his house without misgiving. His wife once wrote to Franklin:

" I know that the man to whom my fate has bound me is a man of merit. I respect him as much as I should and as much as he deserves. I have perhaps always loved him beyond what his heart can return. Twenty-four years difference in our ages, his severe training, with mine perhaps a little too much cared for on the side of pleasing talents, have tightened his heart and expanded mine. My papa, marriages in this country are made for a weight in gold; on one side of the scale the wealth of a young man, on the other that of a girl. When equality is found the matter ends to the satisfaction of the parents. They do not think of considering the taste, the age, or the relations of character. A girl whose heart contains the fire of youth is married to a man who extinguishes it. Yet one requires that the woman be virtuous! My friend, this history is mine, and many others'. I shall strive to prevent its being that of my daughters, but alas, shall I be mistress of their fate? "

Again she wrote:

" It is difficult for a woman who would give her life without hesitation to insure her husband's happiness to see the results of her exertions destroyed by intrigue and falsehood. . . . Adieu, you whom I love so much, my kind papa. Yesterday you called me ' Madame,' and my heart shrank. I examined myself to see whether I had done you any wrong, or if I had failings you would not mention to me. Pardon, my friend, I am not reproaching you; I am accusing myself of a weakness. I was born much too sensitive for my happiness and for that of my friends. Cure me or pity me; if you can, do one or the other. Tomorrow, Wednesday, you will come to tea, will you not? . . ."

The intrigue referred to by Mme. Brillon apparently did not abate, and one day a terror came upon her. She sent Franklin this note:

" . . . It is of the utmost necessity that I should have a long and detailed conversation with you. I want to have you sound the very depths of my soul and know those who have wounded me so cruelly. Perhaps it is important for you to know something which some day may affect you. Will you, can you, receive me the day after tomorrow, Wednesday, at ten o'clock in the morning and close your doors to all others for an hour, so that I may pour forth my soul in yours, and so gain consolation and counsel? Answer, if only a line, at once. It is unnecessary that anyone should know I am writing you, and that I am coming to see you. Adieu, you are my father, and that is why I crave more than ever the certainty of your friendship."

On the day and at the hour appointed, the American plenipotentiary ceased, for an hour, to be an ambassador, admiralty judge, money-raiser, accountant, scientific authority, and maid-of-all-work to a distant Congress, and became a woman's priest.

In the confessional she found the relief she craved. She wrote:

" My soul is calmer, my dear papa, now that it has overflowed in yours, now that it no longer fears lest Mlle. J. take up her quarters with you, and prove a torment to you and your dear son. . . . My husband will perhaps be for a long time still under her influence. Goodby, oh you dear friend, you whom I revere, whom I love. I have read and reread your letter. I shall conform myself to the truth it contains. I shall try to become a worthy pupil of a great philosopher and sage. I shall try to show the best of papas and friends that his daughter does not conceive friendship as consisting merely in the pleasure of seeing him and demonstrating it to him; that she does not wish to be content merely with pleasing him by such attractions as he meets with every day and in a far higher degree in the society of many other women; rather far by the completion and fulfilment of all the virtues which should make her, in all truth, the lawful friend of her good papa were she ugly, were she a man, in a word, were she anything else than in a state of life wherein the senses play their part in the gallantry men show to women. Until tomorrow — tomorrow is Saturday, is it not, dear papa? And you didn't come last Wednesday. . . ."

Though she continually kept her elderly suitor at arm's length, she did not fail to reproach him for fancied neglect. Once, when out of town, she wrote:

" What, not one word, my kind papa? Have you forgot your daughter? You have doubtless encountered so many lovely ladies on your path that they have distracted you. Then remember that friendship, that confidence, that feeling so sweet and true, which your daughter cherishes for you, and consider whether in these twelve days since she left you, her heart ought to approve of you. This is not a rebuke, but you know that it is but a step from reproach to indifference. I neither can nor do I wish to reveal even the appearance of coldness toward you, consequently I cannot help very gently, very tenderly complaining of your neglect."

It was possibly in reply to this letter that Franklin referred to " the kind of avarice that leads you to monopolize all my affections and not allow me any for the agreeable ladies of your country." He concluded by offering to do all she asked provided that she consent to an agreement containing nine articles. The eighth and ninth were as follows: " That when he is with her he shall do everything he pleases," and " that he shall love no other women no matter how agreeable they may be." To the last this footnote was appended: "The other women can go drown themselves."

Madame Brillon's answer to this is not on record, but no doubt it was in a clear but graceful negative. She knew how to keep the sting from her refusals. Her reply to Franklin's proposal regarding a marriage between his grandson, William Temple Franklin, and one of her daughters — she had two, named Cunegonde and Aldegonde — was gentle but plain. There were insuperable obstacles, she said, chief of which was the difference in religious belief. She spoke of the young man whom she liked to call " M. Franklinet " with but faint praise; possibly she read him better than his grandfather; Temple was an efficient worker and secretary as long as he was under Franklin's direction, but in later years he showed himself to have but few of his grandsire's qualities.

In other respects she was ready to obey Franklin's lightest wish, and it is probable that it was she who corrected his state papers and documents into grammatical and dignified French. She once complained of a paper by him that " the corrector of your French spoiled your work." She added this sound advice. " Leave your works as they are. Use words that say things, and laugh at grammarians who by their purity weaken all your sentences."

It is a happy picture that she drew of what took place during Franklin's semi-weekly visits to her home in this letter written from La Thuillerie:

" How are you, my good papa? Never has it cost me so much to love you. Every evening it seems to me that you would be very glad to see me, and every evening I think of you. On Monday, the 21st, I shall come for you. I hope that you will then be well on your feet, and that the teas of

Wednesday and Saturday and that of Sunday morning will recover all their brilliance. I will bring you la bonne évèque. My fat husband will make us laugh, our children will laugh together, our big neighbor will quiz, the Abbés La Roche and Morellet will eat all the butter, Mme. Grand, her amiable niece, and M. Grand will not harm the gathering. Father Pagin will play ' God of Love ' on his violin, I the march on the piano, and you ' Petits Oiseaux ' on the armonica."

But halcyon hours such as these do not go on forever, and at last comes a day when Franklin, feeble with age and gout, packs to go home, and Madame Brillon writes this parting letter:

" I could not bring myself to bid you a final farewell, my good friend. My heart was so overflowing on leaving you that I feared that for you and for me another such grievous experience would only add to the deep sorrow which this separation causes me, without adding further proof of the tender and unalterable friendship I have pledged to you for all time. Every day of my existence memory reminds me that a great man, a sage, once deigned to be my friend. My thoughts accompany him wherever he goes. My heart mourns him unceasingly; unceasingly I shall say, always: ' Eight years I spent in the company of Dr. Franklin. They are passed and I shall never see him more.' Nothing in the world can ever console me for that loss, unless it be the conviction of that peace and happiness you must experience in the bosom of your family, and that fame which you surely enjoy in the land that owes you its liberty. O my friend, my good friend! I pray you may be happy. Tell me that you are, let me hear from you, and if it be sweet for you to recall the woman who loved you most dearly, think of me, think of all those members of my family who were and always must be your best friends. Goodby, my heart fails me, it cannot bear being torn asunder from you; but that it shall never be, my loving papa. You will often realize its presence near you. Question it, and it will answer you."

Chapter XXXI

Franklin and Madame Helvetius

I

AN altogether different sort of person was another feminine friend in whose home Franklin passed many hours of pleasing relaxation. This was Madame Helvetius, widow of the philosopher Claude Adrien Helvetius, who died in 1771, leaving behind a fortune which he had made as one of the French farmers-general. She lived at the suburb of Auteuil, and hence was called by Franklin "Our Lady of Auteuil." Franklin was accustomed to dine with her at least once a week, usually in company with the genial abbés Morellet and de la Roche and the physician Cabanis.

She lived in a handsome house which she had purchased from Quentin de la Tour, painter of the king. Franklin was first taken there by Turgot, the statesman, who had once been a suitor of Mme. Helvetius when she was the Countess Ligniville. Here she was mistress of a salon at which many celebrated men were visitors, including Condorcet, the philosopher. She maintained a regiment of cats and had so much furniture that Franklin once called her home "the House of a Thousand Sofas."

"His conversation," wrote the Abbé Morellet of Franklin, "was exquisite — a perfect good nature, a simplicity of manners, an uprightness of mind that made itself felt in the smallest things, an extreme gentleness, and above all, a sweet serenity that easily became gayety. . . . He seldom spoke long, except in composing tales — a talent in which he excelled, and which he greatly liked in others. His tales always had a philosophical aim; many had the form of apologues, which he himself invented, and he applied those which he had not made with infinite justice."

One of the bagatelles which Franklin wrote for his hostess and which the Abbé quotes, relates to a visit to the Elysian Fields. There Franklin encountered Helvetius himself, who announced that he has consoled himself for his separation from Madame Helvetius by taking another wife. When this new wife appeared, bearing a glass of nectar, " I instantly recognized her," says Franklin in his essay, " as Mrs. Franklin, my old American friend. I reclaimed her, but she said to me coldly, ' I have been your good wife forty-nine years and four months, almost half a century; be content with that.' Dissatisfied with this refusal of my Eurydice, I immediately resolved to quit those ungrateful shades, and to return to this good world to see again the sun and you. Here I am. *Let us avenge ourselves*."

Two pen-pictures of Madame Helvetius have come down to us. One is by Franklin himself in a letter to Cabanis:

" We often talk of you at Auteuil, where everybody loves you. I now and then offend our good lady, who cannot long retain her displeasure, but, sitting in state on her sopha (*sic*), extends graciously her long, handsome arm, says, ' la; baisez ma main; je vous pardonne,' [1] with all the dignity of a sultaness. She is as busy as ever, endeavoring to make every creature about her happy, from the Abbés down thro' all ranks of the family to the birds and Poupon."

In another letter to Cabanis Franklin wrote:

" M. Franklin is sorry to have caused the least hurt to

[1] " There; kiss my hand; I forgive you."

those beautiful tresses that he always regards with pleasure. If that lady likes to pass her days with him, he would like as much to pass his nights with her; and since he has already given many of his days to her, although he had such a small remnant of them to give, she would seem ungrateful to have never given him a single one of her nights, which run continually to pure waste, without promoting the good fortune of anyone except Poupon." [2]

The other picture is by Abigail Adams, the able but acidulous wife of John Adams:

" She entered the room with a careless, jaunty air; upon seeing ladies who were strangers to her, she bawled out, ' Ah! mon Dieu, where is Franklin? Why did you not tell me there were ladies here? ' You must suppose her speaking all this in French. ' How I look! ' said she, taking hold of a chemise made of tiffany, which she had on over a blue lute-string, and which looked as much upon the decay as her beauty, for she was once a handsome woman; her hair was frizzled; over it she had a small straw hat, with a dirty gauze half-handkerchief round it, and a bit of dirtier gauze than ever my maids wore was bowed on behind. She had a black gauze scarf thrown over her shoulders. She ran out of the room; when she returned, the Doctor entered at one door, she at the other; upon which she ran forward to him, caught him by the hand, ' Hélas, Franklin '; then gave him a double kiss, one upon each cheek, and another upon his forehead. When we went into the room to dine, she was placed between the Doctor and Mr. Adams. She carried on the chief of the conversation at dinner, frequently locking her hand into the Doctor's, and sometimes spreading her arms upon the backs of both

[2] One of the Madame's eighteen cats.

the gentlemen's chairs, then throwing her arm carelessly upon the Doctor's neck.

" I should have been greatly astonished at this conduct, if the good Doctor had not told me that in this lady I should see a genuine Frenchwoman, wholly free from affectation or stiffness of behavior, and one of the best women in the world. For this I must take the Doctor's word; but I should have set her down for a very bad one, although sixty years of age, and a widow. I own I was highly disgusted, and never wish for an acquaintance with any ladies of this cast. After dinner she threw herself upon a settee, where she showed more than her feet. She had a little lapdog, who, was, next to the Doctor, her favorite. This she kissed, and when he wet the floor she wiped it up with her chemise. This is one of the Doctor's most intimate friends, with whom he dines once every week, and she with him. She is rich, and my near neighbor; but I have not yet visited her. Thus you see, my dear, that manners differ exceedingly in different countries. I hope, however, to find amongst the French ladies manners more consistent with my ideas of decency, or I shall be a mere recluse."

The statement regarding " manners " by Mrs. Adams, closely paralleling that by Madame Brillon in a letter to Franklin quoted in a previous chapter, would seem to indicate that the good lady believed herself to have come from a country where manners were so different as to be impeccable. But before the word of the pot concerning the behavior of the kettle is accepted as authentic, let us consult an authority on certain urban manners as noted in America during the same period. The writer of this lively letter is Miss Rebecca Franks, of Philadelphia, who is describing for the benefit of her sister Abigail, wife of Andrew Hamilton, a visit to eighteenth century New York:

"Flatbush, August 10, 1781 [3]

" . . . I will do our ladies, that is Philadelphians, the justice to say they have more cleverness in the turn of an eye than the N Y girls have in their whole composition. With what ease have I seen a Chew, a Penn, Oswald, Allen, and a thousand others entertain a large circle of both sexes, and the conversation without the aid of cards not flag or seem the least strained or stupid. Here, or more properly speaking, in N Y, you enter the room with a formal set curtsey and after the how do's, 'tis a fine, or a bad day, and those trifling nothings are finish'd, all's a dead calm till the cards are introduced, when you see pleasure dancing in the eyes of all the matrons and they seem to gain new life. The misses, if they have a favorite swain, frequently decline playing for the pleasure of making love — for to all appearances 'tis the ladies and not the gentlemen that shew a preference nowadays. 'Tis here, I fancy, always leap year. For my part, that am used to quite another mode of behaviour, I cannot help shewing my surprise, perhaps they call it ignorance, when I see a lady single out her pet to lean almost in his arms at an Assembly or play-house . . . and to hear a lady confess a partiality for a man who perhaps she has not seen three times."

II

Those things which to a bridling dame from New England appeared to be coarse vulgarities, were no doubt to Franklin and his grey-haired cronies of the Church mere harmless gallantries with which elderly beaux whiled away the hours when in the company of an elderly flapper. That Madame Helvetius was coarser grained than Madame

[3] From the Pennsylvania Magazine of History and Biography, 1899.

Brillon there is no doubt; and that she was ill-educated and unversed in spelling is proved by her letters to Franklin, but that she had the ability to create an amiable atmosphere in which her guests enjoyed themselves is demonstrated by this letter from the Abbé Morellet to Franklin, written after the latter had returned to Philadelphia:

" I shall never forget the happiness I have enjoyed in knowing you and seeing you intimately. I write to you from Auteuil, seated in your arm chair, on which I have engraved *Benjamin Franklin hic sedebat*,[4] and having by my side the little bureau, which you bequeathed to me at parting with a drawerful of nails to gratify the love of nailing and hammering, which I possess in common with you. But, believe me, I have no need of all these helps to cherish your endeared remembrance and to love you."

After his return home, Madame Helvetius wrote to Franklin about the possibility of meeting one's spouse in heaven. She added: " But I believe that you, who have been a coquin [rogue], will be restored to more than one."

---

[4] Benjamin Franklin sat here.

Chapter XXXII

Franklin and the Countess d'Houdetot

I

A PURELY platonic, though fervent, admirer of Franklin was Sophie Lalive, Countess d'Houde-tot, once the beloved of Jean Jacques Rousseau, and the friend and patron of St. John de Crèvecoeur, the French immigrant to the United States who became the author of *Letters of a Pennsylvania Farmer.* From the first she seems to have been an ardent sympathizer with the American cause, and when at the age of about fifty she met Franklin, she at once joined the circle of those ladies who wrote tender letters to the sage during his entire stay in France; and afterwards, too. She had a passion for planting trees as souvenirs at her home at Sanois, in the valley of Montmorency. She called them her "memorials." She once asked Thomas Jefferson to procure her more than twenty different trees from the United States, which she wanted for her garden. Her letters to Franklin were always expressed in worshipful terms, closing with such expressions as "A thousand tender sentiments to Monsieur Franklin." The following is a specimen:

"You have promised, my dear and venerable doctor, a little visit at Sanois. This is the moment to remind you of it; our path and my garden are in all their beauty and our flowers call you. If it is convenient to come Wednesday, Saturday, Sunday, or some other day, remember that you have promised me to be entirely my guest and to dwell

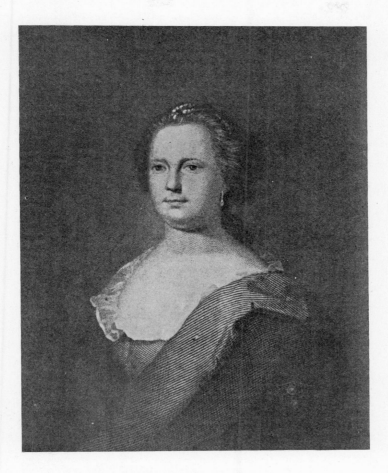

DEBORAH READ FRANKLIN
WIFE OF BENJAMIN FRANKLIN.

under my roof. You will find nowhere else one who will have greater pleasure in seeing you; it will be a memorial the more to embellish and honor my little country retreat, where I conserve with care the memory of all that has drawn my admiration and touched my heart. How much, my dear doctor, have you the right to these distinctions! . . ."

At another time she wrote:

" Permit me to press against my heart, with religious tenderness, the man of my age who appears to me most to merit the respect of the human race."

When Franklin visited Sanois in the spring of 1781, she gave an elaborate *fête champêtre* in his honor. She and her guests met him a half mile from the house and escorted him to the grounds, where, on alighting from his carriage, Franklin was made the center of a circle which recited a verse of welcome. Dinner was then served, to the accompaniment of music. As each glass of wine was poured, the Countess, her son and daughter-in-law, and the Counts Tressau and d'Apeché rose in turn and sang a laudatory verse. Afterwards Franklin was conducted to the garden where he was asked to plant an acacia tree from America. A near-by pillar was inscribed as follows:

> " Sacred tree! the lasting monument
> Of the visit to these scenes
> A Wise Man deigned to pay;
> Of these gardens henceforth the pride,
> Receive, receive the just homage
> Of our vows and of our incense.
> And may'st thou, all down the ages,
> Touched gently by the hand of time.
> Last as long as his name, his laws, and his writings."

Soon after Franklin had returned home, she wrote the following letter in English to Thomas Jefferson, his successor at Paris:

" Sir: I am greatly indebted to you for your polite attention in sending me so early the news of our dear & venerable doctor's happy and safe arrival in his own country — He is become respectable to all nations & peculiarly dear to his own, as well as to his numerous friends and acquaintances. You have relieved me from a great load of uneasiness & afforded me at ye same time a most heartfelt joy — Your elegant account of ye reception he has meet with at Ph^{ia}, has moved me even to tears.

" Antiquity itself does not afford a more pleasing spectacle. This happy event seems to justify a Superintending Providence, which has crowned virtue with a most valuable reward. I shall unite the homage I owe this Great man to that of the two Continents — His knowledge has been immensely useful to both & his virtue singularly so to his own."

The Countess d'Houdetot was one of the few women on whom an American city conferred its freedom. New Haven so honored her on May 10, 1785, along with nine other French " personages."

II

In the American Philosophical Society's great collection of Franklin manuscripts, containing no less than 13,800 pieces, there are many other delicate missives written to the venerable American envoy at Paris, all of them exhaling incense and adoration. Franklin, as we have seen, could not always resist the temptation to love his neighbor's wife as himself; this is a letter from Madame Le Roy, wife of his good friend, the scientist, showing that he had plenty of encouragement:

" You compliment me, my dear Papa, on my courage in having gone up in a balloon. Alas, it only served to make me regret that I could not go very far away in it, for if that vehicle could have transported me towards you, I would have remained near you and would have given you proofs of the consideration and esteem which you have ineffaceably engraved on my heart. . . . I assure you that as long as I have a breath of life I shall love you. I embrace you with all my heart."

Most of the tender notes in this collection are signed, but some are not. This is one of those not signed, apparently written as a New Year greeting:

" Receive, good papa, at the renewal of the year the vows which I have made for your happiness and for the conservation of your days, which are precious to all those persons who have the advantage of knowing you."

And this is signed by the Countess de Golofkin:

" I have a great desire, my dear and good papa, to see you, to embrace you, and to say two words. Let me know at what moment I can be sure of not interrupting you, and receive meanwhile the tender assurance of sentiments which I have vowed to you until the end of my life."

Lest this note be misunderstood, however, it should be added that further correspondence from the little Countess makes it plain that though she may have embraced the good doctor, she was meantime looking over his shoulder. Her real affections were centered on an adventurous Lovelace who had gone off to the wars in America, leaving her a prey to unspeakable terrors. At the news of every battle in America, she came flying down to Franklin. She was simply certain that her beloved had been killed; or at least horribly wounded. Would Franklin please find out at once and advise her?

Chapter XXXIII

Final Days in France

I

WITH all the honors and attentions showered upon him, the remainder of Franklin's stay in France might have passed like a happy dream, had it not been for the constant necessity of raising new funds and of attending to the complicated transactions connected with the outfitting of privateers and the shipping of supplies home.

" The storm of bills which I found coming upon us both," he wrote to John Jay, who was vainly begging money from Spain, " has terrified and vexed me to such a degree that I have been deprived of sleep, and so much indisposed by continual anxiety, as to be rendered almost incapable of writing "; and to Jonathan Williams he wrote: " I, in all these mercantile matters, am like a man walking in the dark. I stumble often, and frequently get my shins broke."

When it wanted money, Congress, with a fine, large disregard for detail, simply drew on Franklin, who meantime had to pay the interest on the French debt and the salaries of all the American agents in Europe. At length Robert Morris, financier of the war, wrote him that he simply must have 25,000,000 francs or go broke. Once more Franklin had to send a humble petition to the Count de Vergennes. The latter's reply was that the great expense under which France labored made such a loan impracticable; but that Louis XVI had resolved to grant the sum of six millions, not as a loan, but as a free gift. It was this gift which enabled Washington to complete his plans for a triumphant end to the war.

Then comes another harassment. John Adams returns to France to conduct the negotiations for peace when Britain shall be ready. Adams, acting independently, at once takes it upon himself to assume charge of all the diplomatic correspondence with Versailles. This promptly gets on the nerves of the Count de Vergennes, and Franklin is kept busy making elaborate explanations. At last Adams, having taken to himself plenty of rope, hangs himself. On being informed that the Count Rochambeau has sailed for America at the head of a strong French fleet, Adams describes his high satisfaction. But a few days later he is moved to write another letter to the Count de Vergennes. He has noted that the king has decided to dispatch this fleet " without having been solicited by the Congress." Adams's pedantic mind cannot let this pass without correction, though it is a detail of no consequence; he points out to the Count that Congress *has* solicited naval assistance.

The Count replies testily. He informs Adams that in future he can treat only with Franklin, who alone has letters of credence to the king. He then asks Franklin to transmit the entire correspondence with Adams to Congress. The result is that Congress cautions Adams, who moves on to Holland.

For this incident Adams never forgave Franklin. Twenty years after the latter's death he wrote that Franklin had " concerted with de Vergennes to crush him." Adams spoke of it as a " vulgar and low intrigue," referring incidentally to Franklin's " extreme indolence and dissipation " and his " passion for women."

II

To amuse himself, between times, with his ancient love for newspaper hoaxes, and incidentally to have some sport with the enemy, Franklin writes and circulates three bogus documents. One is supposed to be a letter from the Count de Schaumberg to the Baron Hohendorf, commanding the Hessian troops hired to George III for service in America, reading in part as follows:

"I am about to send you some new recruits. Don't economize them. Remember glory before all things. Glory is true wealth. There is nothing degrades a soldier like the love of money. He must care only for honor and reputation, but this reputation must be acquired in the midst of dangers. A battle gained without costing the conquerer any blood is an inglorious success, while the conquered cover themselves with glory by perishing with their arms in their hands. Do you remember that of the 300 Lacedemonians who defended the defile of Thermopylae, not one returned? How happy should I be, could I say the same of my brave Hessians! "[1]

The second document is a supposed " Extract of a letter from Captain Gerrish, of the New England Militia." It appears in an imaginary supplement to the *Boston Independent Chronicle*. It describes the taking of booty from the Seneca Indians, among which were eight packages of scalps taken from American soldiers, farmers, women, boys, girls, and infants. Accompanying is an " invoice and explanation " from James Crauford, a trader, to the governor of Canada, with the request that the " peltry " be sent to the King of England. This horrifying hoax deceived not only the English, but the home folks. American news-

[1] Bigelow's Works of Franklin.

papers continued to reprint it as genuine for years afterward.

The third document was written over the signature of Commodore John Paul Jones, who repelled the stigma of pirate applied to him by Sir Joseph Yorke and named as the real pirate King George III.

III

In 1780 occurs the capture of Henry Laurens, envoy to Holland, by the British off Newfoundland. He is taken to the Tower of London, where he is imprisoned for fifteen months, while Franklin vainly attempts to have him exchanged for Gen. Burgoyne and to lighten the rigor of his imprisonment. Laurens is not released before Cornwallis surrenders at Yorktown, October 17, 1781.

When he heard the news of the surrender, Franklin, by now well past most human illusions, must have felt much as he did when he wrote this to Dr. Priestley:

"A young angel of distinction being sent down to this world on some business for the first time, had an old courier-spirit assigned him as a guide. They arrived over the seas of Martinico, in the middle of the long day of obstinate fight between the fleets of Rodney and De Grasse. When, through the clouds of smoke, he saw the fire of the guns, the decks covered with mangled limbs, and bodies dead or dying; the ships sinking, burning, or blown into the air; and the quantity of pain, misery, and destruction, the crews yet alive were thus with so much eagerness dealing round to one another he turned angrily to his guide and said, 'You blundering blockhead, you are ignorant of your business; you undertook to conduct me to the earth, and you have brought me into hell!' 'No, sir,' said the guide, 'I have made no mistake; this is really the earth, and these are

men. Devils never treat one another in this cruel manner;
they have more sense, and more of what men (vainly) call
humanity.' "

Also the Doctor repeated to the Bishop of Asaph his celebrated saying:

" There never was a good war, or a bad peace."

IV

It was about this time that Franklin attained the very
height of his popularity in France. He was besieged by
inventors who wished him to pass on their discoveries and
by eccentric persons with " schemes " to unfold. He was
consulted as an authority on everything from internal ailments to the principles of government. He received a correspondence in nine different languages. One day he got a
curious letter, the first of a series from a writer who would
sign himself only as " The Representative of the Author."
The writer divulged that he had been investigating the
properties of heat and light; he sent his papers and drawings to Franklin with this letter composed in an awkward
English:

" Was it not so material a point to the Author that a candid judgment should be passed upon his work, he would
trust to time alone. But he is certain that many a Accadem-
ical gentleman do not look with pleasure upon his discoveries and will do their utmost to prejudice the whole Body.
Let the cabal be ever so warm, it certainly will be silenced
by the sanction of such a man as Doctor Franklin, and how
far a judgment passed by himself and the Royal Academy
can influence public opinion is well known."

Franklin later learned that the writer was a certain French
physician who had formerly lived in London. His name
was Jean Paul Marat — " Friend of the People " in the

French Revolution and in 1793 stabbed to death, when seated in his bathtub shaped like a shoe, by Charlotte Corday.

Some time later another odd letter was received from a lawyer in the town of Arras. It was as follows:

" Monsieur: A judgment rendered by the èchévins of St. Omer, prohibiting the use of lightning rods, has afforded me the opportunity of pleading before the Council of Artois the cause of a sublime discovéry for which mankind is indebted to you. The desire to aid in uprooting the prejudices opposed to its progress in our province led me to have printed the argument which I made in this case. I venture to hope, monsieur, that you will deign kindly to receive a copy of this work, the object of which was to induce my fellow citizens to accept one of your benefactions. I am happy to have been able to be of service to my province in determining its highest magistrates to receive this important discovery, happier still if I can add to this advantage the honor of securing the patronage of a man whose least merit is to be the most illustrious savant of the world. I have the honor to be with respect, monsieur,

" Your very humble and very obedient servant,
               " De Robespierre,
               " Advocate to the Council of Artois."

The precise little lawyer who thus sought Franklin's help in converting provincial Frenchmen to the use of lightning rods was the Maximilien de Robespierre who eleven years later was regarded as the incarnation of the Great Terror and who was destined to become, in 1794, one of its victims on the scaffold.

A third letter of an unexpected nature came from another famous figure — Turgot, once the right-hand minister of Louis XVI, but afterwards dismissed at the demand of

Marie Antoinette. Turgot asked Franklin to instruct him in an economical method of heating a house. Franklin responded by contriving for him a new type of stove called the " syphon " model.

A book would be required in which to relate all the curious activities of Franklin at this period. For example, he was asked to attend in 1783 one of Montgolfier's first balloon experiments in the garden of the queen's palace. A legend says that some scoffer remarked: " What is the use of a balloon? "

" What," replied Franklin, " is the use of a new-born baby? "

V

In 1782 began the negotiations for peace between the United States and Great Britain. In October Franklin wrote feelingly to John Adams: " *Blessed are the peacemakers,* is, I suppose, to be understood in the other world; for in this they are frequently *cursed.*"

All of Franklin's diplomatic gifts were needed to maintain harmony between the negotiators, for transactions were conducted in an atmosphere of intense suspicion, and more than once John Adams and John Jay were on the verge of creating an ugly breach between the United States and France.[2] The French government was highly nervous for more than one reason, its finance minister, Necker, having already disclosed the appalling drain on its revenues, due partly to the cost of maintaining the horde of parasites clustering around the court at Versailles.

The business of concluding peace occupied two years and a quarter. Preliminary articles were signed in 1782, but the treaty with England was not ratified by Congress until January 14, 1784.

[2] " Mr. Jay likes Frenchmen as little as Mr. Lee and Mr. Izard did. He says they are not a moral people." — Works of John Adams.

Franklin seems to have allowed himself to be persuaded by Adams and Jay to sign the articles with England without consulting the French government. " I am at a loss, sir," wrote the Count de Vergennes, " to explain your conduct, and that of your colleagues on this occasion. You have concluded your preliminary articles without any communication between us, although the instructions from Congress prescribe that nothing shall be done without the participation of the king." The Count also wrote to the French minister in America: " If we may judge of the future from what has passed here under our eyes, we shall be but poorly paid for all that we have done for the United States, and for securing to them a national existence."

And it was at this very moment that Congress was asking, through Franklin, for a gigantic loan! Franklin was compelled to acknowledge that an " indiscretion " had been committed; but he assured the Count that, as regards the king, " no prince was ever more beloved and respected by his own subjects, than the king is by the people of the United States." He got, not the loan, but a free gift of six millions. It was one of the final nails driven into the coffin of the French monarchy by the monarchy itself.

VI

The year 1784 brought Franklin a little more leisure than he had enjoyed for several years, but not a great amount of peace. Gout attacked him more fiercely than ever, and a new ailment, the stone, frequently sent him to bed in severe pain; and there was little relaxation in the demands on his time and services.

In this year the king appointed him on a commission of nine to investigate the operations of Mesmer, whose appearance in Paris from Germany, whence he had fled, had given tremendous circulation to two new terms, " mesmerism," and " animal magnetism." One of the members of this commission was Dr. Guillotin, whose name was afterwards applied to the bloody machine so freely used during the Revolution; not because he was the inventor of it, but because he was an advocate of more humane methods of capital punishment than hanging or shooting. Two other members — Lavoisier, the chemist, and Bailly, the historian of astronomy, the first president of the National Assembly, and the first mayor of Paris — were destined to die beneath this same machine. A fourth associate was Le Roy, one of the best of Franklin's French friends. Some of the experiments made during this investigation took place at Franklin's house at Passy. His was the first name signed to the report. It condemned mesmerism as a fraud. Mesmer decamped to England.

Other events of importance to Franklin occurred in this year. William Franklin, writing from London, asked for a renewal of relations with his father. Franklin sent William's son, Temple, over to " pay his duty," but discouraged William's offer to come to Passy. It is doubtful if he ever quite forgave William for joining the Tories.

Two incidents which Franklin doubtless enjoyed were his success in having John Carroll, his companion on the bitter trip to Canada, appointed as the first Catholic bishop in North America; and his circumvention of the Church of England in refusing ordination to two young Episcopal priests from America. " If the English won't have you," said Franklin, " try the Scotch." The scheme worked, Samuel Seabury, of Connecticut, being the first American to receive consecration at the hands of three Scottish bishops.

He probably also enjoyed writing this oft-quoted letter to Benjamin Webb, an American stranded in France who had appealed to Franklin for help:

" I send you herewith a bill for ten louis d'ors. I do not pretend to give such a sum. I only *lend* it to you. When you shall return to your country with a good character, you cannot fail of getting into business that will in time enable you to pay all your debts. In that case, when you meet with another honest man in similar distress, you must pay me by lending this sum to him; enjoining him to discharge the debt by a like operation, when he shall be able and shall meet with such another opportunity. I hope it may thus go through many hands before it meets with a knave that will stop its progress. This is a trick of mine for doing a deal of good with a little money. I am not rich enough to afford *much* in good works, and so am obliged to be cunning and to make the most of a *little*."

Franklin had already done the same favor three years previously, on the same terms, for one William Nixon, and had enjoined him similarly, closing his letter as follows:

" Let kind offices go round. Mankind are all of a family."

In August, 1784, Thomas Jefferson arrived in Paris to assist Franklin and Adams in completing commercial treaties. He wrote home that " there appeared to me more respect and veneration attached to the character of Dr. Franklin in France, than to that of any other person in the same country, foreign or native."

Franklin, who had several times asked that he be permitted to return home, now renewed his request. Congress, on March 7, 1785, granted the permission, and appointed Thomas Jefferson as plenipotentiary in his stead. Jefferson's remark, at his first meeting with the Count de Vergennes, is historic.

" It is you, monsieur," said the Count, " who replaces Dr. Franklin? "

" I am only his successor, sir; no one can replace him."

Jefferson and Franklin had ever been good friends. In certain traits and beliefs they were markedly similar. In political and economic theory they upheld a kind of democratic individualism, as against John Adams and Alexander Hamilton, who believed that government should be in the exclusive hands of the wealthy and well-born. It was because they differed in principle and viewpoint that Adams and Franklin so often clashed personally.

Franklin was too feeble to go to Versailles to take his leave, but the king bestowed on him a parting gift of his portrait, circled twice with 408 diamonds. Men came to embrace him and young women to kiss him for the last time. The queen's litter was provided to bear him to Havre. On July 12, 1785, he left Passy, which named a street after him, accompanied by his friends Le Veillard, de Chaumont, Mlle. de Chaumont, and his two grandsons. The party proceeded by easy stages, being entertained all the way. They spent three days accepting hospitalities at Havre. When Franklin reached Southampton, the British government graciously exempted his baggage from the usual examination. He was greeted there by William Franklin and by the loyal and affectionate Bishop of St. Asaph and his daughter Catherine.

" We are forever talking of our good friends," wrote the latter in a farewell note. " Something is perpetually occurring to remind us of the time spent with you. We never walk in the garden without seeing Dr. Franklin's room and thinking of the work that was begun in it."

Franklin's ship turned her bow homeward on July 28, 1785. He had been in France nine years. He was 78 years old. He wrote back to Madame Lavoisier that he did not " forget Paris, and the nine years' happiness I enjoyed there in the sweet society of a people whose conversation is instructive, whose manners are highly pleasing, and who, above all the nations of the world, have, in the greatest perfection, the art of making themselves beloved of strangers, and now, even in my sleep, I find that the scenes of all my pleasant dreams are laid in that city or in its neighborhood."

During the voyage Franklin spent most of his time in his cabin, writing. A stranger might have thought he was busy with his memoirs of a country seen in its brilliant decay, or reminiscences of its great men and fascinating women. But when he emerged from his labors he was bearing a paper entitled "The Cause and Cure of Smoky Chimneys."

Chapter XXXIV

"Home Is the Sailor"

I

WHEN Franklin lands in Philadelphia it is at that Market Street wharf from which more than sixty years before he first surveyed the quaint little town. Throngs are waiting for a sight of him, for those persons who are adults now were children when he departed for France; they greet him with tumultuous hurrahs, cannonades and cheers that follow him to his door. The Pennsylvania Assembly and Gen. Washington send him congratulatory letters. He finds Sarah Bache and her seven children well, and writes in his diary: " God be praised and thanked for all his mercies! "

No sooner is he made comfortable than his fellow citizens resume their ancient habit of electing him to office. " They have eaten my flesh," he resignedly writes to a friend, " and seem resolved to pick my bones." He receives a seat on the Philadelphia Common Council and is promptly made its chairman. He is next elected president of the Supreme Executive Council of the State, or, as we would call it today, governor.

His political duties, however, are at first not exacting, and he finds time to add a wing to his house and to turn his garden into a lawn on which he can sit under the mulberry tree and play games with his grandchildren. He also invents a contrivance for reaching the books on the high shelves of his library and a chair which can be unfolded into

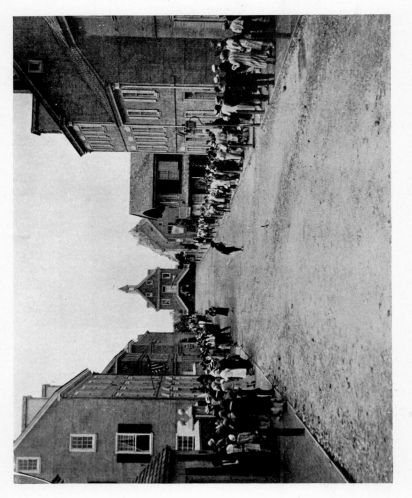

HIGH STREET (NOW MARKET STREET), PHILADELPHIA, IN FRANKLIN'S TIME AS RECONSTRUCTED AT THE SESQUICENTENNIAL EXHIBITION

a step-ladder. At intervals he tries to work on his uncompleted " Autobiography." He strangely rejects an appeal from " crazy John Fitch " for help in his project for running vessels by steam out of the port of Philadelphia, where Robert Fulton is a miniature painter; but takes up the cudgels in behalf of religion against an unknown correspondent, believed to have been Thomas Paine.

" Think," he writes, " how great a portion of mankind consists of weak and ignorant men and women, and of inexperienced, inconsiderate youth of both sexes, who have need of the motives of religion to restrain them from vice, to support their virtue, and to retain them in the practice of it till it becomes *habitual*, which is the great point for its security."

He assists the founding of a college for young Germans at Lancaster, being accompanied there by Hector St. John, formerly St. John de Crèvecoeur, who was, as has been noted, the protégé of the Countess d'Houdetot; he writes several papers, among them the *Retort Courteous* and *Sending Felons to America*, both aimed at Great Britain; he attends the meetings in his house of the American Philosophical Society, the Abolition Society, and the Society for Political Education. He has in mind another society, of which he writes to Dupont de Nemours, the French Encyclopedist, who became one of the ancestors of the American powder-making family of the same name, as follows:

" Would to God I could take with me Messrs. Dupont, Dubourg, and some other French friends, with their good ladies! I might then, by mixing them with my friends in Philadelphia, form a happy society that would prevent my ever wishing again to visit Europe."

Visitors, both from home and abroad, begin to pour upon him, and soon he writes impatiently to Le Veillard in France:

" My time is so cut to pieces by friends and strangers, that I have sometimes envied the prisoners in Bastille."

This is the first indication that Franklin is aware of what has been going on in France since his departure. This letter was written in 1788. The Parisians overran and emptied the Bastille on July 14, 1789, four months after the election of George Washington as first President of the United States.

But meantime there has been pleasanter news from France. Temple Franklin writes his grandfather from Rancocas farm: " All the family (the Chaumonts) send their love to you, and the beautiful Mme. Foucault accompanys hers with an English kiss "; to which our old *galant* rouses himself to reply: " Thanks to Mad. Foucault for her kindness in sending me the kiss. It has grown cold by the way. I hope for a warm one when we meet." Also the Abbé Morellet writes directly to say: " I cannot express to you the pleasure, the transport which I felt at the news of your arrival at Philadelphia, which a friend of Mr. Jefferson has brought me. . . . May your days be prolonged and be free from pain; may your friends long taste the sweetness and charm of your society, and may those whom the seas have separated from you be still happy in the thought that the end of your career will be, as our good La Fontaine says, ' the evening of a fine day.' "

The Abbé also wrote of the arrival of Thomas Paine in France, whither he went, provided with an abundance of introductory letters by Franklin, to sell his newly invented bridge. Among Paine's hostesses in France was Madame Helvetius.

II

In the same year, 1787, the Constitutional Convention assembled in Philadelphia, and Franklin was soon taking an active part in its proceedings. He vainly tried to induce the Convention to accept two of his pet ideas: one was that the nation's President should serve without salary; and the other was that the more important and populous States should have a larger representation in the national legislature than the smaller.

One day he surprised those who had always regarded him as a free-thinker by proposing that prayers should be held every morning before the Convention began business. " The longer I live," said he, " the more convincing proofs I see of this truth: That God governs in the affairs of men." But the delegates were cold; only three of four supported Franklin's plea, and the assembly adjourned without voting on it.

Franklin was now too old and ailing to speak from the floor. He therefore put his arguments into written speeches which were read aloud by his colleague, James Wilson. He urged that Congress should consist of only one House, but when the two-chamber system was adopted, it was his suggestion that in the Senate every State should have equal representation but in the House each State should be represented in proportion to its population. He also proposed that the House should have the exclusive right to originate money bills. He, strangely enough, supported the measure giving the President authority to suspend the laws for certain periods, but vigorously fought the proposal to give votes to property holders exclusively. Madison wrote that " Dr. Franklin expressed his dislike to everything that tended to debase the spirit of the common people," saying, " some of the greatest rogues he was ever acquainted with were the richest rogues." Franklin favored giving Congress the power to impeach the President, and opposed the President's having the right of absolute veto. He supported the measure dealing with treason, which required that it be an overt act witnessed by at least two persons.

When the time came to vote on the adoption of the Constitution, Franklin admitted he was dissatisfied with it, but urged that it be accepted as the best that fallible men could produce. He could not say that even his own objections to it were well founded, and told the story of the French lady who, in a dispute with a sister, said:

" I don't know how it happens, sister, but I meet with nobody except myself that is always in the right."

III

In the same year Franklin was elected governor of Pennsylvania for the third time; he sighed a little but admitted his gratification.

" I seem to have intruded myself into the company of posterity," he said, " when I ought to have been abed and asleep."

In this, his 82nd year, his infirmities were intensified by a fall down the stone steps of his garden. His sufferings from the stone increased, and he began to prepare for death. He rallied, however, and was soon entertaining visitors with his accustomed verve. When J. P. Brissot, deputy for Paris in the French National Assembly and a leader of the Girondins, visited him in 1788, he wrote: " Thanks to God, Franklin still exists! . . . I have just been to see him and enjoy his conversation in the midst of his books, which he still calls his best friends. The pains of his cruel infirmity change not the serenity of his countenance, nor the calmness of his conversation." Brissot, like so many others

among Franklin's friends, soon afterwards died beneath the
blade of "Sainte Guillotine."

It was the next year that the "anvil," as Thomas Jefferson expressed it, began to use violence against the hammer
in France, and there came a letter from Madame Brillon,
saying:

"We are at a critical stage, wherein evil at its apex ought
to (or at least it behooves us to hope so) usher in the good;
if the new order of things which is proposed becomes a
reality, your unsullied prayers (since those of the just alone
are pleasing to the Supreme Being) will be most needful
to us. Pray for us, my good papa. You love France, the
French people; be our saint and if these messieurs did but
resemble you I would become their faithful follower. I
am yours, my dear papa; I revere you, honor you, love you;
not a day passes that my heart does not draw near you in
thought at least; not one wherein I fail to recall your friendship, so precious to me that nothing can ever rob me of it,
and the memory of the days when I enjoyed it more closely,
more intimately, makes one of the shining spots of happiness
in my life."

Franklin seems not to have made much comment on the
progress of the French Revolution; he was perhaps too old,
too preoccupied with home affairs, to have grasped its full
import. It is doubtful if, before he left France, he realized
the nearness of its approach. Jefferson was able to roam
about the country and see the condition of the people in the
scantiness of the peasant's soup-pot and the hardness of his
bed, but Franklin was grown too gouty and heavy for such
ramblings.

In 1789 he diverted himself by writing several papers.
One was his protest against the over-much teaching of Latin
and Greek in schools and colleges. "The best master of

languages," he used to say to his intimates, " is a mistress."
Having by this time joined the fight against slavery, he also
wrote his " Plea for improving the Condition of Free
Blacks "; " An Address to the Public from the Pennsyl-
vania Society for Promoting Abolition of Slavery "; and
" An Account of the Supremest Court of Judicature in
Pennsylvania, namely, the Court of the Press."

His pieces against slavery were followed by one of his
most famous newspaper contributions. It was a supposed
speech by Sidi Mehemet Ibrahim, " a member of the Divan
of Algiers," given in a bogus historical work called " Martin's Account of his Consulship," and was described as
against the petition of a sect " who prayed for the abolition
of piracy and slavery as being unjust."

He also wrote one of his spirited, gossipy letters to Noah
Webster, who gave his name to the spelling book and the
dictionary on which generations of his countrymen have
been reared, concerning the integrity of words.

In the spring of 1790 gout, stone, and a general break-
down forced him to his bed, but at intervals he was able
to see friends. Jefferson visited him and found him cheerful but much emaciated. Franklin listened with close attention to Jefferson's account of what he had seen of the French
Revolution. " I observed," wrote Jefferson, " his face often
flushed." Gen. Washington also came to see him and was
shown a new washing mangle, Franklin's latest invention.

Mary Hewson, the former Polly Stevenson, who had
spent the winter of 1784–1785 with Franklin at Passy, had
meantime arrived in Philadelphia to be with him during
his last days. She left the following account:

" When the pain was not too violent to be amused, he
employed himself with his books, his pen, or in conversation with his friends, and upon every occasion displayed the

clearness of his intellect, and the cheerfulness of his temper. Even when the intervals from pain were so short that his words were frequently interrupted, I have known him to hold a discourse in a sublime strain of piety. I shall never forget one day that I passed with our friend last summer (1789). I found him in bed in great agony; but when that agony abated a little, I asked him if I should read to him. He said yes, and the first book I met with was Johnson's Lives of the Poets. I read the life of Watts, who was a favorite author with Dr. Franklin; and instead of lulling him to sleep, it roused him to a display of the powers of his memory and his reason. He repeated several of Watts' Lyric Poems and descanted upon their sublimity in a strain worthy of them and their pious author.''

About April 1 pleurisy, which had once almost slain him during his boyhood, appeared in his lungs and he became feverish. An abcess developed and he was able to rest only by the aid of laudanum. On the 8th he wrote a letter to Jefferson about the northwestern boundary of the United States. It was in his characteristically clear style. On the 12th he got up so that his bed might be made. When someone remarked that he was going to get well, he answered, " I hope not."

When he had resumed his bed, his breathing became difficult. Finally the abcess in his lungs burst and he gradually sank. April 17 found him unconscious. At 11 o'clock that night, while he lay as if sleeping quietly, a shudder passed through the great frame, and he ceased to breathe.

In Philadelphia the procession to the old Christ Church burial ground was the greatest ever seen in that city. Congress, which had not yet acted on his claims for services and for moneys expended, adopted a badge of mourning for one month. In France Mirabeau, then vainly trying to moderate the revolutionary tempest, delivered before the National Assembly his oft-quoted speech beginning:

"Franklin is dead! The genius that freed America and poured a flood of light over Europe has returned to the bosom of the Divinity." From the entire civilized world came the echo: "Franklin is dead!"

CHAPTER XXXV

Franklin's Will

I

FRANKLIN left an estate estimated at $150,000, in those days a considerable fortune. He owned various houses and lots in Philadelphia and Boston, and tracts of land in Nova Scotia, Georgia, and Ohio. He also held bonds, bank shares, and about $25,000 in cash or quick securities.

His will, dated July 17, 1788, disposed of all his property and remembered all his relatives and closest friends with great exactness. He even marked the catalogue showing how his books were to be disposed of. His old business debts he bequeathed to the Pennsylvania Hospital, which would have preferred something relatively easy to handle, like a wounded bear.

A codicil bequeathed his crab-tree walking stick, " with a gold head curiously wrought in the form of the cap of liberty," given to him by Madame de Forbach, Dowager Duchess of Deux Ponts, to Gen. Washington.

The most curious feature of this codicil, and the one which has caused the most dissension since, was the bequest to the town of Boston and the corporation of Philadelphia of 1000 pounds sterling ($5000) each, " to let out the same upon interest at five per cent. per annum to such young married artificers, under the age of twenty-five years, as have served an apprenticeship in the said town, and faithfully fulfilled the duties required in their indentures, so as to obtain a good moral character from at least two respectable citizens, who are willing to become their sureties, in a bond with the applicants, for the repayment of the moneys so lent, with interest." Loans were not to exceed 60 pounds or be less than 15 pounds, and each borrower was required to pay back, with the yearly interest, one tenth of the principal.

Franklin calculated that the total sum in 100 years would amount to 131,000 pounds for each city. Of this sum the managers were to lay out 100,000 pounds in public works of general utility to the inhabitants. The remaining 31,000 pounds were to be let out in loans as directed for another hundred years, when Franklin calculated that the sum would have grown to 4,661,000 pounds.

Not even Franklin's wisdom, however, was able to foresee the rapid changes in conditions that would ensue during the next century, or to provide for contingencies. The first hundred years under the terms of the will terminated in Boston in 1891, but instead of there being the $655,000 which Franklin counted on, there was actually only $391,-168.68 in the fund. Philadelphia made an even worse showing; there the fund contained less than $100,000. In both cases the funds were tied up for a time by unsuccessful suits brought by the descendants of Franklin. In Philadelphia it was charged that the fund had been partly used for purposes which would not have been approved by its founder, while in Boston there was in its early years evidence of careless administration.

One hundred years is a long time and Franklin is not the first will-maker who has failed to anticipate inevitable and far-reaching changes, or to leave money in such a way that trouble will not ensue.

Only seven years after Franklin's death, the Pennsylvania Hospital asked that it be permitted to return its legacy, having found the debts due Franklin either small, too old, or in other respects uncollectable.

II

Of Franklin's descendants not one is left bearing his own name. William, the only survivor of his two sons, died in England, in 1813, at the age of 82.

William Temple Franklin, his grandson, died in Paris in 1823 and was buried in Père La Chaise Cemetery, where guides earn extra francs from American tourists by pointing out his grave.

Sarah Franklin survived her father eighteen years and was buried beside him. Her numerous male descendants became professional or army and navy men. One of them, Richard Bache, 2nd, a lawyer, became a member of the Texas Senate, where he was the only member casting an adverse vote against union with the United States.

Franklin, however, needed no descendants to keep his name alive. He engraved it so deeply into the history of his time as to be ineffaceable. And this he did, not by industry, frugality, or the other virtues which he so sedulously preached, but by drawing men to him through his gift of being intensely alive, incessantly observant, immensely charitable, and unalterably radiant in the infectious cheer of his disposition.

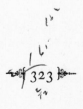